Alcohol and Drug Misuse

This comprehensive textbook provides an accessible and skills-oriented introduction to alcohol and substance misuse for healthcare students and practitioners new to the field.

Divided into five parts, this text explores:

- The context of alcohol and drug misuse and the nature and theories of addiction, including a historical overview and policy initiatives in contemporary society.
- An overview of psychoactive substances and the problems associated with them.
- An exploration of the impact of psychoactive substances on groups, such as culturally and linguistically diverse communities, young people, women, older people, and the homeless.
- An understanding of the generic role responses to substance misuse in a variety of different settings and contexts, including primary care, the community, and hospitals.
- A framework for assessment, care planning, harm reduction approaches, dealing with overdose, intoxication and withdrawals, and psychological and pharmacological interventions.

This new edition is fully updated and includes expanded coverage of performance-enhancing drugs, e-cigarettes, cannabis use, gender disparities in substance use and treatment, public health approaches to substance use, and screening tools for alcohol misuse. *Alcohol and Drug Misuse* is enhanced with activities and learning outcomes throughout.

It is essential reading for nursing, healthcare, and social work students taking substance misuse modules, as well as related post-registration/qualification courses for health and social care professionals.

G. Hussein Rassool is Professor of Islāmic Psychology at the Centre for Islāmic Studies and Civilisations, Charles Sturt University, Australia. He is also Director of Studies at the Department of Islāmic Psychology, Psychotherapy, and Counselling, Al Balagh Academy, and Chair of Al Balagh Institute of Islāmic Psychology Research. He is a Fellow of the International Association of Islāmic Psychology (FIAIP) and the Royal Society of Public Health (FRSPH) and Professional membership of the International Assocaition of Substance Use. He works as a part-time Islāmic psychotherapist. He is one of the leading academics in the areas of Islāmic psychology and psychotherapy and is involved in the development of the first BSc Islāmic psychology at the International Open University. His research interests include psychosocial and spiritual problems in relation to mental health, psychosocial and spiritual interventions, indigenous psychology, Islāmic counselling and psychotherapy, and Islāmic ethics in psychology. He has published over 22 books, as well as over 150 papers and reviews in peer-reviewed journals.

Alcohol and Drug Misuse

A Guide for Health and Social Care Professionals

Third edition

G. Hussein Rassool

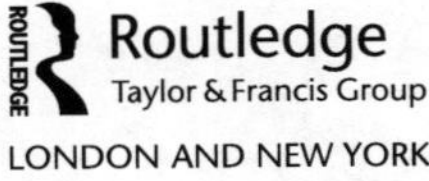

LONDON AND NEW YORK

Designed cover image: Getty Images/Shulz

Third edition published 2025
by Routledge
4 Park Square, Milton Park, Abingdon, Oxon, OX14 4RN

and by Routledge
605 Third Avenue, New York, NY 10158

Routledge is an imprint of the Taylor & Francis Group, an informa business

© 2025 G. Hussein Rassool

The right of G. Hussein Rassool to be identified as author of this work has been asserted in accordance with sections 77 and 78 of the Copyright, Designs and Patents Act 1988.

All rights reserved. No part of this book may be reprinted or reproduced or utilised in any form or by any electronic, mechanical, or other means, now known or hereafter invented, including photocopying and recording, or in any information storage or retrieval system, without permission in writing from the publishers.

Trademark notice: Product or corporate names may be trademarks or registered trademarks, and are used only for identification and explanation without intent to infringe.

First edition published by Routledge 2009
Second edition published by Routledge 2018

British Library Cataloguing-in-Publication Data
A catalogue record for this book is available from the British Library

ISBN: 978-1-032-59871-0 (hbk)
ISBN: 978-1-032-59869-7 (pbk)
ISBN: 978-1-003-45667-4 (ebk)

DOI: 10.4324/9781003456674

Typeset in Berling
by Apex CoVantage, LLC

Dedicated to Idrees Khattab ibn Adam Ibn Hussein Ibn Hassim Ibn Sahaduth Ibn Rosool Ibn Olee Al Mauritiusy.

Knowledge

Knowledge is of two kinds: that which is absorbed and that which is heard. And that which is heard does not profit if it is not absorbed.

Ali Ibn Abi Talib (Radia' Allāh Anhu)

Contents

Tables

Figures

Preface to the third edition

It has been more than five years since the second edition of this book presented readers with a solid foundation and perspective on alcohol and drug misuse. This is the third edition of what has become an indispensable textbook for health and social care professionals at all levels of experience when dealing with alcohol and drug use and misuse. The popular reception of the book and the rapid changes in the global nature and use of psychoactive substances; the emergence of new types of drugs; research on anabolic androgenic steroids and associated image- and performance-enhancing drugs (IPEDs); the use of heroin adulterated with isotonitazene ("iso"); the use of fentanyl; the use of nitrous oxide; the ongoing gender treatment gap; the disparities in drug use and treatment; alcohol use screening tests; low-risk drinking guidelines; new evidence-based healthcare interventions; and the early indications and effects of cannabis legalisation call for a new edition to assist student and healthcare professionals in the care and management of alcohol and drug misuse.

The feedback from students, teachers, and colleagues about the contents of the book and its associated activities will be incorporated in the new edition. Although the structure of the third edition of this book will remain unchanged, there will be significant updating and revision throughout.

- Provision of technical corrections, updates, clarifications in all chapters of the original book
- Updated literature in all chapters substantially and reordered and added to the material in most chapters
- New developments in the field and evidence-based practice
- Updated references and reflective activities

The most obvious changes in this third edition are changes in a few chapters, as stated in the following

- Chapter 1: The global drug scene has been updated Literature from UNODC World Drug Report, and global drug use. Update on HIV, hepatitis. Overview of COVID-19 and substance misuse.
- Chapter 4: Update on bio-psychosocial-spiritual theory.
- Chapter 6: Global policy initiatives and strategy on alcohol and drug. Update on some of the policy changes. Includes early indications and effects of cannabis legalisation. Update on drug laws around the world. Update on the use of medical cannabis
- Chapter 7: Update on alcohol use screening tests and low-risk drinking guidelines.
- Chapter 8: Opiates – insert contents on the use of fentanyl. This drug can be used as an analgesic and is about 100 times more potent than morphine. Global consumption of fentanyl has increased steadily in the last decade. The use of heroin adulterated with isotonitazene ("iso").
- Chapter 9: Cannabis – contents on high-THC cannabis products and potential effects. Cannabis manufacturers are extracting THC to make oils, edibles, wax, sugar-size crystals, and glass-like products called shatter that advertise high THC levels. High-potency cannabis use and mental health consequences and psychotic disorder, like schizophrenia. Update on the use of medical cannabis.
- Chapter 12: New contents on research on anabolic androgenic steroids and associated image- and performance-enhancing drugs (IPEDs).
- Chapter 13: Review and update on the effects of electronic nicotine delivery systems. E-cigarettes are harmful to health.

- Chapter 15: Update on ongoing gender treatment gap and disparities in drug use and treatment.
- Chapter 21: Public health approaches to substance misuse – update on alcohol and drug misuse prevention.
- Chapter 24: Framework for assessment and screening – update on alcohol screening.

I should add some acknowledgements to those I made in the preface to the second edition. I have changed institution, so I should add my thanks to my new colleagues at the Centre for Islāmic Studies and Civilisations, Charles Sturt University, Australia (https://arts-ed.csu.edu.au/centres/cisac/staffns). I am especially grateful for the ongoing encouragement and support of Grace McInnes and the support staff at Routledge. I would also like to thank the reviewers for providing substantial and constructive criticisms in developing this new edition

I am incredibly grateful to my beloved parents, who instilled in me the importance of education. Their unwavering love and guidance have been instrumental in shaping who I am today, and I am truly grateful for their wisdom and encouragement. I am humbled and deeply grateful for the unwavering love and support of Mariam, Idrees Khattab Ibn Adam Ali Hussein Ibn Hussein Ibn Hassim Ibn Sahaduth Ibn Rosool Al Mauritiusy, Adam Ali Hussein, Reshad Hasan, Yasmin Soraya, Isra Oya, Asiyah Maryam, Nabila Akhrif, Nusaybah Burke, Musa Burke, Fatima Azzahra, Dr Najmul Hussein, and Mohammed Ali. Their presence in my life is a blessing, and I am forever indebted to them for their love, support, and inspiration.

I am grateful to acknowledge the invaluable contributions of my teachers, who have played a crucial role in enabling me to deepen my understanding of authentic Islām. Through their guidance and teachings, I have been able to embark on the right path, following the *Creed of Ahlus-Sunnah wa'l-Jamaa'ah*. I sincerely pray to Allāh that He forgives me and accepts my humble effort in authoring this book. May He make it a source of benefit and fruitfulness for all those who find it useful and informative. May this book serve as a means of guidance and understanding for those who seek knowledge and insight.

G. Hussein Rassool
17 March 2024

Preface

Alcohol and drug misuse, their associated sequelae and their intervention strategies are the premises of the book. The increase in the number of individuals with alcohol and drug problems has attracted considerable interest as one of the most important public health challenges. The book focuses on the approaches and intervention strategies that health and social care professionals can use to respond to this new challenge in specialist and non-specialist settings. The book underpins a number of current policy initiatives as applied to current practice and covers practically most aspects relating to alcohol and drug misuse. An added dimension is the coverage of special issues and needs of special populations, prevention and harm reduction, assessment, care planning, dealing with emergencies, and psychological and pharmacological interventions.

The book provides a basic clinical and practical text on areas of clinical issues and practice, interventions, management, and education. It will enable health and social care professionals and students to understand the extent and nature of substance use and misuse and foster the knowledge and skills required in its management to provide effective care to those patients they encounter in their daily practice. In addition, it provides a framework to assist practitioners in dealing with complex issues related to alcohol and drug misuse. It is envisaged that the book will act as an excellent resource for health and social care practitioners who are unfamiliar with the substance misuse field. It will be of relevance to students in medicine, nursing, psychology, social work, and the criminal justice system and those attending undergraduate and postgraduate courses in addiction and mental health studies. The book is practice-oriented and has several activities related to the content of the chapters.

Structure of the book

The book is presented in five parts. Part 1 provides an understanding of alcohol and drug misuse, the nature and theories of addiction, with a historical overview. Policy initiatives and strategy in alcohol and drugs that have shaped the provision and delivery of care are included. Part 2 presents the nature and problems associated with psychoactive substances from alcohol to eco-drugs. Part 3 deals with blood-borne viruses and special populations: Black and minority ethnic groups, young people, women, elderly, and the homeless. Part 3 covers aspects of a synthesis of role, shared care, dual diagnosis in acute inpatient and forensic settings and models of care. Part 4 deals with the generic roles and responses to substance misuse in a variety of different settings and contexts. These include engaging substance misusers in primary care, community, and hospital settings. Subsequent chapters cover prevention and health education, strategies in helping people change and working with diversity. Part 5 focuses on frameworks for assessment, care planning, harm reduction approach, dealing with overdose, intoxication and withdrawals, and psychological and pharmacological interventions.

The book contains a number of activities (true-or-false items, multiple-choice questions and questions requiring short answer) in each chapter. The reader is encouraged to undertake the reflective activities found in each chapter to gain the added value of the contents. This book incorporates some of the knowledge and the skills specification of DANOS (Drugs and Alcohol National Occupational Standards).

Acknowledgements

I would like to thank Eloise and Grace at Taylor & Francis for their support and patience throughout the process of writing and the publication of this book. I am also particularly grateful to Professor James P. Smith, Professor John Strang, Professor A. Hamid Ghodse, Dr Nek Oyefeso, and the Florence Nightingale Research Foundation, for their guidance in my professional development. Special thanks go to Professor Margarita Villar-Luis, Escola De Enfermagem de Ribeirao Preto, Universidade de Sao Paulo, Brazil, for our collaboration and development in publishing, teaching, and research activities in addiction and mental health.

To my patients and students, for teaching me about the practice in the addiction field. Thanks also go to all my brothers at Al-Furqan, Les Guibies, for their friendship and support. I would like to acknowledge the contributions of my teachers, who enabled me, through my own reflective practices, to follow the path. My special thanks also to Mariam for all the help and support during the writing of the book. Finally, I owe my gratitude to my children, Yasmin, Adam, and Reshad, who keep me going and active in various endeavours and taught me about life.

Part 1

Alcohol and drug global policy initiatives

Chapter 1

Demystifying terms

Understanding substance-related concepts and disorders

Learning outcomes

- Provide a brief overview of the global drug scene.
- Explain the meaning of the following terms: *drug, drug dependence, addiction, addictive behaviours, alcohol use disorder, hazardous drinker, harmful drinker, substance use disorder, synthetic drugs*, and *individuals with substance use disorder*.
- Examine the components of the concept of dependence: tolerance, withdrawal symptoms, and physical and psychological dependence.
- Differentiate between commonly used legal and illicit psychoactive substances.

INTRODUCTION

In the 21st century, the use of psychoactive substances, both natural and synthetic, remains a significant aspect of society. These substances, whether stimulants, depressants, hallucinogens, synthetic, or mind-expanding, have profound effects on individuals' cognitive, affective, and behavioural dimensions. While the use of alcohol and drugs has long been woven into the social and psychological fabric of developed countries, a notable trend is the increasing prevalence of substance use in developing countries. Throughout history, societies have co-existed with psychoactive substances, employing them for various purposes, such as ritual ceremonies, medicinal applications, and recreational use. Remarkably, substances like tea, coffee, and tobacco have all been illegal in the United Kingdom (UK) at various points in history (Whitaker, 1987). Over time, factors such as increasing availability and widespread use have led to shifts in societal opinions, resulting in the normalisation of these substances as part of the fabric of society. The perception of which substances are deemed legal or illicit evolves over time and is influenced by economic and political considerations. This dynamic interplay reflects the complex relationship between cultural norms, society, and psychoactive substances, shaping attitudes and policies regarding their use or prohibitions.

Alcohol and drugs pose significant harm on physical, social, psychological, and economic levels, impacting not only individuals but also their families and communities. The associated harms include increased risks of premature death; the potential for blood-borne infections, like hepatitis B, C, and HIV; overdoses; respiratory failure; and various physical and mental health issues. Despite these detrimental effects, the deep-rooted presence of alcohol and drugs in human culture makes it unrealistic to expect these compounds to vanish entirely from society. However, the concern, from a public health perspective, is the rapid proliferation of new "cheap and easy" synthetic drugs in the global landscape, leading to lethal consequences. Estimates of those who inject drugs reveal higher numbers than previously thought, highlighting shortcomings in treatment services and interventions (UNDOC, 2023). Youth populations globally, particularly in various regions, are highly susceptible to drug use and disproportionately affected by substance use disorders. Recent research on the use of controlled drugs for treating mental health conditions indicates their potential efficacy (UNDOC, 2023). However, there is a concern that commercial interests are being prioritised over public health considerations.

Despite efforts involving zero-tolerance approach, policy legislation, increased taxation, penalties for

DOI: 10.4324/9781003456674-2

possession and sale, decriminalisation of certain drug, preventive health education, harm reduction, and anti-drug campaigns, alcohol and drugs persist as significant public health problems. The nature and extent of the global drug and alcohol problem are interwoven with all aspects of sustainable development. This includes social development, economic development, environmental sustainability, the promotion of peaceful and just societies, and the importance of partnerships (UNDOC, 2016). There is an interconnectedness of social and economic inequalities with drug challenges. The World Drug Report (2023) underlines the reciprocal relationship, where these inequalities both drive and are driven by issues related to drugs. The report also brings attention to the environmental destruction and human rights violations associated with illicit drug economies. The nature and dynamics of the drug problem are influenced by these interconnected elements. The global alcohol and drug misuse highlights the multifaceted nature of alcohol- and drug-related challenges, encompassing social, economic, environmental, and human rights dimensions.

GLOBAL DRUG SCENE

The most commonly consumed drugs in the world include alcohol and cannabis/marijuana, followed by opioids and opiates. The UN Office on Drugs and Crime (UNODC, 2022) suggests that cannabis legalisation in certain regions has led to an acceleration in daily cannabis use and associated health impacts. Opioids remain the most lethal group of drugs, accounting for two-thirds of deaths related directly to drugs (mostly overdoses). It is estimated that 0.4% of the global adult population use cocaine (UNDOC, 2023). Methamphetamines remain the second most commonly used drug and the world's dominant illegally manufactured synthetic drug. The UNODC (2023) report provides a global overview of psychoactive substance use across various regions. In Latin and South America, there are significant challenges related to cocaine trafficking and the prevalence of cocaine use disorders. In North America, there are diverse challenges, including the expansion of synthetic drug markets, high prevalence of opioids, methamphetamine manufacture, and the increasing use of stimulants like methamphetamine and cocaine. Fentanyl, a powerful synthetic opioid, contributes to high levels of drug overdose, with the majority of those involving illegally manufactured fentanyl. Non-medical use of pharmaceutical stimulants is higher in the Americas than in other regions. In Europe, there are notable trends in substance misuse, including an expanding cocaine market and an increasing prevalence of amphetamine-type stimulants (ATS) and opiates.

In the Russian Federation and Commonwealth of Independent States (CIS), the region experiences the expansion of opiate use, novel psychoactive substances (NPS), and synthetic drug markets. There is a high prevalence of HIV among people who inject drugs, pointing to significant public health concerns associated with substance use. In the Golden Crescent (Afghanistan, Iran, and Pakistan) and the Middle East, substance misuse challenges encompass the production, trafficking, and use of opiates, reflecting a significant presence of opioids in the region. Opioid use disorder is a significant public health concern in the Middle East and North Africa (MENA) region, impacting as many as 12 Arab countries. Bahrain and Kuwait have notably high rates of opioid use (Wilby & Wilbur, 2017). Concurrently, the MENA region is experiencing a worsening HIV epidemic, with people who inject opioids through non-sterile methods being particularly vulnerable to HIV infection (UNAIDS, 2021).

Additionally, there is a concerning increase in methamphetamine trafficking and use, signifying a diversification of substance use patterns.

In the Indian subcontinent, there is a high prevalence of opioid use and the expansion of the market for amphetamine-type stimulants (ATS), indicating an increased use of stimulant substances. In the Golden Triangle, encompassing parts of Southeast Asia like Myanmar, Laos, and Thailand, the challenges involve the manufacture of methamphetamine, signalling the production and trafficking of synthetic stimulants. Opiates production is also observed in the Golden Triangle, highlighting cultivation and trafficking of opioid substances. In Asia, specifically in Japan, there is a significant and concerning trend of a large methamphetamine market. In Australia, there is a high prevalence of stimulant use, specifically methamphetamine and cocaine. This indicates a significant presence and usage of these substances in the country.

In Africa, particularly West and Central Africa, high cannabis use is driven by prevalence in Nigeria. The subregion also faces notable opioid use, especially the non-medical use of tramadol in North, West, and Central Africa. Other African regions primarily engage in opiates, with rising cocaine use in West and Southern Africa. Synthetic NPS use is reported more in Southern Africa, while East Africa sees widespread khat use. Sub-Saharan Africa experiences diverse substance use patterns, including opioid-related overdoses, methamphetamine and cocaine use, and local manufacture of psychoactive substances. Southern Africa has the highest prevalence of persons who inject drugs and the highest HIV prevalence among this group. Overall, the substance use landscape in Africa is diverse and dynamic.

Novel psychoactive substances (NPS), commonly sold under names like spice, bath salts, and herbal incense, are marked by a constant influx of new substances. These synthetic substances mimic the effects of opiates, benzodiazepines, dissociatives, hallucinogens, and cannabinoids. These drugs navigate existing legal and pharmaceutical regulations by altering their chemical compositions. The psychoactive substances in this category encompass cannabinoids, cathinones, opioids, phenethylamines, tryptamines, benzodiazepines, and arylalkylamines, reflecting a diverse range of chemical compounds. This summary underscores the dynamic and evolving nature of NPS, posing challenges to regulatory frameworks and public health efforts (EMCDDA, 2015; UNDOC, 2016). By the end of 2020, around 209 synthetic cannabinoids and 156 synthetic cathinones had been identified in Europe (EMCDDA, 2021a). Synthetic cannabinoids are typically found in herbal blends or, less typically, in the form of tablets, capsules, and powders, and recently in liquid forms for e-cigarettes (Le Boisselier et al., 2017; Scourfield et al., 2019). Synthetic cathinones are typically found in powder (Brunt et al., 2017). However, there is limited information of the dangers and toxicity of most of the novel synthetic psychoactive drugs.

Alcohol remains our favourite social lubricant and is associated with adverse physical, mental, and behavioural health conditions and social consequences related to its intoxication, toxicity, and dependence. Alcohol and tobacco use is the most prevalent addictive behaviour and causes a large majority of the harm (Gowing et al., 2015). The global impact of the harmful use of alcohol is substantial and is linked to over 200 health conditions, including liver diseases, road injuries, violence, cancers, cardiovascular diseases, suicides, tuberculosis, and HIV/AIDS, highlighting the diverse and extensive negative health outcomes associated with excessive alcohol consumption (WHO, 2018). The number of people using tobacco in the world is declining, despite population growth (WHO, 2019). Tobacco is one of the world's largest preventable causes of premature death, accounting for more than 8 million deaths (WHO, 2021). Tobacco-attributable diseases encompass a range of serious health conditions, such as lung and heart diseases, chronic respiratory diseases, cancers, and diabetes. Importantly, these conditions may contribute to the increased severity of COVID-19, emphasising the heightened risks faced by individuals with a history of tobacco use. Evidence shows that cigarette smokers are more likely to be hospitalised or die from COVID-19 (WHO, 2021). The interplay between tobacco-related health issues and the potential aggravation of COVID-19 highlights the importance of addressing tobacco use in efforts to mitigate the impact of the pandemic. However, it is important to note that "[a]s cigarette sales have fallen, tobacco companies have been aggressively marketing new products – like e-cigarettes and heated-tobacco products – and lobby governments to limit their regulation. Their goal is simple: to hook another generation on nicotine. We cannot let that happen" (Bloomberg, 2021, p. 17).

There are other harmful products, including cigars, water pipe tobacco (hookah), and smokeless tobacco. These alternative tobacco products also pose health risks, contributing to various diseases and health complications. With the rise in the trend in the use of water pipe tobacco smoking (hookah), "e-hookahs," "e-shisha," or "hookah pens" in Western countries, there are new dangers and harms. Hookah smoking that delivers the addictive drug nicotine carries many of the same health risks as cigarettes. However, hookah smoking has been associated with lung cancer, respiratory illness, low birth weight, and periodontal disease (Akl et al., 2010; American Lung Association, 2007; CDC, 2015a; Kadhum et al., 2015).

Polydrug use refers to the consumption of more than one drug, either simultaneously or sequentially, by an individual. This includes both illicit drugs and legal substances, such as alcohol and medicines. Most drug users occasionally engage in polydrug use. The simultaneous consumption of different substances in close proximity can heighten drug toxicity, leading to increased health risks (EMCDDA, 2021b). Psychoactive substances may interact, escalating the potential for risky use of other substances. For instance, alcohol intoxication can impair judgement regarding opioid consumption or the risk of reduced tolerance after treatment or prison. Additionally, combining cocaine and alcohol (Cocaethylene) can elevate toxicological risks. Co-using multiple substances also amplifies the risk of accidents or injuries. Recognising these interactions is crucial in understanding and addressing the complex and compounded dangers associated with polydrug use. Polydrug users are usually admitted for emergency medical treatment due to overdose, and there is a high morbidity rate among this sub-population of drug users.

The non-medical use of prescription drugs, defined as the misuse of these medications, poses a significant global health concern. This involves taking prescription drugs in ways other than prescribed, using someone else's prescription, or taking medication to achieve euphoria or get high (UNDOC, 2011). Common types of psychoactive prescription drugs include opioids (e.g. hydrocodone, oxycodone), central nervous system depressants (e.g. barbiturates, benzodiazepines), and central nervous system stimulants (e.g. amphetamines, methylphenidate) (UNDOC, 2011). This misuse can lead to various health risks and complications, emphasising the importance of addressing and preventing the non-medical use of prescription drugs on a global scale. The over-prescribing of psychoactive substances, mainly opioids, for pain or illness management has led to addictive behaviours and an increase in mortality. It is reported that over-prescribing of opioid pain relievers has been associated with a rise of opioid addiction and overdose deaths (Kolodny, 2015; Rudd et al., 2016). Opioid medications like Vicodin (hydrocodone), OxyContin (oxycodone), and methadone are responsible for the increase in addiction, drug overdose and mortality (CDC, 2015b).

Over-the-counter (OTC) medications are integral to self-medication and play a significant role in health and lay care systems. These drugs are accessible without a prescription and are typically available at pharmacies or supermarkets. OTC medications offer individuals the convenience of managing common health issues independently, contributing to the overall accessibility of healthcare products for various health concerns. Almost 50% of patients use these drugs incorrectly, resulting in increased morbidity and mortality (Costa et al., 2017).

Some commonly misused OTC medications include codeine-based analgesics, cough products containing dextromethorphan, sedative antihistamines, decongestants, and laxatives. Evidence suggests that misuse of OTC drugs occurs, particularly among individuals already struggling with alcohol and drug problems, emphasising the importance of addressing and monitoring their usage (Frei et al., 2010; Hughes et al., 1999).

GLOBAL-SCENE HIV

HIV continues to be a major global public health issue. Some countries report increasing trends in new infections when previously it was on the decline (WHO, 2022). Globally, almost three-quarters (71%) of people living with HIV in 2022 (76% of women and 67% of men living with HIV) had suppressed viral loads (UNAIDS, 2023). Illicit drug users face elevated risks of HIV, hepatitis, and tuberculosis due to compromised judgement and decision-making resulting from alcohol or drug consumption. Substance use can contribute to risky sexual behaviour, such as engaging in unsafe sex, trading sex for drugs, and needle sharing. Injection drug use is a recognised pathway for transmitting blood-borne infections, notably HIV, tuberculosis, and hepatitis B and C. These health concerns underline the need for targeted interventions and support for this high-risk population. Breakthroughs in addressing HIV/AIDS are most prominent in countries demonstrating a political commitment and investing in proven strategies. Successful nations have proactively eliminated societal and structural barriers, such as criminalising laws, gender inequalities, stigma, discrimination, and human rights violations, which jeopardise individuals' health and well-being (UNAIDS, 2023). The key to success lies in concerted efforts to create an environment conducive to health protection and promotion. There are new strategies that have been proposed, with a common vision to end epidemics and advance universal health coverage, primary healthcare and health security, in a world where all people have access to high-quality, evidence-based, and people-centred health services (WHO, 2022).

HIV infection during pregnancy has emerged as a predominant medical complication, and women are particularly vulnerable to HIV due to both biological and socio-cultural factors. The findings of a review on HIV in pregnancy (WHO & Joint United Nations Programme on HIV/AIDS, 1999) indicated that breastfeeding significantly contributes to HIV transmission in developing countries, posing a risk

Activity 1.1 What is a drug?

State by ticking yes or no what you think is/are the definition(s) of a drug.

Definitions	Yes	No
A substance other than food intended to affect the structure or function of the body.*		
A substance intended for use in the diagnosis, cure, mitigation, treatment, or prevention of a disease.*		
A substance used as a medication or in the preparation of a medication.*		
A substance recognised in an official pharmacopoeia or formulary.*		
A substance intended for use as a component of a medicine but not a device or a component, part, or accessory of a device.*		
A substance used in dyeing or chemical operations.		
A commodity that is not saleable or for which there is no demand.*		
Something, and often an illegal substance, that causes addiction, habituation, or a marked change in consciousness.*		
Any substance or chemical that alters the structure or functioning of a living being.**		
A psychoactive substance that affects the central nervous system and alters mood, perception, and behaviour.		

Source: * Encyclopædia Britannica (2007)
** World Health Organization (1981).

Activity 1.2

Questions

- What is drug use and misuse?
- What is meant by the term *alcohol use disorder*?
- What is meant by the term *substance use disorder*?
- Explain the following terms: *dependence, addiction, addictive behaviours.*
- What is meant by *tolerance*?
- What is meant by *physical* and *psychological* dependence?
- Users of psychoactive substances are described as experimental, recreational, or dependent. What do the terms *experimental*, *recreational*, and *dependent* mean? What are their characteristics?

to children. Adverse pregnancy outcomes associated with HIV-positive women include increased rates of spontaneous early abortion, low birth weight, stillbirths, preterm labour, preterm rupture of membranes, and various infectious complications, such as bacterial pneumonia and urinary tract infections. However, the direct attribution of these outcomes to HIV infection remains uncertain. Addressing HIV in pregnancy requires comprehensive strategies to mitigate these risks and improve maternal and child health outcomes.

In fact, these are all potential definitions of a drug. According to WHO (1981), a *drug* is "any substance or chemical that alters the structure or functioning of a living being." Despite the broadness of the concept, which limits its use for clinical and for certain practical purposes, it provides some perspective into its pervasive nature. A *drug*, in the broadest sense, is a chemical substance that has an effect on bodily systems and behaviour. This includes a wide range of prescribed drugs – illegal, over the counter, and socially accepted recreational substances. Defining a drug involves various perspectives, with the term "addiction" adding complexity to the discussion. A common language is crucial for understanding addiction to alcohol and drugs. The concept of a drug is influenced by socio-cultural context and purpose, encompassing elements such as food or chocolate. Drug definitions range from therapeutic use, involving pharmacological preparations for medical purposes, to non-therapeutic use, which refers to the consumption of illegal or socially disapproved substances (Rassool, 1998).

USE OF TERMINOLOGY IN ALCOHOL AND DRUG USE/MISUSE

When using terminology in alcohol and drug use, some of the terms can be perceived as highly stigmatising by people who use alcohol and/or other drugs. Terms such as *addict, alcoholic, substance abusers, problem drug users, alcohol/drug misuse,* and *alcohol/drug abuse* are terminologies that can contribute to negative stereotypes and hinder effective communication. It is important to adopt language that emphasises the person first, rather than reducing them to their condition. For example, saying "a person with a substance use disorder" instead of "a substance abuser" helps humanise individuals and reduce the stigma associated with their struggles. Advocates for mental health and substance use awareness often encourage the use of person-centred language to reduce stigma and foster a more compassionate and inclusive dialogue. However, in this new edition of the book, the terminologies have been modified, when appropriate, to alternatives that are often considered less-stigmatising.

- *Addict/substance or drug abuser*. Individual with a substance use disorder (SUD) or an individual with an opioid use disorder.
- *Alcoholic*. Individual with alcohol use disorder or who misuses alcohol/engages in unhealthy/hazardous alcohol use.
- *Alcohol/drug abuse*. Unhealthy or problematic substance use.
- *Problem alcohol/drug users*. Individuals alcohol/ drug use disorder.
- *Substance abuse*. Use, for illicit drugs; misuse, for prescription medications used other than prescribed.

DRUG USE AND MISUSE

The terms *drug use* and *misuse* are subjective and context-dependent, influenced by cultural, ideological, etiological, and clinical factors and the effect of the substance on the individual. Cultural norms, societal attitudes, and prevailing ideologies shape how these terms are understood. Clinical practices and diagnostic criteria also play a role in determining whether an individual's drug-related behaviour is classified as use or misuse. In the American context, the terms *use* and *misuse* are often used to describe the consumption of drugs in different contexts, particularly when distinguishing between illicit drugs and prescription medications (NIDA, 2021). Drug *use* typically refers to the act of consuming substances that are illegal or controlled by law. Drug *misuse* or substance *misuse* refers to the use of a substance in a way that is not intended or recommended by a healthcare professional, particularly in the case of prescription medications. *Misuse* can include taking a medication in higher doses than prescribed, using it for non-medical purposes, or using someone else's prescription.

In the British context, the terms *drug use* and *misuse* are often employed within the framework of drug policy. *Drug use* generally refers to the consumption of psychoactive substances, whether legal or illegal, for various purposes, including medicinal, recreational, or cultural reasons. Drug or substance *misuse* is typically used to describe the inappropriate or harmful use of substances, particularly in the context of illegal or controlled drugs. The term *drug misuse* may be seen as the use of drug in a socially unacceptable way that is harmful or hazardous to the individual or others (Royal College of Psychiatrists and Royal College of Physicians, 2000). Drug misuse occurs when a psychoactive substance is consumed in an unintended manner, leading to physical, social, and psychological harm. This includes usage outside therapeutic recommendations, causing adverse effects on health or functioning. *Drug misuse* encompasses a spectrum of behaviours ranging from experimental and recreational use to patterns of dependence. The term *substance misuse* is commonly employed as a generic expression to encompass both alcohol and drug misuse, emphasising the broader context of problematic or harmful substance-related behaviours.

WORLD HEALTH ORGANIZATION: LEXICON OF ALCOHOL AND DRUG TERMS

The World Health Organization recommends the use of the following terms, based on the lexicon of alcohol and drug terms (WHO, 1994).

- *Unsanctioned use*. A drug that is not approved by society or a group within society. This term implies that disapproval is accepted as a fact in its own right.
- *Dysfunctional use*. A drug leading to impaired psychological or social functioning. For example loss of employment or marital problems.
- *Hazardous use*. Defined as "a pattern of substance use that increases the risk of harmful consequences for the user . . . hazardous use refers to patterns of use that are of public health significance despite the absence of any current disorder in the individual user." *Hazardous drinkers* are drinking at levels over the sensible drinking limits, either in terms of regular excessive consumption or less-frequent sessions of heavy drinking. *Hazardous drinker* is not a diagnostic label.

Activity 1.3 State whether the category of drug has high, moderate, or no potential for physical or psychological dependence.

Category of drug	Physical dependence	Psychological dependence
Opiates and opioids (e.g. opium, heroin, morphine)		
Stimulants (e.g. amphetamines, cocaine)		
Depressants (e.g. alcohol, benzodiazepines)		
Cannabinoids (e.g. cannabis marijuana)		
Hallucinogens and psychedelics (e.g. LSD, psilocybin)		
Synthetic cathinones (e.g. bath salts – mephedrone, methylone)		
Synthetic opioids (e.g. fentanyl, U-47700)		
Synthetic cannabinoids (e.g. spice, K2)		
Synthetic hallucinogens (e.g. NBOMe compounds; 2C series – 2C-B, 2C-I)		
Synthetic stimulants (e.g. methamphetamine [synthetic version], synthetic cocaine analogues)		
Designer benzodiazepines (e.g. etizolam, flubromazolam)		
Inhalants (nitrous oxide [laughing gas], amyl nitrite [poppers], nitrites, solvents, aerosol sprays, gasoline, household cleaners)		

- *Harmful use*. Defined as "a pattern of use which is already causing damage to health." The damage may be physical (hepatitis following injection of drugs) or mental (depressive episodes due to heavy alcohol misuse). This may involve social consequences, but this is not sufficient to have a diagnosis of harmful use. Harmful drinkers are usually drinking at levels above those recommended for sensible drinking, typically at higher levels than most hazardous drinkers. Unlike hazardous drinkers, harmful drinkers show clear evidence of some alcohol-related harm.

While terms like *unsanctioned use*, *dysfunctional use*, *hazardous use*, and *harmful use* provide a comprehensive perspective on problematic substance use, they are not commonly employed in addiction literature.

TOLERANCE

Tolerance is the body's adaptation to a drug's repeated presence, necessitating higher quantities to achieve desired effects. Tolerance varies across psychoactive substances, developing rapidly with LSD, slowly with alcohol or opiates, and dependent on regular and adequate use. The development and persistence of tolerance to psychoactive substances are influenced by a variety of factors. These include individual characteristics, such as body weight, types of illnesses, stress levels, the strength of the immune system, and age.

Tolerance can decrease rapidly after a period of abstinence, which may occur due to factors like imprisonment or participation in drug treatment programmes. Importantly, if an individual resumes using the same amount or dose of a psychoactive substance after a period of abstinence, there is a heightened risk of overdosing. Furthermore, environmental factors play a role in tolerance, as suggested by evidence indicating that tolerance may be influenced when a person uses drugs in a new or unfamiliar setting (Siegel et al., 1982). This change in environment can contribute to an increased risk of overdose. The interplay of individual and environmental factors stresses the complexity of tolerance development and its implications for the potential dangers associated with resuming drug use after a period of abstinence

Opiate drugs like heroin and morphine may induce tolerance over time and stand out for their common association with both physical and psychological dependence. Physical dependence is prevalent, often leading to withdrawal symptoms upon discontinuation, while psychological dependence is also significant, marked by cravings and emotional reliance. Stimulants like amphetamines cause substantial tolerance. Though generally exhibiting less-pronounced physical dependence compared to opiates, can still induce strong psychological dependence, with users developing cravings and a sense of reliance. Cocaine can lead to psychological dependence without tolerance or moderate physical dependence. Medical use of morphine may result in tolerance and physical dependence without a prominent psychological component.

Depressants, including alcohol and benzodiazepines, commonly result in both physical and psychological dependence. Long-term and heavy use of these substances often lead to physical dependence, characterised by withdrawal symptoms. Psychological dependence is frequently present, as individuals may rely on these substances for mood regulation or anxiety reduction. In contrast, hallucinogens like LSD and psilocybin typically evoke minimal physical dependence, with withdrawal symptoms being uncommon. While psychological dependence on hallucinogens can vary, these substances are generally less associated with compulsive use. Cannabis, characterised by relatively uncommon physical dependence and mild withdrawal symptoms, can still lead to psychological dependence in some individuals, manifesting as a pattern of compulsive use. These distinctions highlight the nuanced interplay between physical and psychological dependence across various drug classes.

Synthetic drugs' potential for physical and psychological dependence exposes varying degrees of risk across different classes. Synthetic cannabinoids exhibit limited evidence for physical dependence, especially with prolonged and frequent use, but some users may develop psychological dependence due to the addictive nature of these substances. Synthetic cathinones, commonly known as bath salts, show limited research on physical dependence, while psychological dependence can occur with chronic use, particularly due to the stimulating effects of these drugs. In contrast, synthetic opioids, including potent substances like fentanyl, pose a high risk for physical dependence, with severe withdrawal symptoms. Additionally, users may develop psychological dependence attributable to the euphoric effects of these synthetic opioids. Synthetic hallucinogens, such as NBOMe compounds, are generally not associated with physical dependence, and their potential for psychological dependence is considered lower compared to substances with more pronounced euphoric effects. Lastly, synthetic stimulants, like methamphetamine analogues, have limited evidence on physical dependence, but the potential for psychological dependence exists due to the stimulating effects. Designer benzodiazepines, such as etizolam, carry a high potential for both physical and psychological dependence, especially with prolonged use, as users may develop reliance on the anxiolytic effects of these synthetic substances. This highlights the diverse risks associated with different categories of synthetic drugs, emphasising the importance of understanding their potential for tolerance and dependence in both physical and psychological aspects.

PHYSICAL DEPENDENCE

Physical dependence is a physiological state that occurs when the body adapts to the regular presence of a substance, such as a psychoactive drug. Alcohol and drugs influence neurotransmitters and brain circuits, particularly those linked to reward and pleasure. Continued substance use leads to the dependence of these circuits on the presence of the substance for normal functioning. Upon cessation, withdrawal symptoms occur due to the disruption of these circuits. The severity and duration of these symptoms are influenced by factors such as the specific substance, duration and quantity of use, and individual characteristics. Physical dependence is not exclusive to illicit substances; it can also develop with the prolonged use of prescribed medications, such as opioids, benzodiazepines, or certain antidepressants. It is characterised by the development of tolerance and the occurrence of withdrawal symptoms upon reducing or discontinuing the substance. The severity of withdrawal symptoms varies, depending on the type or category of drugs. For instance, withdrawal from nicotine may result in relatively slight physiological symptoms, while substances like opiates and depressants can lead to withdrawal experiences ranging from mild to severe. In the case of alcohol withdrawal, symptoms can escalate to hallucinations or epileptic fits, potentially posing life-threatening risks. Dependence can exist without withdrawal, and conversely, withdrawal can occur without dependence, highlighting the complexity of these relationships.

Moreover, it is worth noting that some signs of physical dependence may be psychosomatic reactions not solely triggered by the chemical properties of psychoactive drugs but also influenced by the user's fears, beliefs, and fantasies about the withdrawal process (Plant, 1987). Even in the absence of true physical dependence, many drugs have the potential to elicit withdrawal symptoms or rebound effects when their dosage is reduced, especially during abrupt or rapid withdrawal (Henssler et al., 2019). These can include stimulants like caffeine. This highlights the complex nature of drug interactions with the body and the central nervous system, illustrating that changes in drug exposure have the potential to initiate both physiological and psychological responses. Understanding these withdrawal symptoms is vital for developing effective approaches to manage and cease drug use, especially when a comprehensive physical dependence is not established.

However, it is essential to distinguish physical dependence from addiction. *Physical dependence* involves the body's adaptation to a substance and the occurrence of withdrawal symptoms upon discontinuation, whereas *addiction* encompasses a complex pattern of behaviours involving compulsive drug use despite negative consequences and a loss of control over use. While physical dependence is a component of addiction, not everyone who develops physical dependence becomes addicted, and addiction involves psychological and behavioural elements beyond physical adaptation.

PSYCHOLOGICAL DEPENDENCE

Psychological dependence, often interconnected with physical dependence, plays a pivotal role in addiction. This form of dependence extends beyond psychoactive drugs to include behaviours such as overeating, engaging in sex, gambling, maintaining relationships, or participating in physical activities. The emphasis is on the compulsive urge to continue these behaviours despite potential negative consequences, reflecting a broader understanding of psychological dependence across various aspects of human behaviour. Unlike the biological or physical need for a substance, psychological dependence delves into the emotional and psychological attachment that individuals develop toward it. Psychological dependence involves intense cravings, a preoccupation with using the substance, and a compulsion to continue using despite negative consequences. This can manifest in various ways, from obsessive thoughts about acquiring and using the substance to neglecting responsibilities and experiencing emotional distress when unable to use.

Psychological dependence, a key element in addiction, is influenced by various factors. Firstly, the activation of the brain's reward system by addictive substances plays an important role. This stimulation leads to pleasurable feelings and euphoria, creating a strong association between the substance and enjoyable experiences. Consequently, the reinforcement of this positive connection contributes to cravings and the ongoing use of the substance. Secondly, psychological dependence can emerge as a coping mechanism for individuals dealing with negative emotions, like anxiety, depression, or trauma. Seeking temporary relief through addictive substances reinforces the belief that these psychoactive substances are necessary for managing emotional difficulties. Social and environmental factors also significantly contribute to the development of psychological dependence. Peer pressure, exposure to drug culture, and the easy accessibility of substances elevate the risk, especially in vulnerable individuals, such as young people and adolescents. The influence of external factors highlights the complex interplay between individual choices and the broader social and environmental contexts in shaping patterns of psychological dependence.

DRUG DEPENDENCE OR ADDICTION?

The term *drug dependence* refers to behavioural responses characterised by a compulsion to take a substance. This is driven by the desire to experience its physical or psychological effects or to alleviate the discomfort of its absence. Dependence is often categorised as either physical or psychological. While physical dependence is a common and significant aspect, it is not always necessary for drug dependence. Key features of dependence include tolerance and both psychological and physical dependence. Dependence is comparable to addiction and involves the user's physical and/or psychological adaptation to the presence of a drug. The user would experience negative consequences or withdrawal symptoms if the drug is removed, emphasising the reliance and adaptation that characterise the condition (Royal College of Psychiatrists and Royal College of Physicians, 2000). It has been suggested that there was so much misunderstanding about the concept of dependence, linking dependence with addiction, as this state can be a normal body reaction to a substance (APA, 2013). O'Brien et al. (2006) have argued about the conflation of dependence with addiction. They posited that

> [t]he term "dependence" has traditionally been used to describe "physical dependence," which refers to the adaptations that result in withdrawal symptoms when drugs, such as alcohol and heroin, are discontinued. Physical dependence is also observed with certain psychoactive medications, such as antidepressants and beta-blockers. However, the adaptations associated with drug withdrawal are distinct from the adaptations that result in addiction, which refers to the loss of control over the intense urges to take the drug even at the expense of adverse consequences.
>
> (p. 764)

Furthermore, people can suffer withdrawal without having addiction and have addiction without suffering withdrawal. The author suggested that clinician confusion stems from the terminological overlap between "dependence" (*DSM-IV* sense [akin to addiction]) and the normal physiological response to repeated medication. This confusion can lead to clinicians mistakenly associating tolerance and withdrawal symptoms with addiction, causing patients in pain management scenarios to endure unnecessary suffering. Moreover, the fear of dependence being equated with addiction may discourage patients from seeking proper treatment with opioid medications. In the *Diagnostic and Statistical Manual of Mental Disorders* (APA, 2013), the categories of substance abuse and substance dependence were replaced with a single category: substance use disorder. Originally, the framework of the dependence syndrome was initially applied specifically to alcohol dependence. However, this framework has been broadened to encompass other psychoactive substances. Derived from disease, biological, and behavioural models, the dependence syndrome offers a shared terminology for both academics and clinicians to discuss similar phenomena. Edwards and Gross (1976) outlined seven components of the syndrome, as detailed in Table 1.1.

Table 1.1
The dependence syndrome

- Increased tolerance to the drug.
- Repeated withdrawal symptoms.
- Compulsion to use the drug. (Psychological state known as craving.)
- Salience of drug-seeking behaviour. (Obtaining and using the drug become more important in the person's life.)
- Relief or avoidance of withdrawal symptoms. (The regular use of the drug to relieve withdrawal symptoms.)
- Narrowing of the repertoire of drug-taking. (Pattern of drinking may become an everyday activity.)
- Rapid reinstatement after abstinence.

Source: Adapted from Edwards and Gross (1976).

These components provide a comprehensive overview of the dependence syndrome associated with substance use. The phenomenon includes increased tolerance, indicating a need for higher drug doses over time. Repeated withdrawal symptoms highlight the challenges, both physical and psychological, in discontinuing substance use. The compulsion to use the drug, known as craving, reflects a powerful psychological drive, while the salience of drug-seeking behaviour stresses its growing importance in an individual's life. Additionally, the relief or avoidance of withdrawal symptoms serves as a motivation for regular drug use, potentially leading to a narrowing of the repertoire of drug-taking behaviour, becoming a routine part of daily life. Finally, rapid reinstatement after abstinence signifies a quick return to drug use, emphasising the persistent nature of dependence.

Addiction is not considered a specific diagnosis in the fifth edition of *DSM* (APA, 2013).

By *addiction* we mean the condition of an individual who has a compulsion and dependence on a psychoactive substance (e.g. alcohol or drug) or a behaviour (e.g. gambling, sex, or physical activity). This means that an addictive behaviour is an explanation of why people do certain things and continue to maintain that behaviour despite the consequences. *Addiction* is defined as

> a chronic, relapsing disorder characterised by compulsive drug seeking and use despite adverse consequences.† It is considered a brain disorder, because it involves functional changes to brain circuits involved in reward, stress, and self-control.
>
> (NIDA, 2024)

The American Society of Addiction Medicine (ASAM) (2011) defines *addiction* as a

> primary, chronic disease of brain reward, motivation, memory and related circuitry. Dysfunction in these circuits leads to characteristic biological, psychological, social and spiritual manifestations. This is reflected in an individual pathologically pursuing reward and/or relief by substance use and other behaviours.

In contrast, *drug addiction* "encompasses a relapsing cycle of intoxication, bingeing, withdrawal and craving that results in excessive drug use despite adverse consequences" (Goldstein & Volkow, 2011, p. 652).

The definitions provided characterise addiction as a chronic, relapsing disorder marked by compulsive drug-seeking and drug use despite adverse consequences. Importantly, it is identified as a neuro-pharmacological, brain, and behavioural disorder with physical dependence or psychological dependence. The brain disorder is due to the functional changes in circuits associated with reward, stress, and self-control. These alterations in the brain's functioning can persist even after the individual has ceased drug use, highlighting the lasting impact of addiction. Drug addiction is also viewed as a cyclical pattern involving stages of intoxication, bingeing, withdrawal, and craving. This cycle leads to excessive drug use despite experiencing adverse consequences. This perspective underlines the complex nature of addiction, involving both behavioural patterns and profound physiological changes in the brain.

The concept of addictive behaviour extends beyond the misuse of psychoactive substances to encompass excessive patterns in various activities, such as eating, drinking, drug use, gambling, and sexuality. Individuals facing issues with these behaviours share similar descriptions of the phenomenology of their disorders (Cummings et al., 1980; Orford, 2001).

This approach advocates for a more inclusive diagnostic category, considering both pharmacological and non-pharmacological addictions (Ghodse, 2010). Addictive behaviour can be viewed as a relapsing pharmacological and behavioural disorder of many forms, some of them related to pharmacological substances, such as tobacco, drug, or alcohol, while others are related to an individual's extreme psychological dependence on behaviours, such as gambling, overeating, sexual addiction, and increasingly, social media surfing. This recognition highlights the commonalities in the nature of addictive behaviours, irrespective of the specific substance or activity involved.

SUBSTANCE USE DISORDERS

In the *Diagnostic and Statistical Manual of Mental Disorders* (*DSM-V*) (APA, 2013). Substance use disorders span a wide variety of problems arising from substance use measured on a continuum from mild to severe. Each specific substance is addressed as a separate use disorder (e.g. alcohol use disorder, stimulant use disorder, etc.), but nearly all substances are diagnosed based on the same overarching criteria. Gambling disorder is the sole disorder in a new category on behavioural addictions. This new condition "reflect[s] research findings that gambling disorder is similar to substance-related disorders in clinical expression, brain origin, comorbidity, physiology, and treatment" (APA, 2013). The most common disorders include:

- Alcohol use disorder
- Cannabis use disorder
- Hallucinogen use disorder

Table 1.2
DSM-V diagnostic criteria for substance use disorder

- Eleven diagnostic criteria (some classes of substances have ten criteria).
- Two or more within a 12-month period.
- Must include a pattern of use leading to clinically significant impairment or distress.
  1. Substance often taken in larger amounts or over a longer period of time than intended (impaired control).
  2. A persistent desire or unsuccessful effort to cut down or control use (impaired control).
  3. A great deal of time spent in activities necessary to obtain the substance, use it, or recover from its effects (impaired control).
  4. Craving or strong desire or urge to use (impaired control) (new criteria).
  5. Recurrent use resulting in failure to fulfil major role or obligations at work, school, or home (social impairment).
  6. Continued use despite having persistent or recurrent social/interpersonal problems caused or exacerbated by use (social impairment).
  7. Important social, occupational, or recreational activities given up or reduced because of use (social impairment).
  8. Recurrent use in situations which are physically hazardous (risky use).
  9. Use is continued despite knowledge of having a persistent or recurrent physical/psychological problem likely to have been caused or exacerbated by use (risky use).
  10. Tolerance: the need for markedly increased amounts of substance to achieve intoxication or desired effect, or a markedly diminished effect with continued use of the same amount (pharmacological).
  11. Withdrawal: a characteristic syndrome or use to relieve or avoid withdrawal (pharmacological).
- A maladaptive pattern of substance use leading to clinically significant impairment or distress, as manifested by three or more of the following occurring during the same 12-month period:
  1. Tolerance, as defined by either of the following:
     - Need for markedly increased amounts of the substance to achieve intoxication or desired effect.
     - Markedly diminished effect of continued use of the same amount of the substance.
  2. Withdrawal, as manifested by either of the following:
     - The characteristic withdrawal syndrome for the substance.
     - The same (or a closely related) substance is taken to relieve or avoid withdrawal symptoms.
  3. The substance is often taken in larger amounts or over a longer period than was intended.
  4. A persistent desire or unsuccessful efforts to cut down or control substance use.
  5. A great deal of time is spent in activities necessary to obtain the substance (e.g. visiting multiple doctors or driving long distances), use the substance (e.g. chain-smoking), or recover from its effects.
  6. Important social, occupational, or recreational activities are given up or reduced because of substance use.
  7. The substance use is continued despite knowledge of having a persistent or recurrent physical or psychological problem that is likely to have been caused or exacerbated by the substance (e.g. current cocaine-induced depression or continued drinking despite recognition that an ulcer was made worse by alcohol consumption).

Source: APA (2013).

- Inhalant use disorder
- Opioid use disorder
- Sedative, hypnotic, or anxiolytic use disorder
- Stimulant use disorder
- Tobacco use disorder
- Non-substance-related disorders/gambling disorder

A diagnosis of substance use disorder is based on evidence of impaired control, social impairment, risky use, and pharmacological conditions. In *DSM-V*, mild substance use disorder requires two to three symptoms, four or five symptoms indicate a moderate substance use disorder, and six or more symptoms indicate a severe substance use disorder. The *DSM-V* criteria for substance use disorder are briefly presented in Table 1.2.

ALCOHOL USE DISORDER

Alcohol use disorder (AUD) is classified based on the presence of two or more of the following criteria within 12 months. The criteria, as outlined in the *DSM-V*, to help diagnose the severity of alcohol use disorder based on the number of criteria met by an individual are presented in Table 1.3.

The severity of AUD is determined based on the number of criteria met by a patient. If an individual meets two or three criteria, they are classified as having a mild AUD. Meeting four or five criteria categorises the patient with a moderate AUD. A severe AUD classification is assigned if the patient meets more than six criteria. This classification system helps healthcare professionals assess and categorise the extent of the disorder, allowing for a more tailored and targeted approach to intervention and treatment.

The criteria revolve around the individual's consumption patterns, including taking alcohol in larger amounts or for a longer duration than intended, persistent desires to control use without success, and devoting significant time to obtaining, using, or recovering from the effects of alcohol. Other criteria reflect on the impact of alcohol use on an individual's responsibilities, social relationships, and overall functioning. This includes impaired responsibilities at work, school, or home; continued use despite social or interpersonal problems; and a significant reduction in important activities due to alcohol use. In addition, the criteria address the physiological aspects of alcohol dependence, including the development of tolerance (requiring increased amounts for the desired effect or experiencing reduced effects with the same amount) and the presence of withdrawal symptoms or frequent alcohol consumption to alleviate or prevent withdrawal. These criteria highlight the adaptive changes in the body due to prolonged alcohol use and the potential physical consequences associated with attempts to stop or reduce consumption. Overall, the *DSM-V* criteria offer a structured and comprehensive approach to diagnosing AUD, taking into account both behavioural and physiological aspects.

Table 1.3
Criteria for alcohol use disorder

Key elements	
Excessive use	Alcohol is taken in larger amounts or consumed for a longer duration than intended.
Unsuccessful control	Persistent desire or unsuccessful efforts to reduce or control alcohol use.
Time spent	Significant time spent obtaining, using, or recovering from the effects of alcohol.
Craving	Strong desire or urge to consume alcohol.
Essential responsibilities	Regular alcohol use leads to an inability to meet essential responsibilities at work, school, or home.
Continued use despite problems	Continued alcohol use despite the presence of physical or psychological problems exacerbated by its use.
Social impairment	Alcohol use interferes with social, occupational, or recreational activities, leading to strained relationships and impaired functioning.
Risky use	Continued alcohol use despite being aware of the associated physical or psychological risks. Or use in situations in which it is physically hazardous.
Continued use despite harm	Continued use despite knowing persistent physical or psychological issues caused or exacerbated by alcohol.
Tolerance	Developing tolerance (needing more alcohol to achieve the desired effect) and experiencing withdrawal symptoms when not drinking.
Withdrawal	Presence of typical withdrawal symptoms or frequent alcohol (or benzodiazepine) consumption to alleviate or prevent withdrawal symptoms.

Source: Adapted from APA (2013).

PERSON WITH SUBSTANCE USE DISORDER (SUD)

To prevent stigmatisation, the terms *problem drug user* and *problem drinker* have been replaced with more neutral and clinically accurate language. Individuals who were once labelled as such are now often referred to as individuals with alcohol use disorder or substance use disorder. This shift in terminology aims to destigmatise the condition by framing it as a medical or clinical issue rather than attaching negative labels to individuals. Using person-centred and non-stigmatising language helps promote a more compassionate and understanding approach to addressing the challenges associated with alcohol or substance use.

The historical definition of a problem drug user (ACMD, 1988) has undergone transformation, and the term has been replaced with a more person-centred approach referring to individuals with alcohol use disorder or substance use disorder. This contemporary definition characterises these individuals as facing a range of challenges, including social, psychological, physical, and legal issues stemming from intoxication, regular excessive consumption, dependence, or addiction. Furthermore, there is a growing recognition of the need to expand this definition to include spiritual needs, providing a more inclusive and nuanced perspective on addiction and reinforcing the idea that individuals with alcohol or substance use disorders have diverse and complex needs (Rassool, 2001; Hammond & Rassool, 2006) that extend beyond the purely physical or behavioural aspects. The emphasis is on addressing the holistic needs of the person, moving away from a substance-oriented perspective.

KEY POINTS

- The nature and extent of the global drug and alcohol problem are interwoven with all aspects of sustainable development.
- Alcohol and drugs pose significant harm on physical, social, psychological, and economic levels, impacting not only individuals but also their families and communities.
- Drug use includes a wide range of synthetic, prescribed drugs and illegal, recreational, and socially accepted substances.
- The most commonly consumed drugs in the world include alcohol and cannabis/marijuana, followed by opioids and opiates.
- *Polydrug use* refers to the consumption of more than one drug, either simultaneously or sequentially, by an individual.
- HIV continues to be a major global public health issue.
- The terms *drug use* and *misuse* are subjective and context-dependent, influenced by cultural, ideological, etiological, and clinical factors and the effect of the substance on the individual.
- Addiction is a chronic, relapsing disorder marked by compulsive drug-seeking and drug use despite adverse consequences.
- Substance use disorders span a wide variety of problems arising from substance use measured on a continuum from mild to severe.
- Alcohol use disorder (AUD) is determined based on the number of criteria of *DSM-V* met by an individual.
- Individuals can develop tolerance to a variety of psychoactive substances.
- Dependence has two components: physical and psychological dependence.
- Drugs can produce considerable tolerance and strong psychological dependence with little or no physical dependence.
- The withdrawal symptoms depend on the type or category of drugs.
- The terms *individual with alcohol use disorder* or *substance use disorder* have been used to refer to those experiencing problematic substance use or those individuals in recovery.

References

Advisory Council on the Misuse of Drugs (ACMD). (1988). *Aids and Drug Misuse: Part 1*. London: HMSO.

Akl, E. A., Gaddam, S., Gunukula, S. K., Honeine, R., Jaoude, P. A., & Irani, J. (2010). The effects of waterpipe tobacco smoking on health outcomes: A systematic review. *International Journal of Epidemiology*, 39(3), 834–857. https://doi.org/10.1093/ije/dyq002.

American Lung Association. (2007). *An Emerging Deadly Trend: Waterpipe Tobacco Use* (PDF-222 KB). Washington, DC: American Lung Association.

American Psychiatric Association. (2013). *DSM-V: Diagnostic and Statistical Manual of Mental Disorders* (5th ed.). Washington, DC: American Psychiatric Association.

American Society of Addiction Medicine. (2011). *Public Policy Statement: Definition of Addiction*. https://www.asam.org/docs/default-source/public-policy-statements/1definition_of_addiction_long_4-11.pdf?sfvrsn=a8f64512_4 (accessed 24 June 2024).

Bloomberg, M. R. (2021). WHO Global Ambassador for Noncommunicable Diseases and Injuries Founder, Bloomberg Philanthropies. Cited in WHO. (2021). WHO Report on the Global Tobacco Epidemic 2021: Addressing New and Emerging Products. Geneva: Word Health Organization.

Brunt, T. M., Atkinson, A. M., Nefau, T., Martinez, M., Lahaie, E., Malzcewski, A., Pazitny, M., Belackova, V., & Brandt, S. D. (2017). Online test purchased new psychoactive substances in 5 different European countries: A snapshot study of chemical composition and price. *The International Journal on Drug Policy*, 4, 105–114. https://doi.org/10.1016/j.drugpo.2017.03.006.

CDC. (2015a). *Dangers of Hookah Smoking*. Centers for Disease Control and Prevention. www.cdc.gov/features/hookahsmoking/ (accessed 24 January 2024).

CDC. (2015b). *Multiple Cause of Death 1999–2014*. CDC WONDER Online Database, released 2015. Centers for Disease Control and Prevention. http://wondercdc gov/mcd-icd10 html (accessed 24 January 2024).

Costa, C. M. F. N., Silveira, M. R., Acurcio, F. A., Guerra, A. A., Jr., Guibu, I. A., Costa, K. S., Karnikowski, M. G. O., Soeiro, O. M., Leite, S. N., Costa, E. A., Nascimento, R. C. R. M. D., Araújo, V. E., & Álvares, J. (2017). Use of medicines by patients of the primary health care of the Brazilian unified health system. *Revista de Saude Publica*, 51(Suppl 2), 18s. https://doi.org/10.11606/S1518-8787.2017051007144.

Cummings, C., Gordon, J. R., & Marlatt, G. A. (1980). Relapse: Prevention and prediction. In W. R. Miller (Ed.), *The Addictive Behaviours: Treatment of Alcoholism, Drug Abuse, Smoking and Obesity*. Oxford: Pergamon Press.

Edwards, G., & Gross, M. M. (1976). Alcohol dependence: Provisional description of a clinical syndrome. *British Medical Journal*, 81: 171–173. https://doi.org/10.1136/bmj.1.6017.1058.

EMCDDA. (2015). *New Psychoactive Substances in Europe: An Update from the EU Early Warning System*. Luxembourg: Publications Office of the European Union.

Encyclopædia Britannica. (2007). *Encyclopædia Britannica Ultimate Reference Suite 2005 DVD*. Encyclopædia Britannica, Inc. www.britannica.com/dictionary (accessed 24 June 2024).

European Monitoring Centre for Drugs and Drug Addiction (EMCDDA). (2021a). *European Drug Report 2021: Trends and Developments*. Luxembourg: Publications Office of the European Union.

European Monitoring Centre for Drugs and Drug Addiction (EMCDDA). (2021b). *Polydrug Use: Health and Social Responses*. https://www.emcdda.europa.eu/publications/mini-guides/polydrug-use-heal (accessed 24 January 2024).

Frei, M. Y., Nielsen, S., Dobbin, M. D., & Tobin, C. L. (2010). Serious morbidity associated with misuse of over-the-counter codeine-ibuprofen analgesics: A series of 27 cases. *The Medical Journal of Australia*, 193(5), 294–296. https://doi.org/10.5694/j.1326-5377.2010.tb03911.x

Ghodse, A. H. (2010). *Ghodse's Drugs and Addictive Behaviour: A Guide to Treatment* (4th ed.). Cambridge: Cambridge University Press.

Goldstein, R. Z., & Volkow, N. D. (2011). Dysfunction of the prefrontal cortex in addiction: Neuroimaging findings and clinical implications. *Nature Reviews: Neuroscience*, 12(11) 652–669. https://doi.org/10.1038/nrn3119.

Gowing, L. R., Ali, R. L., Allsop, S., Marsden, J., Turf, E. E., West, R., & Witton, J. (2015). Global statistics on addictive behaviours: 2014 status report. *Addiction*, 110(6), 904-919. https://doi.org/10.1111/add.12899.

Henssler, J., Heinz, A., Brandt, L., & Bschor, T. (2019). Antidepressant withdrawal and rebound phenomena. *Deutsches Arzteblatt International*, 116(20), 355–361. https://doi.org/10.3238/arztebl.2019.0355.

Hughes, G. F., McElnay, J. C., Hughes, C. M., & McKenna, P. (1999). Abuse/misuse of non-prescription drugs. *Pharmacy World and Science*, 21(6), 251–255.

Kadhum, M., Sweidan, A., Jaffery, A. E., Al-Saadi, A., & Madden, B. (2015). A review of the health effects of smoking shisha. *Clinical Medicine*, 15(3), 263–266. https://doi.org/10.7861/clinmedicine.15-3-263.

Kolodny, A., Courtwright, D. T., Hwang, C. S., Kreiner, P., Eadie, J. L., Clark, T. W., & Alexander, G. C. (2015). The prescription opioid and heroin crisis: A public health approach to an epidemic of addiction. *Annual Review of Public Health*, 36, 559–574. https://doi.org/10.1146/annurev-publhealth-031914-122957.

Le Boisselier, R., Alexandre, J., Lelong-Boulouard, V., & Debruyne, D. (2017). Focus on cannabinoids and synthetic cannabinoids. *Clinical Pharmacology and Therapeutics*, 101(2), 220–229. https://doi.org/10.1002/cpt.563.

NIDA. (2021). *Words Matter: Preferred Language for Talking About Addiction*. National Institute on Drug Abuse. https://nida.nih.gov/research-topics/addiction-science/words-matter-preferred-language-talking-about-addiction (accessed 24 January 2024).

NIDA. (2024). *Drug Misuse and Addiction*. National Institute on Drug Abuse. https://nida.nih.gov/publications/drugs-brains-behavior-science-addiction/drug-misuse-addiction (accessed 24 January 2024).

O'Brien, C. P., Volkow, N., & Li, T. K. (2006). What's in a word? Addiction versus dependence in DSM-V. *The American Journal of Psychiatry*, 163(5), 764–765. https://doi.org/10.1176/ajp.2006.163.5.764.

Orford, J. (2001). *Excessive Appetites: A Psychological View of Addictions* (2nd ed.). Chichester: John Wiley & Sons Ltd.

Plant, M. (1987). *Drugs in Perspective*. London: Hodder & Stoughton.

Rassool, G. H. (1998). *Substance Use and Misuse: Nature, Context and Clinical Interventions*. Oxford: Blackwell Science.

Rassool, G. H. (2001). Substance use and dual diagnosis: Concepts, theories and models. In G. H. Rassool (Ed.), *Dual Diagnosis: Substance Misuse and Psychiatric Disorders*. Oxford: Blackwell Science.

Royal College of Psychiatrists and Royal College of Physicians Working Party. (2000). *Drugs: Dilemmas and Choices*. London: Gaskell.

Rudd, R. A., Aleshire, N., Zibbell, J. E., & Gladden, R. M. (2016). Increases in drug and opioid overdose deaths – United States, 2000–2014. *MMWR: Morbidity and Mortality Weekly Report,* 64(50–51), 1378–1382. https://doi.org/10.15585/mmwr.mm6450a3.

Scourfield, A., Flick, C., Ross, J., Wood, D. M., Thurtle, N., Stellmach, D., & Dargan, P. I. (2019). Synthetic cannabinoid availability on darknet drug markets: Changes during 2016–2017. *Toxicology Communications,* 3(1), 7–15. https://doi.org/10.1080/24734306.2018.1563739.

Siegel, S., Hinson, R. E., Krank, M. D., & McCully, J. (1982). Heroin "overdose" death: Contribution of drug-associated environmental cues. *Science,* 216(4544), 436–437. https://doi.org/10.1126/science.7200260.

UNAIDS. (2021). *End Inequalities: End AIDS. Global AIDS Strategy. 2021–2026.* https://www.unaids.org/sites/default/files/media_asset/global-AIDS-strategy-2021-2026_en.pdf (accessed 23 January 2024).

UNAIDS. (2023). *The Path That Ends AIDS 2023 UNAIDS Global AIDS Update.* https://thepath.unaids.org/ (accessed 24 January 2024).

UNDOC (United Nation Office of Drugs and Crime). (2011). *The Non-Medical Use of Prescription Drugs. Policy Direction Issues.* New York: United Nations Office on Drugs and Crime. https://www.unodc.org/documents/drug-prevention-and-treatment/nonmedical-use-prescription-drugs.pdf (accessed 23 January 2024).

UNDOC (United Nation Office of Drugs and Crime). (2016). *World Drug Report 2016.* www.unodc.org/doc/wdr2016/WORLD_DRUG_REPORT_2016_web.pdf (accessed 23 January 2024).

UNDOC (United Nation Office of Drugs and Crime). (2022). *World Drug Report 2022.* https://www.unodc.org/unodc/data-and-analysis/world-drug-report-2022.html (accessed 23 January 2024).

UNDOC (United Nation Office of Drugs and Crime). (2023). *World Drug Report 2023.* https://www.unodc.org/unodc/en/data-and-analysis/world-drug-report-2023.html (accessed 23 January 2024).

Whitaker, B. (1987). *The Global Connection: The Crisis of Drug Addiction.* London: Jonathan Cape.

WHO. (2018). *Global Status Report on Alcohol and Health 2018.* Geneva: World Health Organization. https://iris.who.int/bitstream/handle/10665/274603/9789241565639-eng.pdf?sequence=1 (accessed 23 January 2024).

WHO. (2019). WHO Global Report on Trends in Prevalence of Tobacco Use 2000–2025 (3rd ed.). Geneva: World Health Organization. https://iris.who.int/bitstream/handle/10665/330221/9789240000032-eng.pdf (accessed 23 January 2024).

WHO. (2021). WHO Report on the Global Tobacco Epidemic 2021: Addressing New and Emerging Products. https://iris.who.int/bitstream/handle/10665/343287/9789240032095-eng.pdf?sequence=1 (accessed 23 January 2024).

WHO. (2022). *Global Health Sector Strategies on, Respectively, HIV, Viral Hepatitis and Sexually Transmitted Infections for the Period 2022–2030.* Geneva: World Health Organization.

WHO. (2023). *HIV and AIDS: Key Facts.* https://www.who.int/news-room/fact-sheets/detail/hiv-aids (accessed 24 January 2024).

WHO & Joint United Nations Programme on HIV/AIDS. (1999). *HIV in Pregnancy: A Review.* https://iris.who.int/bitstream/handle/10665/65985/WHO_CHS_RHR_99.15_eng.pdf (accessed 24 January 2024).

Wilby, K. J., & Wilbur, K. (2017). Cross-national analysis of estimated narcotic utilisation for twelve Arabic speaking countries in the Middle East. *Saudi Pharmaceutical Journal,* 25(1), 83–87.

World Health Organization. (1981). Nomenclature and classification of drug- and alcohol-related problems: A WHO memorandum. *Bulletin of the World Health Organization,* 59, 225–242.

World Health Organization (WHO). (1994). *Lexicon of Alcohol and Drug Terms.* Geneva: World Health Organization. https://iris.who.int/bitstream/handle/10665/39461/9241544686_eng.pdf?sequence=1 (accessed 24 January 2024).

Chapter 2

Breaking stereotypes

Developing self-awareness and attitude

Learning outcomes

- Foster increased sensitivity and empathy for individuals grappling with substance use disorder.
- Explore the stigmatisation and stereotypes confronted by those dealing with substance use disorder.
- Compile a list of harmful psychoactive substances.
- Cultivate awareness and enhanced confidence when working with individuals experiencing substance use disorder.

INTRODUCTION

The chapter aims to enhance understanding and empathy towards individuals facing substance use disorder (SUD), by exploring stigmatisation and stereotypes, compiling information on harmful psychoactive substances, and cultivating awareness and confidence in working with those experiencing SUD. The focus lies on reflecting on your own relationship with alcohol and drugs, and other behavioural activities.

ATTITUDE AND STIGMATISATION

Attitudes towards individuals with substance use disorders significantly influence the quality of interaction and effectiveness of the quality of care. While a positive attitude involves feeling good about the work and roles associated with this client group, attitudes can vary widely among individuals. Some may perceive working with individuals struggling with SUD as challenging or may hold beliefs about insufficient sanctions for related issues like drinking and driving. These attitudes encompass emotional, cognitive, and behavioural responses, shaping one's approach and perspective. Understanding and addressing these attitudes are crucial for fostering empathy, effective communication, and support for individuals facing substance use challenges. Nursing literature examines the range of attitudes and emotions nurses may hold towards individuals with substance use disorders, encompassing intolerance, anger, distrust, powerlessness, anxiety, and feelings of manipulation. Additionally, nurses may grapple with frustration, futility, and disappointment, especially regarding patient relapse and recidivism (Tierney, 2016). Factors contributing to these attitudes include lack of knowledge, training, organisational structures, policies, and past experiences (Rassool, 2018). Stigmatisation surrounding SUD manifests in negative attitudes, stereotypes, and discrimination, resulting in social exclusion and diminished opportunities for employment, housing, and healthcare. Individuals with SUD often internalise this stigma, experiencing shame, guilt, and low self-esteem, which hampers their willingness or access to seek treatment. Stigma contributes to treatment barriers, including fear of judgement, lack of culturally competent care, and limited access to generic and specialist addiction services. Moreover, stigma undermines recovery by discouraging help-seeking, amplifying stress and isolation, and perpetuating cycles of addiction and relapse, highlighting its pervasive impact on individuals with SUD.

Attitudes towards individuals with SUD encompass both professional and personal dimensions. Professional attitudes revolve around beliefs concerning one's role in addressing alcohol or drug use

DOI: 10.4324/9781003456674-3

within professional practice, considering factors like role legitimacy and professional responsibilities. Equally, personal attitudes are influenced by emotions and beliefs stemming from the stigmatisation of substance use disorders, including feelings of blame and anger fuelled by societal judgements and stereotypes. These personal attitudes significantly impact how individuals interact with and support those dealing with substance use issues. Understanding the interplay between professional and personal attitudes is crucial for healthcare professionals to provide effective and empathetic care to individuals facing challenges associated with substance use disorders.

Complete the Rassool "attitude towards substance misusers" questionnaire (© Copyright G. Hussein Rassool [2004]). Permission should be obtained from the author for the use of the questionnaire. Reflect about your attitudes towards individuals with alcohol and drug problems.

Positive attitudes towards individuals with substance use disorder encompass compassion,

Activity 2.1 Rassool attitude towards substance misusers questionnaire (RATSMQ-10).

The statements on the following pages reflect several different opinions, beliefs, and viewpoints about substance use and misuse. Please indicate how strongly you agree or disagree with each statement. To complete the instrument, please place a tick in the box that best reflects how strongly you agree or disagree with each statement.

1. Personal use of illicit drug should be legal in the confines of one's home.

Strongly agree	Agree	Uncertain	Disagree	Strongly disagree

2. Individuals with substance use disorder suffer from feelings of inferiority.

Strongly agree	Agree	Uncertain	Disagree	Strongly disagree

3. People who use illicit drug do not respect authority.

Strongly agree	Agree	Uncertain	Disagree	Strongly disagree

4. Heroin is so addictive that no one can really recover once substance use disorder is developed.

Strongly agree	Agree	Uncertain	Disagree	Strongly disagree

5. Rehabilitation of individuals with substance use disorder always fails.

Strongly agree	Agree	Uncertain	Disagree	Strongly disagree

6. Illicit substance use is a monetary and social drain on the community.

Strongly agree	Agree	Uncertain	Disagree	Strongly disagree

7. Compulsory treatment is necessary for those who have alcohol and substance use disorder.

Strongly agree	Agree	Uncertain	Disagree	Strongly disagree

8. Individuals with alcohol use disorder should be referred to a specialist once health problems are identified.

Strongly agree	Agree	Uncertain	Disagree	Strongly disagree

9. Those individuals with alcohol and substance use disorder are unpleasant to work with.

Strongly agree	Agree	Uncertain	Disagree	Strongly disagree

10. Individuals with alcohol and substance use disorder are stigmatised by healthcare professionals.

Strongly agree	Agree	Uncertain	Disagree	Strongly disagree

understanding, and recognition of addiction as a complex medical condition rather than a moral failing. Such attitudes prioritise support and empowerment, aiming to facilitate access to treatment, resources, and a nurturing environment for recovery. They embrace a non-judgemental approach that acknowledges the diverse factors contributing to addiction, including genetics, environment, and psychosocial influences. Moreover, positive attitudes entail advocacy efforts for policy changes, improved treatment accessibility, and educational initiatives to increase awareness about the challenges encountered by individuals with SUD, fostering a more supportive and inclusive society.

HARM: SUBSTANCE USE

Health policy regarding drug and alcohol use primarily aims at reducing the harm caused to individual users, their families, and society at large. This harm encompasses physical, social, psychological, and economic consequences. Currently, harmful substances are regulated based on classification systems based on the United Nations Single Convention, 1971, and in the UK, the Misuse of Drugs Act, 1971. It was designed as a way to control the use of illegal drugs according to their relative harmfulness. The classification system helps in determining the legal status of substances and guides policies related to their production, distribution, and use. A primary objective of classifying illegal drugs is to establish a deterrent effect by aligning legal consequences with the harms attributed to specific substances (Gossop, 2006). The legal frameworks governing controlled drugs aim to balance access for legitimate medical purposes with measures to prevent diversion, misuse, and harm. By establishing clear guidelines, monitoring systems, and accountability mechanisms, these regulations contribute to the safe management and use of controlled drugs within healthcare and social care settings.

Substance use disorder poses a complex threat, encompassing physical, social, psychological, and economic harm. Physically, it contributes to a range of health issues from acute overdose to chronic conditions, like liver disease and infectious diseases. Socially, it strains relationships, leads to social isolation, and subjects individuals to stigma and discrimination. Psychologically, substance use disorder harms mental health disorders and impairs cognitive functioning. Economically, it incurs financial instability, healthcare costs, law enforcement expenses, and productivity losses.

Classifying substances according to the degree of harm they cause is a complex task influenced by various factors, including physical effects, addictive potential, social consequences, and overall societal impact. This exercise examines an individual's notion of a "harmful" drug. You should classify and write each substance according to the relative degree of harm you think it causes.

Activity 2.2 List of substances.

Amphetamines	GHB
Anabolic steroids	Heroin
Alkyl nitrates	Examine
Alcohol	Khat
Barbiturates	LSD
Benzodiazepines	Methadone (street)
Buprenorphine	Solvents
Cocaine	Synthetic drugs
Cannabis	Tobacco
Ecstasy	

You should classify and write each substance in the preceding table according to the relative degree of harm you think it causes. For example, if you think that ecstasy is the most harmful substance in the list, you should write it in the space provided in the following table in the number 1 ranking.

1		11	
2		12	
3		13	
4		14	
5		15	
6		16	
7		17	
8		18	
9		19	
10			

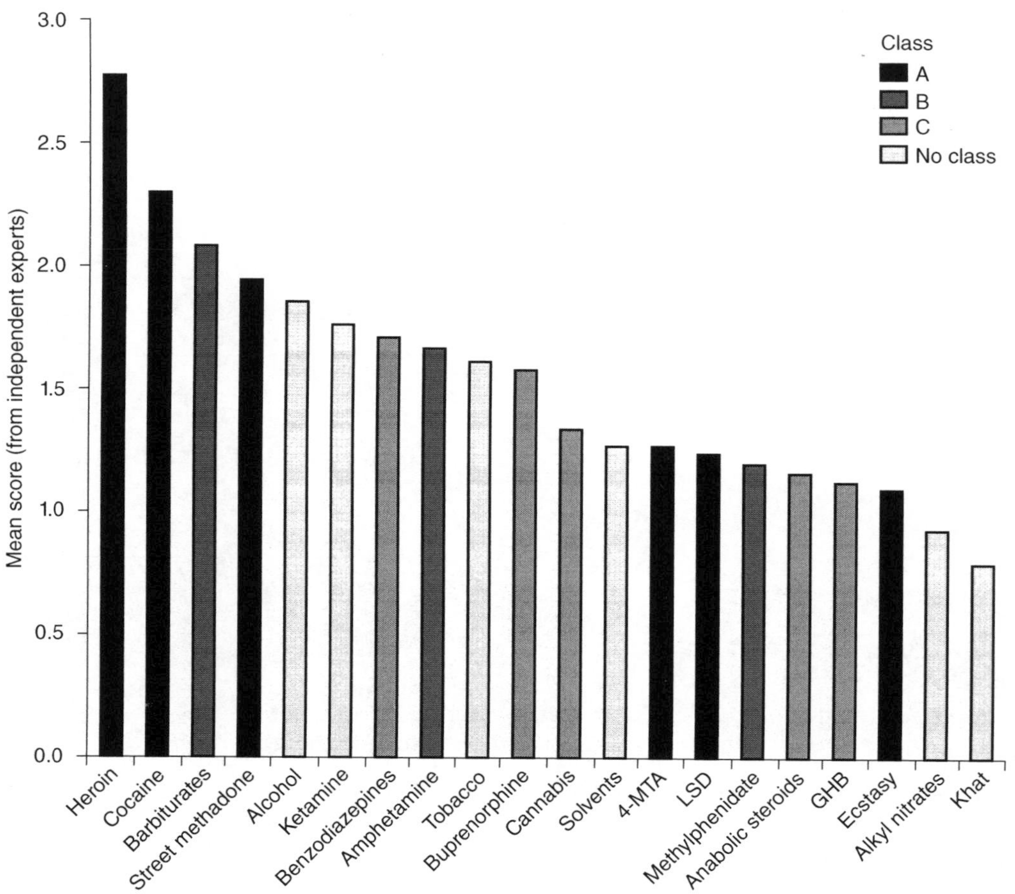

FIGURE 2.1 Mean harm score of 20 psychoactive substances.
Source: Nutt et al. (2007).

A new "matrix of harm" for drugs of abuse has been proposed by Nutt et al. (2007). The study proposes that drugs should be classified by the amount of harm that they do, rather than the sharp A, B, and C divisions in the UK Misuse of Drugs Act. Nutt et al. (2007) identified three main factors that together determine the harm associated with any drug of potential abuse:

- The physical harm to the individual user caused by the drug.
- The tendency of the drug to induce dependence.
- The effect of drug use on families, communities, and society.

The new ranking places alcohol and tobacco in the upper half of the league table, indicating a higher perceived level of harm. This suggests that the new ranking views alcohol and tobacco as more harmful substances than previously thought. Cannabis is ranked lower in the new classification, indicating a perception of lesser harm. Class A drugs (LSD, 4-methylthioamphetamine, ecstasy) are placed lower in terms of perceived harm compared to alcohol and tobacco. Heroin, cocaine, barbiturates, an methadone are consistently ranked among the most harmful in this classification, indicating a consensus regarding their high potential for harm. Now compare your own classification with those of Nutt et al. (2007), as shown in Figure 2.1.

- What are the similarities or differences in comparison?
- Are your ideas of harm of substances based on the media, your personal experience, or the experiences of others?
- Is the notion of harm based on medical, moral, social, or legal criteria?

CONFIDENCE SKILLS

Confidence plays an important role in the effectiveness of nurses and other healthcare professionals when working for individuals with alcohol or substance use disorder. It is a psychological quality that stems from assessing one's capabilities in a given context. Confidence can function as a self-fulfilling prophecy: individuals who lack confidence may refrain from attempting tasks or may experience failure due to their lack of belief, whereas those who possess confidence may succeed primarily because of their self-assurance rather than innate ability. Healthcare professionals often exhibit varying levels of confidence across different aspects of their practice. Confidence typically grows with experience and practice, but it can also be cultivated as an attitude or habit of thought. Taking a positive attitude towards one's abilities can facilitate the development of confidence skills when working with alcohol and drug users.

The process outlined involves completing a questionnaire on intervention confidence skills when working with individuals with alcohol or substance

Activity 2.3 Addiction intervention skills questionnaire (© Rassool, 2004). To complete the instrument, please place a tick in the box that best reflects your confidence level.

	Low confidence	Moderate confidence	High confidence
Providing alcohol use education and prevention information			
Recognising signs and symptoms of alcohol use disorder			
Talking to patients about risks of alcohol use disorder			
Taking an alcohol history			
Referring patients for alcohol treatment			
Providing care for individuals with alcohol use disorder			
Providing drug use education and prevention information			
Recognising signs and symptoms of substance use disorder			
Talking to patients about risks of substance use disorder			
Taking a substance use disorder history			
Refer patients to addiction treatment			
Providing care for patients with substance use disorder			
Giving health risk information on prescribed medication			
Informing smokers about health risks of tobacco smoking			
Providing tobacco education and prevention information			
Knowledge of drug and alcohol services			

use disorders. By initially assessing one's confidence levels before engaging with educational material, individuals can establish a baseline understanding of their perceived abilities in working with individuals with alcohol or substance use disorders. After completing the book or course, participants can then reassess their confidence levels using the same questionnaire. Comparing the two sets of responses enables individuals to gauge any improvements or changes in their intervention confidence skills following the educational intervention.

ACTIVITY 2.4

Disclaimer: Engaging in Activity 2.4, which involves reflecting on your own relationship with alcohol and drugs, can evoke sensitive and potentially distressing emotions. Substance use is a complex and personal topic, and exploring one's experiences may bring forth challenging feelings. It is crucial to approach this activity with caution and self-awareness. If you find that exploring these aspects triggers discomfort or emotional vulnerability, we strongly recommend seeking appropriate support. This may involve reaching out to a mental health professional, counsellor, online help and support, or a trusted individual in your support network who can provide guidance and assistance. Remember that your well-being is paramount, and it is entirely acceptable to refrain from participating in the activity if you feel it may adversely affect your emotional state.

This reflective journaling activity provides individuals with a structured yet flexible approach to explore their coping mechanisms and habits. Participants are encouraged to delve into various aspects of their lives that serve as sources of comfort, whether they be substances, activities, or relationships.

KEY POINTS

- It is important to reflect on our habits and how they may impact our physical and mental health.
- Attitudes and stigma surrounding substance use disorder play significant roles in how individuals with addiction are perceived, treated, and supported within society.
- It is important to develop a positive attitude in order to enhance the quality of care given to those with alcohol or substance use disorder.
- Harm caused by problematic substance use includes physical harms, social harms, psychological harms, and economic harms.
- Working with individuals having alcohol or substance use disorder requires confidence derived from experience and practice.
- By taking a positive attitude, this may enable the development of confidence skills in working with alcohol and drug users.

Activity 2.4 Please answer the following questions, if appropriate.

- What psychoactive substances, if any, do you find yourself relying on for comfort or escape?
- Are there any psychoactive substances you feel you might rely on more than you should?
- Have you ever found yourself relying on substances to cope with difficult emotions or situations?
- Are there any substances you consume regularly that you feel you might be overly dependent on?
- Have you noticed any patterns in your substance use that concern you?
- Are there any activities or behaviours that you find yourself constantly engaging in?
- Do you find yourself engaging in specific activities as a way to distract yourself from other issues?
- Do you feel dependent on certain activities to cope with stress or boredom?
- Have you noticed any changes in your behaviour related to certain activities?
- Are there specific people, behavioural activities you feel you cannot do without?
- Do you find yourself relying heavily on certain relationships or possessions?
- Have you ever felt controlled by your attachment to someone or something?
- Have you ever felt like you could not function without the presence or involvement of certain people or things?

References

Gossop, M. (2006). Classification of illegal and harmful drugs. *BMJ (Clinical Research Ed.)*, 333(7562), 272–273. https://doi.org/10.1136/bmj.38929.578414.80.

Nutt, D., King, L. A., Saulsbury, W., & Blakemore, C. (2007). Development of a rational scale to assess the harm of drugs of potential misuse. *The Lancet*, 369(9566), 1047–1053.

Rassool, G. H. (2018). *Alcohol and Drug Misuse: A Guide for Health and Social Care Professionals*. Oxford: Routledge.

Tierney, M. (2016). Improving nurse's attitudes toward patients with substance use disorders. *American Nurse Today*, 11(11). https://americannursetoday.mydigitalpublication.com/articles/improving-nurse-s-attitudes-toward-patients-with-substance-use-disorders (accessed 25 January 2024).

Chapter 3

From ancient rituals to modern addictions

A history of psychoactive substances

Learning outcomes

- Explore traditional rituals and practices involving psychoactive substances.
- Analyse the impact of psychoactive substances on societies throughout history.
- Trace the evolution and innovation of psychoactive substances.
- Contrast the contemporary usage of a psychoactive substances with historical patterns of consumption.

INTRODUCTION

From the earliest civilisations to the complexities of contemporary society, the use of psychoactive substances has been intertwined with human culture, spirituality, medicine, and commerce. Psychoactive substances have been used for medicinal, religious, cultural, and recreational purposes, as well as social lubrication. Ancient civilisations, such as the Egyptians, Greeks, and Indigenous cultures of the Americas, revered psychoactive plants like peyote, ayahuasca, and cannabis for their claimed abilities to facilitate spiritual enlightenment, divine communication, and therapeutic healing. During the transition from the Middle Ages to the Renaissance, the utilisation of psychoactive substances underwent further development, becoming rooted with practices of alchemy, mysticism, and the emerging disciplines of medicine and pharmacology. Alchemists and herbalists were involved in the creation of potions, elixirs, and tinctures, driven by the elixir of life. They utilised herbal remedies containing substances such as opium, mandrake, and belladonna for various purposes, ranging from pain relief to inducing sleep. This approach illustrates the integration of science, spirituality, and the pursuit of wellness during that historical period.

The historical evolution of psychoactive substance use, spanning from the Renaissance to the present day, reflects dynamic changes in societal norms, scientific advancements, cultural attitudes, policy development, and legal sanctions. In the contemporary era, globalisation, technological progress, and shifting social values have transformed substance use patterns, introducing new synthetic drugs and associated challenges. Despite advancements in understanding and treatment, substance use remains a complex issue with significant implications for health and society. Understanding the historical context of psychoactive substance use enhances our understanding of current attitudes, behaviours, and challenges surrounding their usage in modern times.

ALCOHOL

The word "alcohol" is of Arabic origin, possibly derived from *al-kuḥl*, an early distilled substance, or *al-ġawl*, meaning "spirit" or "demon," akin to liquors being called "spirits" in English. Late Stone Age beer jugs indicate intentionally fermented beverages existed by the Neolithic period (cir. 10,000 BC), potentially preceding bread as a staple. Wine appeared as a finished product in Egyptian pictographs around 4,000 BC (Hanson, 1995). Despite the presence of wine in religious

DOI: 10.4324/9781003456674-4

contexts, both the Old and New Testaments caution against excessive alcohol consumption and drunkenness. In ancient Egypt, alcoholic beverages, overseen by the god Osiris, were integral to life, serving purposes of pleasure, nutrition, medicine, ritual, remuneration, and funerary rites. Drinking bouts and excessive consumption were common in both ancient Egypt and Assyria, often associated with religious rituals and festive celebrations. One of the first mentions of *wine* in the Old Testament, during the time of Abraham, is: "Then Melchizedek king of Salem [Jerusalem] brought out bread and wine-since he was priest of God Most High" (Genesis 14:18). This has significant symbolic and theological implications. However, the use of alcohol is also noted, as seen when Noah became drunk from wine (Genesis 9:21) and in the accounts of Lot (Genesis 19:30–36) and Nabal (Samuel 25:36). Despite the presence of wine in religious contexts, both the Old and New Testaments caution against excessive alcohol consumption and drunkenness. Several verses in the Qur'an address the issue of alcohol, emphasising its harmful effects on individuals and society. For example, in Surah Al-Baqarah (2:219), believers are instructed to avoid alcohol and gambling because they bring more harm than benefit. Additionally, in Surah Al-Ma'idah (5:90), it is stated that intoxicants and gambling are abominations of Satan's handiwork, and believers are advised to abstain from them to attain success.

In ancient Egypt, alcoholic beverages, overseen by the god Osiris, were integral to life, serving purposes of pleasure, nutrition, medicine, ritual, remuneration, and funerary rites. Drinking bouts and excessive consumption were common in both ancient Egypt and Assyria, often associated with religious rituals and festive celebrations. In ancient Greece, mead, made from honey and water, was the first popular alcoholic drink, followed by wine, which became integral to religious rituals, social gatherings, and daily meals. Despite its widespread use, habitual drunkenness was uncommon due to social norms promoting moderation and temperance (Hanson, 1995). Similarly, in China, alcohol, known as *Jiu*, was considered a spiritual nourishment and used across society for inspiration, hospitality, and fatigue relief. Chinese beliefs emphasised moderation in alcohol consumption as prescribed by heaven (Hanson, 1995). In India, alcoholic beverages like Sura, distilled from rice meal, were prevalent between 3,000 BC and 2,000 BC, with specific social contexts governing their use among warriors and peasants (Peele & Grant, 1999).

During the height of the Roman Empire, there was a notable transition from ceremonial to everyday drinking, leading to a rise in chronic drunkenness akin to modern alcoholism (Babor, 1989). Wine became the favoured beverage, often distributed freely or at minimal cost, contributing to occasional excesses at festivals and celebrations. While criticisms of abusive drinking persisted, there was a gradual decline in such behaviour over subsequent centuries (Austin, 1985). Following the collapse of the Roman Empire, brewing and winemaking techniques were preserved by religious institutions, particularly monasteries, in Christian Europe. The early ritualisation of alcohol in Christian rituals, coupled with the church's aversion to mind-altering substances, further solidified alcohol's dominance in European societies (Gossop, 2007). By the millennium, festivities in England revolved around "ales," with ale and beer becoming prominent commodities. The industrial revolution ushered in new beverages, production methods, distribution channels, and drinking customs (Jernigan, 2000). Presently, alcohol consumption across North Africa and the Middle East is particularly low – in many countries, close to zero. At the upper end of the scale, alcohol intake across Europe is higher (Ritchie & Roser, 2024).

During the Middle Ages, distillation, a pivotal development, was pioneered by Muslim chemists like Jabir ibn Hayyan, Al-Kindi, and Al-Razi during the Abbasid caliphate (Al-Hassan & Hill, 1986; Hassan, 2001). Jabir ibn Hayyan, credited with inventing the alembic still, observed the flammable vapour released from heated wine, noting how it was "of little use, but of great importance to science." Al-Razi further described the distillation of alcohol and its medicinal uses (Hassan & Hill, 1986). The introduction of distillation and the concept of pure alcohol were brought into Europe during the 12th century by European authors who translated and popularised the discoveries of Islamic and Persian alchemists (Hassan, 2001). While alcohol has served roles in religious worship, nutrition, hydration, medicine, and social interactions, its purified form has inflicted significant harm, particularly when consumed outside historical and cultural contexts. This discrepancy highlights the potential for distilled alcohol to cause havoc, as noted by Whitaker (1987) concerning North American Indians and Australian Aborigines.

OPIATES AND OPIOIDS

Opium, extracted from the seedpods of the opium poppy, has multifaceted uses and chemical composition. The poppy plant's seeds can be utilised in various culinary applications, while its pods are infused to create traditional sedative drinks. Opium itself is a complex mixture comprising sugars, proteins, fats, and various alkaloids, notably morphine, codeine, noscapine, papaverine, and thebaine. Cultivated in ancient Persia, Egypt, and Mesopotamia, the poppy plant has a rich historical presence, with fossil remains dating back over 4,000 years. Middle Eastern and Asian cultures embraced its use, which eventually spread to Europe through trade routes and expeditions. Hippocrates acknowledged opium's medicinal properties, highlighting its efficacy in treating internal diseases and epidemics. References to opium date back to Assyrian medical tablets from the 17th century BC and Sumerian ideograms from around 4,000 BC, where it was referred to as the "plant of joy" (Berridge & Edwards, 1987). In Egyptian civilisation, opium preparations were promoted for household use, and pharaohs were buried with opium artifacts. By the AD 8th century, opium use had expanded to Arabia, India, and China, with Arab physicians like Ibn-Sina recommending it for various ailments, including diarrhoea and eye diseases.

In England, opium found extensive use as both a narcotic and a hypnotic, evidenced in literary works like Chaucer's *The Canterbury Tales* and Shakespeare's *Othello*. Known by various evocative names such as the "sacred anchor of life" and "milk of paradise," opium gained prominence through figures like Thomas Sydenham, who standardised laudanum, a popular formulation containing opium, saffron, cinnamon, cloves, and Canary wine. Throughout the 19th century, laudanum became a household remedy for minor ailments and discomforts, with opium-based preparations like Godfrey's Cordial and Mrs. Winslow's Soothing Syrup commonly used for sedation, even among infants and young children. Opium's prevalence extended beyond medicinal use, being favoured over alcohol and employed in various forms to combat endemic conditions like malaria, particularly among rural communities, such as those in the Fens of England (Lincolnshire, Norfolk Cambridgeshire, Huntingdonshire, Northamptonshire, and Suffolk). The British Medical Association (cited in *The Good Drug Guide*) estimated that sparsely populated Cambridgeshire and its environs consumed around half of Britain's annual opium imports. This consumption was topped up by the generous use of poppy tea brewed from homegrown poppies.

Meanwhile, the British East India Company's control over the Asian opium trade precipitated conflict with China, leading to the First Opium War in 1839 and subsequent hostilities. The treaties that followed expanded opium markets in China, resulting in widespread addiction among its population by the end of the 19th century. Opium, historically recognised as one of the world's earliest antidepressants, possesses unique qualities distinct from other pain-relieving agents like alcohol, ether, or barbiturates (*The Good Drug Guide*). Unlike these substances, opium does not impair sensory perception, intellect, or motor coordination, allowing pain to be perceived without causing distress. Despite contemporary associations of habitual opioid use with states of stupor and oblivion, Samuel Taylor Coleridge famously described opium's effects as "intensify," highlighting its historical and cultural significance.

Opium, being cheaper than alcohol, became popular among the working classes, who saw it as an effective hangover cure. By the 1870s and 1880s, addiction to opium had become so widespread that a new term, "morphinomania," entered the English language (Brereton, 2020).

Morphine was first isolated from opium in 1805 by a German pharmacist, Wilhelm Sertürner, who named it *morphium*, after Morpheus, the Greek god of sleep and dreams. It carries a meaning for what was, in reality, a dreadful addiction. By the late 19th century, morphine became popular among high society and middle-class professionals. The invention of the hypodermic syringe allowed for the injection of pure morphine, initially believed to be non-addictive and effective in treating opium and morphine addiction. The prevalence of opium-related issues prompted calls for stricter regulation of the sales of opium and its derivatives, laudanum, by the early 19th century. However, it was not until the Pharmacy Act of 1868 that regulations were introduced, classifying opium as dangerous and restricting its sales (Brereton, 2020). However, patented tinctures containing opium as a component remained readily accessible. For example, Mrs. Winslow's Soothing Syrup, employed to relieve teething discomfort in children, persisted in usage in the UK until the late 19th century. Opium remained available for over-the-counter purchase until the implementation of the Dangerous Drugs Act of 1920, and laudanum remained a standard inclusion in home medical supplies well into the 20th century (Brereton, 2020).

However, the quest for a powerful, non-addictive alternative to opium and morphine led to the synthesis of heroin through acetylation of morphine by English pharmacist C. R. Alder Wright in 1874. Wright boiled morphine and acetic acid to produce diacetylmorphine, C17H17NO (C2H3O2). Diacetylmorphine was synthesised and marketed commercially by Bayer in 1898 – heroin. Subsequently, the identification of the active alkaloids of opium and the development of the process of acetylation by which morphine is converted to heroin changed the whole pattern of opiate use, not only in the West, where the discovery was made, but also in the East, where the parent drug originated (Ghodse, 2010).

DEPRESSANT AND HALLUCINOGENS

Cannabis contains cannabinoids like THC and CBD, as well as terpenes, which interact with the brain to produce various effects. While THC, the main psychoactive cannabinoid, exhibits depressant-like effects by slowing down brain functions and inducing relaxation, it does not typically cause drowsiness or impairment like alcohol or benzodiazepines. While not a true hallucinogen, cannabis can lead to mild distortions in perception, especially at high doses, including intensified sensory experiences and altered sense of time or space. Additionally, cannabis can act as a stimulant by increasing heart rate, boosting energy levels, and enhancing creativity and focus in some individuals. The classification of cannabis as either a depressant, hallucinogenic, or stimulant substance depends on factors like dosage, strain, individual reactions like metabolism and brain chemistry, and method of consumption.

Cannabis sativa, also known as cannabis or marijuana, was among the earliest cultivated plants for its non-food properties, primarily valued for its fibre. Originating in Asia around 2,700 BC in China, it was recommended by Emperor Shen Nung for its pharmacological benefits, including pain relief and treating ailments like gout and absent-mindedness (Maisto et al., 2021). Additionally, cannabis was speculated to have been used for countering evil spirits and for its psychoactive properties (Abel, 1980). In India, cannabis was considered a sacred plant and used in religious rituals, while hashish, derived from the resin, was identified among Arabs in the 10th century. The recreational and intoxicating use of cannabis is associated with the Middle East and North Africa, reaching European countries in the 19th century following the Arab invasion of Spain. The exposure of cannabis to Europe was influenced by printed literature detailing personal experiences with hashish. During the mid-19th century, the medical profession began to take interest in cannabis. William O'Shaughnessy, an Irish physician who described its medical applications in India, introduced cannabis to Great Britain (Bloomquist, 1971). In France, a group of writers, intellectuals, and artists, including Charles Baudelaire and Theophile Gautier, described the use and effects of hashish. The establishment of *Le Club des Hachishins* (the Hashish Club) in Paris in the 1840s marked a notable event. French authors such as Charles Baudelaire and Theophile Gautier both described the splendours of their hallucinatory experiences in the use of hashish. Gautier vividly depicted the splendours and various emotional experiences induced by hashish, including mystery, joy, ecstasy, fear, and paranoia (Gautier, 1844/1966).

Despite its initial appeal, cannabis did not immediately gain widespread use in Europe. However, in the 1960s, the cultural movement of the young generation, influenced by trends imported from the United States, contributed to the widespread use of cannabis or hashish for its psychoactive properties in Europe. Over the past decades, cannabis has remained the most frequently used illicit drug globally. While the plant grows naturally worldwide, it is indigenous to Central Asia and the Himalayan region, being cultivated widely in Africa, India, North America, and the Caribbean region. Cannabis prohibition in the early 20th century led to clandestine indoor cultivation, utilising basements, grow tents, roof spaces, and repurposed buildings. This period witnessed the development of technologies like fluorescent lights, hydroponics, and ventilation systems, vital for successful indoor cannabis growth. The increasing legalisation of medical cannabis and decriminalisation, alongside growing acceptance of recreational use, further fuelled the expansion of indoor cultivation. Today, indoor growing spans from small-scale setups in private homes to large-scale commercial facilities, fulfilling the demand for cannabis products in legal markets. However, the environmental impacts of cannabis cultivation include water intensity, indoor air quality concerns, energy consumption leading to greenhouse gas emissions, soil erosion risks, and heavy metal absorption (Zheng et al., 2021).

Hallucinogenic drugs, historically referred to as "phantastica" (Lewin, 1964), and later termed "psychedelics" (Stevens, 1987), have been a subject of intense controversy due to their psychoactive nature. Central and South American indigenous peoples traditionally used naturally occurring psychoactive plants in religious rituals, healing practices, and divination ceremonies. Sacred mushrooms like psilocybin mushrooms, dating back to the Mayan civilisation, and cactus plants like peyote from Mexico have been integral to cultural and religious traditions (Schultes, 1976). Ritualistic use of hallucinogenic mushrooms and morning glory seeds (ergine and isoergine) for healing and divination continues in certain regions of Mexico, reflecting the enduring significance of these substances in indigenous practices.

Hallucinogenic psychoactive plants had minimal impact on European culture until the 1960s, when synthetic hallucinogens like LSD (lysergic acid diethylamide) gained scientific and medical attention. Discovered in 1943 by chemist Albert Hofmann at Sandoz Laboratories in Switzerland, LSD was initially marketed as Delysid in 1947. Initially used in psychotherapy and later explored for various conditions, LSD gained popularity in the 1960s within the emerging hippie subculture for spiritual and mystical experiences. The drug's experimentation peaked in the mid-1960s, popularised by figures like Timothy Leary (Parish et al., 2015). While LSD use declined in the UK during the 1980s, it resurfaced in the late 1980s, particularly in the rave subculture. Concurrently, the drug ecstasy (MDMA), synthesised in 1985 as an appetite suppressant in Germany, gained popularity, leading to increased consumption of both ecstasy and LSD among young people. Hallucinogens are currently being utilised and studied for their potential in treating psychiatric disorders.

STIMULANTS

Caffeine, the world's most popular psychoactive substance, has a rich history dating back to ancient times, when plants containing caffeine were used to create beverages. Coffee, originating from the Ethiopian plateau, has a legendary beginning attributed to the goat herder Kaldi. Initially known to Arab travellers as *qahwa*, meaning "wine," coffee gained popularity and was exported from Ethiopia by Yemeni traders (Ukers, 1935). It was used medicinally and for religious purposes, notably by the Dervishes, to stay awake during long rituals (Ghodse, 2010). Coffee spread from Yemen to major cities like Makkah, Medina, Cairo, Damascus, Baghdad, and Constantinople (Galland, 1992), facilitated by the pilgrimage route to Makkah. Early references to coffee's medicinal benefits date back to the works of the 10th-century Persian botanist and physician Abu Bakr Muhammad ibn Zakariya al-Razi and Ibn Sina, who discussed the medicinal benefits of coffee beans for the stomach (Momin, 2015). In the 15th century, the earliest documented evidence of coffee consumption or knowledge of the coffee tree traces back to Sufi monasteries in Yemen (Weinberg & Bealer, 2001). By 1554, a proliferation of coffee houses emerged within the Ottoman Turkish Empire, serving as hubs for recreation and intellectual exchange, sometimes challenging mosques as a meeting place (McHugo, 2013). Despite initial opposition from Islamic scholars who compared its effects to alcohol, attempts to ban coffee failed. By the 16th century, coffee drinking had spread from the Arab world and Persia to Europe, including Britain.

The introduction of coffee to European societies faced resistance, with some viewing it as a "bitter invention of Satan." Its acceptance required approval from Pope Clement VIII. Coffee houses, known as "intellectual cafés," became popular in major European cities, gradually replacing traditional breakfast beverages like beer and wine. In 1^{8t}h-century England, coffee was considered an alternative to sex and a remedy for alcohol intoxication. In the 1840s, Parisian "Bohemians" shocked public opinion by adopting coffee as a lifestyle drug. In various countries, efforts were made to close down coffee houses, which were perceived as centres of sedition and dissent, and to prohibit coffee consumption altogether (Ghodse, 2010). In the New World, tea remained the preferred beverage, until the Boston Tea Party in 1773, after which Americans shifted to coffee. Thomas Jefferson referred to coffee as "the favourite drink of the civilised world" in 1824. Coffee cultivation spread in Indonesia through Dutch colonists, while the French planted millions of coffee trees in Martinique, which became the parent of coffee trees across the Caribbean and the Americas. By the early 1800s, coffee was being grown in

British colonies all over the world (Smith, 2022). Brazilian coffee owes its origins to French settlers in Pará in the early 18th century. Muslim slaves from West Africa possessed more knowledge about coffee than did their Portuguese masters (Reis, 1993). By the late 18th century, coffee had become one of the world's most profitable export commodities, and Switzerland boasts the highest per-capita consumption of cocoa (James, 1991).

The use of the coca leaf traces back to the Inca civilisations and their descendants, with origins dating to around 300 BC among the Aymara Indians of Bolivia (Grinspoon & Bakalar, 1976). For centuries, Andean Indians in Peru and other South American regions have chewed coca leaves for various purposes, including religious ceremonies, medicine, rituals, burials, and special occasions. Peruvian Indians utilise coca to boost physical strength, alleviate fatigue, and stave off hunger. Following the Spanish conquest of the Inca, the conquistadores promoted coca leaf consumption, believing it enhanced productivity. Eventually, the Spanish monopolised coca production and distribution, utilising it as a means to control the conquered population (Petersen, 1977). In the early 1800s, Europeans began experimenting with the use of coca, and by the 1850s, chemists were able to isolate cocaine, the more potent ingredient in the coca leaf. Sigmund Freud, in his work *On Coca*, advocated for the therapeutic and recreational use of cocaine, believing it to be an aphrodisiac (Byck, 1974) and suggesting it for various medical purposes, such as anaesthesia and treatment for addiction, depression, and asthma. By the 1880s, cocaine was widely available in patent medicines, like Mariani's Coca Wine and Coca-Cola, as well as in cigarettes, nose sprays, and chewing gum (Gossop, 2007).

In the 1980s, the United States (US) experienced a "cocaine epidemic," fuelled partly by the drug's association with glamour and the misconception of its non-addictive nature. Cocaine consumption increased significantly, making it the second most commonly used illicit substance after cannabis. The introduction of coca leaves and other psychoactive substances like coffee, tea, and tobacco to Europe originated from South America, where the coca plant is indigenous to the Andean Highlands of Bolivia, Colombia, and Peru.

In 1887, Romanian chemist Lazar Edeleanu synthesised amphetamine from a compound found in *Ma-Huange*, a plant native to China. By 1932, amphetamine was marketed as a Benzedrine inhaler for treating nasal congestion, mild depression, schizophrenia, alcoholism, and obesity. During the 1930s, amphetamine became widely abused, especially among young people. To achieve a high, individuals would remove the amphetamine strip from Benzedrine inhalers and either dissolve them in coffee or chew and swallow them directly. In 1937, the American Medical Association approved amphetamines in tablet form for treating narcolepsy, post-encephalitic Parkinsonism, and minor depression. Amphetamine gained popularity for treating minor depression and was widely prescribed, as it was believed to be non-addictive (Carson-DeWitt, 2001). However, in 1939, the adverse effects of amphetamines and medications containing them were recognised. During World War II, amphetamines were extensively used by the military to maintain troop functionality under stressful conditions. In the 1950s, doctors over-prescribed amphetamines for various common conditions. Connell's (1958) study revealed the risk of amphetamine psychosis, which could affect anyone given enough of the drug. The use of the stimulant became widespread amongst truck drivers, college student athletes, and sport men and women to enhance their exploits and performances.

In the 1960s, amphetamine misuse surged among youth, sparking a methamphetamine injection epidemic. By the mid-1990s, highly potent forms like "ice," "glass," and "crystal" methamphetamine gained popularity. The history of methamphetamines spans from its synthesis in Japan, in 1919, for medical use to its widespread abuse and illicit production in subsequent decades. Initially prescribed as a nasal decongestant and bronchodilator, methamphetamine gained popularity during World War II for its stimulant effects among soldiers. In the post-war years, its availability over the counter led to widespread misuse, particularly in the United States. By the 1980s and 1990s, illicit production surged, with crystal methamphetamine emerging as a highly potent and addictive form of the drug. The initial amphetamine epidemic stemmed from pharmaceutical industry practices and prescribing habits. The current resurgence of amphetamine misuse is driven by recreational drug trends and heightened illicit supply since the late 1980s (Rasmussen, 2008). More recently, amphetamines have been utilised in treating conditions like narcolepsy (Turner, 2019) and attention-deficit hyperactivity disorder (ADHD) (Castells et al., 2018).

TOBACCO AND SHISHA SMOKING

Tobacco, native to North and South America, was historically utilised for medicinal purposes, such as dressing wounds and alleviating toothaches, due to its perceived healing properties. While nicotine traces have been found in some Old World plants and archaeological remains, habitual tobacco use was not evident in ancient civilisations outside the Americas (Borio, 2007). In South and Central America, tobacco played a significant role in religious and political ceremonies, contributing to the development of intricate rituals surrounding its consumption (www.imperialtobaccocanada.com, 2007). In 1492, Christopher Columbus received dried tobacco leaves as a gift from American Indians, marking the introduction of tobacco to Europe. Its popularity grew due to perceived medicinal properties, as documented in 1571 by Spanish doctor Nicolas Monardes, who claimed tobacco could cure numerous health issues. By the 1600s, tobacco was used as currency and faced emerging health concerns, notably recognised by Sir Francis Bacon in 1610. In 1632, smoking in public became illegal in Massachusetts, United States, reflecting moral beliefs among settlers. Scientific understanding advanced with the discovery of pure nicotine in 1826, leading to increased awareness of tobacco's harmful effects. The tobacco industry expanded globally in the 19th and 20th centuries, with companies like Philip Morris establishing iconic brands like Marlboro. Chewing tobacco gained popularity in the American West, while pipe smoking was introduced to Britain by Sir Walter Raleigh. Throughout history, tobacco's social, economic, and health implications have evolved significantly. During the Crimean War (1854–1856), soldiers were offered cigarettes to overcome the misery of food deprivations. Cigarettes became popular around this time when soldiers brought them back to England from the Russian and Turkish soldiers. In 1875, R. J. Reynolds Tobacco Company was established to produce chewing tobacco (Randall, 1999). It was not until the 1900s that the cigarette became the major tobacco product made and sold. The use of cigarettes exploded during World War I (1914–1918), where cigarettes were called the "soldier's smoke." During World War II (1939–1945), cigarettes were included in a soldier's rations. Tobacco companies sent millions of cigarettes to the soldiers for free, thus developing potential customers when these soldiers came home.

In the 1950s, groundbreaking studies by Richard Doll and A. Bradford Hill linked smoking to lung cancer, prompting awareness of the health risks associated with tobacco. Despite denial from the tobacco industry, subsequent research and reports, such as Doll and Hill's findings in 1954 (Doll & Hill, 2004) and the Surgeon General's report in 1964, led to increased regulation of cigarette advertising and sales in the United States and the UK. The acknowledgement of the smoking–lung cancer link by governments prompted health warnings on cigarette packs in the UK in 1971. During the 1980s and 1990s, the tobacco industry expanded its marketing efforts globally, particularly targeting developing countries. Despite growing evidence of the harmful effects of cigarettes, smoking bans in public places were implemented in the late 1990s. In many developing countries, tobacco consumption has risen notably in recent years, spurred by increased exports from developed nations and expanded domestic cultivation, often at the expense of food production (Tominaga, 1986). The consequences of heightened consumption have led to economic burdens due to increased medical costs and imports of cigarettes and declines in food production and importation. Despite numerous obstacles, effective smoking control measures are imperative in these nations to mitigate health risks, alleviate economic strains, and bolster food security. However, cigarettes remain one of the most heavily marketed products worldwide, indicating ongoing challenges in tobacco control efforts.

Shisha smoking, also known as hookah or water pipe smoking, has a long history dating back several centuries. Shisha is a method of smoking tobacco invented in the 16th century by a physician named Hakim Abul-Fath Gilani (Chattopadhyay, 2000; Maziak, 2013). Hakim Abul-Fath Gilani is credited with discovering a remedy to mitigate the harmful effects of tobacco on health. His insight led to the invention of the hookah, which involves passing tobacco smoke through water. This innovation was believed to reduce the detrimental impacts of tobacco consumption (Chattopadhyay, 2000). The hookah device, with its water-filled base and hoses, became a popular social activity in regions like India and the Arab world, where it was often used in gatherings and ceremonies. Over time, shisha smoking evolved into a cultural tradition in many societies, symbolising hospitality and social interaction. In the late 20th century and early 21st century, shisha smoking gained popularity globally, especially among young people, as hookah lounges and cafés began to proliferate. Shisha smoking has undergone evolution, transitioning from simple tobacco to infused flavours like apple, grape, and mint. The accessibility of shisha smoking has expanded due to the proliferation of shisha-serving venues and more affordable prices. Despite its long history and cultural significance, shisha smoking has raised concerns due to its health risks, including exposure to harmful chemicals and the potential for addiction to tobacco products used in shisha mixtures. Efforts to regulate shisha smoking and raise awareness of its health implications continue in many countries.

SYNTHETIC DRUGS

The mid-20th century witnessed the development of synthetic drugs such as amphetamines, barbiturates, and benzodiazepines, which were widely prescribed for various medical conditions but also became targets for recreational use. In the 20th century, the synthesis of psychoactive substances expanded rapidly, leading to the discovery of LSD in 1938 and MDMA (ecstasy) in 1912, among others. In the latter half of the 20th century and continuing into the 21st century, significant advancements in organic chemistry and pharmacology have facilitated the synthesis of diverse synthetic drugs. These include cannabinoids, synthetic opioids like fentanyl, and novel psychoactive substances (NPS) commonly known as "designer drugs." These novel psychoactive substances were formulated to bypass legal constraints and drug testing protocols.

Synthetic drugs, including new psychoactive substances, emulate the effects of illicit drugs and are categorised into cannabinoids like "spice" and "K2" (synthetic marijuana) and stimulants like bath salts, often imitating cocaine, LSD, and methamphetamine. Spice emerged in London in 2004 and gained traction in the United States by 2008, yet its chemical compounds were originally developed for experimental use decades earlier. These include CP 47,497 from Pfizer Pharmaceuticals in the 1980s, HU-210 from Hebrew University of Jerusalem in 1988, and JWH-018 and others by Professor John W. Huffman of Clemson University in 1995 (www.drugfreeworld.org). Following the ban on these compounds in the United States in 2012, underground chemists developed UR-144 and XLR11 to mimic marijuana's effects, highlighting the ongoing challenge of regulating synthetic drugs.

In 2013, UR-144 and XLR11 were outlawed, yet a new generation of synthetic marijuana emerged by that time. Bath salts, synthetic cathinones, initially synthesised in France in 1928 and 1929 for potential medical use, later gained popularity as antidepressants in the former Soviet Union during the 1930s and 1940s (www.drugfreeworld.org). The khat-like cathinones substances, containing cathinones like cathinone, methcathinone, and cathine, entered the Israeli drug scene as *hagigat* and gathered attention among drug users through internet forums before being introduced in the United States during the 1990s. N-BOMe, a potent synthetic hallucinogen akin to LSD, was discovered in 2003 by chemist Ralf Heim at the Free University of Berlin, derived from the 2C family of phenethylamines (PEA). It emerged as a common recreational drug around 2010 (www.drugfreeworld.org).

The popularity of synthetic drugs is expected to increase further due to their easy accessibility, online marketing, misleading advertising, and chemical compounds that evade detection in standard drug screenings, circumventing local, national, and international laws. These substances present significant challenges for law enforcement and public health agencies in terms of regulation and monitoring, highlighting the urgent need for enhanced measures to address their proliferation and associated risks.

CONCLUSIONS

The historical and cultural evolution of psychoactive substances reflects a complex interplay between medicinal, religious, recreational, and economic factors. Throughout history, substances like cannabis, tobacco, and alcohol have held significant roles in various cultures, often revered for their perceived medicinal or spiritual properties. However, as societies evolved and global trade expanded, the use of these substances underwent transformation. In the case of England, tobacco played a pivotal role in its colonial expansion, with the establishment of lucrative trade networks centred on tobacco production and distribution, being essential to England's economic future (Harrison, 1993). In the 1920s, Britain experienced significant drug panics fuelled by the detection of underground cocaine and heroin usage. These panics facilitated discussions about women, race, sex, and the nation's global position. Historically, the outlawing of drugs was less about their pharmacological effects and more about their association with perceived socially dangerous groups (Kohn, 1992). The Opium Wars, for instance, underline Britain's historical promotion of psychoactive substances like opium to China, leaving lasting impressions on public consciousness. Contrary to popular beliefs, major drug importers and criminal gangs in Britain are predominantly led by White businessmen or criminals with the necessary resources, challenging prevailing stereotypes about drug trade leadership (Clutterbuck, 1995). In modern times, the use of psychoactive substances has shifted primarily towards recreational and social contexts. Furthermore, the multilayered nature of psychoactive substances extends beyond their recreational and economic dimensions. These substances also have profound implications for public health, social justice, and legal frameworks.

Despite efforts such as legalisation, regulation, and harm reduction strategies, little progress has been made in curbing the proliferation of psychoactive substances. The commitment to reduce illicit cultivation and demand for substances like coca, cannabis, and opium by 2008 has not been achieved, with no signs of stability in production, trafficking, or consumption of drugs like cocaine, heroin, cannabis, amphetamines, and novel psychoactive substances. Achieving a "drug-free world," as advocated by the United Nations, remains a daunting challenge, highlighting the persistent complexities and difficulties in addressing global drug issues.

KEY POINTS

- Throughout history, alcohol and drugs have served various purposes, including medicinal, religious, cultural, and recreational, acting as social facilitators.
- Alcohol has been consumed for pleasure, nutrition, medicinal, ritualistic, compensatory, and funerary reasons.
- Opium is a substance extracted from the exudates of opium poppy seedpods.
- Cannabis remains the most commonly used illicit drug globally in recent decades.
- Amphetamines were extensively utilised by the armed forces to sustain troop functionality under stressful conditions and were also employed in treating narcolepsy and hyperactivity in children.
- Cocaine gained immense popularity in the late 19th century and was marketed in various forms, like cigarettes, nose sprays, and chewing gum.
- Morphine was employed in treating opium addiction.
- LSD was primarily used as a supplement in psychotherapy, aiding in treating alcoholism, drug dependence, sexual issues, and psychotic and neurotic disorders.
- Caffeine stands as the world's most preferred and popular psychoactive substance.
- Tobacco was believed to possess healing properties, used for wound dressing, and as a remedy for toothaches.
- Shisha smoking involves inhaling flavoured tobacco through a water pipe, also known as a hookah, and is popular in various cultures worldwide for social and recreational purposes
- *Novel psychoactive substances* (NPS) refer to synthetic or naturally occurring compounds that mimic the effects of traditional drugs like cannabis, cocaine, or ecstasy.
- Despite the anti-drug stance and the "war on drugs," little progress has been made in reducing the proliferation of new psychoactive substances.

Activity 3.1

There is only one correct answer to each of the following multiple-choice questions.

1. During the transition from the Middle Ages to the Renaissance, the utilisation of psychoactive substances:
   a. Declined in popularity
   b. Became solely associated with recreational use
   c. Underwent further development
   d. Was banned by religious authorities
   e. Remained unchanged from previous eras

2. What does the historical evolution of psychoactive substance use reflect?
   a. Static patterns
   b. Dynamic changes
   c. Cultural stagnation
   d. Linear progression
   e. Consistent traditions
3. What is the possible origin of the word "alcohol"?
   a. Greek
   b. Latin
   c. Arabic
   d. French
   e. German
4. Who were some of the Muslim chemists credited with pioneering distillation during the Middle Ages?
   a. Galileo Galilei
   b. Isaac Newton
   c. Marie Curie
   d. Jabir ibn Hayyan, Al-Kindi, and Al-Razi
   e. Albert Einstein
5. How was the introduction of distillation and the concept of pure alcohol into Europe during the 12th century facilitated?
   a. By European chemists
   b. Through indigenous European practices
   c. By Asian alchemists
   d. Through translation and popularisation of Islamic and Persian alchemists' discoveries
   e. By trial-and-error experimentation in European laboratories
6. How are various parts of the poppy plant utilised in different applications?
   a. The seeds are used for medicinal purposes, while the pods are consumed in culinary dishes.
   b. Both the seeds and pods are consumed in traditional sedative drinks.
   c. The seeds are utilised in culinary applications, while the pods are used for medicinal purposes.
   d. The pods are used in culinary applications, while the seeds are consumed in traditional sedative drinks.
   e. Both the seeds and pods are used in medicinal applications.
7. Who played a significant role in popularising opium through the standardisation of laudanum?
   a. Thomas Sydenham
   b. Hippocrates
   c. Galen
   d. Paracelsus
   e. Avicenna
8. What event precipitated the conflict between the British East India Company and China?
   a. The establishment of trade routes
   b. The signing of peace treaties
   c. The First Opium War
   d. The expansion of Chinese markets
   e. The introduction of new agricultural techniques
9. Who first isolated morphine from opium in 1805, and what was it initially named after?
   a. John Dalton, named after the Latin word "mors"
   b. Wilhelm Sertürner, named after Morpheus, the Greek god of sleep and dreams

c. Marie Curie, named after the Greek word "morphē"
d. Alexander Fleming, named after the Roman god "Mars"
e. Albert Hofmann, named after the German word "morgen"

10. Who synthesised heroin through the acetylation of morphine in 1874?
a. Wilhelm Sertürner
b. Thomas Sydenham
c. Alexander Fleming
d. C. R. Alder Wright
e. Marie Curie

11. Which component of cannabis is primarily responsible for its psychoactive effects?
a. Terpenes
b. CBD
c. THC
d. Benzodiazepines
e. Alcohol

12. What term did Richard Evans Schultes, a prominent ethnobotanist, and William Emboden, a pharmacologist, coin in the 1970s to describe plants that affect the human psyche?
a. Psychotropics
b. Hallucinogenics
c. Phantastica
d. Ethnobotanicals
e. Phytopharmaceuticals

13. What is the origin of coffee, according to legend?
a. It was discovered in Ethiopia by a goat herder named Kaldi.
b. It was brought to Ethiopia by Arab traders.
c. It was first cultivated in Yemen.
d. It was discovered by monks in a monastery.
e. It was introduced to Europe by Dutch traders.

14. Who are two notable figures from the Islamic Golden Age who discussed the medicinal benefits of coffee beans?
a. Thomas Sydenham and John Locke
b. Leonardo da Vinci and Michelangelo
c. Abu Bakr Muhammad ibn Zakariya al-Razi and Ibn Sina
d. William Harvey and Andreas Vesalius
e. Galileo Galilei and Nicolaus Copernicus

15. Who advocated for the therapeutic and recreational use of cocaine in his work *On Coca*?
a. Albert Einstein
b. Sigmund Freud
c. Carl Jung
d. Wilhelm Wundt
e. Ivan Pavlov

16. What conditions were amphetamines initially approved to treat by the American Medical Association in 1937?
a. Anxiety and insomnia
b. Schizophrenia and bipolar disorder
c. Narcolepsy, post-encephalitic Parkinsonism, and minor depression
d. Chronic pain and migraines
e. Alzheimer's disease and dementia

17. What were some of the historical medicinal uses of tobacco?
    a. Treating respiratory infections
    b. Dressing wounds and relieving pain
    c. Improving memory and cognitive function
    d. Preventing cardiovascular disease
    e. Alleviating digestive issues
18. Who is credited with inventing the method of smoking tobacco through a water pipe, also known as shisha or hookah?
    a. Albert Einstein
    b. Sigmund Freud
    c. Hakim Abul-Fath Gilani
    d. Leonardo da Vinci
    e. Ibn Sina
19. Which of the following is NOT an example of a synthetic drug mentioned in the passage?
    a. LSD
    b. MDMA (ecstasy)
    c. Cannabis
    d. Fentanyl
    e. Novel psychoactive substances (NPS)

References

Abel, E. L. (1980). *Marijuana: In the First Twelve Thousands Years*. New York: Plenum Press.

Al-Hassan, A. Y. (2001). *The Different Aspects of Islamic Culture, Science and Technology in Islam* (Vol. 4, Part II). Cambridge: Cambridge University Press, UNESCO.

Al-Hassan, A. Y., & Hill, D. (1986). *Islamic Technology: An Illustrated History*. Cambridge: Cambridge University Press, UNESCO.

Austin, G. A. (1985). *Alcohol in Western Society from Antiquity to 1800: A Chronological History*. Santa Barbara, CA: ABC-CLIO.

Babor, T. (1989). *Alcohol-Customs and Rituals*. London: Burke Publishing Company Limited.

Berridge, V., & Edwards, G. (1987). *Opium and the People: Opiate Use in Nineteenth-Century England*. London: Yale University Press.

Bloomquist, E. R. (1971). *Marijuana: The Second Trip* (revised ed.). Beverly Hills, CA: Glencoe Press.

Borio, G. (2007). *Tobacco BBS (212–982–4645)*. www.tobacco.org (accessed 24 June 2024).

Brereton, A. (2020). *Morphinomania in the 19th Century*. Edinburgh: The National Trust for Scotland he National Trust for Scotland. https://www.nts.org.uk/storiesanuscriptia-ca-in-the-19th-century (accessed 27 January 2024).

Byck, R. (Ed.). (1974). *Cocaine Papers by Sigmund Freud*. New York: Stonehill Publishing Company.

Carson-DeWitt, R. (Ed.). (2001). *Encyclopaedia of Drugs, Alcohol and Addictive Behaviour* (2nd ed., Vol. 1 (A-D)). Durham, NC: Palgrave Macmillan.

Castells, X., Blanco-Silvente, L., & Cunill, R. (2018). Amphetamines for attention deficit hyperactivity disorder (ADHD) in adults. *The Cochrane Database of Systematic Reviews*, 8(8), CD007813. https://doi.org/10.1002/14651858.CD007813.pub3.

Chattopadhyay, A. (2000). Emperor Akbar as a healer and his eminent physicians. Bulletin of the Indian Institute of History of Medicine (Hyderabad), 30(2), 151–157.

Clutterbuck, R. (1995). *Drugs, Crime, and Corruption: Thinking the Unthinkable*. Basingstoke, Hampshire: MACMILLAN Press Ltd.

Connell, P. H. (1958). *Amphetamine Psychosis*. Oxford: Oxford University Press.

Doll, R., & Hill, A. B. (2004). The mortality of doctors in relation to their smoking habits: A preliminary report, 1954. *BMJ (Clinical Research Ed.)*, 328(7455), 1529–1533. https://doi.org/10.1136/bmj.328.7455.1529.

Galland, G. (1992). *De l'origine et duanuscris du café: Extrait d'unanuscriptt Arabe de la Bibliothèque du Roi*. Paris: La Bibliothèque, coll. "L'écrivain voyageur".

Gautier, T. (1844/1966). Le club de hasishins. In D. Solomon (Ed.), *The Marijuana Papers*. New York: Bobbs-Merrill, pp. 121–135.

Ghodse, A. H. (2010). *Ghodse's Drugs and Addictive Behaviour: A Guide to Treatment*. Cambridge: Cambridge University Press.

The Good Drug Guide. *The Plant of Joy*. https://www.hedweb.com/opioids/red.html (accessed 27 January 2024).

Gossop, M. (2007). *Living with Drugs*. Aldershot: Ashgate Publishing Limited.

Grinspoon, L., & Bakalar, J. B. (1976). *Cocaine: A Drug and Its Social Evolutions*. New York: Basic Books Inc.

Hanson, D. J. (1995). *History of Alcohol and Drinking Around the World*. Westport, CT: Praeger.

Harrison, L. (Ed.). (1993). *Race, Culture and Substance Problems*. Department of Social Policy and Professional Studies. Hull: University of Hull.

James, J. E. (1991). *Caffeine and Health*. New York: Academic Press.

Jernigan, D. (2000). Applying commodity chain analysis to changing modes of alcohol supply in a developing country. *Addiction, 95*(4), 465–475.

Kohn, M. (1992). *Dope Girls: In the Birth of the British Drug Underground*. London: Lawrence & Wishart.

Lewin, L. (1964). *Phantastica-Narcotic and Stimulating Drugs: Their Use and Abuse*. London: Routledge and Kegan Paul.

Maisto, S. A., Galizio, M., & Connors, G. J. (2021). *Drug Use and Abuse*. Boston, MA: Cengage Learning.

Maziak, W. (2013). The waterpipe: An emerging global risk for cancer. *Cancer Epidemiology, 37*(1), 1–4. https://doi.org/10.1016/j.canep.2012.10.013.

McHugo, J. (2013). *Coffee and Qahwa: How a Drink for Arab Mystics Went Global*. www.bbc.com/news/magazine-22190802 (accessed 27 January 2024).

Momin, A. R. (2015). Coffee in Europe, India and the Americas: A shared legacy of Muslim culture. *The IOS Minaret, 10*(7), 16–31. www.iosminaret.org/vol 10/issue7/Coffee_in_India.php (accessed 27 January 2024).

Parish, B. S., Cameron, S., Richards, M. E., Talavera, F., & Dunayevich, E. (2015). *Hallucinogen Use*. https://emedicine.medscape.com/article/293752-overview (accessed 24 June 2024).

Peele, S., & Grant, M. (Eds.). (1999). *Alcohol and Pleasure: A Health Perspective*. Philadelphia: Brunner/Mazel, p. 102.

Petersen, R. C. (1977). History of cocaine. In R. C. Petersen & R. C. Stillman (Eds.), *Cocaine, Research* (Monograph 13). Washington, DC: National Institute of Drug Abuse, pp. 17–34.

Randall, V. R. (1999). *History of Tobacco*. Boston University Medical Center. http://academic.udayton.edu/health/syllabi/tobacco/history.htm (accessed 27 February 2024).

Rasmussen, N. (2008). America's first amphetamine epidemic 1929–1971: A quantitative and qualitative retrospective with implications for the present. *American Journal of Public Health, 98*(6), 974–985. http://doi.org/10.2105/AJPH.2007.110593.

Reis, J. J. (1993). *Slave Rebellion in Brazil: The Muslim Uprising of 1835 in Bahia*. Trans. A. Brakel. Baltimore: The Johns Hopkins University Press.

Ritchie, H., & Roser, M. (2024). *Alcohol Consumption*. https://ourworldindata.org/alcohol-consumption (accessed 27 January 2024).

Schultes, R. E. (1976). *Hallucinogenic Plants*. New York: Golden Press.

Smith, P. (2022). *The British Empire and Coffee*. https://www.historic-cornwall.org.uk/the-british-empire-and-coffee/ (accessed 27 January 2024).

Stevens, J. (1987). *Storming Heaven: LSD and the American Dream*. New York: Atlantic Monthly Press.

Tobacco History. (2007). www.imperialtobaccocanada.com/ (accessed 28 November 2016).

Tominaga, S. (1986). Spread of smoking to the developing countries. *IARC Scientific Publications, 74*, 125–133.

Turner, M. (2019). The treatment of narcolepsy with amphetamine-based stimulant medications: A call for better understanding. *Journal of Clinical Sleep Medicine: JCSM: Official Publication of the American Academy of Sleep Medicine, 15*(5), 803–805. https://doi.org/10.5664/jcsm.7788.

Ukers, W. (1935). *All About Coffee*. New York: The Tea and Coffee, Trade Journal Company, pp. 9–10.

Weinberg, B. A., & Bealer, B. K. (2001). *The World of Caffeine*. New York: Routledge, pp. 3–4.

What Is Synthetic Drugs? www.drugfreeworld.org/ (accessed 28 January 2024).

Whitaker, B. (1987). *The Global Connection: The Crisis of Drug Addiction*. London: Jonathan Cape Ltd.

Zheng, Z., Fiddes, K., & Yang, L. (2021). A narrative review on environmental impacts of cannabis cultivation. *Journal of Cannabis Research*, 3(1), 35. https://doi.org/10.1186/s42238-021-00090-0.

Chapter 4

Exploring addiction

Models and theoretical perspectives

Learning outcomes

- List the various theories of addiction, including moral, disease, genetic, psychoanalytic, social learning, socio-cultural, and bio-psychosocial models.
- Briefly discuss the various theories of addiction, including moral, disease, genetic, psychoanalytic, social learning, socio-cultural, and bio-psychosocial models.
- Appreciate the importance of holistic approaches to addiction, and consider the interconnectedness of biological, psychological, social, and spiritual dimensions.

Activity 4.1

There is only one correct answer to each of the following multiple-choice questions.

1. Which of the following is not a major theory of addiction?
   a. Genetic
   b. Adaptation
   c. Moral
   d. Psychological
   e. Spiritual
2. Which statement is incorrect regarding the moral theory of addiction?
   a. The moral theory is based on the belief that using alcohol or drug is a sign of moral weakness.
   b. The moral theory accepts that there is a biological basis for addiction.
   c. According to the moral theory, individuals are responsible for their behavioural choices and their own recovery.
   d. "Victim-blaming" approach is evident in this theory.
   e. This theory has been criticised for oversimplifying the complex nature of addiction and stigmatising individuals struggling with substance use disorders.
3. Which statement is incorrect? The disease theory of addiction
   a. Maintains that addiction is a disease due to either the impairment of behavioural and/or neurochemical processes.
   b. Claims that the cause of the disease is not attributed to the genetic/biological make-up of the individual.

DOI: 10.4324/9781003456674-5

c. Holds that alcohol and drug addiction is a unique, irreversible, and progressive disease.
d. Holds that while alcohol or drug addiction cannot be cured, abstinence is the only option.
e. This theory suggests that addiction involves changes in brain structure and function, which may predispose individuals to continued substance use.

4. Which statement is incorrect? The genetic theory of addiction
   a. Puts forward a genetic predisposition to alcohol or drug addiction.
   b. Maintains that early-onset alcoholism is genetically determined.
   c. Is based on evidence mainly from drug research studies.
   d. Incorporates the psychosocial factors in the development of addiction.
   e. Numerous studies have demonstrated that genetic variations can influence a person's susceptibility to addiction by affecting factors such as drug metabolism, brain chemistry, and responses to stress.
5. Which statement is incorrect?
   a. Asians encompass the only race that exhibits Asian flushing.
   b. Acetaldehyde is an important enzyme for alcohol metabolism.
   c. American Indians and Eskimos are genetically identical.
   d. Flushing is common amongst White Europeans.
   e. All of the above.
6. Regarding genetic studies of addiction, which one is incorrect?
   a. Twin studies are the most powerful.
   b. Twins-reared-apart studies are the most powerful.
   c. Family studies are scientifically sound.
   d. Adoption studies are easy to do because good records are kept.
   e. Genetic studies of addiction have revealed that addiction susceptibility is influenced by the interaction of multiple genes.
7. Which statement is incorrect?
   a. Family studies have shown an increased incidence of alcoholism in families.
   b. Adoption studies have not shown any correlation between addiction and genetics.
   c. Twins-reared-apart studies are the most powerful.
   d. Monozygotic twins and dizygotic twin studies show slightly different outcomes.
   e. Animal studies have been used extensively to evaluate the genetic contributions to alcohol addiction.
8. Which one of the following is not considered to be a component in psychological theories?
   a. Psychoanalytical
   b. Genetic
   c. Personality
   d. Social learning
   e. Role modelling
9. Which statement is incorrect? The psychoanalytic theory of addiction
   a. Stems from the belief that addiction stems from unconscious death wishes.
   b. Includes the notions of conflict between a repressed idea and the defence against it.
   c. Proposes that aetiology of alcohol or drug dependence is assumed.
   d. Genetic studies of addiction have revealed that addiction susceptibility is influenced by the interaction of multiple genes to develop from the avoidance of pain or anxiety.
   e. States that use of alcohol or drug (smoking) is related to the "fixation" at the anal stage of development.
10. Which one of the following is not considered in behavioural theories?
    a. The theory makes provision for individual differences (genetic factors).
    b. The use of psychoactive substances is viewed as an acquired behaviour.

c. Behaviour is learned through the process of classical conditioning and operant conditioning.
d. The theory of classical conditioning does not include social factors or the expectations of drug effects.
e. Behavioural theories of addiction typically encompass various psychological perspectives that focus on how behaviours are learned, reinforced, and maintained.

11. Which one of the following is not considered in social learning theories?
   a. The theory is formed and maintained through the process of positive and negative reinforcement.
   b. Behaviour is formed through role-modelling and the need to conform.
   c. In order to understand the effects of alcohol or drug, cognitive processes must be considered in relation to other factors.
   d. An individual's prior experience with alcohol or drug and the social setting in which drinking or drug-taking occurs are least important in the theory.
   e. Social learning theories emphasise the importance of social interactions, reinforcement, and modelling in shaping behaviours.
12. Which one of the following is not considered in socio-cultural theories?
   a. In the systems theory, behaviour is determined and maintained by the ongoing demands of interpersonal systems in which an individual interacts.
   b. In the cultural theory, behaviour is through role-modelling and the satisfaction of a hierarchy of needs.
   c. The availability theory suggests that the greater the availability, the greater the prevalence and severity of substance use problems in society.
   d. Cultural and religious attitudes have been considered to be a defensive shield against alcohol and drug addiction.
   e. The emphasis is on understanding how social and cultural factors influence the development, maintenance, and treatment of addiction.
13. Which one of the following is not considered in bio-psychosocial theories?
   a. In bio-psychosocial theory, behaviour is mainly determined and maintained by genetic factors.
   b. The theory includes genetic inheritance, physiological differences, family, community, peer, or social pressure.
   c. This theory postulates a role for social and spiritual factors in the development of and recovery from addiction.
   d. Supports the concept of a hierarchy of harm reduction outcome goals, including abstinence-related goals.
   e. These theories emphasise the interconnectedness of biological, psychological, and social factors in shaping individuals' experiences and functioning.
14. Which one of the following is incorrect regarding the bio-psychosocial-spiritual theory?
   a. The spiritual theory of addiction is akin to the moral theory of addiction.
   b. The spiritual theory suggests that the individual gets disconnected with religious beliefs and practices.
   c. The spiritual theory of addiction focuses on a spiritual path to recovery.
   d. The spiritual theory of addiction seeks to identify the aetiology of the addictive process.
   e. The spiritual theory of addiction seeks a higher being, which leads to an ultimate lack of meaning and purpose in life.

INTRODUCTION

Various models and theories, including the moral, disease, genetic, psychoanalytic, socio-cultural, and spiritual frameworks, offer valuable perspectives on addictive behaviours. Each model provides unique insights into the multilayered nature of addiction, addressing factors such as moral judgements, neurobiological mechanisms, genetic predispositions, unconscious motivations, societal influences, and spiritual dimensions. These frameworks contribute to a comprehensive understanding of addiction, recognising its diverse causes and manifestations within individuals and societies. However, no single theory or model offers a comprehensive explanation for addiction, as multiple risk factors contribute to individual experiences. Various models of addiction provide different perspectives on its aetiology and treatment. The moral model attributes addiction to moral weakness, while the disease model views it as a chronic brain disorder. Genetic theories focus on genetic predispositions, while psychoanalytic theories emphasise unconscious motivations. Social learning theories highlight environmental influences, and socio-cultural theories underscore cultural norms and societal values. The bio-psychosocial model integrates biological, psychological, and social factors. Additionally, the spiritual model views addiction as a spiritual disease, emphasising the role of spirituality in recovery.

MORAL THEORY

The moral model of addiction attributes addictive behaviour to moral weakness, character flaws, or sinful behaviour rather than genetic or biological factors. According to this perspective, individuals who misuse alcohol or drugs are seen as making conscious choices that deviate from societal norms and moral standards. Addiction is perceived as a result of poor decision-making and lack of self-control, leading to social stigma and labelling of individuals with addiction as morally deficient. The moral model often involves a "victim-blaming" approach, where individuals with addiction are held responsible for their behaviour and stigmatised based on moral judgements rather than receiving support for recovery. The moral model of addiction places responsibility on individuals for their behavioural choices and recovery from addiction. It emphasises social disapproval, moral persuasion, and punishment as means of behavioural control, rather than prevention and treatment. The model's focus on punishment, exemplified by initiatives like the "war on drugs" and "zero tolerance," reflects a less-tolerant and punitive approach. However, the moral model's limited therapeutic value and failure to fully explain addiction have led to its diminishing relevance in understanding addiction and designing effective interventions.

DISEASE THEORY

The disease theory of addiction conceives that addiction is a result of impaired behavioural or neurochemical processes, or a combination of both, leading to changes in brain structure and function. It asserts that addiction is a unique, irreversible, and progressive disease characterised by the inability to control consumption. Advocates of this theory attribute the cause of addiction to a brain disease (Heilig et al., 2021). Once initiated, addiction increases cravings, overriding cognitive or voluntary control (Jellinek, 1960). The model emphasises abstinence as the sole treatment option and promotes access to healthcare and treatment rather than punitive measures. This approach involves adopting the sick role, where individuals are treated as having a disease, and emphasises sustained recovery through total abstinence, often supported by self-help groups such as "AA," "NA," and "GA" (Alcoholics Anonymous, Narcotic Anonymous, Gamblers Anonymous). The disease concept of addictive behaviour is incorporated into the philosophy underpinning the approaches of NA or AA in the adoption of the "Minnesota model" (Cook, 1988). While this model acknowledges the physiological origins of addiction, it tends to overlook the interplay of psychological, socio-cultural, and spiritual factors in the development and maintenance of addictive behaviours.

GENETIC/BIOLOGICAL THEORY

The genetic and biological model of addiction suggests a predisposition to alcohol or drug addiction rooted in genetic factors and biological abnormalities. According to this theory, variations in brain chemistry, brain structure, and genetic make-up contribute to the development of addictive behaviours. Numerous studies have indicated that alcohol or drug addiction may stem from genetic or induced biological abnormalities of physiological, structural, or chemical nature. There is strong evidence that early-onset alcoholism is genetically determined (Gupta et al., 2020). Genetic factors account for 50 to 60% of the variance in risk for developing alcoholism in twin, adoption, and family studies (Foroud et al., 2010). The findings of a meta-analysis of twin and adoption studies showed that the heritability of alcohol use disorder is approximately 50% (Verhulst et al., 2015). Adoption and twin studies consistently highlight a significant genetic predisposition to alcohol use disorder. Research findings reveal that both adoption and twin studies emphasise the substantial genetic influence on the risk of alcoholism, with this influence being equally strong in women as it is in men (Heath, 1995).

However, the findings of the Copenhagen study (Goodwin et al., 1977), one of the best research studies on methodological grounds, showed that there was a fourfold increase in the incidence of alcoholism among male adoptees that were removed from their alcoholic parents soon after birth. While the exact nature of genetic inheritance remains unclear, the review highlights a consistent trend: sons, rather than daughters, are more susceptible to developing alcohol use disorder, as evidenced by all studies evaluated within similar cultural and racial groups. Tsuang et al.'s (1996) study on pairs of twins indicates that the development of dependence on opiates or stimulants is more influenced by genetic factors than shared environmental factors. The research highlights that certain individuals may have a reduced sensitivity to alcoholic beverages, leading them to consume more before experiencing intoxication, potentially contributing to vulnerability in these individuals.

Genetic predispositions, particularly observed among certain racial groups like Eskimos, American Indians, and Asians, manifest in deficiencies in acetaldehyde production enzymes, rendering individuals hypersensitive to alcohol effects and prone to the "Asian flushing" phenomenon. Studies, predominantly focused on alcohol, employ varied methodologies, including interviews, hospital records, and operational definitions of alcohol use disorder, which may impact findings' comparability. While genetic factors play a role in addictive behaviour, psychosocial and environmental influences also significantly shape outcomes. Further investigation is needed to clarify the extent of genetic contributions to addiction development.

PSYCHOLOGICAL THEORIES

Various psychological theories aim to explain the origins of addictive behaviours. These theories offer diverse perspectives on addiction causation, shedding light on its multifaceted nature.

PSYCHOANALYTIC THEORY

Psychoanalytic theory, rooted in Freud's work on the components of the self and their functioning throughout psychosexual development stages, offers insights into addiction causation. Early psychoanalytical perspectives linked alcohol and drug addiction to instinctual gratification (Feniche, 1945) while Glover (1956) suggested that substances were used to manage emotional pain, aggression and rage. Addiction is viewed as a consequence of the dynamic interaction among the id, ego, and superego, along with intrapsychic conflict, with emphasis on the superego's role (Wurmser, 1977). Additionally, another psychodynamic approach conceives addiction as stemming from unconscious death wishes, akin to "slow suicide" (Khantzian, 2013). Levin (1991) further characterises those with addictive problems as unstable, highlighting their reliance on drugs in terms of narcissistic needs.

Psychoanalytic theory is derived from the work of Freud based on the components of the self and their functioning during the stages of psychosexual development. Early psychoanalytical explanation viewed alcohol and drug abuse in terms of instinctual gratification (Feniche, 1945). Glover (1956) went further in suggesting that drugs were used to cope with emotional pain, aggression, and rage. Addiction is also seen as the result of the interplay of the dynamic interaction of the id, ego, and superego and intrapsychic conflict, focusing on the superego's role (Wurmser, 1977). Another psychodynamic approach stems from the belief that addiction stems from unconscious death wishes as a form of "slow suicide" (Khantzian, 1980). Levin (1991) views addicts as precarious, and their reliance on drugs can be viewed in terms of narcissistic need. Other psychoanalytic perspectives (Morgenstern & Leeds, 1993; Khantzian, 1980) explore the conflict between repressed ideas and the defence mechanisms against them, as well as the notion of a deficient ego.

A contemporary psychoanalytic approach (Thombs & Osborn, 2019) perceives addiction as a mechanism against anxiety. According to psychoanalytic theory, adaptive behaviour hinges on the harmonious functioning of the id, ego, and superego, which evolve through psychosexual development stages. Alcohol and drug use, including smoking, are linked to fixation at the oral stage of development. Pathological conditions like alcohol use disorder stem from conflicts during these developmental stages, resulting in destructive interactions among the self's components. The aetiology of alcohol or drug substance disorder is believed to arise from the pursuit of sensual satisfaction (to avoid pain or anxiety), conflicts among the id, ego, and superego, and fixation in the infantile past (Allen, 1996). Alcohol consumption is seen as offering relief from conflicts stemming from oral fixation or repressed homosexuality, as suggested by Freud. Opiate addiction, on the other hand, may be viewed as an attempt to cope with excessively punitive parental standards, leading to feelings of worthlessness (Blatt et al., 1984).

Mental defence mechanisms serve as psychological strategies individuals employ to avoid fully confronting the reality of their situations and to seek relief from emotional or psychological distress. These mechanisms operate within conflicts among the components of the self. Denial, repression, projection, avoidance, isolation of affect, rationalisation, intellectualisation, and displacement are among the behavioural patterns observed in maintaining addictive behaviours. Substance-dependent individuals often exhibit psychodynamic characteristics, such as challenges in affect management, narcissism, object relations, judgement, and self-care (Treece & Khantzian, 1986). These issues may predispose individuals to drug dependence, as they serve as the basis for anxieties or distresses alleviated by consuming psychoactive substances. Addiction entails the gradual integration of drug effects and the perceived need for them into the defensive structure of the ego itself (Treece & Khantzian, 1986).

The psychoanalytic theory of addiction has prompted the development of various approaches to brief psychodynamic psychotherapy, applied across a spectrum of clinical disorders (Crits-Christoph, 1992; Messer & Warren, 1995). While psychodynamic theory has enriched our comprehension of psychological defence mechanisms and therapeutic interventions, its empirical support is limited due to methodological challenges in psychoanalytic studies (Rassool, 2025). Suggestions have been made for integrating brief psychodynamic therapies into comprehensive treatment packages, incorporating both pharmacological and psychosocial interventions for enhanced effectiveness (Center for Substance Abuse Treatment, 1999).

BEHAVIOURAL THEORIES

The behavioural model of addiction focuses on how behaviours are learned and reinforced through conditioning processes. In behavioural theories of addiction, psychoactive substance use is seen as a learned behaviour acquired through processes such as classical conditioning (Pavlovian conditioning), operant conditioning (Skinner), and social learning (Hyman et al., 2006). Addictive behaviour patterns develop through repeated pairing of cues, responses, and reinforcers, a phenomenon observed even in non-human species (Ahmed, 2011; Heinz et al., 2019). That is, positive reinforcement, such as the pleasurable effects of drugs, strengthens the behaviour of substance use, while negative reinforcement, like alleviating withdrawal symptoms, also contributes to its continuation.

Classical conditioning contributes to dependence by associating specific factors with substance use, leading to the desire for drugs based on environmental cues (Tiffany, 1990). Wikler (1948, 1961) emphasised the significant role of classical conditioning in motivating drug use, as illustrated in smoking addiction by West (2013). For example, the sensory experiences associated with smoking, such as the sensation of smoke in the throat and the visual and tactile sensations, acquire reinforcing qualities through their association with the rewarding effects of nicotine. This strengthens the entire behavioural sequence involved in smoking beyond just the nicotine reward itself (West, 2013).

Operant conditioning involves learning through reinforcement, where behaviours are strengthened by positive or negative reinforcements. In the context of psychoactive substance use, positive reinforcement occurs when drugs induce pleasurable sensations, reinforcing continued use. However, classical conditioning theory overlooks individual differences, genetic factors, and social influences, as well as the role of intentions and beliefs not acquired through experience (Vuchinich & Heather, 2003). The effectiveness of cognitive behavioural therapies, including cue-exposure techniques, has been subject to scrutiny (Conklin & Tiffany, 2002). However, the model has been criticised for oversimplifying addiction and not accounting for individual differences, genetic factors, and the role of cognition and social influences in substance use behaviours.

SOCIAL LEARNING THEORY

Social learning theory, rooted in cognitive psychology, elucidates how behaviour is shaped and perpetuated through reinforcement, both positive and negative. It posits that individuals learn from observing others and are influenced by role models and societal norms (Becker, 1966; Bandura, 1977; Barnes, 1990). Becker, Bandura, and Barnes have contributed to the understanding of how behaviour is influenced by reinforcement and social modelling. Studies have highlighted the significant association between exposure to role models, especially in media portrayals, and the adoption of addictive behaviours (Anderson et al., 2009; Kandel & Andrews, 1987; Lovato et al., 2011). Collins and Marlatt's (1981) research highlights the influence of modelling on drinking behaviour, showing how individuals adjust their alcohol consumption to match that of their drinking companions. Their findings suggest that heavy-drinking males are particularly responsive to models exhibiting similar behaviour. Moreover, cognitive social learning theory emphasises the importance of cognitive processes in understanding the impact of alcohol or drug use, highlighting the role of observation and cognitive factors alongside social modelling in shaping behaviour. Social learning theory emphasises the interplay between personal factors, such as expectations and beliefs, and environmental factors, like social settings, in shaping behaviour related to alcohol or drug use. While the theory expounds the role of imitation and role modelling in behavioural outcomes, it falls short in explaining how addictive behaviour can manifest without direct exposure to models. Moreover, evidence supporting the effectiveness of interventions based on social learning theory in addressing addictive behaviours remains limited (West, 2013).

The tension-reduction theory postulates that individuals consume alcohol or drugs to alleviate tension or anxiety, with the substances acting as reinforcers due to their tension-reducing effects (Cappell & Greeley, 1987). The self-awareness model proposed by Hull (1981) explores how psychoactive substances disinhibit social behaviour by diminishing an individual's self-awareness. Meanwhile, the expectancy theory elucidates the cognitive factors influencing the initiation and persistence of substance use despite adverse outcomes (Stacy et al., 1990). This theory stresses the development of beliefs about psychoactive substances from an early age, where "outcome expectancy" links substance use to specific situational contexts. Expectations regarding alcohol consumption have been found to be more predictive of drinking behaviour among adolescents than social background or demographic factors, such as ethnicity, religious affiliation, and parental attitudes. For instance, studies by Christiansen and Goldman (1983) indicate that adolescents believe alcohol can enhance cognitive and motor functioning. Orford (2001) presents the theory of "excessive appetites" within the social learning paradigm suggesting that individuals' levels of involvement in "appetitive activities" are influenced by multiple interacting determinants, including biological, personality, social, and ecological factors.

PERSONALITY THEORY

Psychological theories suggest that individuals with certain personality traits may be more prone to developing addictive behaviours, often referred to as having an "addictive personality." Lang (1983) identified nine characteristics associated with the addictive personality, including impulsive behaviour, difficulty in delaying gratification, sensation seeking, antisocial personality, nonconformist values, sense of alienation, deviant behaviour, heightened feelings of stress, and little regard for society's valued goals. However, Lang (1983) found no singular addictive personality type but noted commonalities among individuals with addictive behaviours. Moreover, research indicates that individuals with traits such as moodiness, irritability, anxiety, impulsivity, and aggression are more likely to experience substance use problems (Courtney, Hanson & Gitterman, 2014). Additionally, hyperactivity, sensation-seeking, antisocial behaviour, and impulsivity have been linked to substance misuse (Sher et al., 1991). These findings indicate the complex interplay between personality traits and addictive behaviours, highlighting the need for comprehensive approaches to addiction prevention and treatment. However, the literature indicates varying degrees of research on traits associated with addiction. Among these traits, narcissism and psychopathy show stronger associations with addiction compared to Machiavellianism (Jauk & Dieterich, 2019). Neuroticism, in particular, has been consistently associated with substance use disorders (Ormel et al., 2013) and a consistent risk factor for internet addiction (Marciano et al., 2020, 2022). *Sensation-seeking* refers to the tendency to seek out novel and thrilling experiences. Sensation-seeking has been found to correlate with engaging in risky behaviours, including substance use. Studies suggest that sensation-seeking and impulsivity-related traits emerged as significant predictors of substance use, with sensation-seeking explaining the majority of the variance in substance use behaviour (Hildebrandt et al., 2021), though the authors indicate that urgency, rather than sensation-seeking, may have a specific association with substance-related problems. It is important to note that while high sensation-seeking can be a risk factor, it does not guarantee that an individual will engage in substance use or develop an addiction. Many other factors, such as environment, genetics, and mental health, also play significant roles in these complex behaviours (substance, personality, set, and setting). The findings of a recent study suggest that high sensation-seeking people have a greater risk of losing control over their drug intake, which makes them more vulnerable to drug addiction (O'Connor et al., 2021). This study, conducted with rats, urges caution in extrapolating animal behaviour to human behaviour.

In essence, the notion of a universal addictive personality lacks empirical support, debunking it as a myth. While certain predisposing factors, including genetic and personality traits like high neuroticism and low conscientiousness, may contribute to addictive behaviours, they do not predict addiction on their own. Research suggests that addiction is influenced by a multitude of factors, and no single personality profile universally characterises individuals with addictions (Griffiths, 2016; Kotov et al., 2010).

PSYCHOPATHOLOGICAL THEORY

Mental health problems and substance use disorder frequently co-exist, leading to comorbidity or dual diagnosis. There are several factors contributing to their intertwined nature. Common risk factors, including genetic predispositions and environmental stressors, may increase the likelihood of developing both substance use disorders (SUDs) and mental disorders. Additionally, individuals with mental disorders may resort to substance use as a form of self-medication, which can exacerbate symptoms over time and contribute to the onset of additional mental health issues. Substance use itself can also lead to changes in brain structure and function, enhancing the rewarding effects of substances and potentially triggering the development of mental disorders (NIDA, 2020). High rates of comorbidity exist between substance use disorders and various mental health conditions. Anxiety disorders, including generalised anxiety disorder, panic disorder, and post-traumatic stress disorder, often co-occur with substance use disorders. Substance use disorders are also prevalent alongside depression, bipolar disorder, attention-deficit hyperactivity disorder (ADHD), psychotic illnesses, borderline personality disorder, and antisocial personality disorder. Individuals with schizophrenia exhibit higher rates of alcohol, tobacco, and drug use disorders compared to the general population (NIDA, 2022). Roughly half of individuals seeking treatment for addiction also experience another significant mental disorder (Miller et al., 2019).

The misuse of psychoactive substances can exacerbate mental health problems by affecting emotions, moods, thought processes, brain chemistry, and behaviour. Research suggests that drug and alcohol misuse can worsen the symptoms of mental health conditions (NAMI, 2016). For instance, regular cannabis use has been associated with a doubled risk of developing psychotic episodes or long-term schizophrenia (Royal College of Psychiatrists, 2022). Moreover, alcohol and drugs can interact with various medications, including antidepressants and anti-anxiety drugs, potentially reducing their effectiveness.

The self-medication theory proposed by Khantzian (1985) suggests that individuals with mental illness may use substances to alleviate distress caused by psychiatric symptoms. Common symptoms such as depression, anxiety, paranoia, and restlessness are often targeted through self-medication with substances like opiates, cannabis, alcohol, or stimulants (Rassool, 2002). These substances may temporarily alleviate symptoms associated with mental illness, providing relief from agitation, anxiety, or depression. The self-medication hypothesis underscores the complex relationship between substance use and mental health, where individuals may turn to substances as a coping mechanism for underlying psychological distress. Furthermore, personality disorders frequently co-occur with substance use disorders, with approximately half of patients diagnosed with a personality disorder also experiencing comorbid substance use disorder. Personality disorders appear to be more prevalent in individuals with drug use disorders compared to those with alcohol use disorders (Walter, 2015). While there is a strong epidemiological association between drug misuse and personality disorder, causality remains unclear, as most studies have focused on comparing drug-dependent individuals with their non-dependent counterparts (Ghodse, 2010). He suggests that certain personality traits may predispose individuals to substance dependence.

SOCIO-CULTURAL THEORIES

Socio-cultural theories of addiction encompass various sub-theories, including systems theory, family interaction theory, anthropological theory, economic theory, gateway theory, and availability theory. Systems theory postulates that behaviour is shaped and sustained by the ongoing dynamics of interpersonal systems within which individuals interact. This framework suggests that behaviours, including addictive behaviours, are influenced by the demands and structures of social systems. Steinglass (1987) supports the notion of alcoholism as a "family disease" or "family disorder," emphasising the interplay of family dynamics in the development and maintenance of addiction. Within family interaction theory, parental deficits arising from parental alcohol use disorder are considered significant aetiological factors. These deficits may manifest as parental absence, family tension, emotional distancing, and rejection, contributing to an environment conducive to addiction development. Additionally, there is evidence suggesting that alcohol may serve an adaptive function within marital relationships by facilitating interaction (Jacob & Leonard, 1988).

The availability theory suggests that the prevalence and severity of substance use problems in society correlate with the accessibility of alcohol and other psychoactive substances. Ghodse (2010) emphasises that drug availability is a prerequisite for misuse and dependence, facilitated by the widespread accessibility of drugs due to modern transportation systems. Factors such as drug availability, cost, social pressures, legal regulations, and marketing practices are identified as significant predictors of addiction development (Henningfield et al., 1991). This theory highlights the role of environmental factors in shaping patterns of substance use and addiction within society. In contrast, the cultural model acknowledges the profound influence of cultural norms and values on individuals' susceptibility to addiction. Cultural and religious attitudes serve as protective factor against alcohol and drug use disorder, with moderate or controlled drinking practices within family settings influencing children's attitudes towards alcohol. Cultural values play a pivotal role in shaping drug-taking and drinking behaviours, guiding social norms and etiquette surrounding substance use. However, migration, social changes, and economic constraints may alter these patterns over time. While psychoactive substances misused by various ethnic groups may not differ significantly from those used by the majority population, preferences for certain substances and modes of consumption are influenced by historical and cultural characteristics specific to each ethnic group, as observed by Oyefeso et al. (2000) and Sangster et al. (2002). Socio-cultural factors profoundly influence alcohol and drug use, encompassing gender, age, occupation, social class, ethno-cultural background, subcultures, alienated groups, family dynamics, and religious affiliation. These factors shape definitions, effects, behaviours, experiences, and choices related to substance use. Recognising these influences is crucial for designing effective interventions tailored to diverse communities and individuals, addressing substance misuse within varying socio-cultural contexts.

BIO-PSYCHOSOCIAL-SPIRITUAL THEORY

The bio-psychosocial model of addiction integrates biological, psychological, spiritual, and sociological perspectives to understand the complex nature of drug and alcohol addiction. Many models of addiction could be criticised for failing to attend sufficiently to social and environmental factors (Copello & Orford, 2002). There have been several attempts to amalgamate the biological, psychological, and sociological theories of drug and alcohol addiction into a mega theory – the bio-psychosocial perspectives (Wallace, 1990). Unlike uni-dimensional theories, this model acknowledges the interplay of various factors in the development and perpetuation of addiction. It incorporates biological factors, such as genetic inheritance and physiological differences, psychological factors like learning, perception, and interpretation of the world, as well as social factors, including family, community, and peer influences. The model also

Table 4.1
Characteristics and focus of the bio-psychosocial-spiritual theory

Characteristics	Focus
The bio-psychosocial theory unifies prior biological, psychological, and social theories of addiction.	Multidimensional and multi-professional approach to addiction.
This theory postulates a role for social and spiritual factors in the development of and recovery from alcohol and substance use disorder and allows for future analysis of these elements.	Recognising the influence of social and spiritual factors in both the development of and recovery from alcohol and substance use disorders.
A conceptual framework that allows attention to be focused on all problems related on a continuum. From experimental users to those who are dependent on psychoactive substances.	Provision of a comprehensive range of services.
Characterises the population of alcohol and substance use disorder as heterogenous.	Meeting individual/holistic needs.
Supports the concept of a hierarchy of harm reduction outcome goals, including abstinence-related goals.	Allows for the delivery of harm reduction services.
Emphasises the role of spirituality and existential meaning in addiction and recovery. Views addiction as a spiritual malady or a disconnection from one's spiritual self or higher power.	Examining one's beliefs, values, sense of purpose, and connection to a higher power or inner self. Engaging in reflection, meditation, prayer, mindfulness, ritual, or other spiritual activities to foster inner growth and healing.
Congruent with other modern theories of health and education.	Diversity of health needs within a population/community. Matching needs to services/treatment. Measuring treatment outcomes on all dimensions.

Source: Adapted from Adult Addictions Services Branch, Alcohol and Drug Services (1996).

recognises the importance of environmental factors, such as social pressure and cultural influences. Additionally, it suggests the inclusion of a spiritual dimension in understanding addiction. By considering these multiple dimensions, the bio-psychosocial model offers a holistic perspective on addiction, emphasising the interaction and temporal ordering of these factors. A summary of the characteristics and focus of the bio-psychosocial-spiritual model is presented in Table 4.1.

The spiritual dimension of the bio-psychosocial-spiritual model of addiction recognises spirituality as broader than religion, encompassing beliefs in God, family, nature, humanism, and the arts. The theory suggests that individuals experience disconnection from religious beliefs or higher beings, resulting in a profound lack of meaning and purpose in life. Re-establishing this spiritual connection, embracing uniquely interpreted universal laws and principles, and finding clarity in the meaning of life and purpose can pave the path towards recovery and a life free from alcohol and drug use disorder. The 12-step programmes have origins in American Protestantism, other spiritual models, including those like Millati Islami Groups, and offer faith-based approaches to treatment and recovery for Muslims that do not rely solely on Christian or theistic beliefs (Rassool, 2025). Al Ghaferia et al.'s (2016) study findings showed that the bio-psychosocial-spiritual model of addiction fit well in the Islamic context. Well-supported scientific evidence demonstrates the effectiveness of 12-step mutual aid groups focused on alcohol and 12-step facilitation interventions (Greene, 2021; SAMSHA, 2016). There is evidence to suggest that there is correlation between increased involvement in Alcoholics Anonymous (AA) and heightened spirituality over time (Kelly et al., 2011). The authors concluded that spirituality plays a crucial role in recovery, and AA facilitates spiritual changes, which contribute to its positive effects on recovery outcomes. AA leads to better alcohol use outcomes, in part by enhancing individuals' spiritual practices, and provides support for individuals with alcohol use disorder.

CONCLUSION

Understanding addiction requires a comprehensive approach that acknowledges its multifaceted nature. Various theories, including biological, social, psychological, pathological, cultural, and spiritual perspectives, offer valuable insights into different aspects of addiction. However, no single theory can fully encapsulate the complexity of addiction. Thus, integrating these diverse perspectives becomes essential to develop effective prevention, harm reduction, and treatment strategies. By synthesising theories and models, professionals can better grasp the interplay between individual motivations, capabilities, and external factors that contribute to addiction (West, 2013). This integrated approach allows for a more holistic understanding of addiction, facilitating tailored interventions that address the unique needs of individuals struggling with alcohol or substance use disorder.

KEY POINTS

- The moral theory posits that alcohol or drug use reflects moral weakness.
- According to the disease theory of addiction, addiction is a disease caused by impairment of behavioural and/or neurochemical processes.
- The genetic theory of addiction suggests a genetic predisposition to alcohol or drug addiction.
- Family studies have indicated a higher incidence of alcoholism within families.
- The psychoanalytic theory of addiction suggests that addiction originates from unconscious death wishes.
- Behaviour is acquired through classical and operant conditioning processes.
- There are strong associations and potential interactions between psychopathology and addictive disorders.
- Social learning theory asserts that understanding the effects of alcohol or drugs requires considering cognitive processes in relation to other factors.
- Socio-cultural theories propose that behaviour is shaped and sustained by the ongoing demands of interpersonal systems.
- In the bio-psychosocial theory of genetic inheritance, physiological differences and various environmental factors like family, community, and social pressures are all considered.
- The spiritual theory of addiction, akin to the moral theory, emphasises a spiritual path to recovery rather than focusing on identifying the aetiology of addiction.

References

Adult Addictions Services Branch, Alcohol and Drug Services British Columbia Ministry for Children and Families. (1996). *The Biopsychosocial Theory: A Comprehensive Descriptive Perspective on Addiction.* http://citeseerx.ist.psu.edu/viewdoc/download?doi=10.1.1.89.1099&rep=rep1&type=pdf (accessed 29 January 2024).

Ahmed, S. H. (2011). The science of making drug-addicted animals. *Neuroscience,* 211, 107–125. https://doi.org/10.1016/j.neuroscience.2011.08.014.

Al Ghaferia, H., Christine Bond, C., & Matheson, C. (2016). Does the biopsychosocial-spiritual model of addiction apply in an Islamic context? A qualitative study of Jordanian addicts in treatment. *Drug and Alcohol Dependence,* 172, 14–20. https://doi.org/10.1016/j.drugalcdep.2016.11.019.

Allen, K. M. (1996). Theoretical perspectives for addictions nursing practice. In K. M. Allen (Ed.), *Nursing Care of the Addicted Client.* Philadelphia: Lippincott.

Anderson, P., de Bruijn, A., Angus, K., Gordon, R., & Hastings, G. (2009). Impact of alcohol advertising and media exposure on adolescent alcohol use: A systematic review of longitudinal studies. *Alcohol and Alcoholism,* 44(3), 229–243. https://doi.org/10.1093/alcalc/agn115.

Bandura, A. (1977). *Social Learning Theory.* Englewood Cliffs: Prentice-Hall.

Barnes, G. (1990). Impact of the family on adolescent drinking patterns. In R. Collins, K. Leonard, & J. Searles (Eds.), *Alcohol and the Family: Research and Clinical Perspectives.* New York: Guilford Press.

Becker, H. (1966). *Outsiders: Studies in the Sociology of Deviance.* New York: The Free Press.

Blatt, S. J., McDonald, C., Sugarman, A., & Wilber, C. (1984). Psychodynamic theories of opiate addiction: New directions for research. *Clinical Psychology Review,* 4(2), 159–189. https://doi.org/10.1016/0272-7358(84)90027-8.

Cappell, H., & Greeley, J. (1987). Alcohol and tension reduction: An update on research and theory. In H. T. Blane & K. E. Leonard (Eds.), *Psychological Theories of Drinking and Alcoholism.* New York: Guildford Press.

Center for Substance Abuse Treatment. (1999). *Brief Interventions and Brief Therapies for Substance Abuse* (Chapter 7, Brief Psychodynamic Therapy (Treatment Improvement Protocol (TIP) Series, No. 34)). Rockville, MD: Substance Abuse and Mental Health Services Administration (US). www.ncbi.nlm.nih.gov/books/NBK64952/.

Christiansen, B. A., & Goldman, M. S. (1983). Alcohol-related expectancies versus demographic/background variables in the prediction of adolescent drinking. *Journal of Consulting and Clinical Psychology,* 51(2), 249–257. https://doi.org/10.1037//0022-006x.51.2.249.

Collins, R. L., & Marlatt, G. A. (1981). Social modelling as a determinant of drinking behavior: Implications for prevention and treatment. *Addictive Behaviors,* 6(3), 233–239. https://doi.org/10.1016/0306-4603(81)90021-6.

Conklin, C. A., & Tiffany, S. T. (2002). Applying extinction research and theory to cue-exposure addiction treatments. *Addiction,* 97(2), 155–167. https://doi.org/10.1046/j.1360-0443.2002.00014.x.

Cook, C. C. (1988). The Minnesota model in the management of drug and alcohol dependency: Miracle, method or myth? Part I. The philosophy and the programme. *British Journal of Addiction,* 83(6), 625–634. https://doi.org/10.1111/j.1360-0443.1988.tb02591.x.

Copello, A., & Orford, J. (2002). Addiction and the family: Is it time for services to take notice of the evidence?. *Addiction (Abingdon, England),* 97(11), 1361–1363. https://doi.org/10.1046/j.1360-0443.2002.00259.x.

Courtney, D. M., Hanson, M., & Gitterman, A. (2014). Chapter 3: Alcoholism and other drug addictions. In A. Gitterman (Ed.), *Handbook of Social Work Practice with Vulnerable and Resilient Populations.* Chichester, West Sussex: Columbia University Press, pp. 54–72. https://doi.org/10.7312/gitt11396-004.

Crits-Christoph, P. (1992). The efficacy of brief dynamic psychotherapy: A meta-analysis. *American Journal of Psychiatry,* 149(2), 151–158.

Feniche, O. (1945). Dynamics of addiction. In J. D. Levin & R. H. Weiss (Eds.), *The Dynamics and Treatment of Alcoholism: Essential Papers (1994).* Northvale, NJ: Aronson, pp. 98–103.

Foroud, T., Edenberg, H. J., & Crabbe, J. C. (2010). Genetic research: Who is at risk for alcoholism. *Alcohol Research & Health: The Journal of the National Institute on Alcohol Abuse and Alcoholism,* 33(1–2), 64–75.

Ghodse, A. H. (2010). *Ghodse's Drugs and Addictive Behaviour: A Guide to Treatment.* Cambridge: Cambridge University Press.

Glover, E. (1956). *On the Early Development of Mind.* New York: International Universities Press.

Goodwin, D. W., Schulsinger, F., Knop, J., Mednick, S., & Guze, S. B. (1977). Alcoholism and depression in adopted-out daughters of alcoholics. *Archives of General Psychiatry,* 34(7), 751–755. https://doi.org/10.1001/archpsyc.1977.01770190013001.

Greene, D. (2021). Revisiting 12-step approaches: An evidence-based perspective. In W. M. Meil & J. A. Mills (Eds.), *Addictions – Diagnosis and Treatment.* IntechOpen. https://doi.org/10.5772/intechopen.95985 (accessed 29 January 2024).

Griffiths, M. (2016). There's no such thing as an "addictive personality" – here's why. *The Conversation.* https://theconversation.com/theres-no-such-thing-as-an-addictive-personality-heres-why-55275 (accessed 29 January 2024).

Gupta, I., Dandavate, R., Gupta, P., Agrawal, V., & Kapoor, M. (2020). Recent advances in genetic studies of alcohol use disorders. *Current Genetic Medicine Reports,* 8(2), 27–34. https://doi.org/10.1007/s40142-020-00185-9.

Heath, A. C. (1995). Genetic influences on alcoholism risk: A review of adoption and twin studies. *Alcohol Health and Research World,* 19(3), 166–171.

Heilig, M., MacKillop, J., Martinez, D., Rehm, J., Leggio, L., & Vanderschuren, L. J. M. J. (2021). Addiction as a brain disease revised: Why it still matters, and the need for consilience. *Neuropsychopharmacology: Official Publication of the American College of Neuropsychopharmacology,* 46(10), 1715–1723. https://doi.org/10.1038/s41386-020-00950-y.

Heinz, A., Beck, A., Halil, M. G., Pilhatsch, M., Smolka, M. N., & Liu, S. (2019). Addiction as learned behavior patterns. *Journal of Clinical Medicine,* 8(8), 1086. https://doi.org/10.3390/jcm8081086.

Henningfield, J. E., Cohen, C., & Slade, J. D. (1991). Is nicotine more addictive than cocaine? *British Journal of Addiction,* 86(5), 565.

Hildebrandt, M. K., Dieterich, R., & Endrass, T. (2021). Disentangling substance use and related problems: Urgency predicts substance-related problems beyond the degree of use. *BMC Psychiatry,* 21, 242. https://doi.org/10.1186/s12888-021-03240-z.

Hull, J. G. (1981). A self-awareness model of the causes and effects of alcohol consumption. *Journal of Abnormal Psychology,* 90(6), 586–600. https://doi.org/10.1037//0021-843x.90.6.586.

Hyman, S. E., Malenka, R. C., & Nestler, E. J. (2006). Neural mechanisms of addiction: The role of reward-related learning and memory. *Annual Review of Neuroscience,* 29, 565–598. https://doi.org/10.1146/annurev.neuro.29.051605.113009.

Jacob, T., & Leonard, K. (1988). Alcohol-spouse interaction as a function of alcoholism subtype and alcohol consumption interaction. *Journal of Abnormal Psychology,* 97(2), 231–237.

Jauk, E., & Dieterich, R. (2019). Addiction and the dark triad of personality. *Frontiers in Psychiatry,* 10, 662. https://doi.org/10.3389/fpsyt.2019.00662.

Jellinek, E. M. (1960). *The Disease Concept of Alcoholism.* New Haven: Hillhouse Press.

Kandel, D. B., & Andrews, K. (1987). Processes of adolescent socialization by parents and peers. *The International Journal of The Addictions,* 22(4), 319–342. https://doi.org/10.3109/10826088709027433.

Kelly, J. F., Stout, R. L., Magill, M., Tonigan, J. S., & Pagano, M. E. (2011). Spirituality in recovery: A lagged mediational analysis of alcoholics anonymous' principal theoretical mechanism of behavior change. *Alcoholism, Clinical and Experimental Research,* 35(3), 454–463. https://doi.org/10.1111/j.1530-0277.2010.01362.x.

Khantzian, E. J. (1980). An ego/self-theory of substance dependence: A contemporary psychoanalytical perspective. In D. J. Littieri, M. Sayers, & H. W. Pearson (Eds.), *Theories on Drug Abuse: Selected Contemporary Perspectives.* Washington, DC: DHSS ADM, pp. 84–967.

Khantzian, E. J. (1985). The self-medication hypothesis of addictive disorders: Focus on heroin and cocaine dependence. *American Journal of Psychiatry,* 142(11), 1259–1264.

Khantzian, E. J. (2013). Addiction as a self-regulation disorder and the role of self-medication. *Addiction,* 108(4), 668–669. https://doi.org/10.1111/add.12004.

Kotov, R., Gamez, W., Schmidt, F., & Watson, D. (2010). Linking 'big' personality traits to anxiety, depressive, and substance use disorders: A meta-analysis. *Psychological Bulletin*, 136(5), 768–821. http://dx.doi.org/10.1037/a0020327.

Lang, A. R. (1983). Addictive personality: A viable construct? In P. K. Levison, D. R. Gerstein, & D. R. Maloff (Eds.), *Commonalities in Substance Abuse and Habitual Behavior*. Lexington, MA: Lexington Books, pp. 157–236.

Levin, J. D. (1991/1994). Alcoholism and regression/fixation to pathological narcissism. In J. D. Levin & R. H Weiss (Eds.), *The Dynamics and Treatment of Alcoholism: Essential Papers*. Northvale, NJ: Aronson, pp. 370–385.

Lovato, C., Watts, A., & Stead, L. F. (2011). Impact of tobacco advertising and promotion on increasing adolescent smoking behaviours. *Cochrane Database of Systematic Reviews*, 10, CD003439.

Marciano, L., Camerini, A.-L., & Schulz, P. J. (2022). Neuroticism and internet addiction: What is next? A systematic conceptual review. *Personality and Individual Differences*, 185, 111260, February. https://doi.org/10.1016/j.paid.2021.111260.

Marciano, L., Camerini, A.-L., & Schulz, P. J. (2020). Neuroticism in the digital age: A meta-analysis. *Computers in Human Behavior Reports*, 2, Article 100026. https://doi.org/10.1016/j.chbr.2020.100026.

Messer, S. B., & Warren, C. S. (1995). *Models of Brief Psychodynamic Therapy: A Comparative Approach*. New York: Guilford Press.

Miller, W. R., Forchimes, A. A., & Zweben, A. (2019). *Treating Addiction: A Guide for Professionals* (2nd ed.). New York: Guilford Press.

Morgenstern, J., & Leeds, J. (1993). Contemporary psychoanalytic theories of substance abuse: A disorder in search of a paradigm. *Psychotherapy: Theory, Research, Practice, Training*, 30(2), 194–206. https://doi.org/10.1037/0033-3204.30.2.194.

NAMI. (2016). *Dual Diagnosis*. National Alliance on Mental Illness.www.nami.org/Learn-More/Mental-Health-Conditions/Related-Conditions/Dual-Diagnosis#sthash.3m0mpCm1.dpuf (accessed 24 June 2024).

National Institute of Mental Health. (2020). *Common Comorbidities with Substance Use Disorders Research Report*. Bethesda, MD: National Institutes on Drug Abuse (US), April. https://www.ncbi.nlm.nih.gov/books/NBK571451/ (accessed 29 January 2024).

NIDA. (2022). *Part 1: The Connection Between Substance Use Disorders and Mental Illness*. https://nida.nih.gov/publications/research-reports/common-comorbidities-substance-use-disorders/part-1-connection-between-substance-use-disorders-mental-illness (accessed 29 January 2024).

O'Connor, S. L., Aston-Jones, G., & Morgan, M. H. (2021). The sensation-seeking trait confers a dormant susceptibility to addiction that is revealed by intermittent cocaine self-administration in rats. *Neuropharmacology*, 195, 108566. https://doi.org/10.1016/j.neuropharm.2021.108566.

Orford, J. (2001). *Excessive Appetites: A Psychological View of Addictions* (2nd ed.). Oxford: John Wiley & Sons Ltd.

Ormel, J., Jeronimus, B. F., Kotov, R., Riese, H., Bos, E. H., Hankin, B., Rosmalen, J. G. M., & Oldehinkel, A. J. (2013). Neuroticism and common mental disorders: Meaning and utility of a complex relationship. *Clinical Psychology Review*, 33(5), 686–697. https://doi.org/10.1016/j.cpr.2013.04.003.

Oyefeso, A., Ghodse, H., Keating, A., Annan, J., Phillips, T., Pollard, M., & Nash, P. (2000). *Drug Treatment Needs of Black and Minority Ethnic Residents of the London Borough of Merton* (Addictions Resource Agency for Commissioners (ARAC) Monograph Series on Ethnic Minority Issues). London: ARAC.

Rassool, G. H. (2002). *Dual Diagnosis: Substance Misuse and Psychiatric Disorders*. Oxford: Blackwell Science.

Rassool, G. H. (2025). *Islāmic Counselling and Psychotherapy: From Theory to Practice*. 2nd Ed. Oxford: Routledge.

Royal College of Psychiatrist. (2022). *Cannabis and Mental Health for Children and Young People*. https://www.rcpsych.ac.uk/mental-health/parents-and-young-people/cannabis-and-mental-health-information-for-young-people (accessed 29 January 2024).

SAMHSA (Substance Abuse and Mental Health Services Administration (US)); Office of the Surgeon General (US). (2016). *Facing Addiction in America: The Surgeon General's Report on Alcohol, Drugs, and Health* (Chapter 5, Recovery: The Many Paths to Wellness) [Internet]. Washington, DC: US Department of Health and Human Services, November. https://www.ncbi.nlm.nih.gov/books/NBK424846/.

Sangster, D., Shiner, M., Sheikh, N., & Patel, K. (2002). *Delivering Drug Services to Black and Minority Ethnic Communities* (DPAS/P16). London: Home Office Drug Prevention and Advisory Service (DPAS).

Sher, K., Walitzer, K., Wood, P., & Brent, E. (1991). Characteristics of children of alcoholics: Putative risk factors, substance use and abuse, and psychopathology. *Journal of Abnormal Psychology*, 100(4), 427–448.

Stacy, A., Widaman, K., & Marlatt, G. (1990). Expectancy models of alcohol use. *Journal of Personal and Social Psychology*, 58(5), 918–928.

Steinglass, P. (1987). A systems view of family interaction and psychopathology. In T. Jacob (Ed.), *Family Interaction and Psychopathology: Theories, Methods, and Findings*. New York: Plenum, pp. 25–65.

Thombs, D. L., & Osborn, C. I. (2019). *Introduction to Addictive Behaviors*. New York: Guilford Publications.

Tiffany, S. T. (1990). A cognitive model of drug urges and drug-use behavior: Role of automatic and nonautomatic processes. *Psychological Review*, 97, 147–168. https://doi.org/10.1037/0033-295X.97.2.147.

Treece, C., & Khantzian, E. J. (1986). Psychodynamic factors in the development of drug dependence. *Psychiatric Clinics of North America*, 9(3), 399–412.

Tsuang, M. T., Lyons, M. J., Eisen, S. A., Goldberg, J., True, W., Lin, N., Meyer, J. M., Toomey, R., Faraone, S. V., & Eaves, L. (1996). Genetic influences on DSM-III-R drug abuse and dependence: A study of 3,372 twin pairs. *American Journal of Medical Genetics*, 67(5), 473–477. https://doi.org/10.1002/(SICI)1096-8628(19960920)67:5<473::AID-AJMG6>3.0.CO;2-L.

Verhulst, B., Neale, M. C., & Kendler, K. S. (2015). The heritability of alcohol use disorders: A meta-analysis of twin and adoption studies. *Psychological Medicine*, 45(5), 1061–1072. https://doi.org/10.1017/S0033291714002165.

Vuchinich, R. E., & Heather, N. (2003). *Choice, Behavioral Economics and Addiction*. Cambridge: Pergamon.

Wallace, J. (1990). The new disease model of alcoholism. *Western Journal of Medicine, 15*(5), 502.

Walter, M. (2015). Chapter 10: Co-occurring addictive and psychiatric disorders. In G. Dom & F. Moggi (Eds.), *Co-Occurring Addictive and Psychiatric Disorders.* Berlin and Heidelberg: Springer, pp. 137–148.

West, R. (2013). *Models of Addiction: European Monitoring Centre for Drugs and Drug Addiction.* Luxembourg: Publications Office of the European Union, p. 38. https://doi.org/10.2810/99994.

Wikler, A. (1948). Recent progress in research on the neurophysiologic basis of morphine addiction. *The American Journal of Psychiatry,* 105(5), 329–338. https://doi.org/10.1176/ajp.105.5.329.

Wikler, A. (1961). On the nature of addiction and habituation. *British Journal of Addiction, 57*(2), 73–79.

Wurmser, L. (1977/1994). Psychodynamics in compulsive drug use. In J. D. Levin & R. H. Weiss (Eds.), *The Dynamics and Treatment of Alcoholism: Essential Papers.* Northvale, NJ: Aronson, pp. 176–204.

Chapter 5

Exploring addiction

Understanding nature, patterns, administration, and risks

Learning outcomes

- Discuss the drug and alcohol experiences in relation to the "substance," "set," and "setting."
- State the reasons people take drug or alcohol.
- Describe the pattern of alcohol or drug use.
- Describe the various routes of drug administration.
- Identify the risks of injecting behaviour.

Activity 5.1

Please circle or tick the correct answer. There is only one correct answer for each statement.

1. When discussing drug and alcohol experiences, which of the following factors are considered as part of the "set" and the "setting"?
   a. The type of substance
   b. The individual's mindset and expectations
   c. The physical environment
   d. Both b and c
   e. All of the above
2. What are some common reasons people may take drugs or alcohol?
   a. To experience pleasure or euphoria
   b. To alleviate pain or stress
   c. To enhance social interactions
   d. All of the above
   e. None of the above
3. Which of the following best describes the pattern of alcohol or drug use?
   a. It remains constant over time.
   b. It fluctuates depending on external factors.
   c. It gradually decreases with age.
   d. It follows a linear progression from experimentation to addiction.
   f. None of the above is correct.
4. What are the various routes of drug administration?
   a. Oral ingestion
   b. Inhalation

DOI: 10.4324/9781003456674-6

   c. Injection
   d. All of the above
   e. None of the above

5. What are the risks associated with injecting behaviour?
   a. Transmission of blood-borne diseases like HIV and hepatitis
   b. Damage to veins and arteries
   c. Overdose due to rapid drug absorption
   d. All of the above
   e. None of the above
6. When considering drug and alcohol experiences, which of the following refers to the physical surroundings or environment?
   a. Substance
   b. Set
   c. Setting
   d. None of the above
   e. All of the above
7. Which of the following is NOT a common reason people take drugs or alcohol?
   a. Social pressure
   b. Religious experiences
   c. Curiosity
   d. Boredom
   e. None of the above
8. How does the pattern of alcohol or drug use typically change over time?
   a. It remains constant.
   b. It becomes more sporadic.
   c. It increases gradually.
   d. It decreases gradually.
   e. None of the above is correct.
9. Which route of drug administration involves injecting substances directly into the bloodstream?
   a. Oral ingestion
   b. Inhalation
   c. Intravenous injection
   d. All of the above
   e. None of the above
10. Which of the following is NOT a risk associated with injecting behaviour?
    a. Transmission of infectious diseases.
    b. Tissue damage.
    c. Slow onset of drug effects.
    d. Overdose.
    e. All of the above are risks associated with injecting behaviour.
11. In the context of drug and alcohol experiences, what does "set" refer to?
    a. The physical environment
    b. The type of substance consumed
    c. The individual's mindset and expectations
    d. Both a and b
    e. None of the above

12. What is the term used to describe the progression of drug or alcohol use from experimentation to dependence?
 a. Tolerance
 b. Addiction
 c. Escalation
 d. Substance abuse disorder
 e. None of the above

INTRODUCTION

Chapter 4 examines various theories surrounding alcohol and substance misuse disorder, acknowledging that no single theory can fully elucidate addiction. In this context, Gossop (2013) appropriately points out that the belief in fixed and predictable effects of specific drugs is a misconception, as individual experiences vary significantly. The discussion underlines the importance of considering both set (personality, mindset, attitudes, and expectancies) and setting (context and environment) in alcohol and drug experiences. While these factors are significant across all substances, they particularly come into play with psychoactive substances, like LSD, ecstasy, ketamine, and hallucinogenic mushrooms. Key topics covered include the motivations behind drug and alcohol use, patterns of use and misuse, and the various routes of drug administration. By examining these aspects, this chapter aims to provide a comprehensive understanding of substance experiences and the factors that contribute to them.

THE DRUG EXPERIENCE

The effects of psychoactive substances, or "drug experiences," are influenced by a complex interplay of pharmacological and non-pharmacological factors. Pharmacological factors encompass the chemical properties, dosage, and route of administration of the drug, all of which determine its mode of action in the body. Different drugs exhibit diverse effects due to their unique pharmacological profiles. Non-pharmacological factors, such as the individual's personality traits, biological make-up, gender, age, and drug tolerance, also significantly shape drug experiences (Rassool, 2018). Personal characteristics can affect how an individual responds to psychoactive substances, with factors like drug tolerance influencing sensitivity to the drug's effects. Additionally, the context or setting in which the drug is used plays a crucial role in shaping the drug experience. Environmental factors, such as the social context, surroundings, and emotional state can influence the subjective effects of the drug. For instance, individual reactions to substances like coffee and cannabis vary based on factors like medical conditions and personality traits. It highlights that some individuals may experience adverse effects even from small doses of substances, while others may benefit. Medical conditions such as angina pectoris or glaucoma can interact with substance effects (ISDD, 1996). Personality traits like introversion or extroversion can influence how individuals respond to drugs (Gossop, 2013).

The psychological state of drug users significantly influences the effects and risks associated with drug and alcohol use. Anxiety disorders, including generalised anxiety disorder, obsessive-compulsive disorder, panic disorder, and social phobia, can reinforce or be reinforced by substance use (Scharff, 2024). Individuals experiencing low mood, anxiety, or depression are more prone to disturbing experiences when using psychoactive substances. Their psychological state may intensify, leading to increased anxiety, disorientation, and potentially aggressive behaviour. An anxiety disorder may lead to using alcohol or other substances to self-medicate or alleviate anxiety symptoms (ADDA, 2024). Those with psychological disorders like anorexia nervosa or bulimia can worsen due to the use of psychoactive substances. Moreover, pre-existing health issues, such as cardiovascular disease, hypertension, asthma, epilepsy, diabetes mellitus, or liver disease, can exacerbate the effects of psychoactive substances, making them more hazardous. Overall, the psychological and physical health conditions of drug users significantly impact the safety and consequences of substance use.

In addition, the psychological set, including knowledge, attitude, and expectations about a drug, which can shape the drug experience. Beliefs and expectations can lead to self-fulfilling prophecies, where the desired effects of a substance are experienced. Additionally, the setting or context of drug use, encompassing the physical environment, cultural influences, and legal framework, also impacts the drug experience. All three of the interrelated factors, pharmacological properties, individual differences, and context of use, influence the individual experiences of drug-taking. The understanding of the interaction between drugs and the brain is not merely a chemical process but a complex phenomenon. It involves the drug itself, the individual's unique characteristics, and the messages and influences from the surrounding environment (Royal College of Psychiatrists, 1987). These external factors strongly shape the nature and significance of the drug experience, highlighting the intricate interplay between pharmacology, personal factors, and environmental contexts in determining drug effects and perceptions.

THE ALCOHOL EXPERIENCE

Alcohol holds significant cultural influence globally, often introduced to young people through parental consumption and accessible social settings, like bars, clubs, and parties. Factors influencing youths' first experiences with alcohol include parental drinking habits and attitudes, occasional sips allowed during special occasions, exposure to alcopops, religious beliefs, and peer pressure to appear "cool" at events like birthday parties. The most common age for a first drink in the UK was 12 to 13, usually when with an adult and celebrating a special occasion (Bremner et al., 2021). Furthermore, young people are more inclined to drink, drink frequently, and drink excessively under certain circumstances. These include receiving less supervision from parents or

Activity 5.2

Questions regarding why people start taking alcohol or drugs and why people continue to use alcohol or drugs. Please provide short answers.

- What role does social influence and peer pressure play in initiating alcohol or drug use?
- How does curiosity and experimentation contribute to the initiation of alcohol or drug use, particularly among adolescents?
- In what ways do individuals use alcohol or drugs as coping mechanisms for stress, trauma, or emotional pain?
- What are the perceived benefits or pleasures associated with alcohol or drug use that motivate individuals to start using psychoactive substances?
- How do environmental factors such as family influence, cultural attitudes, and media portrayal contribute to the initiation of alcohol or drug use?
- How does physical dependence and withdrawal symptoms influence continued alcohol or drug use?
- What role does psychological dependence play in continuing alcohol or drug use among individuals?
- In what ways do alcohol or drugs serve as a means of escapism or avoidance for individuals?
- How does social and peer pressure contribute to continued alcohol or drug use within social circles or communities?
- What factors contribute to the development of tolerance to alcohol or drugs, and how does this impact continued use?
- How do individuals' coping mechanisms, or their lack, influence their tendency to continue using alcohol or drugs?
- What role do habitual behaviour and routine play in perpetuating ongoing alcohol or drug use?
- How do social and environmental factors contribute to the maintenance of alcohol or drug use patterns over time?

close adults, spending multiple evenings per week with friends who drink, being exposed to family members who drink heavily, having positive attitudes and expectations towards alcohol, and having easy access to alcohol (Bremner et al., 2021). These factors collectively contribute to increased alcohol consumption among young individuals. Some individuals have an initially unfavourable experience with alcohol, citing distaste for beverages like beer and feelings of light-headedness or dizziness. The effects of alcohol typically manifest within 10 to 20 minutes and vary based on factors such as age, body size, stomach contents, drink quantity and speed, physical conditions, alcohol type, tolerance, gender, and mood. Similar to drug experiences, individual experiences with alcohol are shaped by interrelated factors, including the type and amount of drink, individual differences, and the context of use.

WHY DO PEOPLE USE DRUG OR ALCOHOL?

Psychoactive substances induce temporary changes in the nervous system, leading to feelings of euphoria or "high." These changes involve an increase in certain neurotransmitters, notably dopamine, associated with pleasure. Research suggests that even the sight and smell of favourite foods can elevate dopamine levels, akin to what addicts experience during drug craving (Volkow et al., 2002). When individuals consume substances like cocaine or tobacco, dopamine levels in the brain rise, resulting in euphoria. While other neurotransmitters like serotonin, norepinephrine, and GABA (gamma-aminobutyric acid) may play roles in addiction, dopamine appears to be essential in the process.

The use of illicit psychoactive substances is not necessarily linked to personal problems, contrary to popular belief. Individuals may be drawn to these substances for reasons similar to alcohol, often finding the initial experience pleasurable. Throughout history and across cultures, drug use for pleasure has been evident. Environmental factors significantly influence substance use, with drug and alcohol misuse thriving in areas marked by multiple deprivation, unemployment, and poor infrastructure. On the contrary, a less-stressful, privileged environment may offer protection against addiction and relapse during recovery (Nader & Czoty, 2005). However, substance use is not limited to urban deprivation; factors like curiosity, youth culture, peer pressure, and media influence also promote drug use. Research indicates that cigarette advertising, for instance, encourages young people to start smoking with teenagers being influenced by various forms of tobacco marketing. Research has shown that non-smoking adolescents who showed higher awareness of tobacco advertising or were more receptive to it were found to be more likely to experiment with cigarettes or become smokers during follow-up periods (Lovato et al., 2011). People may use or continue to use drugs or alcohol for various reasons, including the influence of role models, peer pressure, and societal norms. Self-medication for mental health issues, relief from stress, combating boredom, addiction to prescribed medications, and coping with traumatic events are common motivations. This highlights the diverse and complex factors that contribute to substance use behaviours. The reasons people use and continue to use psychoactive substances are listed in Table 5.1.

The initial reasons for starting drug use may differ from the motivations behind continued use. While initial use may stem from various factors, including curiosity or social influences, continued substance use is often driven by physiological and psychological dependence rather than rational decisions. Reasons for continued use may include dependence, chaotic patterns of use, fear of withdrawal symptoms, social exclusion, mental health issues, and other psychosocial and environmental factors (Rassool, 2018). Many individuals struggling with alcohol and drug misuse may manage short periods of abstinence without experiencing withdrawal symptoms but find it difficult to maintain long-term abstinence.

PATTERNS OF SUBSTANCE USE: EXPERIMENTAL, RECREATIONAL, AND DEPENDENCE/ADDICTION

The progression of addiction spans from no use to dependence, with individuals moving through stages such as no use, experimental use, recreational use, problematic use, and addiction. These stages reflect varying degrees of involvement with alcohol or drugs, from abstaining to experiencing negative consequences and addiction. Individuals may transition between stages and may also engage in patterns like binge drinking or chaotic use. Table 5.2 depicts the characteristics of experimental, recreational, and dependent/addiction substance users.

Table 5.1
Why people use and continue to use psychoactive substances

Use psychoactive substance	Continue to use psychoactive substance
Curiosity: Some people try alcohol or drugs out of curiosity.	Physical dependence: Continued use of alcohol or drugs can lead to physical dependence.
Experimentation: Experiment with the effects (altered states of consciousness), especially during adolescence.	Withdrawal symptoms: In physical dependence, individuals experience withdrawal symptoms when they try to stop using, prompting them to continue using to avoid discomfort.
Perceived benefits or pleasure: The perceived benefits or pleasure associated with alcohol or drug use, such as relaxation, euphoria, or enhanced social experiences, can motivate individuals to start using substances.	Psychological dependence: Individuals may develop psychological dependence on alcohol or drugs, relying on them to cope with emotional difficulties or to feel a sense of pleasure or relief.
Social influence: Individuals may start using alcohol or drugs to fit in with social circles.	Tolerance development: Over time, individuals may develop tolerance to the effects of alcohol or drugs, requiring higher doses to achieve the desired effects, which can lead to continued use and escalation of substance consumption.
Peer pressure: Peer groups where substance use is normalised or encouraged.	Social pressure: Social norms within social circles or communities where substance use is prevalent can contribute to continued alcohol or drug use.
Environmental factors: Exposure to family members or friends who use substances.	Peer pressure: Peer pressure within social circles or communities where substance use is prevalent can contribute to continued alcohol or drug use.
Cultural attitudes and media influence: They can contribute to the initiation of alcohol or drug use.	Social and environmental factors: Continued exposure to social environments or situations where alcohol or drug use is common, coupled with easy access to substances, can perpetuate ongoing use.
Coping mechanism for stress and trauma: People may turn to alcohol or drugs as a way to cope with stress, trauma, or emotional pain, seeking relief from difficult emotions or life circumstances.	Lack of effective coping mechanisms: Individuals may lack alternative coping mechanisms or healthy strategies for managing stress, emotions, or life challenges.
Escapism and avoidance: Alcohol or drugs may serve as a means of escaping from reality or avoiding problems, providing temporary relief from stress, anxiety, or other challenging emotions.	Habitual behaviour and routine: Long-term alcohol or drug use can become ingrained in daily routines and habits, making it difficult for individuals to envision life without substance use.
	Addiction to prescribed medications: Addiction on prescribed medications can lead to continued use, even when it is no longer medically necessary.

Experimental users are individuals who have tried drugs, legal or illicit, on a few occasions, typically motivated by curiosity, social experiences, and anticipation of effects. This initial stage of drug use often brings pleasure due to minimal consequences and low tolerance. There is no consistent pattern in substance use, and the choice of substance is influenced by factors like availability, social marketing, and peer influence. Experimental use is part of adolescent exploration and risky behaviour, with no significant change in lifestyle or social integration. However, it poses a high risk for infections, medical complications, or overdose due to indiscriminate use of substances. The likelihood of further engagement or disengagement from substance use remains uncertain at this stage.

Recreational users commonly engage with substances like alcohol, caffeine, nicotine, cannabis, amphetamine, LSD, and ecstasy. Experimental users may or may not transition to recreational use of illicit psychoactive substances, spanning all societal strata. In recreational use, pleasure and relaxation are primary motivations, with strict adherence to usage patterns, often limited to specific occasions like weekends. Users typically have a preferred drug, understanding its effects and methods of consumption. Drug or alcohol use supplements social and recreational activities but does not typically result in adverse medical or social consequences, akin to controlled drinking. Recreational users perceive health damage and legal risks as main hazards, while they see gaining "time-out" from stress and achieving leisure and relaxation

Table 5.2
From experimental users to addiction

Experimental	Users: Have used drugs, legal or illicit, on a few occasions. Motivations: Curiosity, anticipation of effects, and availability drive initial drug or alcohol use. Lack of pattern: No consistent pattern in the use of psychoactive substances. Indiscriminate choice: Drug misuse is indiscriminate, influenced by factors like availability, reputation, subculture, fashion, and peer influence. Short-lived experience: Experimental use of illicit substances is typically short-lived. Risk factors: Experimental users face the highest risk for infections (if injecting), medical complications, or overdose due to indiscriminate use. Transition: Experimental users may or may not become recreational users.
Recreational	Recreational use: Pleasure and relaxation are prime motivations, with strict adherence to usage patterns. Preference: Recreational users typically have a preferred drug, method of use, and appreciation of effects. Integration: Drug or alcohol use complements social and recreational activities for recreational users. Consequences: Typically, no adverse medical or social consequences arise from recreational use. Escalation: Evidence suggests some Muslim participants escalate from experimentation to dependence.
Dependence/addiction	Progression: User has moved to regular and problematic use/addiction. Polydrug use: May become a multiple-drug user or polydrug user. Dependence: Psychological and/or physical dependence may be present. Frequency: More frequent and regular use, but less controlled. Obsession: Alcohol and drug use obsession supersedes all other interests, including work activities and relationships. Injection: Injecting drugs is common. Consequences: Frequent use leads to problems like intoxication, infections from sharing needles, and other medical complications. Problems: Personal, social, psychological, and legal issues may arise in this group.

Source: Adapted from Rassool (2021).

as primary benefits. Despite this, recreational users generally avoid "hard drugs" based on their personal risk-and-pleasure assessments. However, recreational users are at high risk for infections, especially from drugs acting as sexual stimulants. These substances may lower inhibition, increase sexual drive, and lead to risky sexual behaviour, increasing the likelihood of HIV and other blood-borne infections. However, there is a concerning rise in the recreational use of "designer drugs," "legal highs," or "research chemicals," termed "new psychoactive substances" (NPS), which represent synthetic alternatives to traditional illegal drugs use (Baumann, 2016).

Individuals with alcohol or substance use disorder have progressed to regular and problematic use of psychoactive drugs, often becoming polydrug users. They exhibit high tolerance and experience psychological and/or physical dependence, distinguishing them from experimental and recreational users. Their substance use is frequent, regular, and less controlled, continuing despite negative consequences. Obtaining the substance becomes more important than the quality of the experience, displacing social activities. Injecting drugs is common, leading to intoxication, infections from needle sharing, and other medical complications. Personal, social, psychological, and legal problems often accompany this group.

BINGE DRINKING

The term "binge drinking" has gained popularity recently, referring to consuming a large amount of alcohol in a single drinking session, which poses significant health risks. The National Institute on Alcohol Abuse and Alcoholism (NIAAA, 2024) defines *binge drinking* as reaching a blood alcohol concentration (BAC) of 0.08% or more, typically occurring when a woman consumes four or more drinks or a man consumes five or more drinks, within about two hours. Research indicates that youths can reach the same BAC with fewer drinks, with girls needing as few as three drinks and boys requiring three to five drinks, depending on factors such as age and size (Chung et al., 2018). In an examination of the lay understanding of the causes of binge drinking in the UK and Australia, the findings of a study (Keatley et al., 2017) found that drinking culture, peer pressure, and low alcohol cost were perceived as direct causes of binge drinking in both UK and Australian participants. Specifically, low alcohol cost was most frequently associated with binge drinking in the UK, while drinking culture held greater prominence in Australian perceptions. Supermarket discounts and the overall low cost of alcohol were identified as indirect causes of binge drinking in both samples.

The World Health Organization (WHO, 2020) views binge or excessive drinking as a significant health problem requiring worldwide attention. The report states that "[f]ar too many people, their families and communities suffer the consequences of the harmful use of alcohol through violence, injuries, mental health problems and diseases like cancer and stroke." (WHO, 2020, p. 85). Conditions associated with excessive alcohol consumption include cancer, epilepsy, cardiovascular diseases, and digestive diseases. Binge drinking is associated with a myriad of health and social problems, including greater risks of injury and death (Caamaño-Isorna et al., 2017); antisocial and illegal behaviour, such as drink-driving, assault, stealing, and damaging property (Yang et al., 2016); dementia (Harris, 2023); prediction of problem gambling behaviour (Zhai et al., 2017); and among young women, a greater risk of sexual assault (Luke, 2009). The findings of a review on binge drinking and emotional responses indicate that binge drinking is associated with heightened negative emotional states, including increased severity of depressive and anxiety symptoms (Lannoy et al., 2021). Binge drinking poses significant health risks, and it is important to recognise its harmful effects.

ROUTES OF DRUG ADMINISTRATION (HOW PEOPLE TAKE DRUGS)

The absorption and effects of psychoactive drugs are influenced by their route of administration. Common routes include oral ingestion, smoking, inhalation, and injection. Orally administered drugs, in liquid or tablet form, are most common but act slower. Injection is preferred for rapid drug

Table 5.3
Modes and key characteristics of drug use

Administration	Modes	Characteristics
Oral	Swallowing a substance in pill, capsule, liquid, or edible form	Slow onset of effects due to absorption through the gastrointestinal tract, relatively safe and convenient, commonly associated with prescription medications and recreational drugs like ecstasy or LSD
Injecting (intravenous or intramuscular)	Introducing a drug directly into the bloodstream or muscle tissue using a syringe	Rapid onset of effects, intense high, and increased risk of overdose, infections, and transmission of blood-borne diseases (e.g. HIV, hepatitis)
Inhalation	Breathing in vapours, smoke, or aerosols of a substance into the lungs	Rapid onset of effects due to direct absorption into the bloodstream via the lungs, associated with substances like tobacco, marijuana, cocaine (crack), and inhalants (e.g. solvents, aerosol sprays)
Nasal (snorting or insufflation)	Inhaling powdered drugs through the nostrils.	Moderate onset of effects, as the drug is absorbed through the nasal mucosa, commonly associated with cocaine, amphetamines, and prescription medications like opioids (crushed pills)
Transdermal	Absorbing drugs through the skin via patches, creams, or gels	Slow and steady release of medication into the bloodstream; used for sustained pain relief (e.g. fentanyl patches), hormone replacement therapy, and nicotine replacement therapy
Rectal	Inserting a drug-containing suppository into the rectum	Efficient absorption due to the rich network of blood vessels in the rectal mucosa; used for medications when oral or intravenous routes are not feasible or practical
Sublingual or buccal	Placing drugs under the tongue (sublingual) or against the cheek (buccal) for absorption through the oral mucosa	Rapid onset of effects, as the drug bypasses first-pass metabolism in the liver, commonly used for medications like sublingual nitroglycerine (for angina) and sublingual or buccal formulations of opioids (e.g. buprenorphine)

Table 5.4
Complications of injecting

Equipment	Drug	Injecting sites	Effects
Tools used for injecting drugs, including needles, syringes, and other paraphernalia. Inadequate sterilisation or sharing of equipment	Drug being injected. Levels of potency and purity. Drugs may contain harmful additives or contaminants	Typically veins in the arms, hands, or legs. Veins can lead to vein damage, thrombosis (blood clots), and collapsed veins over time. Muscle tissue (intramuscular injection) can cause abscesses, infection, and tissue damage. Injecting into arteries or accidentally injecting air can lead to serious complications such as embolism or tissue death.	Repeated use of needles can cause tissue damage, scarring, and vein collapse, making future injections more difficult and increasing the risk of infection. Overdose, poisoning, infection, thrombosis embolism, respiratory depression, cardiovascular complications. Transmission of blood-borne infections, such as HIV/AIDS, hepatitis B, and hepatitis C. Long-term effects may include addiction, chronic health conditions, and social or legal problems.

action, often seen with drugs of misuse like heroin. Smoking is typical for drugs like cannabis, crack cocaine, and heroin, while some drugs like cocaine and amphetamine are taken intranasally. Identical drugs can yield different outcomes based on administration route. For instance, naloxone, an opiate antagonist, given intravenously treats overdose, whereas oral administration targets constipation. Figure 5.1 depicts the modes and key characteristics of drug use.

Various routes of drug administration exist, each presenting unique characteristics and risks. Oral ingestion, the most prevalent method, involves swallowing drugs, resulting in gradual absorption into the bloodstream. Unlike smoking or injecting, oral consumption typically carries no societal stigma. Smoking is another effective route, with drugs like tobacco or heroin inhaled for rapid absorption. Cannabis is commonly smoked in joints, often mixed with tobacco. Inhalation, or sniffing, enables drug absorption through the mucous membranes of the nose and mouth, providing quick responses, especially evident with crack cocaine. Suppositories, although less common for illicit drugs, allow for rectal administration of water-soluble substances like cocaine, amphetamine, and ecstasy, posing risks due to rectal tissue sensitivity and potentially fatal complications.

Injecting drugs, while less widespread, presents significant hazards, including the risk of overdose and infections like hepatitis B and HIV. Injection methods encompass intramuscular, subcutaneous, and intravenous routes. The rapid onset of drug effects with intravenous administration contributes to its prevalence, with heroin, cocaine, amphetamines, and certain sedatives commonly injected. Despite its effectiveness, injecting poses severe health risks, including abscesses, gangrene, and thromboses. Overall, the choice of administration route affects the speed and intensity of drug effects and carries varying degrees of risk, emphasising the importance of understanding and addressing the implications of each method for public health interventions. Table 5.4 summarises the complications of injecting.

KEY POINTS

- Pharmacological properties, individual differences, and the context of use influence individual experiences with drug-taking substance use.
- Continued substance use among alcohol and drug users is driven more by physiological and psychological dependence rather than rational decisions.
- Drug or alcohol use patterns may vary over time for some individuals.
- Young people are often introduced to alcohol drinking in households where parents drink and where alcohol is accessible.
- Experimental use of illicit psychoactive substances is typically short-lived, with many individuals limiting consumption to socially acceptable drugs.

- Common drugs used by recreational users include alcohol, caffeine, nicotine, cannabis, LSD, and ecstasy.
- Dependent users have progressed to regular and problematic drug use or have become multiple drug users.
- Binge drinking involves drinking with the intention of becoming drunk.
- Routes of administration include oral ingestion, smoking, inhalation, suppository use, and injection.
- Injecting drugs, while less common, is the most hazardous route of administration, associated with a higher risk of overdose and infections.

References

ADDAS. (2024). *Substance Use*. Anxiety & Depression Association of America. https://adaa.org/understanding-anxiety/co-occurring-disorders/substance-abuse (accessed 30 January 2024).

Baumann, M. H. (2016). The changing face of recreational drug use. *Cerebrum: The Dana Forum on Brain Science*, 2016, cer-01-16.

Bremner, P., Burnett, J., Nunney, F., Ravat, M., & Mistral, W. (2021). *Young People, Alcohol and Influences*. London: Joseph Rowntree Foundation. https://www.jrf.org.uk/sites/default/files/migrated/migrated/files/young-people-alcohol-summary.pdf (accessed 30 January 2024).

Caamaño-Isorna, F., Moure-Rodríguez, L., Doallo, S., Corral, M., Rodriguez Holguín, S., & Cadaveira, F. (2017). Heavy episodic drinking and alcohol-related injuries: An open cohort study among college students. *Accident; Analysis and Prevention*, 100, 23–29. https://doi.org/10.1016/j.aap.2016.12.012.

Chung, T., Creswell, K. G., Bachrach, R., Clark, D. B., & Martin, C. S. (2018). Adolescent binge drinking. *Alcohol Research: Current Reviews*, 39(1), 5–15.

Gossop, M. (2013). *Living with Drugs* (7th ed.). Farham, Surrey: Ashgate Publishing Company.

Harris, E. (2023). Binge drinking, other substance use up in midlife adults. *JAMA*, 330(11), 1030. https://doi.org/10.1001/jama.2023.16111.

ISDD. (1996). *Drug Abuse Briefing*. London: Institute for the Study of Drug Dependence.

Keatley, D. A., Ferguson, E., Lonsdale, A., & Hagger, M. S. (2017). Lay understanding of the causes of binge drinking in the United Kingdom and Australia: A network diagram approach. *Health Education Research*, 12(1), 33–47. https://doi.org/10.1093/her/cyw056.

Lannoy, S., Duka, T., Carbia, C., Billieux, J., Fontesse, S., Dormal, V., Gierski, F., López-Caneda, E., Sullivan, E. V., & Maurage, P. (2021). Emotional processes in binge drinking: A systematic review and perspective. *Clinical Psychology Review*, 84, 101971. https://doi.org/10.1016/j.cpr.2021.101971.

Lovato, C., Watts, A., & Stead, L. F. (2011). Impact of tobacco advertising and promotion on increasing adolescent smoking behaviours. *The Cochrane Database of Systematic Reviews*, 2011(10), CD003439. https://doi.org/10.1002/14651858.CD003439.pub2.

Luke, K. P. (2009). Sexual violence prevention and technologies of gender among heavy-drinking college women. *Social Service Review*, 83(1), 79–109.

Nader, P. W., & Czoty, M. A. (2005). PET imaging of dopamine D2 receptors in monkey models of cocaine abuse: Genetic predisposition versus environmental modulation. *American Journal of Psychiatry*, 162, 1473–1482.

National Institute of Alcohol Abuse and Alcoholism. (2024). *Understanding Binge Drinking* https://www.niaaa.nih.gov/publications/brochures-and-fact-sheets/binge-drinking (accessed 30 January 2024).

Rassool, G. H. (2018). *Alcohol and Drug Misuse. A Guide for Health and Social Care Professionals* (2nd ed.). Oxford: Routledge.

Rassool, G. H. (2021). *Mother of All Evils; Addictive Behaviours from an Islamic Perspective*. London: Islamic Psychology Publishing (IPP) & Institute of Islamic Psychology Research (ERIIPR). Amazon/Kindle.

Royal College of Psychiatrists. (1987). *Drug Scenes: A Report on Drugs and Drug Dependence*. London: Royal College of Psychiatrists.

Scharff, C. (2014). *Anxiety and addiction: Part I, the Connection*. https://www.anxiety.org/why-people-look-to-substance-abuse-to-escape-anxiety (accessed 30 January 2024).

Volkow, N. D., Wang, G. J., Fowler, J. S., Logan, J., Jayne, M., Franceschi, D., Wong, C., Gatley, S. J., Gifford, A. N., Ding, Y. S., & Pappas, N. (2002). Nonhedonic food motivation in humans involves dopamine in the dorsal striatum and methylphenidate amplifies this effect. *Synapse*, 44(3), 175–180.

World Health Organization. (2020). *Who Global Status Report on Alcohol and Health 2018*. Geneva: World Health Organization. https://www.who.int/substance_abuse/publications/global_alcohol_report/en (accessed 30 January 2024).

Yang, O., Zhao, X., & Srivastava, P. (2016). Binge drinking and antisocial and unlawful behaviors in Australia. *Economic Record*, 92(297), 222–240.

Zhai, Z., Yip, S., Steinberg, M., Wampler, J., Hoff, R., Krishnan-Sarin, S., Potenza, M., Zhai, Z. W., Yip, S. W., Steinberg, M. A., Hoff, R. A., & Potenza, M. N. (2017). Relationships between perceived family gambling and peer gambling and adolescent problem gambling and binge drinking. *Journal of Gambling Studies*, 33(4), 1169–1185.

Chapter 6

Global policy initiatives and strategy on alcohol and drugs

Learning outcomes

- Have an understanding on the international conventions on narcotics drugs.
- Explain the terms *decriminalisation*, *depenalisation*, and *legalisation*.
- Critically examine the arguments for and against legalisation or decriminalisation of cannabis.
- Examine the alternative drug policies in countries with the legalisation and decriminalisation of cannabis.
- Discuss the evidence of the benefits of access to medicinal cannabis.
- Outline the global drug policy programme.
- Outline the global alcohol strategy.
- Outline the global tobacco strategy.

Activity 6.1

Please circle or tick the correct answer. There is only one correct answer for each statement.

1. Which of the following international conventions primarily addresses narcotics drugs?
   a. Convention on Psychotropic Substances
   b. Single Convention on Narcotic Drugs
   c. Convention on Biological Diversity
   d. Convention on the Rights of the Child
   e. None of the above
2. What does decriminalisation of drugs refer to?
   a. Legalising drug production and distribution
   b. Removing criminal penalties for drug possession
   c. Strict enforcement of drug laws
   d. Establishing drug rehabilitation programmes
   e. None of the above
3. Which term describes the policy approach of reducing or eliminating criminal penalties for drug possession?
   a. Depenalisation
   b. Legalisation
   c. Criminalisation
   d. Regulation
   e. None of the above

DOI: 10.4324/9781003456674-

4. What is the primary argument for the legalisation of cannabis?
   a. Increase government revenue
   b. Reduce drug-related crime
   c. Protect public health
   d. Undermine drug cartels
   e. None of the above
5. In which countries has cannabis been legalised for recreational use?
   a. Canada and Australia
   b. Uruguay and Portugal
   c. Netherlands and Spain
   d. United States and United Kingdom
   e. None of the above
6. Which term refers to the process of making cannabis available for medical purposes?
   a. Legalisation
   b. Decriminalisation
   c. Medicalisation
   d. Depenalisation
   e. None of the above
7. What is the primary objective of the global drug policy programme?
   a. Eradicate drug use entirely
   b. Reduce demand for illicit drugs
   c. Eliminate drug trafficking
   d. Promote harm reduction strategies
   e. None of the above
8. Which organisation leads the global alcohol strategy?
   a. World Health Organization (WHO)
   b. United Nations Office on Drugs and Crime (UNODC)
   c. International Narcotics Control Board (INCB)
   d. United Nations Children's Fund (UNICEF)
   e. None of the above
9. What is the main focus of the global tobacco strategy?
   a. Reduce tobacco-related mortality and morbidity
   b. Increase tobacco production
   c. Promote tobacco advertising
   d. Expand tobacco exports
   e. None of the above
10. Which country was the first to legalise the production and sale of cannabis for recreational use?
    a. Canada
    b. Uruguay
    c. Netherlands
    d. Portugal
    e. None of the above
11. Which term describes the policy approach of reducing legal penalties for drug possession without fully legalising the substance?
    a. Depenalisation
    b. Legalisation
    c. Criminalisation

d. Regulation
e. None of the above

12. What evidence supports the benefits of access to medicinal cannabis?
    a. Reduction in opioid overdose deaths
    b. Improvement in chronic pain management
    c. Treatment of epilepsy in children
    d. All of the above
    e. None of the above

INTRODUCTION

Despite the sustained political focus and considerable resources in strategies dedicated to addressing alcohol and substance disorders, they persist as chronic public health concerns. The evolving landscape of alcohol and substance use, including emerging trends, such as proliferation of new psychoactive substances, presents additional challenges for policymakers, healthcare professionals, and communities. The international drug control system has had its fair share of criticism. The Global Commission on Drug Policy (2011) stated that

> [t]he global war on drugs has failed, with devastating consequences for individuals and societies around the world. Fifty years after the initiation of the UN Single Convention on Narcotic Drugs . . . fundamental reforms in national and global drug control policies are urgently needed.
>
> (p. 2)

This highlights a widely recognised sentiment among experts and policymakers regarding the failure of the global war on drugs. The declaration emphasises the devastating consequences of current drug control policies on individuals and societies worldwide. Despite half a century passing since the initiation of the UN Single Convention on Narcotic Drugs, the Commission argues that fundamental reforms in both national and global drug control policies are urgently required. The call for fundamental reforms suggests a shift towards evidence-based and harm reduction–oriented policies that prioritise public health, human rights, and social justice over punitive measures.

Many developed and developing nations have addressed prominent alcohol and drug issues through diverse policies and initiatives aimed at tackling this significant public health challenge. A recognised approach in reducing the supply and eliminating the cultivation of illicit drugs involves alternative and sustainable development strategies, coupled with balanced drug control policies (UNDOC, 2015, 2016). This acknowledgement signifies a shift towards comprehensive, multifaceted approaches to combatting substance use on a global scale. By prioritising sustainable development initiatives and implementing balanced alcohol and drug control policies, nations aim to address the underlying socio-economic factors contributing to substance-related issues, while effectively managing drug production and distribution. This chapter focuses on selected policy issues which are important in the understanding of the larger context of alcohol and drugs.

INTERNATIONAL DRUG CONTROL TREATIES

The international control of psychoactive substances is governed by key conventions: the Single Convention on Narcotic Drugs (UNDOC, 1961), the Convention on Psychotropic Substances (1971), and the United Nations Convention against Illicit Traffic in Narcotic Drugs and Psychotropic Substances (1988). These conventions aim to prevent drug use and trafficking through coordinated international efforts. They regulate the cultivation, distribution, and use of various substances for medical and scientific purposes while targeting illicit drug trade and related activities like money laundering. Oversight of the international drug control system is provided by organisations such as the Commission on Narcotic Drugs, the United Nations Office on Drugs and Crime (UNODC), and the International Narcotics Control Board (INCB).

The three major international drug control treaties provide a framework for countries to regulate psychoactive substances, yet each nation has the flexibility to interpret and implement them within their own legal systems. While these treaties form the legislative foundation of the United Nations drug control system and encourage common efforts among states, criticism has emerged regarding their effectiveness (Ghodse, 2008). The European Parliament (2002), for instance, has argued that the policy of drug prohibition, based on these conventions, contributes to increasing harm inflicted by illegal drug production, trafficking, and use on society, the economy, and public institutions. Despite criticisms, many countries remain signatories to the treaties, although some exploit technicalities to bend the laws to their advantage.

The international drug policy framework, governed by various conventions and institutions, faces criticism and challenges due to its rigidity and enforcement-oriented approach. Measures such as non-enforcement, decriminalisation, and medicalisation are viewed as softer challenges to the existing treaties, allowing countries to comply with technical legalities while implementing de facto policy changes that align better with their desired objectives (Haase et al., 2012). However, institutions overseeing drug policies have been resistant to reform, maintaining strong prohibition strategies and law enforcement focus as the primary means to achieve control system objectives. Tensions have arisen between national policy practices and the rigid framework of UN drug treaties, particularly concerning liberalisation, decriminalisation, and legalisation, notably in cannabis regulation. Uruguay's pioneering move to regulate cannabis in 2014 illustrates this shift, allowing residents limited rights to purchase, grow, and possess the substance. However, existing conventions operate under a "one size fits all" approach, failing to address the complexities of diverse societies and a multi-ethnic world adequately. Calls for modernising the treaty system to accommodate contemporary contexts and evolving perspectives on drug policy have been voiced by organisations like the Count the Costs. They advocate for reforms guided by evidence and human rights principles, unhindered by legal constraints imposed by outdated drug control treaties. This suggests a growing recognition of the need for flexibility and adaptability in international drug policy to better address the complex realities and diverse needs of contemporary societies.

CURRENT APPROACH TO DRUGS STRATEGIES

The current global approach to substance use disorders varies across countries and can be characterised along a continuum between purely public health approaches and purely law enforcement approaches. At one end of the continuum are countries that prioritise public health approaches. These nations emphasise prevention, treatment, and harm reduction strategies aimed at reducing the negative health consequences of substance use. Public health–focused policies often include initiatives such as education campaigns, access to treatment and rehabilitation services, needle exchange programmes, and supervised injection sites. The primary goal is to promote the well-being of individuals struggling with substance use disorders while minimising the societal impact of drug-related harms. At the other end of the continuum are countries that adopt predominantly law enforcement approaches. These nations prioritise the enforcement of drug laws, criminalisation of drug possession and trafficking, and punitive measures against drug offenders.

Law enforcement–focused policies often involve aggressive policing tactics, strict penalties for drug-related offenses, and incarceration of individuals involved in the drug trade. The primary objective is to deter drug use through legal sanctions and to control the supply of illicit substances through enforcement measures. Many countries fall somewhere along the spectrum between these two extremes, adopting a combination of public health and law enforcement approaches in their drug policies (Johnson et al., 2022). These countries recognise the importance of addressing both the health and social dimensions of substance use disorders while balancing concerns related to public safety and drug-related crime. A global movement is emerging to adopt more humane and evidence-based policies towards drugs and individuals who use them (Johnson et al., 2022). However, the dominant strategy for addressing drug use worldwide continues to focus on reducing the drug supply through law enforcement efforts, despite its high cost and limited effectiveness, as observed both in the United States and internationally (Babor et al., 2018; Wood et al., 2010).

In many countries, the phenomena of the so-called "war on drugs" has remained unmovable for the past few decades despite its obvious limitations.

The "war on drugs" originated from a policy aimed at safeguarding public health and combating addiction to narcotic drugs by reducing their production, supply, and use. Prohibition was seen as a means to achieve a drug-free society with a zero-tolerance approach. This strategy, though initially American (Health, 1996), became a global metaphor. Despite its widespread adoption, the war on drugs has persisted for decades with limited success, remaining entrenched in many countries despite its evident shortcomings. The debate over drug policy revolves around the effectiveness of prohibition versus alternative approaches like legalisation or decriminalisation. Advocates of prohibition contend that enforcement measures have successfully reduced illicit drug use, although they now emphasise public health and prevention efforts (Count the Costs). However, there is a global divergence in public sentiment regarding the continuation of prohibition versus the exploration of new approaches. Moreover, globally, geo-politics have played a significant role in maintaining the status quo of the existing drug policies.

DRUG DECRIMINALISATION, DEPENALISATION, AND LEGALISATION ISSUES

The debate over legalising and decriminalising non-medical use of psychoactive substances is gaining momentum in several countries. It is important to understand the distinctions between decriminalisation, depenalisation, and legalisation. Decriminalisation entails treating possession and use of illicit drugs as civil rather than criminal offenses, removing their status as criminal acts. According to the European Monitoring Centre for Drugs and Drug Addiction (EMCDDA, 2001), *decriminalisation* means that certain drug-related acts no longer constitute criminal offenses, particularly those related to demand, such as acquisition, possession, and consumption, though some sanctions may still apply. *Depenalisation* refers to the abolition or reduction of the penal sanction for personal consumption. The term *legalisation* refers to the removal of all drug-related offences from criminal law: use, possession, cultivation, production, trading, etc. (Blickman & Jelsma, 2009). That means "drug production, possession, and consumption are all legal, and there is no penalty whatsoever for participating in these activities" (Greenwald, 2009, p. 2).

Supporters of drug legalisation and decriminalisation, often driven by anti-prohibitionist movements, contend that drug prohibition has led to more harm than good in society. They argue that the "war on drugs" has failed to effectively address addiction to psychoactive substances while contributing to various social and public health problems. Proponents advocate for alternative approaches that prioritise harm reduction, public health initiatives and treatment over punitive measures. They believe that legalising or decriminalising drugs can lead to reduced stigma, improved access to healthcare and support services for individuals struggling with substance use disorder, and a more effective allocation of resources towards addressing underlying issues associated with addiction. Opponents of drug legalisation argue that maintaining prohibition is necessary to prevent increased addiction and associated public health risks. They highlight concerns about negative social consequences, including higher crime rates and decreased productivity, as well as the potential for drug legalisation to serve as a gateway to more harmful substances. Critics also stress the importance of law enforcement efforts in targeting drug trafficking networks and regulating drug markets. Overall, they emphasise the need to maintain existing drug policies to mitigate the potential risks and negative outcomes associated with drug legalisation. The arguments that are in opposition to drug legalisation and promote the continued prohibition of all drugs and arguments for drug policy reform are presented in Table 6.1.

It is important to note that allowing a free market of controlled psychoactive substances for non-medical purposes would lead many countries signatories to the Single Convention on Narcotics and the Convention on Psychotropic Substances to violate international treaties. These treaties impose restrictions on the production, distribution, and use of such substances. Allowing a free market would contradict the principles and obligations outlined in these agreements, potentially undermining global efforts to regulate and control psychoactive substances to prevent abuse, addiction, and related societal harms. However, drug control strategies can have several negative effects (UNDOC, 2008), including the creation of a criminal black market where illegal drug trade prospers. Additionally, these strategies can lead to "policy displacement," redirecting limited resources from health initiatives to enforcement efforts. Moreover, enforcement efforts often result

Table 6.1
Key arguments for prohibition and drug policy reform

Prohibitionists	Drug policy reform
Success of the "war on drugs" (Wilson, 1990)	Prohibitions increased in non-drug-related violence (Miron & Zwiebel, 1995).
Risks for public health, social well-being, and international drug control system (INCB, 1992)	Depenalisation in the Netherlands did not increase the levels of cannabis use (MacCoun & Reuter, 1997).
Drug use and systemic violence (Markowitz, 2000)	Removal of the prohibition against possession itself (decriminalisation) does not increase cannabis use (MacCoun & Reuter, 2001).
Prohibition discouraging drug use (Weatherburn & Jones, 2001)	Cannabis is not a stepping stone to using cocaine or heroin (Golub & Johnson, 2001; Morral et al., 2002; van Ours, 2003).
Failed experiment with legalisation in Alaska (U.S. Department of Justice, 2003)	Some legal drugs, including alcohol and tobacco and prescribed and over-the-counter drugs, cause more harm than scheduled or controlled drugs (MacCoun & Reuter, 2001; WHO, 2002; Nutt et al., 2007; Grayling, 2016).
Cannabis as a gateway drug (Lynskey, 2003); Swedish drug policy (UNODC, 2007; Ministry of Health and Social Affairs Sweden, 2008)	Medical use of psychoactive substances in the treatment of chronic depression, post-traumatic stress disorder, and alcohol use disorder (Pekkanen, 1992; Brown, 2007).
Legalisation compromising public health and public safety (Kerlikowske, 2010)	Exacerbated many public health problems (Rolles, 2010).
Public opinion against legalisation, health concerns, success of prohibition (Drug Free Australia, 2024)	Multiple sclerosis (Rog, 2010), neuropathic pain in multiple sclerosis (Rog et al., 2005), rheumatoid arthritis (Blake et al., 2006), peripheral neuropathic pain (Nurmikko et al., 2007), pain associated with advanced cancer (Johnson et al., 2010).
Health arguments and cannabis use (Hall & Degenhardt, 2009; Asbridge et al., 2012; Meier et al., 2012, 2016; Smith et al., 2014; WHO, 2016)	

in "geographical displacement," merely shifting drug production, transit, and supply to different locations rather than eliminating them altogether. Similarly, "substance displacement" occurs when enforcement measures do not eradicate drug use but merely push users toward different substances. Finally, drug control strategies can contribute to stigmatisation and discrimination against drug users, deterring them from seeking treatment and support services.

One of the primary arguments against the legalisation or decriminalisation of certain psychoactive substances is the concern that it would diminish the social stigma associated with illicit drug use. Critics fear that such actions would convey a message of "laissez-faire" and complete tolerance, potentially leading to a significant increase in drug use. Additionally, they argue that legalising or decriminalising drugs could act as a gateway to harder substances, with cannabis often cited as an example. Morality and religious values also play a role in opposing drug policy reform, as drug use, whether legal or illicit, is often perceived as morally wrong and harmful. Proponents of drug policy reform view substance use disorder as a public health issue rather than a criminal one. They argue that prohibition leads to physical and psychosocial harm for individuals, families, and society at large. Advocates emphasise the need for a legally regulated market to mitigate the demand for illicit drugs and encourage individuals with substance use disorders to seek treatment without fear of legal repercussions from the criminal justice system.

Six models for drug policy reform have been identified, ranging from depenalisation to decriminalisation, with various degrees of legal and social interventions (Hughes et al., 2019). Each model presents distinct advantages and challenges. For instance, depenalisation is straightforward to implement but may exacerbate disparities in access to justice. In contrast, decriminalisation with targeted health and social referrals requires more resources but offers potential reductions in both criminal justice burdens and drug-related harms. Overall, the models represent different approaches to addressing drug policy, each with its own implications for society, justice, and public health.

DRUG POLICIES AROUND THE WORLD

On a global scale, countries exhibit diverse approaches to drug policy, reflecting cultural, legal, and social norms. Drug policies vary globally due to differences in cultural, legal, and social norms. What is deemed socially acceptable in one country might incur severe penalties, including death, in another (DrugAbuse.net, 2017). Some nations prioritise strict punitive measures, enforcing law enforcement, and criminalisation, while others emphasise harm reduction strategies and public health interventions. This variation extends to the legalisation and decriminalisation of specific drugs, particularly cannabis. While certain countries have adopted policies allowing for personal use of cannabis, focusing on public health rather than punishment, others maintain stringent regulations. These policies often entail diversion programmes, drug courts, and access to harm reduction services. The legalisation and decriminalisation of cannabis represent a subset of broader drug policy discussions, highlighting the complexities and divergent perspectives shaping global responses to substance use and related health crises. This is a brief summary of the legalisation and decriminalisation of cannabis in selected countries and treatment interventions or other drugs.

In Europe, various countries have adopted distinct approaches to drug policy and decriminalisation. Portugal pioneered the decriminalisation of possession, selling, and personal use of all drugs, transitioning from criminal prosecution to a focus on harm reduction, treatment, and rehabilitation for substance users. Individuals found with illegal drugs are referred to the Committee for the Dissuasion of Addiction, staffed by legal, psychological, and social work professionals. Offenders undergo assessment and, if deemed dependent, are directed to treatment centres. This shift reframed drug use as a health concern rather than a criminal offense (Drug Science, 2022), signifying a significant change in addressing substance abuse and addiction. Switzerland implements some of the most liberal drug policies globally, prioritising prevention, therapy, harm reduction, and prohibition (Drug Science, 2022). Switzerland gained international attention for its government-sponsored "safe rooms," where heroin addicts can inject with clean needles in a non-threatening environment. Switzerland has decriminalised cannabis use and provides a range of supportive services, including housing, job programmes, needle exchanges, and methadone programmes, for those individuals with substance use disorder. Meanwhile in the Czech Republic, drug possession laws allow individuals to grow up to five marijuana plants, possess an ounce of cannabis, a gram of cocaine, one and a half grams of heroin, or two grams of methamphetamine. Additionally, possession limits include 40 psychedelic mushrooms, five peyote plants, and five tablets of LSD. The treatment packages include harm reduction programmes, aluminium foil to drug users for heroin smoking, counselling, and free tests for infectious diseases.

Germany's drug policies are recognised as some of the strictest in Europe, with severe penalties for the sale or possession of large drug quantities (Drug Science, 2022). However, the country does not pursue criminal action for small-scale possession or the use of several narcotics, including cannabis. The treatment intervention packages include public health measures, harm reduction, supervised "drug rooms," and counselling services. Since 1996, the Netherlands has tolerated the sale of small quantities of drugs in coffee shops, provided they adhere to specific criteria. These include restrictions on advertising, the prohibition of hard drug sales, maintaining public order around the coffee shop, and refraining from selling to minors or in large quantities per transaction (maximum 5 grams) (EMCDDA, 2019). In 2013, restrictions were placed on "cannabis tourism" from participating in cannabis use in the "coffee shops," thus restricting admittance and sales to residents of the Netherlands, though local adjustments in implementation are permitted. In the Netherlands, harm reduction activities are comprehensive and include methadone substitution therapy, needle and syringe exchange programmes, outreach work, low-threshold facilities, and centres for "social addiction care."

In the United Kingdom (UK), drug laws are structured under the Misuse of Drugs Act of 1971, which categorises drug-related offenses into three classes: Class A, Class B, and Class C, with Class A representing the most dangerous drugs and Class C the least dangerous. While possession laws in the UK may be more lenient compared to those in the United States, possession with intent to sell can lead to severe penalties, including the possibility of life imprisonment. The Psychoactive Substances Act (2016) is a piece of legislation enacted in the UK to address the sale, production, and distribution of psychoactive substances (synthetic cannabinoids, mephedrone, and 25i-NBOMe. The Act covers "legal highs" derived from food, plants, herbs, and remedies causing psychoactive effects but exempts caffeine, alcohol, nicotine, and medicine. The Act aims to prohibit the production, supply, importation, and exportation of such substances, excluding those explicitly exempted under the legislation. The law defines *psychoactive substances* broadly as substances capable of producing a psychoactive effect on a person, affecting mental functioning or emotional state. The Act seeks to prevent the harmful effects of these substances and protect public health by introducing strict controls and penalties for those involved in their production and distribution. It is reported that while the Psychoactive Substances Act successfully reduced the prevalence of new psychoactive substances (NPS), it failed to decrease overall drug use (DrugAbuse.net, 2017). Moreover, drug-related deaths have increased annually since its implementation, including deaths from NPS. Some individuals who had turned to NPS as a supposedly safer alternative reverted to more harmful traditional drugs. Vulnerable populations like prisoners and the homeless, who relied on NPS such as spice, were driven into illegal markets due to the Act's restrictions (DrugAbuse.net, 2017).

The United States (US) enforces strict penalties for drug possession and sale, contributing to a significant portion of the country's prison population being individuals with drug-related issues. Marijuana laws are changing at a rapid pace across all 50 states. Several states in the United States have implemented various policies regarding marijuana legalisation, medical marijuana, and decriminalisation. Some states have a combination of legalisation, medical use, and decriminalisation (DISA, 2024). In Colorado, adults over 21 can buy and possess up to 1 ounce of cannabis and grow six plants privately. Tourists and residents can make single transactions for up to 28 grams. In Washington, adults can privately possess 1 ounce of cannabis and specific amounts of marijuana-infused products without facing criminal or civil penalties. However, public cannabis consumption is subject to fines. Canada legalised medical cannabis in July 2001 and expanded legalisation to include adult recreational use in October 2018. Similar to alcohol and tobacco, the country regulates cannabis distribution and consumption, with designated safe areas and licensed producers. Strict penalties are in place for selling cannabis to minors or driving while impaired.

Uruguay made history by becoming the first country to legalise the cultivation, consumption, and sale of marijuana, breaking the International Convention on Drug Control. The government oversees the production and distribution of cannabis, setting a fixed price per gram to undercut the black market. It sells cannabis for $1 per gram, significantly impacting drug trafficking. Citizens and residents can purchase up to 40 grams monthly from pharmacies or join cannabis clubs for cultivation. Individuals are allowed to grow up to six plants themselves. Additionally, personal use of most psychedelic mushrooms is legal. While heroin and cocaine use is not illegal, selling or distributing these drugs incurs legal sanctions.

Uruguay's approach has drawn international attention and sparked discussions about alternative drug policies worldwide. It represents a significant departure from traditional prohibitionist strategies, emphasising regulation and harm reduction instead. However, challenges remain in implementing and evaluating the effectiveness of this groundbreaking policy.

In Australia, laws regarding the use and possession of illicit drugs primarily fall under the jurisdiction of states and territories, rather than the Commonwealth government. As of 2016, in most states and territories, drug use and possession constitute criminal offenses punishable by up to two years in prison (Hughes, 2014). In Australia, cannabis use, possession, cultivation, and sale are illegal nationwide, but penalties for cannabis offenses vary across states and territories. There is growing support in Australia for shifting from a law enforcement approach to drug use to a health-oriented response. Many programmes across the country operate outside formal legislation and are focused on diversion, cautions, and fines rather than criminal charges for drug possession (Alcohol & Drug Foundation, 2023). While all Australian states and territories have some form of in-practice decriminalisation, only three (Australian Capital Territory, South Australia, and the Northern Territory) have in law decriminalisation (Alcohol & Drug Foundation, 2023). Under the Australian Capital Territory's laws, individuals can possess up to 50 grams of dried cannabis or grow up to two cannabis plants per person (or four per household) for personal use. In other states and territories, cannabis offenses remain criminal, and offenders may receive cautions, attend Cannabis Intervention Sessions (CIS), or be directed to diversion programmes. A Cannabis Intervention Session (CIS) is a one-to-one therapeutic intervention with a trained alcohol and drug counsellor.

Many other countries are already leading the way for drug policy reform, and many countries have decriminalised drug use in various ways. These include France, Germany, Austria, Spain, Belgium, Italy, Denmark, Estonia, Ecuador, Armenia, India, Brazil, Peru, Colombia, Argentina, Mexico, Paraguay, Costa Rica, and Jamaica. Currently, there is a bill in Ireland that proposes to decriminalise the personal use of cannabis.

The policy effect of decriminalisation of cannabis has been a subject of interest in numerous studies (Bernard et al., 2020). The data from Portugal's decriminalisation framework indicate resounding success across various metrics. Drug usage has decreased in absolute terms, particularly in certain key demographic segments (Greenwald, 2009). Decriminalising cannabis has reduced enforcement costs without increasing cannabis use. In the United States, decriminalisation has redirected resources towards combating trafficking and other illicit drugs, with no significant rise in cannabis use or related issues (Single et al., 2000). Researchers at the Finnish Institute for Health and Welfare (Unlu et al., 2020) conducted a study evaluating the impact of decriminalisation policies across various settings. The study analysed reports, peer-reviewed articles, and critical response papers, revealing substantial evidence of reduced infectious diseases and drug-related deaths among individuals who use drugs in countries with decriminalisation policies. Decriminalisation of drug use promotes a supportive atmosphere for seeking help and treatment, aids in integrating drug users into society, and improves educational and employment prospects. It also reduces the strain on the criminal justice system, leading to lower policing and imprisonment expenses. Nonetheless, apprehensions about potential rises in drug use hinder the widespread acceptance of decriminalisation policies. However, the findings of a particular study indicated that legal reforms were commonly not correlated with alterations in substance use across a range of metrics (Scheim et al., 2020).

MEDICINAL CANNABIS

The use of cannabis for both recreational and medicinal purposes can be traced back 6,000 years (Nkard, 2021). The term *medical marijuana* refers to using the whole, unprocessed marijuana plant or its basic extracts to treat symptoms of illness and other conditions (NIDA, 2018). The two main cannabinoids from the marijuana plant with medical interest are THC (delta-9-tetrahydrocannabinol) and CBD. THC is marijuana's main mind-altering ingredient that makes people "high." THC is known to increase appetite and reduce nausea. Additionally, THC may alleviate pain, inflammation, and muscle control problems. CBD, short for cannabidiol, is one of the many cannabinoids found in the cannabis plant. Unlike THC, CBD is non-psychoactive, meaning, it does not produce a "high" sensation commonly associated with marijuana use.

The therapeutic use of marijuana and cannabinoids has a history spanning over 4500 years (Earleywine, 2002). Substantial evidence supports the effectiveness of cannabis or cannabinoids in treating pain in adults, chemotherapy-induced nausea and vomiting, and spasticity associated with multiple sclerosis. Moderate evidence indicates potential benefits for secondary sleep disturbances. However, evidence supporting improvement in appetite, Tourette's syndrome, anxiety, post-traumatic stress disorder, cancer, irritable bowel syndrome, epilepsy, and various neurodegenerative disorders is described as limited, insufficient, or absent (Abrams, 2018). There are consistent findings indicating its effectiveness in lowering intraocular pressure associated with glaucoma. Evidence also supports its efficacy in alleviating pain, spasticity, nausea, vomiting, weight loss, and loss of appetite in various medical conditions (Hasan, 2023).

The legislation of cannabis for medical use has been gaining ground globally. In the United States, the FDA (the US Food and Drug Administration) approved a CBD-based liquid medication called Epidiolex® for the treatment of two forms of severe childhood epilepsy, Dravet syndrome and Lennox–Gastaut syndrome (NIDA, 2018, p. 3). Two FDA-approved drugs, dronabinol and nabilone, contain THC and are utilised to treat chemotherapy-induced nausea and to increase appetite in patients experiencing extreme weight loss due to AIDS. In addition, nabiximols (Sativex®), a mouth spray containing THC and CBD, has been approved in the UK, Canada, and several European countries. It is used to address muscle control problems associated with multiple sclerosis (MS), although it has not received FDA approval in the United States. Scientists are exploring the potential of marijuana and its extracts in clinical trials to address symptoms associated with various illnesses and conditions, including those affecting the immune system, inflammation, pain, seizures, substance use disorders, and mental disorders (NIDA, 2018). A detailed analysis funded by the National

Institute on Drug Abuse (Bachhuber et al., 2015) revealed that legally protected medical marijuana dispensaries, in addition to medical marijuana laws, were linked to several positive outcomes: decrease in opioid prescribing, reduction in self-reports of opioid misuse, and decline in treatment admissions for opioid addiction.

However, there are concerns regarding the use of therapeutic cannabis and herbal cannabis–based preparations, including the risk of dependence, although it is lower compared to benzodiazepines, opiates, cocaine, or nicotine (Joy et al., 1999). Additionally, medical marijuana use is not correlated with subsequent use of other illicit drugs. According to the National Institute on Drug Abuse (NIDA) (2016), limited information exists regarding the long-term effects of marijuana use among individuals with health-related vulnerabilities, such as older adults or those with conditions like cancer, AIDS, cardiovascular disease, multiple sclerosis, or other neurodegenerative diseases. Further research is necessary to determine if individuals with compromised health due to disease or treatment, such as chemotherapy, are at heightened risk for adverse health outcomes from marijuana use. Studies have shown that chronic use of marijuana can, in rare instances, result in cannabinoid hyperemesis syndrome, characterised by severe nausea, vomiting, and dehydration (Galli et al., 2011). This syndrome typically affects individuals under 50 years of age with a long history of marijuana use. Sufferers may seek frequent emergency room visits, but symptoms often resolve upon cessation of marijuana use.

The use of medical marijuana presents implications for healthcare professionals across medicine, psychiatry, and pharmacology. Recommendations for prescribing and treatment should align with accepted standards of medical responsibility. This involves conducting a comprehensive review of the patient's substance use history, physical condition, co-occurring medical and psychiatric conditions, and family history. Healthcare professionals should collaborate with patients to develop a treatment plan and document medical marijuana use in the patient's record. Healthcare professionals have a responsibility to educate patients about the potential risks and benefits of medical marijuana use. This includes providing information about the physical and psychological effects of cannabis, potential drug interactions with other medications the patient may be taking, and precautions to ensure safe use. Patients should be informed not to drive or operate machinery after using medical marijuana and to store it securely to prevent accidental ingestion by children or pets. Healthcare professionals should regularly monitor patients who are using medical marijuana to assess treatment efficacy, monitor for any adverse effects or complications, and make adjustments to the treatment plan as needed. Regular follow-up appointments provide an opportunity to address any concerns or questions the patient may have and to ensure that the treatment remains appropriate and effective.

GLOBAL DRUG POLICY PROGRAMME

There are ongoing conflicts among countries regarding global drug policy strategies, particularly concerning the legalisation or decriminalisation of cannabis. This has prompted calls from policymakers, academics, healthcare and social care professionals, individuals within the criminal justice system, and civil society groups for a re-evaluation of the current approach to addressing drug-related issues. The recommendation of the World Drug Report 2022 (UNODC, 2022) emphasises ensuring access to essential medicines during humanitarian responses, maintaining continuity of evidence-based care for drug use disorders and related infectious diseases, and preventing negative coping behaviours, especially among children and youth, through family and psychosocial support. The approach aims to leave no one behind by improving data collection, tailoring interventions to specific demographics, and closing treatment gaps without stigma or discrimination. Furthermore, a whole-of-society approach is advocated, involving multiple sectors and industries, to strengthen evidence-based prevention efforts.

The United Nations General Assembly Special Session (United Nations, 2016) held a review of the drug control system. The previous special session on drugs was held in 1998, focused on the total elimination of drugs from the world. Heads of state, government officials, and representatives of member states express their commitment to addressing the global drug problem through a joint document. They reaffirm their dedication to the goals and objectives outlined in the three international drug control conventions. Their concerns include the health and welfare of humanity, particularly focusing on the individual and public health–related, social, and safety issues associated with narcotic drugs and psychotropic substances. There is a specific emphasis on preventing substance use among children and young people, combating drug-related crime, and preventing and treating substance abuse while also countering illicit cultivation, production, manufacturing, and trafficking of drugs.

The final Outcome Document of the joint commitment to address the world drug problem delineated seven key operational areas: demand reduction and related measures; access to controlled substances for medical and scientific purposes; supply reduction and related measures; human rights and cross-cutting issues; evolving trends and emerging challenges; international cooperation; and sustainable or alternative development. Regarding "harm reduction," specific references were made in the Outcome Document concerning the use of naloxone and overdose prevention, "medication-assisted therapy programmes" (opioid substitution therapy), and "injecting equipment programmes" (needle and syringe programmes). The UN's 2016 Outcome Document, while containing references to harm reduction measures like naloxone use and medication-assisted therapy programmes, has been criticised for reaffirming the unrealistic goal of achieving a "society free of drug abuse." This language, described as outdated and dangerous by the International Drug Policy Consortium (2016), was reluctantly accepted by progressive member states in exchange for the inclusion of harm reduction provisions. The failure of the document to enact substantive drug reform policies has left members of the Global Commission on Drug Policy disillusioned. Arbour (2016) observed that countries interested in pursuing policies such as cannabis legalisation or drug decriminalisation face a dilemma: they must either denounce international conventions, a significant step that may influence other countries to renege on commitments, or pretend compliance despite non-compliance.

The Global Commission on Drugs (2021) recommends that a new international drug control strategy is needed to empower national and local governments to test drug regulation models prioritising citizen health and safety while undermining transnational criminal networks' influence and profits. The success of the reform movement in the next decade relies on rallying around a positive agenda that promotes a healthy, sustainable future with economic opportunities for everyone. Key principles of this global reform agenda include decriminalising drug use and possession for personal use, guaranteeing access to essential controlled medicines, investing in drug use prevention, offering accessible non-compulsory treatments and harm reduction services, introducing alternatives to incarceration for small-scale nonviolent participants in the illegal drug market, and gradually regulating all drug markets to safeguard marginalised and vulnerable populations.

GLOBAL ALCOHOL STRATEGY

The global alcohol strategy refers to a comprehensive approach aimed at addressing the challenges associated with alcohol consumption on a global scale. This strategy typically involves collaboration among governments, international organisations, public health agencies, and other stakeholders to develop policies and initiatives to reduce harmful alcohol use and its related consequences. Key components of a global alcohol strategy may include public awareness campaigns, regulation of alcohol marketing and advertising, implementation of evidence-based interventions for prevention and treatment, taxation policies, and monitoring of alcohol-related trends and outcomes. The overarching goal of a global alcohol strategy is to promote responsible alcohol consumption, protect public health, and mitigate the social, economic, and health burdens associated with alcohol misuse. The World Health Organization (WHO, 2010) aims to mitigate the health, psychological, and social impacts stemming from the harmful use of alcohol. *Harmful use* is characterised as drinking behaviour that leads to negative health and social consequences for the individual, their immediate environment, and society overall. It encompasses patterns of drinking linked to heightened risks of adverse health outcomes.

The global strategy to reduce the harmful use of alcohol, outlined by the World Health Organization (WHO, 2010), aims to achieve several objectives:

1. Raise global awareness about the health, social and economic harms associated with alcohol consumption.
2. Enhance the knowledge base on effective interventions to prevent and reduce alcohol-related harm.
3. Provide increased technical support for the prevention and management of alcohol use disorders and associated health conditions.

4. Strengthen partnerships and improve coordination among stakeholders to mobilise resources for prevention efforts.
5. Enhance monitoring and surveillance systems at various levels and improve the dissemination and application of information for advocacy, policy development, and evaluation purposes.

(p. 8)

Additionally, the strategy includes guiding principles for the development and implementation of alcohol policies. The guiding principles are presented in Table 6.1.

The global alcohol strategy emphasises concerted efforts in public health advocacy and partnership to support governments and key stakeholders in reducing harmful alcohol use. Priority areas include technical support, capacity building, knowledge dissemination, and resource mobilisation. At the national level, a focus is placed on mitigating harm to vulnerable populations, such as children, adolescents, women of childbearing age, pregnant and breastfeeding women, indigenous peoples, and other minority or low-socio-economic status groups. Governments are tasked with formulating, implementing, monitoring, and evaluating public policies to address harmful alcohol use. Establishing a national alcohol council ensures a cohesive approach to alcohol policies. Many countries have implemented stricter blood alcohol concentration limits and developed national alcohol policies following the recommendations of the global strategy. The strategy outlines ten target areas for policy options and interventions, including leadership, awareness, health services response, community action, drink-driving policies, alcohol availability, marketing regulations, reducing negative consequences of drinking, addressing illicit alcohol, and enhancing monitoring and surveillance. Since the endorsement of the global strategy in 2010, member states' commitment to reducing the harmful use of alcohol has been further strengthened by the global alcohol action plan 2022–2030 (WHO, 2021) to strengthen implementation of the global strategy to reduce the harmful use of alcohol.

Evidenced-based measures for the management of alcohol use disorder include screening and brief interventions (Anderson et al., 2009), community interventions (Ramstedt et al., 2013), and regulating serving practices in bars and restaurants (Trolldal et al., 2013). These also include the models of care implemented in primary care settings that can enhance treatment uptake, including both psychosocial interventions and pharmacotherapy (Rombouts et al., 2020). The global strategy aims to address the harmful impacts of alcohol consumption worldwide, yet evidence suggests that evidence-based policies have been overshadowed by those favoured by the alcohol industry (McCambridge et al., 2014). Despite extensive knowledge of the health implications of alcohol use, policy responses have often been fragmented and fail to adequately address the magnitude of health and social development impacts (Institute of Alcohol Studies, 2013).

Table 6.2
Guiding principles for the development and implementation of alcohol policies

1. Public policies and interventions to prevent and reduce alcohol-related harm should be guided and formulated by public health interests and based on clear public health goals and the best available evidence.
2. Policies should be equitable and sensitive to national, religious, and cultural contexts.
3. All involved parties have the responsibility to act in ways that do not undermine the implementation of public policies and interventions to prevent and reduce harmful use of alcohol.
4. Public health should be given proper deference in relation to competing interests, and approaches that support that direction should be promoted.
5. Protection of populations at high risk of alcohol-attributable harm and those exposed to the effects of harmful drinking by others should be an integral part of policies addressing the harmful use of alcohol.
6. Individuals and families affected by the harmful use of alcohol should have access to affordable and effective prevention and care services.
7. Children, teenagers, and adults who choose not to drink alcoholic beverages have the right to be supported in their non-drinking behaviour and protected from pressures to drink.
8. Public policies and interventions to prevent and reduce alcohol-related harm should encompass all alcoholic beverages and surrogate alcohol.

Source: WHO (2010).

TOBACCO STRATEGY

Tobacco use continues to be the leading global cause of preventable death, and measures are in place to combat the harms caused by tobacco smoking. The global strategy defines key priorities to advance the implementation of the WHO FCTC through 2025 (WHO, 2023). "It empowers Parties to work with the health and non-health sectors in promoting a coordinated and focused whole-of-government, whole-of-society approach to achieve policy coherence, both domestically and internationally." The global tobacco control strategy is governed by the

WHO Framework Convention on Tobacco Control (WHO FCTC, 2003), a treaty signed by countries covering 90% of the world's population. The treaty outlines a comprehensive set of obligations aimed at implementing both supply- and demand-side measures to combat the global tobacco epidemic. This strategy encompasses various initiatives and policies designed to reduce tobacco consumption and its associated health risks on a global scale. The WHO Framework Convention on Tobacco Control (WHO FCTC, 2003) is a landmark treaty negotiated by the World Health Organization, which established legally binding obligations for its parties to focus on reducing both the supply and demand for tobacco products. With 180 parties committed to prioritising tobacco control and minimising its harms, the WHO FCTC has played a pivotal role in guiding global tobacco control policy. Since its inception, significant progress has been noted across all regions and income levels, reflecting the effectiveness of the treaty. In 2008, WHO identified six evidence-based tobacco control measures, known as MPOWER:

- Monitor tobacco use and prevention policies.
- Protect people from tobacco smoke.
- Offer help to quit tobacco use.
- Warn about the dangers of tobacco.
- Enforce bans on tobacco advertising, promotion, and sponsorship.
- Raise taxes on tobacco.

The MPOWER package, recognised as a comprehensive strategy to combat the tobacco epidemic, has seen widespread adoption globally. According to reports, nearly 20% of the world's population is covered by two or more MPOWER measures at the highest level, indicating significant implementation progress (WHO, 2015). Since 2012, numerous countries have enacted robust tobacco control practices, including comprehensive smoke-free laws for indoor public places and workplaces, the provision of smoking cessation services, implementation of health warning labels on cigarette packs, complete bans on tobacco advertising, promotion, and sponsorship (TAPS) activities, and substantial increases in cigarette taxes exceeding 75% of the retail price. These efforts reflect a concerted commitment to reducing tobacco use and its associated harms on a global scale.

Despite some significant changes as a result of the Framework Convention on Tobacco Control, more needs to be done to implement all of its provisions in order to reduce the burden of tobacco smoking as a public health problem. It has been suggested that tobacco cessation remains uncommon in mos low- and middle-income countries.

> Barriers exist in low- and middle-income countries to implementing affordable tobacco-cessation initiatives such as advice from health-care professionals, text messages and cheap pharmacotherapy. Using lower-level health-care workers for cessation support, integrating cessation into health-care programmes, subsidising pharmacotherapy and collaborating with international stakeholders to disseminate text messages could overcome these barriers.
>
> (Peer & Kengne, 2018, p. 1,390)

However, the proposed solutions offer practica approaches to address these barriers. By leveragin lower-level healthcare workers for cessation support integrating cessation services into existing health care programmes, subsidising pharmacotherapy, an collaborating with international stakeholders to dis seminate text messages, countries can enhance th availability and affordability of cessation interven tions. These strategies recognise the importance o adapting interventions to local contexts while lever aging international expertise and resources.

The tobacco industry poses a significant obstacl to reducing the prevalence of tobacco smoking. On approach advocated is to neutralise the strategie employed by the tobacco industry (Jha & Alleyn 2015). By doing so, it could pave the way for highe taxation and more robust tobacco control mea sures in the coming decade. However, during thes challenges, the Framework Convention on Tobacc Control (FCTC) serves as a crucial platform for th global anti-tobacco movement. It sets the agend and provides guiding principles and accountabilit for policymakers worldwide.

With the rise in e-cigarette usage, 68 countrie have implemented legal regulations governing va ious aspects of e-cigarettes, including sales, adve tising, packaging, product regulation, taxation, an usage (Kennedy et al., 2017). These regulation encompass areas such as age restrictions, healt warnings, nicotine concentration, and vape-fre zones (Institute for Global Tobacco Control, 2016 Some countries have prohibited the importatio distribution, commercialisation, and advertising o e-cigarettes, while others permit their use withou nicotine. Water tobacco smoking, or *shisha* smokin falls under the purview of the WHO Internation Framework Convention on Tobacco Control. Partie to the treaty are obligated to integrate water pip tobacco use into their tobacco control policies. Th recognition highlights the global effort to addre emerging forms of tobacco consumption and underscores the importance of comprehensive regulation to mitigate their public health impacts. For a detailed overview of the legal status of electronic cigarettes worldwide, a comprehensive resource can be found at www.ecigarette-politics.com/electronic-cigarettes-global-legal-status.html.

The WHO study group on tobacco product regulation (Tob Reg) (2015) has suggested that regulators should take actions, including:

- Water pipes themselves, as well as parts and accessories, should also be taxed.
- Water pipes, water pipe tobacco, parts, and accessories should be prohibited or restricted from being sold tax- or duty-free.
- Water pipe cafés or lounges must not be exempted from clean indoor air laws.
- Indoor water pipe smoking in public areas should be prohibited, and smoking allowed only outside.
- Water pipe venues should not be allowed within large shopping areas, such as indoor malls.
- Water pipe tobacco and water pipe smoke should be tested by the same stringent standards that are applied to cigarette tobacco.
- Legislation should ensure that water pipe tobacco is not exempt from testing and regulation of contents and emissions.
- Effective measures should be in place to disseminate information to the public about the toxicity and emissions of water pipe tobacco smoke, health warnings.
- Comprehensive education and public awareness programmes on the dangers of water pipe smoking should be implemented.

Governments, ministries of health, and communities are urged to take decisive and effective measures to address the harmful and addictive nature of water pipe smoking. Strong actions are necessary to protect the public from both direct water pipe smoking and exposure to second-hand water pipe smoke. This call emphasises the importance of implementing comprehensive strategies and regulations to combat the health risks associated with water pipe tobacco products (Control and Prevention of Waterpipe Tobacco Products, 2014).

CONCLUSION

Numerous strategies and policies, both at national and global levels, have been established to address the harms caused by drug and alcohol use. Some countries have adopted new drug and harm reduction policies in addition to enforcement and legal sanctions. A few jurisdictions have moved towards decriminalisation of cannabis and legalised medical marijuana. The United Nations Office on Drugs and Crime (UNODC, 2015) recognises that treatment and rehabilitation of illicit drug users are more effective than punishment. However, the direction of drug reform remains a contentious issue. There are several questions that need reflection and discussion regarding the legalisation of non-medical use of psychoactive substances. This includes considerations about public health, social impacts, regulatory frameworks, and harm reduction strategies, amidst diverse cultural and legal contexts. Ghodse (2008) lists some of the questions to demonstrate the complexities implicit in the proposals for legalisation. For example:

- Which drugs should be legalised?
- What potency levels would be permitted?
- How to deal with the adverse consequences?
- Would there be age limits for the use of legalised drugs?
- Where would the drugs be sold?

The drug policy debate, especially regarding cannabis reform, is complex and involves both factual and value-based considerations. Steiner (2024) highlights the clash between societal values and non-sanctioned drug use, reflecting a strong negative stance from the dominant social order. Drug policy discussions are complicated by insufficient knowledge about new psychoactive substances. Regarding cannabis reform, Hill (2014) emphasises the importance of distinguishing between medical and recreational use. Clear separation highlights the need for cannabis to be administered under controlled conditions for medical purposes, conveying the message that like any therapeutic drug, cannabis can have adverse effects if misused. This distinction is crucial in educating the public about responsible cannabis consumption. Implementing a global alcohol strategy faces significant challenges, particularly in countering the influence of the global alcohol industry on public health policies. Monteiro (2011) highlights the globalisation of the alcohol industry, which has concentrated power among a few major producers, notably beer producers. These industry giants wield considerable influence over national policies, prioritising commercial interests that often conflict with public health objectives.

Addressing these challenges requires strong political engagement at both national and international levels, along with a united response from the global health community. Effective health promotion efforts necessitate advocacy for evidence-based policies and the countering of strategies employed by the alcohol and tobacco lobby. This collaborative approach is vital for promoting public health and mitigating the adverse effects associated with alcohol consumption.

KEY POINTS

- United Nations entities overseeing the international drug control system include the Commission on Narcotic Drugs, the United Nations Office on Drugs and Crime (UNODC), and the International Narcotic Control Board (INCB).
- Despite persistent political attention and considerable investment, alcohol and drug dependence are evolving into chronic health conditions.
- Long-term strategies for reducing drug supply and eliminating illicit drug cultivation emphasise alternative and sustainable development alongside balanced drug control policies.
- The prevailing global drug approach revolves around three major international drug control treaties, primarily focusing on prohibition.
- Decriminalisation entails treating possession and consumption of illicit drugs as civil, not criminal, offenses.
- Legalisation involves removing all drug-related offenses from criminal law, including use, possession, cultivation, production, and trading.
- Drug prohibition is deemed more harmful to society than beneficial, indicating the failure of the "war on drugs" policy.
- Opposition against legalising or decriminalising certain psychoactive substances argues that it could diminish the social stigma associated with illicit drug use.
- Proponents of drug policy reform view substance use as a public health issue.
- Several countries have implemented alternative drug policies by legalising or decriminalising cannabis.
- *Medical marijuana* refers to using the entire unprocessed marijuana plant or its basic extracts to treat diseases or symptoms.
- Concerns exist regarding therapeutic and herbal cannabis–based preparations due to the largely unregulated market and potential for misuse.
- Utilising medical marijuana as a therapeutic intervention poses implications for healthcare professionals in medicine, psychiatry, and pharmacology.
- One of WHO's objectives is to minimise the health, psychological, and social burden from harmful alcohol consumption.
- Establishing a national alcohol council ensures a coherent approach to alcohol policies.
- WHO has identified six evidence-based tobacco control measures, known as "MPOWER," to reduce tobacco use effectively.
- The tobacco industry remains a significant obstacle to reducing tobacco smoking prevalence.
- With the rising use of e-cigarettes, numerous countries have enacted legal provisions to regulate them.
- Water tobacco smoking, or *shisha* smoking, falls under the WHO International Framework Convention on Tobacco Control.
- Implementing comprehensive education and public awareness programmes on water pipe smoking dangers is crucial.
- Various strategies and policies at national and global levels have been established to address the harms of drug and alcohol use.
- Effective health promotion efforts require strong political activity at both national and international levels, along with a unified response from the global health community, to counteract the influence of the alcohol lobby.

References

Abrams, D. I. (2018). The therapeutic effects of cannabis and cannabinoids: An update from the national academies of sciences, engineering and medicine report. *European Journal of Internal Medicine*, 49, 7–11. https://doi.org/10.1016/j.ejim.2018.01.003.

Alcohol and Drug Foundation. (2023). *Decriminalisation in Australia*. https://adf.org.au/insights/decriminalisation-australia/ (accessed 1 February 2024).

Anderson, P., Chisholm, D., & Fuhr, D. C. (2009). Effectiveness and cost-effectiveness of policies and programmes to reduce the harm caused by alcohol. *Lancet*, 373(9682), 2234–2246. https://doi.org/10.1016/S0140-6736(09)60744-3.

Arbour, L. (2016). Cited in Godfrey, W. (2016). Global commission slams UNGASS 2016 outcome that strains the credibility of international law. *The Influence*. http://theinfluence.org/global-commission-slams-an-ungass-2016-outcome-that-strains-the-credibility-of-international-law/ (accessed 1 February 2024).

Asbridge, M., Hayden, J. A., & Cartwright, J. L. (2012). Acute cannabis consumption and motor vehicle collision risk: Systematic review of observational studies and meta-analysis. *BMJ,* 344, e536. http://dx.doi.org/10.1136/bmj.e536.

Babor, T. F., Caulkins, J. P., Edwards, G., Fischer, B., Foxcroft, D., Humphreys, K., & Medina-Mora, M. E. (2018). *Drug Policy and the Public Good* (2nd ed.). Oxford: Oxford University Press. https://doi.org/10.1093/oso/9780198818014.001.0001.

Bachhuber, M. A., Saloner, B., & Barry, C. L. (2015). What ecologic analyses cannot tell us about medical marijuana legalization and opioid pain medication mortality – reply. *JAMA Internal Medicine,* 175(4), 656–657. https://doi.org/10.1001/jamainternmed.2014.8027.

Bernard, C. L., Rao, I. J., Robison, K. K., & Brandeau, M. L. (2020). Health outcomes and cost-effectiveness of diversion programs for low-level drug offenders: A model-based analysis. *PLoS Medicine,* 17(10), e1003239. https://doi.org/10.1371/journal.pmed.1003239.

Blake, D. R., Robson, P., Ho, M., Jubb, R. W., & McCabe, C. S. (2006). Preliminary assessment of the efficacy, tolerability and safety of a cannabis-based medicine (Sativex) in the treatment of pain caused by rheumatoid arthritis. *Rheumatology,* 45(1), 50–52. https://doi.org/10.1093/rheumatology/kei183.

Blickman, T., & Jelsma, M. (2009). *Drug Policy Reform in Practice: Experiences with Alternatives in Europe and the US.* Transnational Institute, July. http://www.mamacoca.org/docs_de_base/Consumo/Tom%20Blickman%20Martin%20JelsmaDrug%20Policy%20Reform%20In%20Practice.pdf (accessed 31 January 2024).

Brown, D. J. (2007). Psychedelic healing? *Scientific American,* 18(6), 60–65.

Control and Prevention of Waterpipe Tobacco Products. (2014). *(Decision FCTC/COP6(10)). Conference of the Parties to the WHO Framework Convention on Tobacco Control, Sixth Session, Moscow, Russian Federation.* Geneva: World Health Organization, 13–18 October.

Count the Costs. *50 Years on the War on Drugs.* www.countthecosts.org; https://transformdrugs.org/assets/files/PDFs/count-the-costs-development-and-security.pdf (accessed 30 January 2024).

DISA. (2024). *Marijuana Legality by State,* Updated 1 February 2024. https://disa.com/marijuana-legality-by-state (accessed 1 February 2024).

DrugAbuse.net. (2017). *Laws Around the World.* https://www.drugabuse.net/drug-policy/drug-laws-around-the-world/comment-page-1/ (accessed 31 January 2024).

Drug Free Australia. (2024). *Drug Free Australia's Arguments Against Drug Legalisation.* https://www.drugfree.org.au/images/pdf-files/library/Drug-Free-Australia/Taskforce_Arguments_for_Prohibition.pdf (accessed 31 January 2024).

Drug Science. (2022). *Drug Policy Explained: Legalisation, Decriminalisation, and Prohibition.* https://www.drugscience.org.uk/drug-policy-explained-legalisation-decriminalisation-and-prohibition/ (accessed 31 January 2024).

Earleywine, M. (2002). *Understanding Marijuana.* Oxford: Oxford University Press.

EMCDDA (European Monitoring Centre for Drugs and Drug Addiction). (2001). *Decriminalisation in Europe? Recent Developments in Legal Approaches to Drug Use.* EMCDDA. https://www.emcdda.europa.eu/drugs-library/decriminalisation-europe-recent-developments-legal-approaches-drug-use-eldd-comparative-study_en (accessed 31 January 2024).

EMCDDA (European Monitoring Centre for Drugs and Drug Addiction). (2019). *The Netherlands, Country Drug Report 2019.* Luxembourg: Publications Office of the European Union. https://www.drugpolicyfacts.org/region/netherlands (accessed 31 January 2024).

European Parliament. (2002). *Recommendation on the Reform of the Conventions on Drugs.* https://www.europarl.europa.eu/doceo/document/B-5-2002-0541_EN.html (accessed 30 January 2024).

Galli, J. A., Sawaya, R. A., & Friedenberg, F. K. (2011). Cannabinoid hyperemesis syndrome. *Current Drug Abuse Reviews,* 4(4), 241–249. https://doi.org/10.2174/1874473711104040241.

Ghodse, H. (Ed.). (2008). *International Drug Control in the 21st Century.* Aldershot, Hampshire: Ashgate.

The Global Commission on Drug Policy. (2011). *War on Drugs: A Report on the Global Commission on Drug Policy.* www.globalcommissionondrugs.org/wp-content/themes/gcdp_v1/pdf/Global_Commission_Report_English.pdf (accessed 30 January 2024).

The Global Commission on Drug Policy. (2021). *Time to End Prohibition.* https://www.globalcommissionondrugs.org/wp-content/uploads/2021/12/Time_to_end_prohibition_EN_2021_report.pdf (accessed 1 February 2024).

Golub, A., & Johnson, B. D. (2001). Variation in youthful risks of progression from alcohol and tobacco to marijuana and to hard drugs across generations. *American Journal of Public Health,* 91(2), 225–232. https://doi.org/10.2105/ajph.91.2.225.

Grayling, A. C. (2016). Morality and non-medical drug use. *BMJ,* 355, i5850. http://dx.doi.org/10.1136/bmj.i5850 (accessed 31 January 2024).

Greenwald, G. (2009). *Drug Decriminalization in Portugal: Lessons for Creating Fair and Successful Drug Policies.* Washington, DC: Cato Institute.

Haase, H. J., Eyle, N. E., & Schrimpf, J. R. (2012). *US Drug Reform? Committee on Drugs and the Law.* https://www2.nycbar.org/pdf/InternationalDrugControlTreatiesArticle.pdf (accessed 30 January 2024).

Hall, W., & Degenhardt, L. (2009). Adverse health effects of non-medical cannabis use. *Lancet,* 374(9698), 1383–1391.

Hasan, K. M. (2023). Cannabis unveiled: An exploration of marijuana's history, active compounds, effects, benefits, and risks on human health. *Substance Abuse: Research and Treatment,* 17. https://doi.org/10.1177/11782218231182553.

Health, D. B. (1996). The war on drugs as a metaphor in American culture. In W. Bickel & R. DeGrandpre (Eds.), *Drug Policy and Human Nature Drug Policy and Human Nature: Psychological Perspectives on the Prevention, Management, and Treatment of Illicit Drug Abuse.* New York: Plenum, pp. 279–299.

Hill, K. P. (2014). Medical marijuana: More questions than answers. *Journal of Psychiatric Practice,* 20(5), 389–391. https://doi.org/10.1097/01.pra.0000454786.97976.96.

Hughes, C. (2014). *Drugs and the Law: What You Need to Know.* Sydney: National Drug and Alcohol Research Centre.

Hughes, C., Stevens, A., Hulme, S., & Cassidy, R. (2019). *Models for the Decriminalisation, Depenalisation and Diversion of*

Illicit Drug Possession: An International Realist Review. A paper for the 2019 International Society for the Study of Drug Policy Conference. https://harmreductioneurasia.org/wp-content/uploads/2019/07/Hughes-et-al-ISSDP-2019-Models-for-the-decriminalisation-depenalisation-and-diversion-of-illicit-drug-possession-FINAL.pdf.

INCB. (1992). Legalisation of internationally controlled drugs. Cited in H. Ghodse (Ed.). (2008). *International Drug Control in the 21st Century.* Aldershot, Hampshire: Ashgate, pp. 3, 27–40.

Institute for Global Tobacco Control. (2016). *Country Laws Regulating E-cigarettes: A Policy Scan.* Baltimore, MD: Johns Hopkins Bloomberg School of Public Health. http://globaltobaccocontrol.org/e-cigarette/country-laws-regulating-e-cigarettes (accessed 24 June 2024).

Institute of Alcohol Studies. (2013). *Draft Global Strategy to Reduce Harmful Use of Alcohol Summary of the Report.* London: The Institute of Alcohol Studies.

International Drug Policy Consortium. (2016). *The 2016 Commission on Narcotics Drugs and Its Special Segment on Preparations for the UNGASS on the World Drug Problem.* Report of Proceedings. https://dl.dropboxusercontent.com/u/566349360/library/CND-proceedings-document-2016_ENGLISH.pdf (accessed 24 June 2024).

Jha, P., & Alleyne, S. G. (2015). Effective global tobacco control in the next decade. *CMAJ: Canadian Medical Association Journal = Journal de l'Association Medicale Canadienne,* 187(8), 551–552. https://doi.org/10.1503/cmaj.150261.

Johnson, J. R., Burnell-Nugent, M., Lossignol, D., Ganae-Motan, E. D., Potts, R., & Fallon, M. T. (2010). Multicenter, double-blind, randomized, placebo-controlled, parallel-group study of the efficacy, safety, and tolerability of THC:CBD extract and THC extract in patients with intractable cancer-related pain. *Journal of Pain and Symptom Management,* 39(2), 167–179.

Johnson, K., Pinchuk, I., Melgar, M. I. E., Agwogie, M. O., & Salazar Silva, F. (2022). The global movement towards a public health approach to substance use disorders. *Annals of Medicine,* 54(1), 1797–1808. https://doi.org/10.1080/07853890.2022.2079150.

Joy, J. E., Watson, S. J., & Benson, J. A. (Eds.). (1999). *Marijuana and Medicine: Assessing the Science Base.* Washington, DC: The National Academies Press. https://doi.org/10.17226/6376.

Kennedy, R. D., Awopegba, A., De León, E., & Cohen, J. E. (2017). Global approaches to regulating electronic cigarettes. *Tobacco Control,* 26(4), 440–445. https://doi.org/10.1136/tobaccocontrol-2016-053179.

Kerlikowske, R. G. (2010). *Why Marijuana Legalization Would Compromise Public Health and Public Safety.* Presentation delivered at the California Police Chiefs Association Conference, San Jose, CA, 4 March. https://wfad.se/latest-news/articles/why-marijuana-legalization-would-compromise-public-health-and-public-safety/ (accessed 31 January 2024).

Lynskey, M. (2003). Escalation of drug use in early-onset cannabis users vs co-twin controls. *JAMA,* 289(4), 427–433.

MacCoun, R. J., & Reuter, P. (1997). Interpreting Dutch cannabis policy: Reasoning by analogy in the legalization debate. *Science,* 278(5335), 47–52.

MacCoun, R. J., & Reuter, P. (2001). Evaluating alternative cannabis regimes. *The British Journal of Psychiatry,* 178(2), 123–128. https://doi.org/10.1192/bjp.178.2.123.

Markowitz, S. (2000). *An Economic Analysis of Alcohol, Drugs and Violent Crime in the National Crime Victimization Survey* (Working Paper 7982). National Bureau of Economic Research. www.nber.org/papers/w7982.

McCambridge, J., Kypri, K., Drummond, C., & Strang, J (2014). Alcohol harm reduction: Corporate capture of a key concept. *PLOS Medicine,* 11(12), e1001767. http://doi.org/10.1371/journal.pmed.1001767.

Meier, M. H., Caspi, A., Ambler, A., Harrington, H., Houts, R. Keefe, R. S., McDonald, K., Ward, A., Poulton, R., & Moffitt T. E. (2012). Persistent cannabis users show neuropsychological decline from childhood to midlife. *Proceedings of the National Academy of Sciences of the United States of America,* 109(40), E2657–E2664. https://doi.org/10.1073/pnas.1206820109.

Meier, M. H., Caspi, A., Cerdá, M., Hancox, R. J., Harrington H., Houts, R., Poulton, R., Ramrakha, S., Thomson, W. M. & Moffitt, T. E. (2016). Associations between cannabis use and physical health problems in early midlife: A longitudinal comparison of persistent cannabis vs tobacco users. *JAMA Psychiatry,* 73(97), 731–740. https://doi.org/10.1001/jamapsychiatry.2016.0637.

Ministry of Health and Social Affairs Sweden. (2008). *The Swedish Action Plan on Narcotic Drugs 2006–2010.* www.politicheantidroga.gov.it/media/327726/swedish.pdf (accessed 11 December 2016).

Miron, J. A., & Zwiebel, J. (1995). The economic case against drug prohibition. *The Journal of American Perspectives,* 9(4) 175–192.

Monteiro, M. G. (2011). The road to a World Health Organization global strategy for reducing the harmful use of alcohol *Alcohol Research and Health,* 3(2), 257–260.

Morral, A. R., McCaffrey, D. F., & Paddock, S. M. (2002). *Using Marijuana May Not Raise the Risk of Using Harder Drugs* Santa Monica, CA: RAND Corporation. https://www.rand.org/content/dam/rand/pubs/research_briefs/2005/RB6010.pdf (accessed 31 January 2024).

NIDA. (2018). *Marijuana as Medicine.* National Institute on Drug Abuse. https://nida.nih.gov/sites/default/files/df-marijuana-medicine.pdf/ (accessed 1 February 2024).

NIDA. (2021). *What Are Marijuana's Effects on Other Aspects of Physical Health?* https://nida.nih.gov/publications/research-reports/marijuana/what-are-marijuanas-effects-on-other-aspects-of-physical-health (accessed 1 February 2024)

Nkard, B. L. (2021). *The History and Use of Marijuana in the Society.* https://dualdiagnosis.org/marijana-treatment/reefer-madness-look-evolution-marijuana-society/ (accessed February 2024).

Nurmikko, T. J., Serpell, M. G., Hoggart, B., Toomey, P. J., Morloin B. J., & Haines, D. (2007). Satvex successfully treats neuropathic pain characterised by allodynia: A randomised, double-blind placebo-controlled clinical trial. *Pain,* 1(2), 10–220.

Nutt, D., King, L. A., Saulsbury, W., & Blakemore, C. (2007) Development of a rational scale to assess the harm of drugs of potential misuse. *The Lancet,* 369(9566), 1047–1053.

Peer, N., & Kengne, A.-P. (2018). Tobacco cessation in low- and middle-income countries: Some challenges and opportunities *Addiction,* 13(8), 1390–1391. https://doi.org/10.1111/add.14214.

Pekkanen, S. (1992). Experts tell FDA some hallucinogens may aid alcoholics, terminally ill and psychiatric patients

Newsletter of the Multidisciplinary Association for Psychedelic Studies, 3, 3.

Ramstedt, M., Leifman, H., Müller, D., Sundin, E., & Norström, T. (2013). Reducing youth violence related to student parties: Findings from a community intervention project in Stockholm. *Drug and Alcohol Review,* 32(6), 561–565. https://doi.org/10.1111/dar.12069.

Rog, D. J. (2010). Cannabis-based medicines in multiple sclerosis – a review of clinical studies. *Immunobiology,* 215(8), 658–672. https://doi.org/10.1016/j.imbio.2010.03.009.

Rog, D. J., Nurmikko, T. J., Friede, T., & Young, C. A. (2005). Randomized, controlled trial of cannabis-based medicine in central pain in multiple sclerosis. *Neurology, 65*(6), 812–819. https://doi.org/10.1212/01.wnl.0000176753.45410.8b.

Rolles, S. (2010). An alternative to the war on drugs. *BMJ,* 41, c3360. http://dx.doi.org/10.1136/bmj.c3360.

Rombouts, S. A., Conigrave, J. H., Saitz, R., Haber, P., & Morley, K. C. (2020). Evidence based models of care for the treatment of alcohol use disorder in primary health care settings: A systematic review. *BMC Family Practice,* 21, 260. https://doi.org/10.1186/s12875-020-01288-6.

Scheim, A. I., Maghsoudi, N., Marshall, Z., Churchill, S., Ziegler, C., & Werb, D. (2020). Impact evaluations of drug decriminalisation and legal regulation on drug use, health and social harms: A systematic review. *BMJ Open,* 10(9), e035148. https://doi.org/10.1136/bmjopen-2019-035148.

Single, E., Christie, P., & Ali, R. (2000). The impact of cannabis decriminalisation in Australia and the United States. *Journal of Public Health Policy,* 21(2), 157–186.

Smith, M. J., Cobia, D. J., Wang, L., Alpert, K. I., Cronenwett, W. J., Goldman, M. B., Mamah, D., Barch, D. M., Breiter, H. C., & Csernansky, J. G. (2014). Cannabis-related working memory deficits and associated subcortical morphological differences in healthy individuals and schizophrenia subjects. *Schizophrenia Bulletin,* 40(2), 287–299. https://doi.org/10.1093/schbul/sbt176.

Steiner, W. G. (2024). *Social and Ethical Issues of Drug Abuse.* https://www.britannica.com/topic/drug-use/Social-and-ethical-issuesof-drug-abuse (accessed 24 June 2024).

Trolldal, B., Brännström, L., Paschall, M. J., & Leifman, H. (2013). Effects of a multi-component responsible beverage service programme on violent assaults in Sweden. *Addiction,* 108(1), 89–96. https://doi.org/10.1111/j.1360-0443.2012.04004.x.

United Nations. (2016). *General Assembly. Resolution Adopted by the General Assembly on 19 April 2016. S-30/1. Our Joint Commitment to Effectively Addressing and Countering the World Drug Problem. Thirtieth Special Session. Agenda Item8.* A/RES/S-30/1. https://www.unodc.org/documents/postungass2016/outcome/V1603301-E.pdf (accessed 1 February 2024).

Unlu, A., Tammi, T. T., & Hakkarainen, P. (2020). *Drug Decriminalization Policy: Literature Review: Models, Implementation and Outcomes.* Finnish Institute for Health and Welfare. https://www.julkari.fi/bitstream/handle/10024/140116/URN_ISBN_978-952-343-504-9.pdf?sequence=1&isAllowed=y (accessed 1 February 2024).

UNDOC. (2008). *World Drug Report 2008.* United Nations Office on Drugs and Crime. www.unodc.org/documents/wdr/WDR_2008/WDR_2008_eng_web.pdf (accessed 31 January 2024).

UNDOC. (2015). *World Drug Report 2015.* Vienna: United Nations Office on Drugs and Crime (UNDOC), United Nations Publication.

UNDOC. (2016). *World Drug Report 2016.* Vienna: United Nations Office on Drugs and Crime (UNDOC), United Nations Publication.

UNODC. (1961). *Single Convention on Narcotic Drugs, 1961.* United Nations Office on Drugs and Crime. www.unodc.org/unodc/en/treaties/single-convention.html (accessed 31 January 2024).

UNODC. (2007). *Sweden's Successful Drug Policy: A Review of the Evidence.* Vienna: United Nations Office on Drugs and Crime (UNDOC).

UNODC. (2022). *World Drug Report 2022.* Vienna: The United Nations Office on Drugs and Crime, United Nations Publication.

U.S. Department of Justice Drug Enforcement Administration. (2003). *Speaking Out Against Drug Legalization.* U.S. Department of Justice. https://web.archive.org/web/20060627082607/www.usdoj.gov/dea/demand/speakout/speaking_out-may03.pdf (accessed 31 January 2024).

Van Ours, J. C. (2003). Is cannabis a stepping stone for cocaine? *Journal of Health Economics,* 22(4), 539–554.

Weatherburn, D., & Craig Jones, C. (2001). *Does Prohibition Deter Cannabis Use? Contemporary Issues in Crime and Justice* (No. 58). Sydney: NSW Bureau of Crime Statistics and Research. www.bocsar.nsw.gov.au/Documents/CJB/cjb58.pdf.

WHO. (2002). *The World Health Report 2002 -Reducing Risks, Promoting Healthy Life.* Geneva: World Health Organization.

WHO. (2003). *World Health Organization Framework Convention on Tobacco Control* (WHO FCTC). Geneva: World Health Organization.

WHO. (2010). *Global Strategy to Reduce the Harmful Use of Alcohol.* Geneva: World Health Organization.

WHO. (2015). *Report on the Global Tobacco Epidemic 2015: Raising Taxes on Tobacco.* Geneva: World Health Organization.

WHO. (2016). *The Health and Social Effects of Nonmedical Cannabis Use.* https://www.who.int/publications/i/item/9789241510240 (accessed 1 January 2024).

WHO. (2021). *Global Strategy to Reduce the Harmful Use of Alcohol First Draft.* World Health Organization. https://cdn.who.int/media/docs/default-source/alcohol/action-plan-on-alcohol_first-draft-final_formatted.pdf?sfvrsn=b690edb0_1&download=true (accessed 1 February 2024).

WHO. (2023). *Global Strategy to Accelerate Tobacco Control: Advancing Sustainable Development Through the Implementation of the WHO FCTC 2019–2025.* https://fctc.who.int/who-fctc/overview/global-strategy-2025 (accessed 2 February 2024).

Wilson, J. Q. (1990). Against the legalization of drugs. *Journal Narc Officer,* 6(5), 13, 18–22.

Wood, E., Werb, D., Kazatchkine, M., Kerr, T., Hankins, C., Gorna, R., Nutt, D., Des Jarlais, D., Barré-Sinoussi, F., & Montaner, J. (2010). Vienna declaration: A call for evidence-based drug policies. *Lancet,* 376(9738), 310–312. https://doi.org/10.1016/S0140-6736(10)60958-0.

Part 2

Psychoactive substances

Chapter 7

Alcohol

Learning outcomes

- Describe the pattern and extent of alcohol use.
- Discuss the harms caused by alcohol misuse.
- Describe briefly the metabolism of alcohol.
- Describe the effects of alcohol on the human body and how these changes affect behaviours.
- Describe the health problems that are associated with excessive alcohol use.
- Explain what is meant by binge drinking.
- Recognize the effects of binge drinking on drinkers.
- Describe the dangers of alcohol/drug interactions.
- Determine what medications interact harmfully with alcohol.
- Discuss why women's low-risk limits are different from men's.
- State what *sensible drinking* means.
- Calculate the strengths of a range of alcoholic drinks.

Activity 7.1

Provide a true-or-false answer for each of the statements listed, and provide some reasons you choose your particular answer.

Statements	True	False
Alcohol functions as a central nervous system depressant.		
Alcoholism ranks among the four most severe public health issues.		
Providing an alcoholic drink to a child under 5 years of age is illegal.		
Cannabis poses more significant problems among young people globally.		
Men and women metabolise alcohol at different rates.		
Carbonated drinks accelerate alcohol absorption.		
Alcohol elimination rates vary among individuals.		
Food in the stomach slows down alcohol's effects.		
Different alcoholic drinks contain distinct types of alcohol.		
Combining alcohol with drugs can be dangerous.		
Drinking water with alcohol does not prevent hangovers.		

DOI: 10.4324/9781003456674-

Black coffee does not aid in sobering up after excessive drinking.		
Alcohol initially affects moral judgement before physical coordination.		
Alcohol can disrupt sleep patterns and increase stress levels.		
Excessive alcohol intake impacts respiration and heart rate.		
More alcohol is not necessarily better for heart health.		
An average mixed drink contains about twice as much alcohol as a pint of beer.		
A pint of beer does not have the same alcohol content as a double whisky.		
Alcopops have the same alcohol content as beer.		
Alcohol consumption correlates with increased likelihood of casual sex, leading to unwanted pregnancies and sexually transmitted diseases.		
Pregnant women risk harming their baby even with moderate alcohol consumption.		
The legal breath/alcohol limit for driving in the UK is 35 micrograms per 100 millilitres of breath.		

Activity 7.2

Please choose one correct answer to the following multiple-choice questions.

1. What term describes the typical pattern of alcohol use in a given population?
   a. Binge drinking
   b. Alcohol dependence
   c. Alcohol misuse
   d. Alcohol consumption
   e. None of the above
2. Which of the following is a harm caused by alcohol misuse?
   a. Increased alertness
   b. Improved memory
   c. Liver damage
   d. Reduced heart rate
   e. None of the above
3. What is the primary organ responsible for metabolising alcohol in the human body?
   a. Liver
   b. Kidney
   c. Stomach
   d. Pancreas
   e. None of the above
4. How does alcohol consumption affect behaviour?
   a. Increases aggression
   b. Improves decision-making
   c. Reduces anxiety

d. Enhances coordination
e. None of the above

5. Which of the following health problems is associated with excessive alcohol use?
   a. Reduced risk of cardiovascular disease
   b. Improved cognitive function
   c. Lower blood pressure
   d. Liver cirrhosis
   e. None of the above
6. What is *binge drinking*?
   a. Drinking alcohol in moderation
   b. Drinking large amounts of alcohol in a short period
   c. Drinking only on weekends
   d. Drinking alcohol with meals
   e. None of the above
7. How does binge drinking affect drinkers?
   a. Increases risk of alcohol dependence
   b. Reduces the risk of accidents
   c. Improves overall health
   d. Decreases cognitive impairment
   e. None of the above
8. What is a danger of alcohol–drug interactions?
   a. Decreased risk of side effects
   b. Increased effectiveness of medications
   c. Risk of overdose or adverse reactions
   d. Improved treatment outcomes
   e. None of the above
9. Which medications can interact harmfully with alcohol?
   a. Antibiotics
   b. Painkillers
   c. Antidepressants
   d. All of the above
   e. None of the above
10. Why are women's low-risk limits for alcohol consumption different from men's?
    a. Women have higher tolerance to alcohol.
    b. Women metabolise alcohol faster.
    c. Women have a smaller volume of blood.
    d. Women are less prone to alcohol-related harms.
    e. None of the above is correct.
11. What does *sensible drinking* mean?
    a. Drinking alcohol excessively
    b. Drinking alcohol irresponsibly
    c. Drinking alcohol in moderation
    d. Drinking alcohol alone
    e. None of the above
12. Which of the following is a measure of the strength of alcoholic drinks?
    a. Volume
    b. Colour

c. Aroma
d. Alcohol by volume (ABV)
e. None of the above

13. What effect does alcohol have on coordination and balance?
 a. Improves coordination
 b. Has no effect on balance
 c. Impairs coordination and balance
 d. Enhances cognitive function
 e. None of the above
14. How does alcohol affect sleep patterns?
 a. Improves sleep quality
 b. Increases sleep duration
 c. Disrupts sleep patterns
 d. Induces deep sleep
 e. None of the above
15. What is the legal blood alcohol concentration (BAC) limit for driving in most countries?
 a. 0.08%
 b. 0.02%
 c. 0.1%
 d. 0.05%
 e. None of the above
16. Which enzyme is primarily responsible for breaking down alcohol in the liver?
 a. Alcohol oxidase
 b. Alcohol dehydrogenase
 c. Alcohol hydroxylase
 d. Alcohol esterase
 e. Alcohol androgens
17. What is defined as a pattern of alcohol use that involves problems controlling drinking, being preoccupied with alcohol, continuing to use alcohol even when it causes problems, having to drink more to get the same effect (tolerance), or experiencing withdrawal symptoms when one stops drinking?
 a. Social drinking
 b. Moderate drinking
 c. Alcohol use
 d. Alcohol use disorder
 e. Controlled drinking

INTRODUCTION

Alcohol is deeply ingrained in the social and cultural fabric of Judeo-Christian societies and stands as the most widely used psychoactive drug globally. It is actively promoted across various cultural, social, and religious contexts and supports national economies through taxation. However, alcohol is often not recognised as a psychoactive substance with addictive potential, despite its severe consequences by laypeople. Public health issues linked to alcohol consumption have reached alarming levels, making it one of the most significant health risks worldwide. Alcohol consumption patterns vary globally, with Europe showing high consumption rates while Africa bears a heavy burden of alcohol-related disease and injury (WHO, 2018). Heavy episodic drinking (HED) is prevalent in Eastern Europe and some sub-Saharan African countries, with rates exceeding 60% among current drinkers. Among

15- to 19-year-olds, current drinking rates are highest in the WHO European Region, followed by the Region of the Americas and the Western Pacific (WHO, 2018). Alcohol is often consumed alongside or before/after other psychoactive substances, and its comorbidity with tobacco dependence is well-documented.

The harmful use of alcohol contributes to over 200 disease and injury conditions globally, resulting in approximately 3 million deaths each year, which accounts for 5.3% of all deaths worldwide. Alcohol consumption also contributes to 5.1% of the global burden of disease and injury, as measured in disability-adjusted life years (DALYs) (WHO, 2022). In addition to health impacts, alcohol misuse leads to significant social and economic losses for individuals and society. It causes premature death and disability, and approximately 13.5% of total deaths among people aged 20–39 are attributed to alcohol. There is a clear causal relationship between alcohol misuse and incidence or outcomes of infectious diseases, such as tuberculosis and HIV. Alcohol consumption by an expectant mother may cause foetal alcohol syndrome (FAS) and preterm birth complications (WHO, 2022). In addition, alcohol use is estimated to be responsible for approximately 20 to 30% of global cases of oesophageal cancer, liver cancer, liver cirrhosis, homicide, epileptic seizures, motor vehicle accidents, alcohol-related injuries, crime, violence, teenage pregnancy, decreased workplace productivity, and homelessness. Alcohol use disorder (AUD) prevalence varies across regions and populations globally due to a complex interplay of cultural, social, economic, and environmental factors. The alcohol global strategy (WHO, 2010) aims to improve health and social outcomes for individuals, families, and communities by significantly reducing morbidity and mortality resulting from the harmful use of alcohol and its associated social consequences. It seeks to foster local, regional, and global efforts to prevent and mitigate the harmful effects of alcohol consumption. The strategy emphasises the importance of tailoring interventions to national circumstances to effectively address alcohol-related issues worldwide.

TYPES OF ALCOHOLIC BEVERAGES

Alcohol beverages encompass a diverse range of types, including spirits like gin, vodka, rum, and whisky, which are distilled drinks. The most popul types of alcohol beverage are beer, cider, wine, an spirits. Beer includes a number of different alcoholi beverages, including lager beers, ales, wheat beer and fruit beers. *Spirits* are distilled alcoholic drink and include gin (juniper berries), vodka (distillatio of grains or potatoes), rum (sugar cane), whisky (fer mented grain), tequila (blue agave plant), absinth (number of different flowers), Ouzo (Greek drink plant anise), Poitín (Irish drink – potatoes/raisins) and brandy (distilling wine). Liqueurs are flavoure spirits infused with various ingredients, includin certain woods, herbs, nuts, fruits, spices, cream, o flowers, into either water or alcohol and sweetene with sugar. Wine also has different types, dependin on the kind of grapes. These include red wine (re or black grapes), rose wine (red grapes), white win (white grapes), champagne (sparkling wine), an fortified wines (including sherry and port). Cider i made from fermented apple juice.

PATTERN OF ALCOHOL USE

Various individual and societal factors influence the levels and patterns of alcohol consumption among young adults. In Western civilisation, alcohol drinking is culturally ingrained and often perceived as acceptable and even encouraged. For young adults alcohol is integrated into leisure activities, and they tend to mimic older adult behaviours as part of their developmental phase, further perpetuating drinking norms. These patterns of also use will be determined by a number of factors related to the individual, the type of drink, and their environment. Demographic factors like age and proximity to alcohol outlets, along with social factors such as family background, socio-economic status, and religious influence, collectively shape alcohol consumption patterns within communities and among individuals (Khamis et al., 2022). There are different levels of alcohol use that can be categorised as non-user (abstention), experimentation (use for novelty or curiosity), social/recreational use (infrequent use – no established pattern), misuse (continued use despite negative consequences), binge drinking and addiction (compulsion to use, inability to stop use, chaotic use, physical and psychological dependence). Harrington et al. (2014) identified eight distinct profiles of alcohol users, presented in Table 7.1.

Table 7.1
Profile of alcohol users

Number of drinks	Times per week	Characteristics
3–4	2–3 times per week (weekend)	Unmarried women. Highest rate of personality disorder. Social drinking. No alcohol-related problems. Less likely to seek treatment.
3–4	2 times per week (weekends)	Youngest group of alcohol users. Moderate weekly cyclical pattern of alcohol use. Social drinking. Intense drinking.
4–5	1–2 times per week (weekends)	No distinct daily or cyclical pattern of alcohol use. Risk of problem drinking.
4–5	1–2 times per week (anytime)	Women. Moderate to strong daily pattern of use. Pre-contemplation stage of readiness to change alcohol use.*
5–6	3–4 times per week (weekends)	Moderate to strong daily pattern. High rate of lifetime alcohol dependence. Highest frequency of attendance to alcohol treatment services. Action stage of readiness to change alcohol use.*
6–7	4 times per week (throughout)	Lifelong dependence on alcohol. Alcohol-related problems. Contemplation stage of readiness to change alcohol use.*
7	4 times per week (anytime)	Unmarried men. Mostly older White men. Lifetime alcohol dependence. Contemplation stage of readiness to change alcohol use.*
9–10	3–4 times per week (on/off)	Most problematic drinkers. Greatest alcohol dependence. Highest rate of alcohol-related problems. High frequency of attendance to treatment services. Action or contemplation stage.*

*Prochaska, J., & DiClemente, C. (1983). Stages and processes of self-change of smoking: Toward an integrative model of change. *Journal of Consulting and Clinical Psychology*, 51(3), 390–395.

Source: Adapted from Harrington et al. (2014).

According to Harrington et al. (2014), the findings of the study showed that individuals with very similar quantities of alcohol consumption can have different patterns of drinking behaviour. This indicates that a one-size-fits-all approach to intervention strategies in clinical settings may be ineffective. Tailoring services to the specific needs of alcohol users is crucial.

The price of alcohol made both a quantitative and a qualitative difference to the way young adults drank. Heavy drinkers are much less responsive to price in terms of quantity, but they are more inclined to adapt their choices by substituting with cheaper alcohol options when the price of alcohol increases (Pryce et al., 2019).

BINGE DRINKING

Binge drinking is a normal mode of consumption among 18- to 24-year-old men and women.

Binge drinking is defined as consuming five or more drinks on an occasion for men or four or more drinks on an occasion for women (CDCP, 2022). In the UK, *binge drinking* refers to the consumption of a large amount of alcohol in a short period with the intention of getting drunk. For men, binge drinking typically involves consuming more than eight units of alcohol in a single session, while for women, it involves consuming more than six units (National Health Service, 2014). In the United States, binge drinking is most common among younger adults aged 18–34, with higher prevalence among men than women. The prevalence is among individuals with higher household incomes, non-Hispanic White ethnicity, and those residing in the Midwest (Bohm et al., 2021). Europe has earned a reputation as the global hub of heavy alcohol consumption (binge drinking), with the highest rates of alcohol-related deaths occurring within the region. According to the OECD (2023), Romania and the

Table 7.2
Binge drinking and health problems

Problems	Examples
Harm	Blackouts and overdoses (NIAAA, 2024).
Unintentional injuries	Motor vehicle crashes, falls, burns, and alcohol poisoning.
Violence	Homicide, suicide, intimate partner violence, and sexual assault.
Sexually transmitted diseases	HIV. Gonorrhoea was nearly five times higher among women who binge (Hutton et al., 2008).
Pregnancy	Unintended pregnancy and poor pregnancy outcomes, including miscarriage and stillbirth (Naimi et al., 2003).
Foetal alcohol spectrum disorders (FASD)	Intrauterine exposure to alcohol is the most common nonheritable cause of intellectual disability. FAS is a relatively prevalent alcohol-related birth defect (Popova et al., 2018).
Sudden infant death syndrome (SIDS)	Intrauterine alcohol exposure is associated with SIDS (Friend et al., 2004; Iyasu et al., 2002).
Chronic diseases	High blood pressure, stroke, heart disease, and liver disease.
Cancer	Breast (among females), liver, colon, rectum, mouth, pharynx, larynx, and oesophagus (Strebel & Terry, 2021).
Memory and learning problems	Reduced impulse control and decision-making deficits (Townshend et al., 2014).
Risk of emotional and mental health problems	Depression and anxiety.
Physical and psychological dependence	Dependence and alcohol use disorder.

UK stand out as prominent heavy episodic drinkers among developed nations. Denmark leads the list for both men and women in terms of binge drinking, indicating significant alcohol misuse. Conversely, Turkey, Italy, and Greece report the lowest rates of binge drinking within the region.

Binge drinking is commonly associated with a higher risk for serious bodily harm, such as injuries, alcohol poisoning, and acute organ damage. Heavy drinking is considered a risk factor for longer-term conditions, such as liver cirrhosis and cardiovascular disease. It has been identified that engaging in binge drinking can serve as the initial stage leading to the development of a severe and persistent alcohol dependence (Hall & Finch, 2023). A number of health consequences that occur as a result of binge drinking are presented in Table 7.2.

METABOLISM OF ALCOHOL

Ethyl alcohol, also known as ethanol (C2H5OH), is a colourless and flammable liquid with a distinct odour and a burning taste. As a psychoactive substance, alcohol depresses the central nervous system and provides calories. Unlike food, alcohol does not require digestion for absorption. Beverages with higher alcohol concentrations, like whisky or brandy, and carbonated drinks, such as cham pagne, are absorbed more rapidly into the blood stream. Alcohol absorption primarily occurs in th mouth, oesophagus, stomach, and initial part of th small intestine. The rate of absorption varies widel among individuals due to differences in physiolog stomach contents, and situational factors. Onc absorbed, alcohol is carried to the liver, where i undergoes metabolism. The enzyme acetaldehyd dehydrogenase breaks down alcohol into acetalde hyde, which is further converted to acetic acid. O average, the liver can metabolise one drink equiva lent per hour, with acetic acid rapidly converted t carbon dioxide and water. However, alcohol inte feres with the body's nutrient absorption and util isation, contributing to malnutrition and vitami deficiencies in heavy drinkers.

Gender differences significantly impact ho alcohol affects the body. Women can become mor intoxicated than men even with the same alcoh intake, partly due to their different fat distributio and lower water content, resulting in less dilutio and greater alcohol potency. Factors like pre-men strual status, birth control pills, and hormon replacement therapy (oestrogen) influence alcoh absorption rates in women. As women metabolis alcohol less effectively than men, they are mor susceptible to the consequences of drinking. Th has important implications for clinicians in understanding and addressing alcohol consumption levels among women.

EFFECTS OF ALCOHOL

Initially, small amounts of alcohol induce feelings of relaxation, euphoria, and reduced inhibition, accompanied by slight impairments in thinking processes and motor functions. With increased consumption, cognitive, perceptual, and behavioural impairments escalate in proportion to the amount of alcohol ingested. Symptoms may include slurred speech, poor coordination, unsteady gait, pupil movement irregularities (nystagmus), impaired judgement, insomnia, hangover, and blackouts, characterised by memory loss following heavy alcohol consumption. The lethal dose of alcohol varies based on body size and physiology, with death possible from excessive consumption or alcohol withdrawal. Chronic alcohol use can lead to significant memory problems and cognitive decline. In women, menstrual disorders and fertility problems have been associated with harmful drinking. Women seem to be more susceptible to the influence of alcohol just prior to or during their menstrual cycle than any other time during their cycle. However, the existing research on alcohol consumption across the menstrual cycle spanning over 40 years reveals significant limitations. The findings from the reviewed studies are diverse, with most studies either reporting increased premenstrual alcohol consumption or no change in alcohol consumption throughout the cycle (Carroll et al., 2015). Overall, the lack of standardised methodologies undermines the reliability and generalisability of the findings in this area of research. A summary of the problems associated with alcohol intoxication and harmful drinking is presented in Table 7.3.

One of the health consequences associated with alcohol consumption of more than one drink a day during pregnancy is foetal alcohol spectrum disorder (May et al., 2013). *Foetal alcohol spectrum disorder* (FASD) is a comprehensive term encompassing a variety of neurological and behavioural issues that may impact individuals born to mothers who consumed alcohol during pregnancy (Dozet et al., 2023). Foetal alcohol spectrum disorder stands as a significant cause of non-genetic mental handicap in the Western world, and notably, it is entirely preventable. Foetal alcohol syndrome, a subset of FASD, arises from pre-natal alcohol exposure and can lead to permanent brain damage in infants, resulting in neurological impairments affecting executive functions. The impact of the amount, frequency, or timing of alcohol consumption during pregnancy on foetal development remains uncertain. Foetal alcohol syndrome is typified by characteristics such as low birth weight, facial abnormalities, speech impairments, heart and eye disorders, genital deformities, and behavioural challenges. Importantly,

Table 7.3
Problems associated with alcohol intoxication and harmful effects

Alcohol intoxication	
Physical	Accidents. Acute alcohol poisoning. Cardiac arrhythmia. Foetal damage. Failure to take prescribed medications. Gout. Gastritis. Hepatitis, HIV (through sexual behaviour). Impotence. Pancreatitis. Stroke.
Psychological	Anger. Anxiety. Amnesia. Attempted suicide. Depression. Impaired relationships. Insomnia. Suicide.
Social	Absenteeism. Aggression. Assault. Burglary. Child neglect/abuse. Domestic violence. Drinking and driving. Family arguments. Football hooliganism. Homicide. Public drunkenness. Unwanted pregnancy. Unsafe sex.
Harmful drinking	
Physical	Brain damage. Breast cancer. Cirrhosis. Cancer of mouth, larynx, oesophagus. Cardiomyopathy. Diabetes. Fatty liver. Gastritis. Hepatitis. Hypertension. Infertility. Neuropathy. Nutritional deficiencies. Obesity. Pancreatitis. Reactions to other drugs. Sexual dysfunction.
Psychological	Attempted suicide. Amnesia. Anxiety. Depression. Delirium tremens. Dementia. Gambling. Hallucinosis. Misuse of other drugs. Personality changes. Suicide. Withdrawal fits.
Social	Divorce. Family problems. Financial liability. Fraud. Habitual conviction for drunkenness. Homelessness. Poor social behaviour. Unemployment. Vagrancy. Work difficulties.

Source: Adapted from the Royal College of General Practitioners (1986). Alcohol: Our favourite drug. London: Tavistock Publications.

Table 7.4
Foetal alcohol spectrum disorders: signs and symptoms

Physical effects	Behavioural and cognitive effects
• Low body weight	• Hyperactive behaviour
• Poor coordination	• Difficulty with attention
• Sleep and sucking problems as a baby	• Poor memory
• Vision or hearing problems	• Difficulty in school (especially with math)
• Problems with the heart, kidneys, or bones	• Learning disabilities
• Shorter-than-average height	• Speech and language delays
• Small head size	• Intellectual disability or low IQ
• Abnormal facial features, such as a smooth ridge between the nose and upper lip (philtrum)	• Poor reasoning and judgement skills

Source: Adapted from NIAAA (2024).

there is no safe level of alcohol consumption during pregnancy. Table 7.4 presents the signs and symptoms of foetal alcohol spectrum disorders.

WERNICKE'S ENCEPHALOPATHY AND KORSAKOFF'S PSYCHOSIS

Wernicke's encephalopathy is a condition caused by alcohol consumption and thiamine (vitamin B1) deficiency. Thiamine is crucial for normal growth, heart function, and nervous system health. Heavy drinkers often have poor nutrition, leading to vitamin deficiencies aggravated by alcohol-induced stomach inflammation, hindering vitamin absorption. Wernicke's encephalopathy symptoms include unsteady gait (ataxia), jerky eye movements, drowsiness, and confusion, which can be challenging to diagnose due to variable presentation. Untreated, it can lead to brain damage or death, but prompt thiamine treatment can reverse symptoms in a few hours. If Wernicke's encephalopathy is untreated or is not treated soon enough, Korsakoff's psychosis may follow. Korsakoff's psychosis may develop gradually, resulting in severe memory impairment. However, many other abilities may remain intact. Korsakoff's differs from most dementias, in which there is often damage to a large area of the cortex (the outer part of the brain). The major symptoms of Korsakoff's syndrome are:

- Anterograde and retrograde amnesia, or severe memory loss
- Confabulation (invented events to fill gaps in memory)
- Apathy
- In some cases, talkative and repetitive behaviou in others

Other problems associated with heavy alcohol con sumption include peripheral neuropathies (lack o sensation or pain in the limbs), "alcohol dementia, and physical, immunological, and psychologica disorders. There appears to be a strong associa tion between the degree to which an individual i dependent on alcohol and the severity of the prob lems experienced by the individual, and this is inde pendent from the amount of alcohol consumed.

ALCOHOL USE DISORDER

Alcohol use disorder (AUD) is a medical conditio characterised by an impaired ability to stop or con trol alcohol use despite adverse social, occupationa or health consequences (NIDA, 2024). AUD encompass a spectrum of conditions characterise by problematic patterns of alcohol consumption including alcohol dependence and addiction. Thes disorders are among the most prevalent menta health issues worldwide (Rehm et al., 2013). Ris factors for alcohol use disorder (AUD) (NIIAAA 2024) include:

- *Early onset of drinking.* Starting drinking befor age 15 significantly increases the risk of develop ing AUD, especially among females. Those wh delay drinking until age 21 or later have lowe risk.
- *Genetics and family history.* Genetics play a sub stantial role in AUD, accounting for about 60% o the risk. Family history of alcohol problems can als contribute to the likelihood of developing AUD.

Table 7.5
Questions to assess for symptoms of alcohol use disorder

Signs and symptoms	Questions
Loss of control over drinking	• Had times when you ended up drinking more, or longer, than you intended? • More than once wanted to cut down or stop drinking, or tried to but could not? • Continued to drink even though it was causing trouble with your family or friends?
Preoccupation with drinking	• Wanted a drink so badly you could not think of anything else? • Spent a lot of time drinking, being sick from drinking, or getting over other after-effects? • Continued to drink even though it was making you feel depressed or anxious or adding to another health problem? • Or after having had an alcohol-related memory blackout?
Negative consequences of drinking	• Found that drinking – or being sick from drinking – often interfered with taking care of your home or family? Or caused job troubles? Or school problems? • Given up or cut back on activities you found important, interesting, or pleasurable so you could drink? • More than once gotten into situations while or after drinking that increased your chances of getting hurt (such as driving, swimming, using machinery, walking in a dangerous area, or unsafe sexual behaviour)?
Tolerance and withdrawal	• Found that your usual number of drinks had much less effect than before? • Found that when the effects of alcohol were wearing off, you had withdrawal symptoms, such as trouble sleeping, shakiness, restlessness, nausea, sweating, a racing heart, dysphoria (feeling uneasy or unhappy), malaise (general sense of being unwell), feeling low, or a seizure? Or sensed things that were not there?

Source: Adapted from NIAAA (2024).

- *Mental health conditions*. Conditions like depression, post-traumatic stress disorder (PTSD), and attention-deficit hyperactivity disorder (ADHD) are often comorbid with AUD and increase the risk of its development.
- *History of trauma*. Individuals with a history of childhood trauma are at increased vulnerability to AUD, highlighting the impact of adverse experiences on alcohol use behaviours.

These are questions that are commonly used as part of screening tools to assess for symptoms of AUD. Table 7.5 presents the questions that can be used to assess for symptoms of alcohol use disorder.

WITHDRAWAL SYMPTOMS

Alcohol use disorder involves both physical and psychological dependence. Alcohol withdrawal syndrome is a set of symptoms that individuals have when they suddenly stop drinking alcohol, following continuous and heavy consumption. Severe withdrawal symptoms can be life-threatening, necessitating medical supervision. Symptoms can be categorised into physical, emotional, and cognitive/psychological manifestation (see Table 7.5). Drinkers who have gone through withdrawal before are more likely to have withdrawal symptoms each time they stop drinking. Some individuals have the forms of syndrome, including tremors, seizures, and hallucinations, typically occurring within 6 to 48 hours after the last alcoholic drink. Withdrawals can be mild, moderate, or severe (see Table 7.6). For most problem drinkers, alcohol withdrawal will not progress to the severe stage of delirium tremens (confusion and hallucination). When an individual has severe withdrawal symptoms, this can be a life-threatening condition and requires supervision under medical care. Here are the mild, moderate, and severe withdrawal symptoms categorised into physical, emotional, and cognitive/psychological categories (Table 7.6).

CONTROLLED DRINKING

The effect of alcohol on an individual varies with age, diet, weight, health, gender, culture, and religious belief. Over two decades ago, the Royal College of Physicians in the UK established recommendations for "sensible" weekly alcohol consumption which are still endorsed today. Different countries offer varying recommendations for alcohol consumption. The UK advises a maximum of 14 units per week spread over at least three days, with "some" alcohol-free days. Belgium suggests that up to 21 drinks per week for men and 14 for women is low risk. In

Table 7.6
Mild, moderate, and severe withdrawal symptoms

	Physical symptoms	Emotional symptoms	Cognitive/psychological symptoms
Mild to moderate psychological symptoms	Feeling of shakiness Fatigue	Feeling of anxiety Irritability or easily excited Emotionally volatile Rapid emotional changes Depression Bad dreams	Difficulty with thinking clearly
Mild to moderate physical symptoms	Headache Sweating (palms and face) Nausea Vomiting Loss of appetite Paleness Rapid heart rate (palpitations) Enlarged, dilated pupils Skin clammy Abnormal movements Tremor of hands Involuntary movements of the eyelids	Irritability or easily excited Emotionally volatile Rapid emotional changes Depression	Difficulty with thinking clearly Bad dreams Insomnia
Severe symptoms	Delirium tremens Elevated temperature Convulsions Blackouts	Agitation Fear, suspicion, and anger Suicidal behaviour	Hallucinations (visual or tactile) Clouding of consciousness Disorientation of time and place Paranoid delusions

Source: Adapted from Finn and Crabbe (1997).

Ireland, the recommendation is up to 17 drinks for men and 11 for women, with two alcohol-free days weekly. France and Australia recommend no more than 10 standard drinks a week, but France also advises no more than 2 drinks per day and at least one alcohol-free day weekly. Meanwhile, the United States recommends no more than two drinks per day for men and one for women. The 2020–2025 Dietary Guidelines for Americans Department of Agriculture and US Department of Health and Human Services (2020) suggest that adults of legal drinking age should either refrain from alcohol or drink in moderation. *Moderation* is defined as limiting alcohol intake to 2 drinks or fewer per day for men, and 1 drink or fewer per day for women, on days when alcohol is consumed. The guidelines strongly advise against individuals who do not drink currently to start for any reason. Moreover, for those who opt to drink, the recommendation highlights that consuming less alcohol is more beneficial for health outcomes compared to drinking more. Countries use different definitions for what constitutes a standard drink, adding to the complexity of alcohol consumption guidelines. In the United States, a standard drink contains 14 grams of alcohol, while in Australia, it is 10 grams, and in the UK, it is approximately 8 grams of ethanol.

The Dietary Guidelines advise certain group to avoid alcohol completely, including pregnan women, individuals under 21, those with certai medical conditions or on specific medications, an those recovering from alcohol use disorder or unabl to control their drinking. For lactating womer while moderate alcohol consumption (up to 1 stan dard drink per day) is generally considered safe, it i recommended to wait at least two hours after a sin gle drink before nursing or expressing breast milk Consulting a healthcare provider is encouraged fo personalised advice regarding alcohol consump tion during lactation. For pregnant women or thos who are breastfeeding or planning a pregnancy, nc drinking is the safest option. Having alcohol-fre days each week is recommended to reduce alcohc consumption. Following a heavy drinking episode, i is advised to have two consecutive alcohol-free day This practice helps prevent the development of tol erance to alcohol and allows the body to reverse an tendency towards tolerance. Failure to control o reset tolerance may lead to increased risky drinking which is detrimental to health. Controlled drinkin also entails personal assessment of risks and respon sibilities associated with drinking, such as avoid ing alcohol consumption when driving, operatin machinery, or taking certain medications.

ALCOHOL CONSUMPTION: BENEFITS OR HARMS?

Alcohol consumption has been linked to both benefits and harms, particularly concerning cardiovascular health and mortality. While some studies suggest that moderate alcohol intake may offer protective effects on heart health, recent research challenges this notion. A study by Karady et al. (2016) found that alcohol consumption, regardless of type, had neither harmful nor protective effects on the arteries of the heart. Additionally, a meta-analysis conducted by Stockwell et al. (2016) revealed that low-volume alcohol consumption does not provide a net mortality benefit when compared to lifetime abstention or occasional drinking.

However, the World Health Organization (Anderson et al., 2023) has stated that there is no safe amount of alcohol consumption that does not affect health. The idea of identifying a "safe" level of alcohol consumption requires scientific evidence demonstrating that below a certain threshold, there is no risk of illness or injury associated with alcohol intake. However, current evidence cannot pinpoint such a threshold where the carcinogenic effects of alcohol do not manifest in the human body. There is a lack of studies demonstrating that the potential benefits of light and moderate drinking on cardiovascular diseases and type 2 diabetes outweigh the cancer risk associated with these levels of alcohol consumption for individual consumers (Anderson et al., 2023). In other words, the potential positive effects of alcohol consumption on certain health conditions are not sufficient to offset the increased risk of developing cancer associated with even light or moderate drinking. This underlines the conclusion that any level of alcohol consumption carries inherent health risks.

ALCOHOL AND DRUG INTERACTIONS

The interactions between alcohol and prescribed medications, over-the-counter drugs, and illicit substances can lead to severe health complications, including trauma, illness, and even death. These interactions may increase the risk of liver damage, heart problems, internal bleeding, impaired breathing, and depression. Even moderate alcohol consumption can exacerbate these risks. Weathermon and Crabb (1999) noted that such interactions can alter the metabolism or activity of medications and alcohol, leading to potentially serious medical consequences. For instance, the sedative effects of alcohol and sedative medications can compound each other, significantly impairing an individual's ability to drive or operate machinery.

Alcohol–medication interactions can be categorised into two types: pharmacokinetic interactions and pharmacodynamic interactions. In pharmacokinetic interactions, alcohol disrupts the activity or metabolism of the drug by affecting its absorption, distribution, metabolism, or excretion. In pharmacodynamic interactions, alcohol amplifies the effects of the medication on the central nervous system. These interactions can lead to decreased medication effectiveness or increased drug toxicity, potentially causing harm. Various categories of prescribed medications, over-the-counter drugs, and illicit substances, including opioids, antidepressants, benzodiazepines, antibiotics, antihistamines, antipsychotics, muscle relaxants, pain medications, anti-inflammatory agents, and coagulants, can interact with alcohol. Consumers of alcohol should be cautioned about the potential health risks associated with combining alcohol and medications, whether they are prescribed, over-the-counter, or illicit drugs. This combination has the potential to lead to health-related complications and even mortality. Individuals who are prescribed multiple medications should be particularly aware of the dangers of mixing alcohol with their medications. Providing clear health warnings about the risks of alcohol–medication interactions can help raise awareness and prevent adverse health outcomes.

UNDERSTANDING BLOOD ALCOHOL CONCENTRATION

Blood alcohol concentration (BAC) is basically the amount of alcohol in your bloodstream and is typically expressed as a percentage. Your BAC depends on how much alcohol you consume. The more you drink, the higher your BAC. Several factors can influence an individual's BAC, including, but not limited to:

- Number of alcohol drinks
- Duration/speed of consumption
- Body type/weight
- Gender
- If food is present in the stomach
- If other medications are present in the body
- Level of fatigue

Table 7.7
Blood alcohol levels and effects

BAC	Potential effects
0.02–0.04%	Light to moderate drinkers begin to feel some effects and mildly relaxed; some light headedness; minor impairment of judgement
0.05–0.07%	Lower inhibitions; euphoric; exaggerated emotions; minor impairments of reasoning and memory
0.08–0.10%	Euphoric; slight impairments of balance, speech, vision, reaction time, and hearing; judgement reduced; reasoning and memory impaired; self-control impaired; fatigue
0.11–0.15%	State of drunkenness; judgement and perception severely impaired; lack of physical control; gross motor impairment; blurred vision; slurred speech; balance, vision, hearing, and reaction time impaired; anxiety and depression more pronounced
0.16–0.19%	Very drunk; nausea and vomiting may occur; dizziness; increased motor impairment; judgement further impaired; strong state of depression
0.20–0.24%	Disorientation to time and place; confused; increased nausea and vomiting; may need assistance to stand or walk; unreceptive to pain; blackouts likely
0.25%	Physical, mental, and sensory functions severely impaired; increased risk of asphyxiation from chocking or vomiting; accidents very likely
0.30%	Stupor; little comprehension of surroundings; may pass out suddenly
0.35%	Coma; alcohol poisoning
+0.40%	Possible death due to respiratory arrest (likely in 50% of drinkers)

Source: Adapted from National Institute on Alcohol Abuse and Alcoholism and University of Wisconsin-Eau Claire (www.uwec.edu/CASE/students/moderation.htm).

BAC can be measured with a breathalyser or by analysing a sample of blood. It is measured by the number of grams of alcohol in 100 millilitres of blood. For example, a BAC of 0.08, the US legal limit for driving for those over 21, means you have 0.08 grams of alcohol in every 100 millilitres of blood. Blood alcohol levels and their effects on behaviours are presented in Table 7.7.

WHAT IS A UNIT OF ALCOHOL?

One unit of alcohol = half a pint of ordinary-strength beer, lager, or cider (3–4% alcohol by volume [ABV]) = a small pub measure of spirits (40% ABV) = a standard pub measure (50 millilitre) of fortified wine, such as sherry or port (20% ABV) = a small glass of ordinary-strength wine (12% ABV) = a standard pub measure of spirits (40% ABV).

The exact number of units in a particular drink can be calculated by multiplying the volume of the drink (number of millilitres) by the % ABV and dividing by 1,000.

For example, the number of units in a strong beer of 500 ml with a 6% ABV = 500 × 6.0 ÷ 1,000 = 3 units.

Another way of calculating units is as follows: the percentage alcohol by volume (% ABV) of a drink equals the number of units in 1 litre of that drink.

For example, strong beer at 6% ABV has six units in 1 litre. If you drink half a litre (500 millilitres) – just under a pint – then you have had three units.

KEY POINTS

- Alcohol has become one of the most important risks to health globally.
- Alcohol consumption can lead to not only alcohol use disorder and dependence but also a risk of developing more than 200 diseases, including liver cirrhosis and some cancers.
- Alcohol is absorbed in the mouth, the oesophagus, and the stomach. This adds to the problem of poor malnutrition or vitamin deficiencies in heavy alcohol drinkers.
- Women do not metabolise alcohol as effectively as men, and they are more vulnerable to the consequences of alcohol drinking.
- A *blackout* is a memory impairment that occurs in anyone who drinks a large amount of alcohol in one session.
- Chronic alcohol use may result in significant memory problems and cognitive impairment.
- Foetal alcohol syndrome is caused by pre-natal alcohol exposure and can cause permanent damage to the baby's brain, resulting in neurological impairment of the executive functions.

- Alcohol withdrawal syndrome is a set of symptoms that individuals have when they suddenly stop drinking alcohol following continuous and heavy consumption.
- There are a variety of alcohol types, different brands, and mixing ingredients.
- Level of alcohol use: non-user (abstention), experimentation (use for novelty or curiosity), misuse social/recreational use (infrequent use – no established pattern), misuse (continued use despite negative consequences), binge drinking (people episodically drink excessively), and addiction (compulsion to use, inability to stop use, chaotic use, physical and psychological dependence).
- Binge drinking is drinking lots of alcohol in a short space of time or drinking to get drunk and is commonly associated with a higher risk for serious bodily harm, such as injuries, alcohol poisoning, and acute organ damage.
- The potential positive effects of alcohol consumption on certain health conditions are not sufficient to offset the increased risk of developing cancer associated with even light or moderate drinking.
- Consumers of alcohol should be cautioned about the potential health risks associated with combining alcohol and medications, whether they are prescribed, over-the-counter, or illicit drugs
- The interactions between prescribed medications, over-the-counter drugs, and illicit drugs and alcohol can lead to trauma, illness, and even death.
- Blood alcohol concentration (BAC) is basically the amount of alcohol in your bloodstream and is typically expressed as a percentage.

The following list shows the number of units of alcohol in common drinks:

- A pint of ordinary-strength lager (Carling Black Label, Fosters) – 2 units
- A pint of strong lager (Stella Artois, Kronenbourg 1664) – 3 units
- A pint of ordinary bitter (John Smith's, Boddingtons) – 2 units
- A pint of best bitter (Fuller's ESB, Young's Special) – 3 units
- A pint of ordinary-strength cider (Woodpecker) – 2 units
- A pint of strong cider (Dry Blackthorn, Strongbow) – 3 units
- A 175-millilitre glass of red or white wine at 13% strength – 2.3 units
- A pub measure of spirits – 1 unit
- An alcopop (Smirnoff Ice, Bacardi Breezer, WKD, Reef) – around 1.5 units

Activity 7.3

Safe drinking – how much do I drink?

Counting units of alcohol can help us keep track of the amount we are drinking. The labels of many bottled drinks will tell you how many units of alcohol are in the bottle. One way of getting a picture of your drinking is to keep a drinking diary for a week or month. When you have an alcoholic drink, please fill in the diary.

DAY	WHEN	WHERE	DRINKS
Sunday			
Monday			
Tuesday			
Wednesday			
Thursday			
Friday			
Saturday			

Activity 7.4

How much do I drink?

Fill in the average number of drinks you have in a day (a 24-hour period), and calculate the number of units by using the calculations given in the text.

Alcoholic drinks	Volume	ABV	Total	Units
Bitter	1 pt	4.7%		
Stout	1 pt	4.5%		
Cider	1 pt	6.2		
Alcopop	275 ml	5%		
Low-strength beer or lager	1 pt	3.5–4%		
Wine (large)	250 ml	12%		
Wine (small)	125 ml	12%		
Fortified wine (sherry/port)	50 ml	20%		
Spirits	35 ml	40%		

Volume (ml) × strength in % ABV ÷ 1,000 =

References

Anderson, B. O., Berdzuli, N., Ilbawi, A., Kestel, D., Kluge, H. P., Krech, R., Mikkelsen, B., Neufeld, M., Poznyak, V., Rekve, D., Slama, S., Tello, J., & Ferreira-Borges, C. (2023). Health and cancer risks associated with low levels of alcohol consumption. *The Lancet Public Health,* 8(l), e1–e84. https://doi.org/10.1016/S2468-2667(22)00317-6.

Bohm, M. K., Liu, Y., Esser, M. B., Mesnick, J. B., Lu, H., Pan, Y., & Greenlund, K. J. (2021). Binge drinking among adults, by select characteristics and state – United States, 2018. *MMWR, Morbidity and Mortality Weekly Report,* 70(41), 1441–1446. https://doi.org/10.15585/mmwr.mm7041a2.

Carroll, H. A., Lustyk, M. K., & Larimer, M. E. (2015). The relationship between alcohol consumption and menstrual cycle: A review of the literature. *Archives of Women's Mental Health,* 18(6), 773–781. https://doi.org/10.1007/s00737-015-0568-2.

CDCP. (2022). *Binge Drinking.* Division of Population Health, National Center for Chronic Disease Prevention and Health Promotion, Centers for Disease Control and Prevention. https://www.cdc.gov/alcohol/fact-sheets/binge-drinking.htm (accessed 3 February 2024).

Dozet, D., Burd, L., & Popova, S. (2023). Screening for alcohol use in pregnancy: A review of current practices and perspectives. *International Journal of Mental Health and Addiction,* 21(2), 1220–1239. https://doi.org/10.1007/s11469-021-00655-3.

Finn, D. A., & Crabbe, J. C. (1997). Exploring alcohol wit drawal syndrome. *Alcohol Health Research World,* 21(2 149–156.

Friend, K. B., Goodwin, M. S., & Lipsitt, L. P. (2004). Alco hol use and sudden infant death syndrome. *Development Review,* 24(3), 235–251. https://doi.org/10.1016/ dr.2004.06.001.

Hall, S., & Finch, N. (2023). Binge drinking. In D. B. Coope (Ed.), *Alcohol Use: Assessment, Withdrawal Managemen Treatment and Therapy.* Cham: Springer. https://do org/10.1007/978-3-031-18381-2_16.

Harrington, M., Velicer, W. F., & Ramsey, S. E. (2014). Typo ogy of alcohol users based on longitudinal patterns of drin ing. *Addictive Behaviors,* 39(3), 607–621.

Hutton, H. E., McCaul, M. E., Santora, P. B., & Erbelding, E. J. (2008 The relationship between recent alcohol use and sexual beha iors: Gender differences among sexually transmitted disease *Alcoholism: Clinical and Experimental Research,* 32(11), 2008 2015. https://doi.org/10.1111/j.1530-0277.2008.00788.x

Iyasu, S., Randall, L. L., Welty, T. K., Hsia, J., Kinney, H. C Mandell, F., McClain, M., Randall, B., Habbe, D., W son, H., & Willinger, M. (2002). Risk factors for sudde infant death syndrome among northern plains Indian

JAMA, 288(21), 2717–2723. https://doi.org/10.1001/jama.288.21.2717.

Karady, J., Szilveszter, B., Drobni, Z. D., Kolossvary, M., Bartykowszki, A., Karolyi, M., Jermendy, A., Panajotu, A., Bagyura, Z., Merkely, B., & Maurovich-Horvat, P. (2016). *Alcohol Consumption Shows No Effect on Coronary Arteries*. Radiological Society of North America annual meeting held from Nov. 27 to Dec. 2 in Chicago. http://press.rsna.org/timssnet/media/pressreleases/14_pr_target.cfm?ID=1918 (accessed 22 December 2016).

Khamis, A. A., Salleh, S. Z., Ab Karim, M. S., Mohd Rom, N. A., Janasekaran, S., Idris, A., & Abd Rashid, R. B. (2022). Alcohol consumption patterns: A systematic review of demographic and sociocultural influencing factors. *International Journal of Environmental Research and Public Health*, 19(13), 8103. https://doi.org/10.3390/ijerph19138103.

May, P. A., Blankenship, J., Marais, A. S., Gossage, J. P., Kalberg, W. O., Joubert, B., Cloete, M., Barnard, R., De Vries, M., Hasken, J., Robinson, L. K., Adnams, C. M., Buckley, D., Manning, M., Parry, C. D., Hoyme, H. E., Tabachnick, B., & Seedat, S. (2013). Maternal alcohol consumption producing fetal alcohol spectrum disorders (FASD): Quantity, frequency, and timing of drinking. *Drug and Alcohol Dependence*, 133(2), 502–512. https://doi.org/10.1016/j.drugalcdep.2013.07.013.

Naimi, T. S., Lipscomb, L. E., Brewer, R. D., & Gilbert, B. C. (2003). Binge drinking in the preconception period and the risk of unintended pregnancy: Implications for women and their children. *Pediatrics*, 111(5 Pt 2), 1136–1141.

NIAAA. (2024). *Understanding Binge Drinking*. National Institute on Alcohol Abuse and Alcoholism. https://www.niaaa.nih.gov/publications/brochures-and-fact-sheets/binge-drinking (accessed 3 February 2024).

NIDA. (2024). *Alcohol's Effects on Health*. Research-Based Information on Drinking and Its Impact. https://www.niaaa.nih.gov/publications/brochures-and-fact-sheets/understanding-alcohol-use-disorder (accessed 2 February 2024).

OECD. (2023). *Health at a Glance 2023: OECD Indicators*. Paris: OECD Publishing. https://doi.org/10.1787/7a7afb35-en.

Popova, S., Lange, S., Probst, C., Gmel, G., & Rehm, J. (2018). Global prevalence of alcohol use and binge drinking during pregnancy, and foetal alcohol spectrum disorder. *Biochemistry and Cell Biology = Biochimie et Biologie Cellulaire*, 96(2), 237–240. https://doi.org/10.1139/bcb-2017-0077.

Prochaska, J., & DiClemente, C. (1983). Stages and processes of self-change of smoking: Toward an integrative model of change. *Journal of Consulting and Clinical Psychology*, 51(3), 390–395.

Pryce, R., Hollingsworth, B., & Walker, I. (2019). Alcohol quantity and quality price elasticities: Quantile regression estimates. *The European Journal of Health Economics: HEPAC: Health Economici in Prevention and Care*, 20(3), 439–454. https://doi.org/10.1007/s10198-018-1009-8.

Rehm, J., Marmet, S., Anderson, P., Gual, A., Kraus, L., Nutt, D. J., Room, R., Samokhvalov, A. V., Scafato, E., Trapencieris, M., Wiers, R. W., & Gmel, G. (2013). Defining substance use disorders: Do we really need more than heavy use? *Alcohol and Alcoholism*, 48(6), 633–640. https://doi.org/10.1093/alcalc/agt127.

Royal College of General Practitioners. (1986). *Alcohol: Our Favourite Drug*. London: Tavistock Publications.

Stockwell, T., Zhao, J., Panwar, S., Roemer, A., Naimi, T., & Chikritzhs, T. (2016). Do "moderate" drinkers have reduced mortality risk? A systematic review and meta-analysis of alcohol consumption and all-cause mortality. *Journal of Studies on Alcohol and Drugs*, 77(2), 185–198.

Strebel, J., & Terry, M. B. (2021). Alcohol, binge drinking, and cancer risk: Accelerating public health messaging through counter marketing. *American Journal of Public Health*, 111(5), 812–814. https://doi.org/10.2105/AJPH.2021.306233.

Townshend, J. M., Kambouropoulos, N., Griffin, A., Hunt, F. J., & Milani, R. M. (2014). Binge drinking, reflection impulsivity, and unplanned sexual behavior: Impaired decision-making in young social drinkers. *Alcoholism, Clinical and Experimental Research*, 38(4), 1143–1150. https://doi.org/10.1111/acer.12333.

U.S. Department of Agriculture and U.S. Department of Health and Human Services. (2020). *Dietary Guidelines for Americans, 2020–2025* (9th ed.). www.dietaryguidelines.gov.

Weathermon, R., & Crabb, D. W. (1999). Alcohol and medication interactions. *Alcohol Research and Health*, 23(1), 40–54.

WHO. (2010). *Global Strategy to Reduce the Harmful Use of Alcohol*. Geneva: World Health Organization.

WHO. (2018). *Global Status Report on Alcohol and Health 2018*. Geneva: World Health Organization.

WHO. (2022). *Alcohol: Key Facts*. World Health Organization. https://www.who.int/news-room/factsheets/detail/alcohol#:~:text=The%20Global%20strategy%20to%20reduce%20the%20harmful%20use,and%20social%20burden%20is%20a%20public%20health%20priority (accessed 2 February 2024).

Chapter 8

Opiates and opioids

Learning outcomes

- Discuss the therapeutic and non-therapeutic uses of heroin.
- Briefly describe the mechanism of action of heroin.
- Describe heroin's effects on the different modes of administration.
- Discuss the sought-after effects of heroin use.
- List the adverse effects of heroin use.
- List the withdrawal symptoms associated with heroin use.
- Discuss the reasons methadone is used for opiate-dependent users.
- List the withdrawal symptoms associated with methadone use.
- Discuss the benefits and risks of prescribing methadone to treat opiate dependence.

Activity 8.1

There is only one correct answer to the following multiple-choice questions.

1. What are the therapeutic uses of heroin?
   a. Pain relief
   b. Anxiety reduction
   c. Cough suppression
   d. All of the above
   e. None of the above
2. Which of the following best describes the mechanism of action of heroin?
   a. Blocks opioid receptors in the brain
   b. Activates opioid receptors in the brain
   c. Inhibits serotonin reuptake
   d. Increases dopamine levels
   e. None of the above
3. How does the mode of administration affect heroin's effects?
   a. Intravenous administration produces the quickest and most intense effects.
   b. Oral administration results in slow onset but prolonged effects.
   c. Smoking heroin produces rapid effects similar to intravenous administration.
   d. All of the above.
   e. None of the above.

DOI: 10.4324/9781003456674-1

4. What are the sought-after effects of heroin use?
   a. Euphoria
   b. Pain relief
   c. Sedation
   d. All of the above
   e. None of the above
5. What are the adverse effects of heroin use?
   a. Respiratory depression
   b. Nausea and vomiting
   c. Constipation
   d. All of the above
   e. None of the above
6. What withdrawal symptoms are associated with heroin use?
   a. Anxiety
   b. Muscle aches
   c. Sweating
   d. All of the above
   e. None of the above
7. Why is methadone used for opiate-dependent users?
   a. To manage withdrawal symptoms
   b. To reduce cravings
   c. To prevent relapse
   d. All of the above
   e. None of the above
8. What withdrawal symptoms are associated with methadone use?
   a. Anxiety
   b. Insomnia
   c. Muscle cramps
   d. All of the above
   e. None of the above
9. What are the benefits of prescribing methadone to treat opiate dependence?
   a. Reduction in drug cravings
   b. Decrease in illicit drug use
   c. Lower risk of overdose
   d. All of the above
   e. None of the above
10. What are the risks of prescribing methadone to treat opiate dependence?
    a. Potential for abuse
    b. Respiratory depression
    c. QT prolongation
    d. All of the above
    e. None of the above
11. What non-therapeutic uses are associated with heroin?
    a. Recreational drug use
    b. Addiction
    c. Crime
    d. All of the above
    e. None of the above

12. How does heroin affect cognitive function?
    a. Improves memory
    b. Enhances decision-making
    c. Impairs cognitive function
    d. All of the above
    e. None of the above
13. What route of administration is associated with the highest risk of overdose?
    a. Intravenous injection
    b. Smoking
    c. Oral ingestion
    d. Intranasal administration
    e. None of the above
14. What are the long-term effects of chronic heroin use?
    a. Liver damage
    b. Kidney failure
    c. Infectious diseases (e.g. HIV, hepatitis)
    d. All of the above
    e. None of the above
15. What factors contribute to heroin addiction?
    a. Genetic predisposition
    b. Environmental factors
    c. Peer pressure
    d. All of the above
    e. None of the above
16. Methadone is considered to be the best substitute drug for opiate-dependent drug users because?
    a. It is easy to administer and long-acting.
    b. It has less withdrawal effects.
    c. It is manufactured in tablet form.
    d. It is easy to administer and short-acting.
    e. All of the above are correct.
17. Methadone maintenance treatment involves:
    a. Daily dispensing of methadone
    b. Monthly injections of methadone
    c. Weekly counselling sessions only
    d. Use of methadone as needed
    e. None of the above
18. Which statement is not true? There is evidence to suggest that oral methadone substitution treatment can help to:
    a. Reduce the use of heroin
    b. Avoid the risks of overdose
    c. Reduce death rates
    d. Increase blood-borne infections
    e. None of the above
19. Drug consumption rooms (DCRs) typically provide which of the following services?
    a. Legal counselling
    b. Hairdressing services
    c. Sterile injecting equipment

d. Tax preparation assistance
e. Veterinary care

20. Supervised injection Facilities aim to:
    a. Increase drug use and addiction rates
    b. Reduce the spread of infectious diseases
    c. Promote illegal drug trafficking
    d. Encourage unsafe drug use practices
    e. Provide free recreational activities

INTRODUCTION

The term *opiate* refers to any psychoactive substance of either natural or synthetic origin that has an effect similar to morphine. *Opium* is the raw exudates of the opium poppy (*Papaver somniferum*) which is scraped from the scored seed head of the poppy, which contains a number of alkaloids, including morphine and codeine. Opium appears either as dark-brown chunks or in powder form and is generally eaten or smoked. The words *opiate* and *opioid* are used interchangeably. *Opiate* refers to natural drugs which produce the characteristic opiate effects, whereas *opioid* refers to synthetic substances derived from or resembling the substances in the poppy plant. Opioids act like opiates on the same receptors in the brain and are mainly used to relieve pain. Some of the common opioid drugs are codeine, heroin (diacetylmorphine), pethidine, methadone, morphine, and diconal. Morphine and codeine are extracted from opium, and heroin is manufactured chemically from morphine. Raw opium is treated with lime and other compounds to leave partially refined morphine. With the addition of acetic anhydride, this produces a base form of diamorphine (heroin). This crude base form of the drug is what makes up the bulk of the global market.

The main source of street heroin can vary depending on various factors, such as geopolitical dynamics, production trends, and trafficking routes. Historically, much of the world's heroin has been derived from the Golden Crescent countries of Southwest Asia: Afghanistan, Iran, and Pakistan; Southeast Asia (primarily Myanmar [Burma]), with significant crops also in Laos, Thailand, China, Vietnam, and Cambodia; and Latin America: Mexico and Colombia. The Golden Crescent countries and Southeast Asian countries are two regions accounting for the vast majority of opium destined for conversion to illicit heroin. Heroin of Southwest Asian origin is consumed locally, but most of the bulk is exported to Europe. Golden Triangle countries, such as the Republic of the Union of Myanmar, Laos, and Thailand, create the traditional heroin that is consumed in Australia. Latin America remains the primary supplier of heroin to the United States. Afghanistan, in particular, has been a major producer of opium, which is used to manufacture heroin. The country has historically been a significant source of the world's heroin due to its vast opium poppy cultivation.

PHARMACOLOGY OF OPIOIDS

Opioid drugs act in receptors (mu opioid receptors [MORs]) that are found within the central nervous system and peripheral tissues. There are naturally occurring chemicals called neurotransmitters, and many of the actions of opiates are related to alteration of the release of endogenous neurotransmitters. Neurotransmitters are natural chemicals that enable communication between neurons in the body. They facilitate the transmission of signals across the nervous system through chemical synapses. These substances are essential for a wide range of bodily functions and play a vital role in shaping everyday life and physiological processes (Rizo, 2018). Opioid receptors, including mu (μ), kappa (κ), delta (Δ), and sigma (σ) receptors, are normally stimulated by naturally occurring peptides, like endorphins, enkephalins, and dynorphins. These peptides are produced in response to painful stimuli. For example, kappa receptor activation produces a range of physiological processes depending on their location, including stress, mood, reward, pain, inflammation, and remyelination (Dalefield et al., 2022).

Opioids are divided into pure agonist, antagonists, and mixed agonists/antagonists, with varying effects on these receptors. Most of the most common opioids are agonists. Agonists stimulate opioid

Table 8.1
Common opiates – comparison chart

Drug	Trade/street name	Equivalent dose	Duration	Abuse potential
Opium	Omnopon	10–20 mg	4–5 hrs	Moderate-high
Morphine	Generic	10 mg	4–5 hrs	High
Codeine	Generic	120 mg	4–5 hrs	Low
Diamorphine	Heroin	3 mg	3–4 hrs	High
Buprenorphine	Temgesic	0.2–0.6 mg	6–8 hrs	Low
Dihydrocodeine	DF118	30 mg	4–5 hrs	Moderate
Dipipanone	Diconal	10 mg	4–5 hrs	High
Dextromoramide	Palfium	5–10 mg	4–5 hrs	High
Methadone	Physeptone	10 mg	3–12 hrs	High
Dextropropoxyphene	Co-Proxamol	60–120 mg	4–5 hrs	Low
Pethidine	Generic	50–150 mg	2–4 hrs	High
Pentazocine	Fortral	30–50 mg	3–4 hrs	Low-moderate

Source: www.idmu.co.uk/opiates2003.htm.

receptors and are agents that produce analgesia. It is the opposite of an antagonist, which blocks an action and diminishes analgesia. Mixed agonists/antagonists have the functions to either stimulate some opioid receptors or block other receptors. Pure agonist drugs include morphine, heroin, methadone, fentanyl, codeine, hydrocodone, hydromorphone, and oxycodone. Mixed agonists/antagonists include etazocine, nalbuphine, butorphanol, and buprenorphine. The most important antagonists include naloxone, naltrexone, buprenorphine (+naloxone), Narcan, and narcon. Opioids come in two main types: short-acting (immediate release) and long-acting (extended release). Short-acting opioids typically take effect within 15 to 30 minutes, peaking between 1.5 and 2 hours. Examples include codeine, Tylenol with codeine, and Demerol (meperidine). Long-acting opioids release slowly into the body and may last between 8 and 12 hours or longer. Common long-acting opioids include methadone, OxyContin, morphine, hydromorphone, fentanyl, buprenorphine, and oxymorphone. A key characteristic of all opioids is the development of tolerance and physical dependence over time. A comparison of common opiates and their abuse potential is presented in Table 8.1.

HEROIN

Heroin is a fine white powder in its purest form and, depending on its form, can be smoked, injected, or snorted. Brown heroin (Golden Crescent) is the result of the first stage of purification of impure diacetylmorphine and is diamorphine-based. It is less refined and is easier to smoke because it burns at a lower temperature. White heroin (Golden Triangle) is diamorphine hydrochloride–based and requires the addition of some kind of acid to make it soluble in water. Being a salt, white heroin burns at a much higher temperature than brown heroin, so it is not effective for smoking. There are different street names for heroin, depending on geographical location and street culture.

Heroin comes in various colours, names, origins, and purities. In the UK, brown heroin is prevalent, and smoking heroin, often termed "chasing the dragon" on foil, is common. In contrast, in the United States, black tar heroin, a dark, sticky substance of Mexican origin, is prominent. Black tar heroin is cheaper and quicker to produce compared to white or brown heroin, but its heroin content is typically low. Another variant, "cheese heroin," combines black tar heroin with Tylenol, an over-the-counter cold medication. Heroin from different regions exhibits distinct characteristics: Southeast Asian heroin is white, powdered, water-soluble, and acidic; Southwest Asian heroin is a brown coarse powder with poor water solubility but good heat stability; Colombian heroin is off-white to light brown, powdered, and acidic, with good water solubility; Mexican heroin is dark-brown to black, solid, of lower purity, and requires heat to dissolve in water despite its acidity.

Illicit drugs are often adulterated with various substances for different purposes. These include benign substances like sugars, compounds that enhance or mimic the effects of the drug (e.g. quinine in heroin), and substances that aid in the administration of the drug (e.g. caffeine in heroin and cocaine to facilitate smoking) (Cole et al., 2011). Some of the adulterants that have been reported in heroin include sugars, procaine, salicylate, caffeine, paracetamol, mannitol, glucose, phenobarbital, lidocaine, methaqualone, citric acid, piracetam, lysine acetylsalicylate, ascorbic acid, phenolphthalein acetic acid, methanol, acetone, ethanol, benzene, acetaldehyde, bupivacaine, griseofulvin, diazepam, and many others. Most adulterants, including bacterial infections, occur before importation, usually as the result of manufacturing, production, or storage techniques. It is stated that

> adverse health effects or deaths due to adulterated drugs are commonly due to poisoning, poor manufacturing techniques, poor storage or packaging, or related to the effects of other substances sold as the illicit drug. Bacterial infections attributed to illicit drug adulteration were most common amongst injecting drug users (particularly heroin and cocaine injectors).
>
> (Cole et al., 2011)

Heroin is usually sold in small quantities, and the cost of street drugs like heroin is wildly divergent in different parts of the world. The price of heroin depends on the type of heroin, its purity, its availability, and its accessibility. The average heroin addict will use between 150 milligrams and 250 milligrams per day. The mean daily dose of heroin intravenously (when used alone, without methadone on the side) was 491.7 milligrams (Uchtenhagen et al., 1999). Traditionally, heroin is sold as crystalline or powder, but there have been reports of "ready-to-use" heroin sold in preloaded syringes and homemade drugs in solution. The injected opiates are purchased in liquid form ("*shirka*") and in preloaded syringes containing "*khanka*" (an opiate produced from poppy straw) and "Vint" (a stimulant – ephedrine and methamphetamine) (Bobkov et al., 2005; Gyarmathy et al., 2010). Heroin users should be made aware of the relative and inherent risks associated with this type of drug use and the potential health effects that may arise from adulteration, bacterial, and blood-borne infections (sharing equipment).

Legal status

From a legal perspective, opium poppies and their derivatives are regulated under the UN Single Convention on Narcotic Drugs of 1961. However, while opium poppy seeds are commonly used in cooking and poppy pods are utilised in dry flower arrangements, opium itself is grown for pharmaceutical purposes under strict government licenses globally. Notably, heroin was not specifically included as a controlled substance in the UN 1971 International Convention on Psychotropic Substances. Therefore, from an international treaty standpoint, heroin is not explicitly banned, which is a significant legal distinction. Heroin is classified as a controlled substance and is illegal for production, distribution, sale, and possession in most countries around the world. The legal status may vary slightly from one country to another in terms of penalties associated with possession, trafficking, and production

The legislation for the use of opiates, mainly heroin, is regulated by national jurisprudence. Several countries have authorised heroin-assisted treatment (HAT) programmes to address long-term heroin addiction. These programmes, implemented in countries such as the UK, Switzerland, the Netherlands, Germany, and Canada, involve prescribing pharmaceutical-grade heroin to individuals who have not responded to traditional treatments like methadone maintenance therapy. In the UK, diamorphine is available by prescription, though it is a restricted Class A controlled drug. Heroin prescription has been a part of Britain's approach to drugs since the 1920s, dubbed as "The British System." The Home Office licenses doctors to prescribe diamorphine to those who do not respond to alternatives like methadone or morphine. In Australia, diamorphine is classified as a Schedule 9 substance under the Poisons Standard. Schedule 9 substances are classified as substances and preparations for therapeutic use that are prohibited from being sold, supplied, or used except under certain circumstances, such as for research or medical purposes, under strict controls. In Canada, diamorphine is classified as a controlled substance under the Controlled Drugs and Substances Act (CDSA). It is listed as a Schedule I substance, which means it is considered to have a high potential for abuse, no accepted medical use, and a lack of accepted safety under medical supervision. In the United States, diamorphine is classified as a Schedule I controlled substance under the Controlled Substances Act (CSA).

As a Schedule I substance, heroin is considered to have a high potential for abuse, no accepted medical use in treatment in the United States, and a lack of accepted safety for use under medical supervision.

Therapeutic uses

Opiates have various therapeutic uses, including pain relief, treatment of diarrhoea and vomiting, and cough suppression. Morphine is commonly used for acute pain caused by conditions like heart attacks, sickle cell crises, surgeries, fractures, burns, and terminal illnesses. Methadone is often prescribed to heroin addicts for maintenance or withdrawal purposes. While opiates like pethidine, morphine, dihydrocodeine, and methadone can be highly addictive, occasional heroin use does not necessarily lead to withdrawal symptoms. Oral administration is the most preferred route, but opioids can also be administered sublingually, buccally, rectally, subcutaneously, intramuscularly, and transdermally. Transdermal fentanyl, for instance, offers continuous opioid administration for chronic pain without the need for pumps or needles.

Non-therapeutic uses

Heroin is the most commonly used opiate, and it is consumed through various methods, including swallowing, smoking, sniffing, or injecting subcutaneously or intravenously. Diverted pharmaceutical opiates and opioids may also be used for injection, oral consumption, or as suppositories. Subcutaneous injection, known as "skin popping," involves injecting heroin solution into the layers of skin, typically in the arms or thighs. Intravenous injection, or "mainlining," entails injecting heroin directly into a vein. Smoking heroin, often referred to as "chasing the dragon" or "booting," involves heating the drug on silver foil and inhaling the resulting smoke through a rolled tube of paper or foil. In some cases, heroin tablets are crushed and injected. Heroin powder intended for injection is typically acidified with lemon juice or other acids, heated with water, and filtered before injection. Additionally, liquefied heroin may be sniffed using a nasal spray bottle, a practice known as "shabanging."

The effects of heroin depend on the method of administration. Orally ingested heroin is metabolised into morphine before crossing the blood–brain barrier, resulting in effects similar to those of or morphine. Intravenous injection produces a rus and euphoria within 30 to 60 seconds, while intr muscular or subcutaneous injection takes three t five minutes to take effect. Snorting heroin leads t onset within three to five minutes, while smokin it results in almost immediate but mild effects th strengthen with prolonged use, occurring within to 11 seconds. Some individuals misuse fentan patches by ingesting the gel or injecting it, whic poses significant risks, including fatalities reporte from chewing or aspirating the transdermal patc A number of fatalities involving chewing and asp rating the transdermal patch have been reporte (Carson et al., 2010; ISMP, 2012).

Controlled use of heroin

Limited literature exists on occasional and co trolled heroin users, who use the drug with info mal controls or constraints on their behavio While heroin use often leads to addiction, there a instances of individuals who use heroin occasional or in a controlled manner. These users may impo restrictions, such as using only on weekends, nev on workdays, never alone, or never in the presen of children. In some cases, controlled heroin use ca continue indefinitely with minimal physical har to the user. It is common for those close to su users to be unaware of their drug use. This phenon enon highlights the complexity of drug use patter and the diverse ways in which individuals intera with substances like heroin. Previous studies ha provided clear evidence that some people are ab to have controlled patterns of heroin use (Shew et al., 1998; Shewan & Dalgarno, 2005; Zinber 1984).

A report from the Joseph Rowntree Found tion (Warburton et al., 2005) found that among sample of 123 heroin users, nearly all were eith employed or studying, had higher socio-econom status compared to those in treatment samples, a enjoyed better housing conditions. The heroin-u ing careers of respondents varied: some engaged mid- or long-term non-dependent use, while othe transitioned from dependent and problematic use non-dependent patterns. A third group maintaine controlled dependence over the mid- to long ter Users were cautious about where and with who they used heroin, often avoiding individuals deep entrenched in the heroin subculture or engaged criminal activities. These findings underscore the diverse experiences and strategies employed by heroin users, challenging stereotypical perceptions of drug use. The findings suggest that heroin users employ various strategies to avoid dependence or maintain control over their drug use. Non-dependent users often adhere to self-imposed rules to limit the frequency of heroin use. Dependent users aim to manage the amount of heroin consumed regularly to prevent interference with their daily work and social activities. Contrary to common beliefs, the research indicates that heroin use does not inevitably lead to dependence, and some individuals are able to regain control over their heroin use. This highlights the complexity of drug use behaviours and challenges stereotypes associated with heroin addiction. More research is needed.

Sought-after effects

In moderate doses, opiates produce generally mild physical effects, primarily the analgesic effect. Faster-acting opiates generate a more intense "high" that may diminish over time. Heroin, with its very short duration of action, produces an exceptionally intense high, inducing a relaxed detachment from pain and anxiety, along with feelings of calm, pleasure, and profound well-being. The depressant effects of heroin reduce nervous system activity, including reflex functions like coughing, respiration, and heart rate. Additionally, they dilate blood vessels, creating a sensation of warmth. Opiates, including heroin, offer potent relief from both physical and psychological pain. Methadone, with effects similar to those of heroin, may be prescribed to prevent opiate withdrawal symptoms. Notably, methadone tincture cannot be injected, reducing the risks associated with injection behaviours.

Adverse effects

Users of heroin often experience nausea or vomiting during initial use or after periods of abstinence. Heroin dependence develops with repeated use over weeks, and sudden withdrawal leads to symptoms such as anxiety, muscle pains, sweating, diarrhoea, and goosebumps. Tolerance to heroin develops rapidly, requiring larger doses to achieve the same effect. After a period of abstinence, tolerance decreases quickly, increasing the risk of overdose with the usual dose. Overdose can lead to respiratory and cardiac arrest and death if immediate medical attention is not received. While overdoses can result in stupor, coma, or death, they typically do not affect motor skills or sensation. Opiate users may appear detached or withdrawn, with contracted pupils. While pharmaceutical heroin is not highly toxic to human organs, street heroin adulterants may pose greater risks, particularly when injected. Injection carries the risk of vein damage, collapse, local infections, abscesses, circulatory issues, ulcers, thrombosis, infections in heart valves, and systemic infections. Sharing injecting equipment increases the risk of blood-borne viruses, such as hepatitis B and C and HIV. Unsterile injections and adulterated street drugs are major contributors to complications. Heroin injection is a risk factor for contracting hepatitis B and C, HIV, and septicaemia.

Mechanism of action

When opiates are injected, swallowed, or smoked, they enter the bloodstream and rapidly affect the brain. In the brain, the drug is converted into monoacetylmorphine and morphine. It is the morphine molecule that binds with opioid receptors, specialised proteins on nerve cells' surfaces that detect the body's own opiate-like substances, known as endorphins. This binding produces the subjective effects of the heroin high, resulting in an extreme sense of well-being centred in the gut. Heroin use reduces or stops the production of endorphins in the brain, leading to dependence on heroin. Cessation of heroin results in uncomfortable withdrawal symptoms, including pain, even without physical trauma. Withdrawal syndrome typically begins six to eight hours after the last heroin dose.

Opiate-related overdose

Drug overdose, primarily from opioids, is the leading cause of accidental death among opioid users. Mortality from overdose of prescription painkillers and heroin is significant, contributing to a record number of deaths annually. Opioid misuse, often combined with benzodiazepines, stimulants, or alcohol, drives these fatalities. Opioids account for the majority (69%) of drug overdose deaths globally. Multiple ongoing opioid overdose epidemics exist worldwide, with one driven by synthetic opioid fentanyl in the United States and Canada, and another in North Africa, West Africa, the Near and Middle East, and South-West Asia due to the non-medical use of synthetic opioid tramadol (Penington Institute, 2022, UNDOC, 2022). Stimulants are the second most reported category of drugs consumed across Europe. Deaths involving amphetamines have increased in several European countries, and substances like amphetamine, MDMA, and methamphetamine are among the most commonly reported in acute drug toxicity presentations at European hospitals. While some cases are related to new psychoactive substances, deaths directly linked to these substances are rare in countries with relevant data (EMCDDA, 2022).

There are a number of risk factors associated with opioid overdose (see Table 8.2). Some of the risk factors associated with opioid overdose are modifiable, including injection drug use, use of alcohol, use of benzodiazepines/sedatives, and use of cocaine (WHO, 2023). Other risk factors are not modifiable, including male gender, a history of prior overdose, and a history of imprisonment or arrest (Wilder et al., 2016).

To address the ongoing epidemic of opioid deaths, comprehensive harm reduction strategies are essential. Naloxone is an important antidote fo opioid overdose, effectively reversing its effects i administered promptly. However, access to naloxone has been limited to health professionals in man countries, including ambulances. Some countrie like Australia, Canada, Italy, the UK, and Ukrain have made naloxone available over the counter i pharmacies without a prescription (WHO, 2023 Programmes worldwide have demonstrated tha providing naloxone to individuals likely to witnes opioid overdose, along with training on its use an resuscitation techniques, significantly reduces opioid-related deaths (WHO, 2023). This approach i particularly impactful for individuals with opioi use disorders, including those leaving prison, wh face elevated overdose risks in the first four week post-release. In addition to expanding naloxon availability to reverse opioid overdoses, efforts t address the opioid epidemic involve various measures: improving health education to raise awareness about opioid risks, and increasing access t treatment, rehabilitation, and aftercare service Training healthcare professionals in managing opoid overdose and educating physicians and psychitrists about rational opioid prescribing practices ar critical components.

Table 8.2
Risk factors associated with opioid overdose

- Male gender*
- Older age*
- History of opioid use disorder*
- History of prior overdose
- Reduced tolerance (following detoxification, release from imprisonment or detention, cessation of treatment)
- Injecting opioids*
- People who use prescription opioids, in particular those taking higher doses, without medical supervision*
- High prescribed dosage of opioids (more than 100 mg of morphine or equivalent daily)*
- Using opioids in combination with alcohol and/or other substances or medicines that suppress respiratory function, such as benzodiazepines, barbiturates, anaesthetics, or some pain medications*
- Multiple prescriptions, including benzodiazepines*
- Polydrug user (use of alcohol, benzodiazepines/sedatives, and cocaine with opioids)
- Use of opioids with medical conditions such as HIV, liver or lung disease*
- Household members of people in possession of opioids (including prescription opioids)
- Mental health problems*
- Lower socio-economic status*

*Risk factors for overdoses with prescribed opioids.

Source: Adapted from WHO (2023); Wilder et al. (2016).

Opiate withdrawal syndrome

Opiate withdrawal symptoms vary in severit depending on the level of physical and psycholog cal dependence. The severity and duration of witl drawal from heroin are influenced by factors such a dosage amount, drug type, method of consumptio and underlying medical conditions. Heroin with drawal typically occurs after sustained daily use fo at least two to three weeks. Symptoms may appea 6 to 12 hours after discontinuation, peak in inter sity within two to three days, and persist for five t ten days. Occasional or controlled heroin use ma not result in withdrawal symptoms. The time fram for withdrawal can fluctuate based on toleranc levels and the amount of the last consumed dos Opioid withdrawal symptoms encompass dru craving, restlessness, irritability, dysphoria, loss o appetite, anxiety, insomnia, diarrhoea, aches, trem ors, excessive sweating, muscular spasms, sneezin and yawning. The severity of symptoms depends o the individual's level of dependence. Withdraw typically follows a timeline, with symptoms peak ing within two to three days and subsiding over fiv

Table 8.3
Opiate withdrawal symptoms

Early withdrawal symptoms	Late withdrawal symptoms
• Agitation	• Nausea and vomiting
• Muscle aches	• Dilated pupils
• Excessive sweating	• Diarrhoea
• Lacrimation (eyes tearing up)	• Goosebumps
• Trouble falling and staying asleep	• Stomach cramps
• Excessive yawning	• Depression
• Anxiety	• Drug cravings
• Nose running	• Rapid heartbeat
• Sweats	• High blood pressure
• Racing heart	
• Hypertension	

to ten days. Newborns exposed to opioids in utero may experience withdrawal symptoms, including digestive issues, poor feeding, dehydration, vomiting, and seizures.

METHADONE

Methadone is a synthetic opioid used therapeutically as an analgesic and in the treatment of opiate addiction. Methadone maintenance treatment is the most employed agent used in substitution treatment for heroin addiction around the world and is still regarded as the most effective. Methadone is utilised as a treatment for heroin addiction in numerous countries worldwide, including the United States, Canada, UK, Australia, France, Germany, Spain, Italy, Sweden, Netherlands, Switzerland, Portugal, Norway, Denmark, Hong Kong, the Republic of China (Taiwan), Malaysia, Indonesia, and several others. In many countries, substitution therapy by methadone is forbidden by law and strictly controlled. Methadone maintenance programmes form part of comprehensive harm reduction strategies to address opioid addiction and reduce associated risks. These programmes aim to stabilise individuals, alleviate withdrawal symptoms, and minimise cravings, thereby supporting recovery from heroin dependence.

Methadone, similar to heroin or morphine, can help break the cycle of dependence on opiates by occupying opioid receptors in the brain. This action stabilises individuals undergoing treatment for heroin addiction, allowing them to change their lifestyles and behaviours. Methadone is highly regarded as a substitute drug for opiate-dependent users due to its ease of administration and long-lasting effects. Typically prescribed as a liquid syrup for oral consumption, methadone is also available in tablet and injectable forms. It is considered nearly as effective when taken orally as it is when administered via injection. For most patients, individualised dose optimisation in methadone maintenance treatment (MMT) generally entails daily doses ranging from 60 to 120 milligrams of methadone (WHO, 2009), and this approach is associated with increased retention in treatment and reduced illicit opioid use (Chalabianloo et al., 2021; Fareed et al., 2010). However, studies have shown that factors beyond dose, such as patient expectations, medication preferences, overall physical and mental health conditions, and improvements in psychosocial functioning can influence treatment satisfaction (Bart, 2012; Muller et al., 2018). The effectiveness of methadone maintenance therapy has been shown in several studies. Methadone maintenance enhances treatment retention and diminishes heroin use in individuals with opioid dependence compared to non-pharmacological alternatives (Mattick et al., 2009). However, it does not lead to improvements in criminal activity or mortality rates when compared with non-pharmacological maintenance approaches. Treatment with methadone was associated with reductions in overdose and serious opioid-related acute care use compared with other treatments (Wakeman et al., 2020).

The duration of methadone maintenance therapy varies from person to person. According to NIDA (2018), the length of methadone treatment should be a minimum of 12 months. However, depending on the complex needs of the patients, some may require treatment on a long-term basis. Methadone's effects last significantly longer than those of heroin or morphine, with a typical half-life of 24 hours or more. This extended duration allows individuals in methadone maintenance programmes to take it once daily without experiencing withdrawal symptoms. While methadone reduces cravings and blocks the euphoric effects of heroin, it does not produce the same rush. However, tolerance and dependence can develop with repeated doses, albeit at varying rates for different physiological effects. Withdrawal symptoms from methadone are slower to develop and less acutely severe compared to morphine and heroin, but they are prolonged, lasting for several weeks or more. Some heroin users find quitting methadone to be more challenging than quitting heroin itself. The withdrawal symptoms of methadone are:

- Nausea and vomiting
- Increased lacrimation
- Rhinorrhoea
- High temperature
- Tremor
- Chills
- Sneezing
- Tachycardia

Patients wishing to discontinue methadone treatment should do so gradually under medical supervision to prevent withdrawal symptoms. Engaging in risky behaviour such as consuming excessive methadone doses or combining it with other depressants, alcohol, or heroin can lead to overdose or death, posing significant dangers to those struggling with opiate use disorder.

DRUG CONSUMPTION ROOMS AND SUPERVISED INJECTION FACILITIES

In recent years, there has been increasing advocacy for the establishment of drug consumption rooms (DCRs) or supervised injection facilities (SIFs), particularly in areas where drug use and related harms are prevalent. Advocates argue that these facilities can help reduce the risk of overdose deaths, prevent the spread of diseases such as HIV and hepatitis, and provide avenues for individuals to access support and treatment services. However, the implementation of DCRs/SIFs in several countries faces various legal, political, social, and religious challenges. The issue remains contentious, and while some voluntary and non-governmental organisations in those countries support the idea, there is not yet a nationwide consensus or legislative framework in place to establish such facilities. Drug consumption room (DCRs) refers to "supervised injecting facilities, are fixed or mobile spaces in which people who inject drugs are provided with sterile injection equipment and can use illicit drugs under the supervision of trained staff" (EMCDDA, 2023). Drug consumption room have been operating in Europe for the last thre decades and currently operate in Switzerland, Germany, the Netherlands, Spain, Denmark, Norwa Luxembourg, France, Belgium, and Portugal. Outside the European Union, countries like Canad and Australia have implemented DCRs or simila programmes.

Drug consumption rooms (DCRs) offer supervised environments for individuals to use drug safely. They provide sterile injecting equipmen overdose intervention, counselling, and basic medical care. Clients receive training in safer drug us and are referred to social, healthcare, and treatmen services. Some DCRs promote opioid agonist treatment. Additional amenities like tea, coffee, phon access, and hygiene facilities may be available. European DCRs are adding smoking rooms, where user can smoke crack or heroin (EMCDDA, 2023; Josep Rowntree Foundation, 2006). Drug consumptio rooms (DCRs) are facilities designed to provide supervised and hygienic environment for individuals to consume pre-obtained controlled drugs. Thes rooms are distinct from "crack houses" and "shooting galleries," which typically lack supervision an may involve the purchase of drugs on-site. Additionally, DCRs differ from places where prescribe heroin is consumed under supervision. The primar purpose of DCRs is harm reduction. By providin a supervised environment, DCRs aim to minimis the risks associated with drug consumption, such a overdose and transmission of infectious diseases lik HIV/AIDS and hepatitis.

Evidence suggests that DCRs do not increas drug use or the frequency of injecting. On the contrary, they serve as pathways to treatment facilities and help decrease local drug-related crim (ECMDDA, 2016). Thus, DCRs offer a harr reduction approach that effectively addresse public health concerns associated with substanc use disorder. Studies indicate that while the healt of people who inject drugs (PWID) typicall declines over time, DCRs or supervised injectio facilities (SIFs) have been effective in reducin injecting-related harms (Tran et al., 2021). Overall, DCRs/SIFs play a crucial role in mitigatin the negative health impacts associated with dru injecting, providing a supportive environment fc individuals seeking assistance and treatment fc their substance use.

The benefits and risks of prescribing heroin t treat opiate dependence are presented in Table 8.

Table 8.4
Benefits and risks of prescribing heroin to treat opiate use disorder

Benefits	Risks
• Engaging people who are not attracted by other treatments (such as methadone), and retaining them in treatment for longer. • Helping people stop or reduce their illicit heroin use. • Ensuring that people dependent on heroin can use a drug of known quality and strength. • Reducing health problems such as overdose or using unsafe injecting practices. • Reducing acquisitive crime to support drug habits. • Providing a stepping stone to a gradual change from heroin use to methadone, and from injecting to oral use.	• Prolonging the time that heroin users are drug-dependent and injecting by removing the motivation to stop using or injecting drugs. • Adverse health consequences as a result of continued heroin injecting, including risk of overdose, infections, abscesses, and blood-borne viruses. • Heroin users presenting for treatment coming to expect heroin, thus making other therapeutic interventions less attractive. • The potential for prescribed heroin being diverted into the illicit market.

Source: Adapted from Stimson and Metrebian (2001).

KEY POINTS

- The term *opiate* refers to any psychoactive substance of natural origin that has an effect similar to morphine.
- *Opioid* refers to synthetic substances derived from or resembling the substances in the poppy plant.
- There is a tradition in the UK to prescribe injectable methadone or injectable heroin to opiate addicts as treatment for their addition, and this approach is known as "The British System."
- The body responds to heroin in the brain by reducing (and sometimes stopping) production of the endogenous opioids (endorphins) when heroin is present.
- Some of the common opiate drugs are codeine, heroin (diacetylmorphine), pethidine, methadone, morphine, and diconal.
- The routes of administration for opiates are oral, subcutaneous, intramuscular, intravenous, rectal, transdermal, and transmucosal.
- Agonists stimulate opioid receptors and are agents that produce analgesia.
- An antagonist blocks an action and diminishes analgesia.
- Mixed agonists/antagonists have the functions to either stimulate some opioid receptors or block other receptors.
- Heroin is a fine white powder in its purest form and, depending on its form, can be smoked and/or injected.
- Illicit drugs are more commonly adulterated with benign substances such as sugars, quinine, and caffeine.
- The medical applications of opiates include effective relief of pain, treatment for diarrhoea and vomiting, and as a cough suppressant.
- Heroin is swallowed, smoked, sniffed, or injected either subcutaneously or intravenously.
- Many studies have provided clear evidence that some people are able to have controlled patterns of heroin use.
- Drug overdose is the leading cause of accidental death amongst opioid users.
- There are a number of risk factors associated with opioid overdose. Some are modifiable, and others are not modifiable.
- In moderate doses, opiates produce a range of generally mild physical effects apart from the analgesic effect. It induces euphoria, which may wear off, but its use is continuous to avoid withdrawal symptoms.
- Heroin dependence develops after repeated use over several weeks, and sudden withdrawal leads to anxiety, nausea, muscle pains, sweating, diarrhoea, and goose flesh.
- The withdrawal syndrome from heroin may become apparent 8 to 24 hours after the discontinuation of sustained use of the drug.
- Methadone maintenance is commonly used as a form of treatment for opiate addiction because it produces similar effects to heroin or morphine.
- Methadone is considered to be the best substitute drug for opiate-dependent drug users because it is easy to administer and long-acting.
- Heroin comes in various colours, names, origins, and purities.
- Drug overdose, primarily from opioids, is the leading cause of accidental death among opioid users.

- Individuals with opiate use disorder take extra methadone above the recommended dose or mix it with other depressants, alcohol, or even heroin, engaging in behaviour that is very dangerous and may result in overdose or death.
- *Drug consumption room* refers to any room specifically set up for the supervised, hygienic consumption of pre-obtained controlled drugs.
- Evidence suggests that DCRs do not increas drug use or the frequency of injecting. On th contrary, they serve as pathways to treatmen facilities and help decrease local drug-relate crime.
- There are benefits and risks of prescribing heroi to treat opiate use disorder.

References

Bart, G. (2012). Maintenance medication for opiate addiction: The foundation of recovery. *Journal of Addictive Diseases*, 31(3), 207–225. https://doi.org/10.1080/10550887.2012.694598.

Bobkov, A. F., Selimova, L. M., Khanina, T. A., Zverev, S. Y., Pokrovsky, V. V., Weber, J. N., Bobkov, E. N., & Rylkov, A. V. (2005). Human immunodeficiency virus type 1 in illicit-drug solutions used intravenously retains infectivity. *Journal of Clinical Microbiology*, 43(4), 1937–1939.

Carson, H. J., Knight, L. D., Dudley, M. H., & Garg, U. (2010). A fatality involving an unusual route of fentanyl delivery: Chewing and aspirating the transdermal patch. *Legal Medicine*, 12(3), 157159.

Chalabianloo, F., Fadnes, L. T., Høiseth, G., Ohldieck, C., Vold, J. H., Aas, C., Løberg, E. M., Johansson, K. A., & Bramness, J. G. (2021). Subjective symptoms and serum methadone concentrations: What should guide dose adjustments in methadone maintenance treatment? A naturalistic cohort study from Norway. *Substance Abuse Treatment, Prevention, and Policy*, 16(1), 39. https://doi.org/10.1186/s13011-021-00367-w.

Cole, C., Jones, L., McVeigh, J., Kicman, A., Syed, Q., & Bellis, M. A. (2011). Adulterants in illicit drugs: A review of empirical evidence. *Drug Testing and Analysis*, 3(2), 89–96. https://doi.org/10.1002/dta.220.

Dalefield, M. L., Scouller, B., Bibi, R., & Kivell, B. M. (2022). The kappa opioid receptor: A promising therapeutic target for multiple pathologies. *Frontiers in Pharmacology*, 13, 837671. https://doi.org/10.3389/fphar.2022.837671.

EMCDDA. (2022). *European Drug Report Trends and Development 2022*. Luxembourg: Publications Office of the European Union.

EMCDDA. (2023). *Spotlight on . . . Drug Consumption Rooms*. https://www.emcdda.europa.eu/spotlights/drug-consumption-rooms_en (accessed 15 February 2024).

Fareed, A., Casarella, J., Amar, R., Vayalapalli, S., & Drexler, K. (2010). Methadone maintenance dosing guideline for opioid dependence, a literature review. *Journal of Addictive Diseases*, 29(1), 1–14. https://doi.org/10.1080/10550880903436010.

Gyarmathy, V. A., Neaigus, A., Li, N., Ujhelyi, E., Caplinskiene, I., Caplinskas, S., & Latkin, C. A. (2010). Liquid drugs and high dead space syringes may keep HIV and HCV prevalence high – a comparison of Hungary and Lithuania. *European Addiction Research*, 16(4), 220–228. https://doi.org/10.1159/000320287.

ISMP. (2012). A top-10 list: Protecting young children from medicine mishaps. *Safe Medicine*, 10(6), 1–3.

Joseph Rowntree Foundation. (2006). *Drug Consumption Rooms – Summary Report of the Independent Working Group*. York: Joseph Rowntree Foundation.

Mattick, R. P., Breen, C., Kimber, J., & Davoli, M. (2009). Methadone maintenance therapy versus no opioid replacement therapy for opioid dependence. *The Cochrane Database of Systematic Reviews*, 2009(3), CD002209. https://doi.org/10.1002/14651858.CD002209.pub2.

Muller, A. E., Bjørnestad, R., & Clausen, T. (2018). Dissatisfaction with opioid maintenance treatment partly explains reported side effects of medications. *Drug and Alcohol Dependence*, 187, 22–28. https://doi.org/10.1016/j.drugalcdep.2018.02.018.

NIDA. (2018). *Principles of Drug Addiction Treatment. A Research-Based Guide* (3rd ed.). https://archives.nida.nih.gov/publications/principles-drug-addiction-treatment-research-based-guide-third-edition (accessed 14 February 2024).

Penington Institute. (2022). *Global Overdose Snapshot*. https://www.penington.org.au/overdose/overdose-projects-campaigns/global-overdose-snapshot/ (accessed 14 February 2024).

Rizo, J. (2018). Mechanism of neurotransmitter release coming into focus. *Protein Science: A Publication of the Protein Society*, 27(8), 1364–1391. https://doi.org/10.1002/pro.3445.

Shewan, D, & Dalgarno, P. (2005). Low levels of negative health and social outcomes among non-treatment heroin users in Glasgow (Scotland): Evidence for controlled heroin use? *British Journal of Health Psychology*, 10(1), 33–48.

Shewan, D., Dalgarno, P., Marshall, A., Lowe, E., Campbell, M., Nicholson, S., Reith, G., McLafferty, V., & Thomson, K. (1998). Patterns of heroin use among a non-treatment sample in Glasgow (Scotland). *Addiction Research*, 6(3), 215–234.

Stimson, G. V., & Metrebian, N. (2001). *Prescribing Heroin: What Is the Evidence?* London: Joseph Rowntree Foundation.

Tran, V., Reid, S. E., Roxburgh, A., & Day, C. A. (2021). Assessing drug consumption rooms and longer term (5 year) impacts on community and clients. *Risk Management and Healthcare Policy*, 14, 4639–4647. https://doi.org/10.2147/RMHP.S244720.

Uchtenhagen, A., Dobler-Mikola, A., Steffen, T., Gutzwiller, F., Blattler, R., & Pfeifer, S. (1999). *Prescription of Narcotics for*

Heroin Addicts: Main Results of the Swiss National Cohort Study (Vol. 1). Basel: Karger. https://doi.org/10.1159/isbn.978-3-318-00369-7.

UNDOC. (2022). *World Drug Report 2022*. Vienna: United Nations Office on Drugs and Crime.

Wakeman, S. E., Larochelle, M. R., Ameli, O., Chaisson, C. E., McPheeters, J. T., Crown, W. H., Azocar, F., & Sanghavi, D. M. (2020). Comparative effectiveness of different treatment pathways for opioid use disorder. *JAMA Network Open*, 3(2), e1920622. https://doi.org/10.1001/jamanetworkopen.2019.20622.

Warburton, H., Turnbull, P. J., & Hough, M. (2005). *Occasional and Controlled Heroin Use Not a Problem?* London: Joseph Rowntree Foundation. www.jrf.org.uk.

WHO. (2009). *Clinical Guidelines for Withdrawal Management and Treatment of Drug Dependence in Closed Settings*. Geneva: World Health Organization.

WHO. (2023). *Opioid Overdose*. https://www.who.int/newsroom/fact-sheets/detail/opioid-overdose (accessed 14 February 2024).

Wilder, C. M., Miller, S. C., Tiffany, E., Winhusen, T., Winstanley, E. L., & Stein, M. D. (2016). Risk factors for opioid overdose and awareness of overdose risk among veterans prescribed chronic opioids for addiction or pain. *Journal of Addictive Diseases*, 35(1), 42–51. http://doi.org/10.1080/10550887.2016.1107264.

Zinberg, N. E. (1984). *Drug, Set and Setting: The Basis for Controlled Intoxicant Use*. New Haven, CT and London: Yale University Press.

Chapter 9

Cannabis and synthetic cannabis

Learning outcomes

- Discuss the therapeutic and non-therapeutic uses of cannabis.
- Briefly describe the mechanism of action of cannabis.
- Describe cannabis effects on the different modes of administration.
- Discuss the sought-after effects of cannabis.
- Discuss the psychological and physical effects of cannabis.
- Discuss the effects of synthetic cannabis.
- Discuss cannabis as a gateway drug.
- List the symptoms of the amotivational syndrome

Activity 9.1

There is only one correct answer to the following multiple-choice questions.

1. What is THC?
   a. A cannabis cigarette
   b. The psychoactive ingredient in cannabis
   c. A cannabis pressure group in favour of legalisation
   d. Treatment for cannabis
   e. Amotivational syndrome
2. The effects of cannabis last for a maximum of how long?
   a. 14 hours
   b. 48 hours
   c. 4 hours
   d. 24 hours
   e. 36 hours

   A common form of cannabis is:
   a. Marijuana
   b. Hashish
   c. Hash oil
   d. Only a
   e. All of the above

DOI: 10.4324/9781003456674-1

3. What is the name of the active chemical in cannabis?
   a. Delta-9 ethanol dehydrogenase
   b. Delta-Fos-9
   c. Delta-9 tetrahydrocannabinol
   d. Delta gamma
   e. Alpha gamma
4. Which of the following statements is the truest?
   a. Cannabis has little effect on an ability to drive a car.
   b. Cannabis is less damaging on the ability to drive a car than alcohol is.
   c. It is safe to get in a car if the driver has been smoking cannabis.
   d. Cannabis impairs coordination and judgement, resulting in an inability to drive.
   e. None of the above is correct.
5. How does the risk of lung cancer for a cannabis smoker compare to a tobacco smoker's risk?
   a. Cannabis causes little risk of lung cancer.
   b. Cannabis contains more of the cancer-causing chemical benzopyrene than tobacco.
   c. Cannabis contains less of the cancer-causing chemical benzopyrene than tobacco.
   d. Cannabis contains the same amount of the cancer-causing chemical benzopyrene as tobacco.
   e. None of the above is correct.
6. Can cannabis use affect your mental health?
   a. No.
   b. Yes.
   c. A risk factor, especially if predisposed to schizophrenia.
   d. If you take another psychoactive substance.
   e. All of the above are correct.
7. How does cannabis affect the brain?
   a. THC affects memory and learning.
   b. Changes in the sensory information processing.
   c. The information processing centre of the brain is suppressed.
   d. All of the above.
   e. Only a and b are correct.
8. Cannabis is:
   a. Physically addictive
   b. Psychologically addictive
   c. More addictive than tobacco
   d. More addictive than alcohol
   e. None of the above
9. Cannabis:
   a. Is a gateway drug
   b. Is not a gateway drug
   c. Leads to heroin use
   d. Leads to dependence
   e. None of the above
10. Cannabis is:
   a. A central nervous system stimulant
   b. A central nervous system depressant
   c. Not an appetite stimulant
   d. Not a bronchodilator
   e. A stimulant and hallucinogen

11. When cannabis is smoked:
    a. The onset of the effect takes between 1 and 2 hours.
    b. The onset of the effect takes between 2 and 3 hours.
    c. The onset of the effect is almost immediate.
    d. The onset of the effect may last several hours.
    e. None of the above is correct.
12. Large doses of potent cannabis:
    a. When swallowed, can cause "toxic psychosis"
    b. When smoked, can cause "toxic psychosis"
    c. Raises the blood pressure
    d. Decreases the risk of heart attack
    e. Only a and d are correct
13. Research suggests that:
    a. There is a link between cannabis use and pregnancy.
    b. Cannabis smoke contains less chemicals than tobacco.
    c. Cannabis does not affect the foetus.
    d. There is no link between cannabis use and pregnancy.
    e. None of the above is correct.
14. The scientific name for cannabis is . . .
    a. Cannabis sativa
    b. Cannabis
    c. Candy floss
    d. Cannabis B
    e. CBD
15. The majority of young people who enter drug treatment have problems associated with:
    a. Cocaine
    b. Heroin
    c. Ecstasy
    d. Cannabis
    e. Alcohol
16. The chemical in cannabis that causes the user to feel "high" is:
    a. Dopamine
    b. *Cannabis sativa*
    c. Tetrahydrocannabinol (THC)
    d. Serotonin
    e. Acetylcholine
17. THC, the active ingredient in marijuana, acts on the brain by:
    a. Coating the nervous system
    b. Binding to specific receptors
    c. Causing brain tissue to grow
    d. Decreasing fat tissue in the brain
    e. None of the above
18. Memory problems associated with marijuana use are due to THC's actions in which part of the brain?
    a. Cerebellum
    b. Hippocampus
    c. Cerebrum
    d. Basal ganglia
    e. None of the above

19. Cannabis affects the brain function of first-time users differently than it does experienced users because:
    a. It causes a decrease in blood flow to the brain.
    b. It causes an increase in blood flow to the brain.
    c. It affects different parts of the nervous system.
    d. It affects some parts of the nervous system.
    e. None of the above.
20. Which statement is true?
    a. Men are more likely than women to become daily users of cannabis.
    b. Women are more likely than men to become daily users of cannabis.
    c. There is no difference between the prevalence rates of women and men.
    d. Cannabis is healthier than tobacco.
    e. None of the above is correct.

INTRODUCTION

Globally, cannabis is by far the most widely cultivated, trafficked, and abused illicit drug. Cannabis legalisation in parts of the world appears to have accelerated daily use and related health impacts, according to the UN Office on Drugs and Crime (UNODC, 2022). Cannabis, derived from the Indian hemp plant, holds the distinction of being the most commonly used psychoactive substance globally. It boasts a rich history of medicinal, recreational, and industrial applications. The plant's various parts, including the flowers, have been utilised to create a wide array of products. Industrially, the fibrous stalks are prized for producing textiles like clothing and durable rope. The term *marijuana* is widely used in American culture, though it originated from the Spanish word "marijhuana" to associate the plant with Mexican immigrants and reinforce negative connotations (Serrano, 2013). Despite its different forms of consumption, cannabis remains a popular relaxant or mild intoxicant among users. There exist over 200 slang terms for cannabis, reflecting its widespread presence in society. These street names vary across regions and countries, illustrating the diversity of cannabis culture. Some of the popular monikers include "ganja," "pot," "weed," and "hashish." Additionally, names may be influenced by the geographic origin of the product, such as "Afghan" or "Moroccan." The sheer breadth of slang terms highlights the global use of cannabis.

Cannabis, derived from the bushy plant *Cannabis sativa*, contains psychoactive substances primarily found in the flowers, notably THC (Δ9-delta-9-tetrahydrocannabinol) and CBD (cannabidiol). THC is the principal active chemical in cannabis, and the plant contains around 60 different cannabinoids. While THC is concentrated in the flowers, seeds, leaves, and stems contain fewer psychoactive elements. Cannabidiol (CBD) is a non-intoxicating cannabis compound known for its medicinal benefits, including anti-seizure, antioxidant, neuroprotective, anti-inflammatory, analgesic, anti-tumour, anti-psychotic, and anti-anxiety properties. CBD can also counteract the psychoactive effects of THC, making it a significant component in medical cannabis treatments (NIDA, 2015). Hashish, a potent form of cannabis, boasts a higher THC content than regular marijuana, resulting in a stronger effect. However, it also contains higher levels of CBD, which can alter or mitigate the impact of THC. Produced from resinous trichomes on cannabis plants, hashish is compressed into blocks, sticks, or balls. Hash oil, another variant, ranges in colour from amber to dark brown and is applied in small quantities to cigarettes before smoking. Varieties like "skunk" are distinguished by their strong odour, while "sinsemilla" refers to seedless buds cultivated without male plants. "Netherweed" contains two to three times the typical amount of THC, enhancing its potency.

The illicit cultivation of cannabis mainly yields two products: herbal cannabis (also known as marijuana) and cannabis resin (also known as hashish or charas) (EMCDDA, 2022). Based on data provided by various international organisations, several countries stand out as major cultivators of marijuana plants. Morocco leads as the largest producer of psychoactive marijuana plants, particularly concentrated in the Rif region. Mexico, with a long-standing tradition in cannabis cultivation, is poised to become a significant producer following recent regulatory changes. Afghanistan, known for its hashish production, has a history of cannabis cultivation but has been surpassed by other countries. Paraguay is recognised as the largest producer of pressed marijuana, exporting to South America and legally exporting medical cannabis to various countries. India is the largest producer of *charas*, a type of hashish. Cannabis is usually retailed in ounces (28 grams) or fractions of ounces: 1/4 ounce (7 grams), 1/2 ounce (14 grams). Generally, about 1/2 a gram of resin is used to make a couple of joints. The retail price around the world varies depending on whether it is sold in herbal (grass) or resin form.

Cannabis is commonly consumed through smoking, often rolled into cigarettes, known as joints, and sometimes mixed with tobacco. Pipes or bongs are also used for smoking cannabis. Smoking offers rapid effects and dose regulation. Cannabis is also found in blunts, which are cigars emptied of tobacco and filled with cannabis or rolled with tobacco paper. Vaping cannabis involves using vaporisers or e-cigarettes with raw cannabis or THC oil, offering alternative consumption methods for oils, waxes, and dry herbs. A variation known as "dabbing" involves vaping concentrated cannabis extracts like butane hash oil, honey oil, wax, budder, or shatter (Al-Zouabi et al., 2018). These methods offer an alternative to traditional smoking and allow users to inhale cannabis without combustion, potentially reducing harmful by-products associated with smoking. Smoking marijuana is harmful to health due to the release of carbon monoxide and other harmful by-products during combustion, which can damage the respiratory system. It is reported that cannabis users perceive vaporisation as a safer alternative to smoking (Lee et al., 2016). There is evidence for harm reduction potential for cannabis vaping. Using cannabis vaporisers can decrease carbon monoxide emissions, chronic respiratory symptoms, and exposure to toxins compared to smoking cannabis, while maintaining similar subjective effects and blood THC concentration (Chaiton et al., 2022). Alternatively, cannabis can be consumed in various forms, such as edibles, like space brownies, cookies, or muffin made with hashish. Some users also brew cannabi tea or prepare cannabis-infused drinks.

MECHANISM OF ACTION

Cannabis contains two primary active ingredient THC and CBD, both classified as cannabinoid These substances interact with abundant receptor throughout the brain and body, producing psycho active effects. The brain naturally produces its ow cannabinoid, anandamide, which plays roles in pai sensation, immune system regulation, and memor THC is absorbed into the bloodstream through th lungs (if smoked) or the stomach and intestines (i eaten), and it distributes to areas high in fat conten such as the brain and testes. Physiologically, TH acts as a hypno-sedative, anti-convulsant, and anal gesic. When THC is consumed orally, the onset c effects typically occurs between one and two hour lasting around four hours, but may lead to unwante psychedelic experiences. Inhaled cannabis enters th bloodstream more quickly than ingested forms. Syn thetic cannabinoids, which act on the same recep tors as THC, may have stronger binding capabiliti and produce more potent effects (NIDA, 2015 However, their effects on behaviour can be unpre dictable and may result in fatal poisonings.

LEGAL STATUS

Cannabis was prohibited in Britain in 1925 due to i association with "harder" drugs like heroin and opiu within the International Opium Convention. How ever, in recent times, many developed and developin nations have been flouting or hesitating to enforc UN conventions prohibiting cannabis use, posse sion, and supply. Different countries have establishe their own regulations regarding cannabis, includin allowances for small-scale recreational and medic use. Uruguay became the first country to legalis the sale, cultivation, and distribution of cannabi Malta has become the first EU country to legalis the cultivation and personal use of cannabis. Whil some nations have adopted more lenient stances o cannabis, the majority of countries worldwide sti consider its cultivation, production, supply, storag possession, or smoking to be criminal offenses. Th complex issues surrounding cannabis legalisation an decriminalisation are explored further in Chapter 6

THERAPEUTIC USE

Therapeutic use of cannabis involves utilising its components, primarily THC and CBD, for medical purposes. It serves as an appetite stimulant for patients experiencing anorexia due to conditions like HIV/AIDS or cancer. Additionally, it functions as an antiemetic agent, relieving severe nausea and vomiting induced by chemotherapy. Cannabis also acts as an analgesic, alleviating pain associated with conditions such as cancer or neuropathy. Moreover, it serves as a muscle relaxant, aiding in the management of spasticity caused by multiple sclerosis (Pagano et al., 2022) or spinal cord injury, and as an anticonvulsant to reduce seizures in treatment-resistant epilepsy among children and young adults. Furthermore, cannabis has shown potential in lowering intraocular pressure in glaucoma patients. Synthetic cannabis extracts have been explored as therapeutic options for Alzheimer's disease, with evidence suggesting that small doses of THC may slow the production of beta-amyloid proteins, associated with the progression of Alzheimer's (Cao et al., 2014). The therapeutic use of cannabis remains a topic of ongoing research and debate. While some studies suggest potential benefits, others highlight concerns about side effects, long-term safety, and the risk of dependence.

SOUGHT-AFTER EFFECTS

Cannabis users commonly experience desired effects, such as talkativeness, cheerfulness, relaxation, and enhanced appreciation of sound and colour. Smoking cannabis initially induces relaxation and a mellow feeling, often accompanied by haziness and light-headedness. Users may become more attuned to their senses, commonly referred to as being "high" or "stoned." Notably, cannabis is renowned for stimulating appetite, leading to cravings for sweet food, a phenomenon known as "getting the munchies." Evidence suggests that cannabis increases both the desire to eat and the palatability of food (Kirkham, 2009).

SHORT-TERM USE

The active chemical in cannabis typically ceases to have noticeable effects after about four hours, but traces can linger in urine and hair for much longer periods. Cannabis reduces blood pressure, inducing intense relaxation, while increasing heart rate, potentially leading to feelings of paranoia or panic. Common effects include talkativeness, laughter, relaxation, and heightened sensitivity to sound and colour. Unlike alcohol, cannabis does not cause hangovers. However, it impairs concentration and manual dexterity, making tasks like driving hazardous. The onset of effects occurs within minutes of smoking and lasts for one to several hours, depending on dosage. Expectations, motivation, and mood influence the user's experience. While short-term effects are not inherently dangerous and may dissipate in a relaxed setting with low cannabis consumption, there is a risk of triggering mental health issues.

LONG-TERM USE

Cannabis use alongside tobacco significantly impacts heart and lung health, potentially leading to bronchitis, respiratory issues, and increased risk of lung cancer due to high concentrations of cancer-causing agents like benzopyrene. Individuals with respiratory or heart disorders face heightened risks with cannabis use. Additionally, cannabis can exacerbate asthma and pose risks for those with cardiovascular problems. Research indicates that THC, the active component in cannabis, can impair immune system function at high doses. Regular cannabis use may reduce sperm count in men, suppress ovulation in women, and potentially affect foetal development during pregnancy, leading to cognitive issues in children. While cannabis can alleviate muscle spasms, it can also cause short-term memory problems by interfering with the hippocampus, impacting memory function. Some users may experience temporary hallucinations and delusions, resolving within hours or days.

Substantial evidence from both animal research and human studies suggests that exposure to marijuana during development can lead to long-term or potentially permanent adverse changes in the brain (NIDA, 2023a). This indicates that the developing brain is particularly vulnerable to the effects of marijuana, and exposure during this critical period can alter brain structure, function, and development. These changes may have implications for cognitive function, emotional regulation, and behaviour later in life. The causal relationship between chronic cannabis use and psychiatric disorders has been an area of interest. Considerable debate has been whether cannabis use causes psychotic symptoms and whether cannabis use may precipitate psychosis in predisposing individuals to acquire a psychotic disorder. Frequent and prolonged cannabis use can have detrimental effects on mental and physical health. Chronic use is associated with mood disorders, exacerbation of psychotic disorders, cannabis use disorders, withdrawal syndrome, neurocognitive impairments, and cardiovascular and respiratory diseases (Karila et al., 2014). The review conducted by Radhakrishnan et al. (2014) suggests that cannabis may act as a contributing factor in the development of psychosis, particularly in individuals with pre-existing genetic or other vulnerabilities. This implies that while cannabis use itself may not directly cause psychosis in all individuals, it can potentially interact with underlying genetic or environmental factors to increase the risk of psychosis emerging.

Di Forti et al. (2012) conducted a study indicating that cannabis users carrying a specific variant of the AKT1 gene (rs2494732) have a significantly higher risk of developing psychotic disorders, particularly among daily cannabis users, compared to infrequent or non-users. However, the relationship between cannabis use and symptoms of mood and anxiety disorders remains inconclusive. Lai et al. (2015) conducted a systematic review and meta-analysis, revealing a significant association between substance use disorder and comorbid mood disorders, with depression being the most prominently correlated, followed by anxiety. On the contrary, Danielsson et al. (2016) found no statistically significant relationship between depression and subsequent cannabis use, or vice versa. Despite efforts to control confounding variables, various studies have shown mixed results, with some indicating a reduction in the relationship between cannabis use and mood disorders, while others suggest a strengthen ing. Troup et al. (2016) emphasised the difficult in drawing conclusions from large-scale studies du to vast differences in cannabis use patterns and cul tural factors surrounding cannabis.

Heavy users of cannabis, especially those wit personality disturbances or psychiatric issues, ma experience temporary exacerbation of symptom perceptual distortions, and heightened anxiety c panic if used during anxious or depressive state Regular use, particularly of potent varieties, like cer tain forms of skunk, can lead to psychotic symptom Long-term effects of cannabis use remain debate due to the scarcity of large longitudinal studies, bu research indicates significant abnormalities in ke brain regions related to emotion and motivatio among young adult recreational users (Gilman et al 2014). While physical dependence on cannabis uncommon, regular use may create a psychologic dependence, with some individuals relying on it as social lubricant. Cannabis withdrawal is a well-docu mented phenomenon observed in about half of reg ular and dependent cannabis users following sudde cessation or substantial reduction in THC-containin cannabis products (Connor et al., 2022). The clinic importance of cannabis withdrawal lies in its poter tial to trigger relapse to cannabis use. Individua with concurrent mental health issues and polysul stance use may experience complicated withdrawa This highlights the need for comprehensive unde standing and management of withdrawal sympton to support individuals in their efforts to discontinu cannabis use effectively. Table 9.1 provides summa ries of the acute and long-term effects of cannabis.

Table 9.1
Acute and long-term effects of cannabis

Acute effects (intoxication)	Long-term effects
• Pleasant feeling of relaxed euphoria	• Impaired learning and coordination
• Heightening or alteration of the senses	• Sleep problems
• Reddening of the conjunctivae of the eyes	• Potential for marijuana addiction
• Reduction in body temperature	• Impairments in learning and memory, with potential loss of IQ
• Increased heart rate and blood pressure	• Increased risk of chronic cough, bronchitis
• Impaired short-term memory	• Increased risk of other drug and alcohol use disorders
• Impaired coordination and balance	• Increased risk of schizophrenia in people with genetic vulnerability
• Anxiety, paranoia, and panic reactions (some users)	• Mood disorders
• Psychosis (at high doses)	• Exacerbation of psychotic disorders in vulnerable people
• Impaired attention, judgement, and other cognitive functions	• Neurocognitive impairments

SYNTHETIC CANNABIS (CANNABINOIDS)

Synthetic cannabinoids, also known as synthetic cannabis, are psychoactive (mind-altering) substances designed to mimic or produce similar effects to cannabis. Synthetic cannabinoids are included in a group of drugs called "new psychoactive substances" (NPS). Synthetic cannabis products are marketed under different brand names and are often labelled "not for human consumption." They have various brand names, including Spice, K2, Black Mamba, and AK-47, among others. There are a variety of herbal "incense" that can be smoked, or liquid "incense" that can be used in vaporisers and e-cigarettes. Some of the newer substances marketed as synthetic cannabis fail to accurately replicate the effects of THC (delta-9-tetrahydrocannabinol), the active compound in natural cannabis. The packaging of synthetic cannabinoids can be misleading, often labelled as "herbal" despite containing synthetic psychoactive materials (Alcohol & Drug Research Foundation, 2023). Ingredient lists may be incomplete or inaccurate, heightening the risk of overdose. Additionally, chemical compositions tend to differ between batches, leading to varying effects even with identical packaging. These inconsistencies underline the dangers associated with the consumption of synthetic cannabinoids and highlight the need for increased awareness and regulation in their production and distribution.

It is essential to note that the composition of synthetic cannabinoids can change rapidly as manufacturers alter their chemical formulas to evade legal restrictions. Consequently, the dangers associated with these substances are often heightened due to the lack of quality control and consistency in their production. Due to their chemical variability and unpredictability, synthetic cannabinoids pose significant health risks and have been associated with numerous adverse effects, including seizures, psychosis, and even death in some cases (see Table 9.2).

Table 9.2
Physical and psychological effects of synthetic cannabinoids

Physical effects	
Increased heart rate	Palpitations and chest pain
Elevated blood pressure	Hypertension and associated complications
Nausea and vomiting	
Dizziness and loss of coordination	Increased risk of accidents and injuries
Respiratory issues	Difficulty breathing or respiratory depression
Headaches	Headaches and migraines
Seizures (in severe cases)	Triggers seizures, posing a significant health risk
Cardiovascular disease	Prolong use may increase risk of cardiovascular disease (Davidson et al., 2017; Pacher et al., 2018)
Other	Acute kidney injury, abdominal pain, miosis, mydriasis, xerostomia, hyperthermia, fatigue, rhabdomyolysis (Cohen & Weinstein, 2018b)
Psychological effects	
Anxiety and panic attacks	Intense feelings of anxiety and panic, which may be accompanied by paranoia and hallucinations
Depersonalisation	For some users, experience of a sense of detachment from reality, or depersonalisation
Impaired cognition	Impaired cognitive function, leading to confusion, disorientation, and difficulty concentrating; executive function deficits of working memory and attention (Cohen & Weinstein, 2018a)
Mood swings	May experience rapid and unpredictable changes in mood, ranging from euphoria to dysphoria; negative mood, manic behaviour, depression, and suicidal ideation (Cohen & Weinstein, 2018a)
Addiction	High potential for addiction and dependence, leading to compulsive drug-seeking behaviour and withdrawal symptoms upon cessation
Psychosis	In high doses (synthetic cannabinoids), can lead to psychotic symptoms, including delusions, catatonia, paranoia, auditory and visual hallucinations, and perceptual alterations (Cohen & Weinstein, 2018b; Seely et al., 2012; Tournebize et al., 2017)

CANNABIS AS A GATEWAY DRUG

The debate over the causal relationship between cannabis use and the subsequent use of harder drugs, as proposed by the "gateway theory," continues. Some research suggests that marijuana use is likely to precede use of other licit and illicit substances (Secades-Villa et al., 2015) and the development of addiction to other substances. While people who smoke cannabis are more likely to use other drugs, it is also observed that those who smoke tobacco and drink are more prone to trying cannabis. Fergusson et al. (2006) found that regular or heavy cannabis use is associated with an increased risk of using and becoming dependent on other illicit drugs, supporting the gateway hypothesis. However, the exact causal mechanisms underlying this relationship remain unclear. Nkansah-Amankra and Minelli (2016) suggest that tobacco smoking may be a better predictor of concurrent illicit hard drug use than cannabis. Additionally, factors such as age, wealth, employment status, and psychological stress have been identified as contributors to the "gateway" phenomenon (Van Gundy & Rebellon, 2010). The RAND Study (Morral et al., 2002) highlights that associations between cannabis and hard drug use may exist even without a direct gateway effect. Instead, differences in the ages of cannabis and hard drug use initiation, as well as variations in individuals' willingness to experiment with drugs, could contribute to these associations. The notion of marijuana serving as a "gateway drug" is supported by research findings; however, it is essential to note that most cannabis users do not progress to using other, more potent substances (NIDA, 2023b). Additionally, cross-sensitisation, where exposure to one substance increases sensitivity to another, is not exclusive to cannabis. In summary, while cannabis may be associated with a progression to other substances in some cases, the majority of users do not transition to harder drugs, and cross-sensitisation occurs with substances beyond marijuana.

AMOTIVATIONAL SYNDROME

The concept of amotivational syndrome in relation to the long-term effects of cannabis remains a controversial entity in the literature. *Amotivational syndrome* is "a behaviour pattern characterised by loss of drive and initiative" (APA, 2018). According to the World Health Organization, amotivational syndrome is characterised by a collection of features linked to substance use, including apathy, decreased effectiveness, reduced ability to execute complex or long-term plans, low tolerance for frustration, impaired concentration, and difficulty in maintaining routines. These symptoms collectively contribute to a lack of drive and engagement in goal-directed activities, impacting various aspects of daily life, including work, school, and social interactions. These symptoms collectively contribute to a diminished motivation and engagement in goal-directed activities, often associated with substance use.

The existence of this condition is controversial. While cannabis use has been historically associated with amotivational syndrome, research on the direct causal relationship remains inconclusive. Research findings indicate that cannabis intake, but not alcohol or tobacco use, is significantly associated with decreased initiative and persistence over time (Lac & Luk, 2018). This suggests that cannabis use may uniquely contribute to reduced motivation and engagement in goal-directed activities, supporting the concept of the cannabis amotivational syndrome. Other factors, such as personality traits, co-occurring mental health disorders, and environmental influences, may contribute to the development of amotivational symptoms.

KEY POINTS

- Cannabis is the most commonly used psychoactive substance in the world and has a long history of medicinal, recreational, and industrial use.
- *Cannabis sativa*, and the part that contains the "psychoactive" substance, is found primarily in the flowers (buds) due to the presence of the cannabinoid substances THC (Δ^{9}- delta-9-tetrahydrocannabinol) and CBD (cannabidiol).
- Herbal cannabis, also known as marijuana or grass, is a weaker preparation of dried plant material.
- Taking oral cannabis may produce undesired psychedelic experiences. Cannabis that is inhaled gets into the bloodstream quicker than when eaten.
- Vaping cannabis is done by placing raw cannabis or THC oil in a vaporiser or e-cigarette.
- Synthetic cannabinoids are psychoactive (mind-altering) substances designed to mimic or produce similar effects to cannabis.

- The physiological properties of THC: acts like hypno-sedative, has an anti-convulsant activity, and is an analgesia.
- Currently, several developed and developing countries in which UN conventions prohibit the use, possession, and supply of cannabis are being increasingly flouted or are reluctant to enforce the convention.
- Cannabis is currently used as a therapeutic product throughout the world.
- The active chemical in cannabis will normally stop having an effect after about four hours.
- Cannabis lowers the blood pressure, which is why some users experience an intense feeling of relaxation.
- Considerable debate has been whether cannabis use causes psychotic symptoms and whether cannabis use may precipitate psychosis in individuals predisposed to acquiring a psychotic disorder.
- On the basis of current research, cannabis cannot be said to provide as clear a withdrawal pattern as other drugs of misuse, such as opiates.
- Generally, people who smoke cannabis are more likely to use other drugs, and people who smoke tobacco and drink are also more likely to try cannabis.
- *A motivational syndrome* is a constellation of features said to be associated with substance use, including apathy, loss of effectiveness, diminished capacity to carry out complex or long-term plans, low tolerance for frustration, impaired concentration, and difficulty in following routines.

Activity 9.2

Questions

- What are the therapeutic uses of cannabis?
- What experiences are sought after by users of cannabis?
- List the short-term effects of cannabis.
- List the long-term effects of cannabis.
- What are the physical and psychological effects of synthetic cannabinoids?
- What is meant by "gateway drug"?
- What is "amotivational syndrome"?

References

Alcohol and Drug Research Foundation (2023). *Synthetic Cannabinoids*. https://adf.org.au/drug-facts/synthetic-cannabinoids/ (accessed 15 February 2024).

Al-Zouabi, I., Stogner, J. M., Miller, B. L., & Lane, E. S. (2018). Butane hash oil and dabbing: Insights into use, amateur production techniques, and potential harm mitigation. *Substance Abuse and Rehabilitation*, 9, 91–101. https://doi.org/10.2147/SAR.S135252.

American Psychological Association (APA). (2018). *APA Dictionary of Psychology*. https://dictionary.apa.org/amotivational-syndrome (accessed 4 March 2024).

Cao, C., Li, Y., Liu, H., Bai, G., Mal, J., Lin, X., Sutherland, K., Nabar, N., & Cai, J. (2014). The potential therapeutic effects of THC on Alzheimer's disease. *Journal of Alzheimer's Disease, 42*(3), 973–984.

Chaiton, M., Kundu, A., Rueda, S., & Di Ciano, P. (2022). Are vaporizers a lower-risk alternative to smoking cannabis? *Canadian Journal of Public Health = Revue Canadienne de Sante Publique,* 113(2), 293–296. https://doi.org/10.17269/s41997-021-00565-w.

Cohen, K., & Weinstein, A. M. (2018a). Synthetic and non-synthetic cannabinoid drugs and their adverse effects – a review from public health prospective. *Frontiers in Public Health, 6,* 162. https://doi.org/10.3389/fpubh.2018.00162.

Cohen, K., & Weinstein, A. (2018b). The Effects of cannabinoids on executive functions: Evidence from cannabis and synthetic cannabinoids – a systematic review. *Brain Sciences,* 8(3), 40. https://doi.org/10.3390/brainsci8030040.

Connor, J. P., Stjepanović, D., Budney, A. J., Le Foll, B., & Hall, W. D. (2022). Clinical management of cannabis withdrawal. *Addiction,* 117(7), 2075–2095. https://doi.org/10.1111/add.15743.

Danielsson, A.-K., Lundin, A., Allebeck, P., & Agardh, E. (2016). Cannabis use and psychological distress: An 8-year prospective population-based study among Swedish men and women. *Addictive Behaviors, 59,* 18–23. https://doi.org/10.1016/j.addbeh.2016.03.005.

Davidson, C., Opacka-Juffry, J., Arevalo-Martin, A., Garcia-Ovejero, D., Molina-Holgado, E., & Molina-Holgado, F. (2017). Spicing up pharmacology: A review of synthetic cannabinoids from structure to adverse events. *Advances in Pharmacology (San Diego, Calif.)*, 80, 135–168. https://doi.org/10.1016/bs.apha.2017.05.001.

Di Forti, M., Iyegbe, C., Sallis, H., Kolliakou, A., Falcone, M. A., Paparelli, A., Sirianni, M., La Cascia, C., Stilo, S. A., Marques, T. R., Handley, R., Mondelli, V., Dazzan, P., Pariante, C., David, A. S., Morgan, C., Powell, J., & Murray, R. M. (2012). Confirmation that the AKT1 (rs2494732) genotype influences the risk of psychosis in cannabis users. *Biological Psychiatry*, 72(10), 811–816. https://doi.org/10.1016/j.biopsych.2012.06.020.

EMCDDA (European Monitoring Centre for Drugs and Drug Addiction and Europol). (2022). EU Drug Market: Cannabis-In-Depth Analysis. https://www.emcdda.europa.eu/publications/eu-drug-markets/cannabis_en (accessed 15 February 2024).

Fergusson, D. M., Boden, J. M., & Horwood, L. J. (2006). Cannabis use and other illicit drug use: Testing the cannabis gateway hypothesis. *Addiction*, 101(4), 556–569. https://doi.org/10.1111/j.1360-0443.2005.01322.x

Gilman, J. M., Kuster, J. K., Lee, S., Lee, M. J., Kim, B. W., Makris, N., van der Kouwe, A., Blood, A. J., & Breiter, H. C. (2014). Cannabis use is quantitatively associated with nucleus accumbens and amygdala abnormalities in young adult recreational users. *Journal of Neuroscience*, 34(16), 5529–5538. https://doi.org/10.1523/JNEUROSCI.4745–4713.2014.

Karila, L., Roux, P., Rolland, B., Benyamina, A., Reynaud, M., Aubin, H. J., & Lançon, C. (2014). Acute and long-term effects of cannabis use: A review. *Current Pharmaceutical Design*, 20(25), 4112–4118. https://doi.org/10.2174/13816128113199990620.

Kirkham, T. C. (2009). Cannabinoids and appetite: Food craving and food pleasure. *International Review of Psychiatry*, 21(2), 163–171.

Lac, A., & Luk, J. W. (2018). Testing the amotivational syndrome: Marijuana use longitudinally predicts lower self-efficacy even after controlling for demographics, personality, and alcohol and cigarette use. *Prevention Science: The Official Journal of the Society for Prevention Research*, 19(2), 117–126. https://doi.org/10.1007/s11121-017-0811-3.

Lai, H. M., Cleary, M., Sitharthan, T., & Hunt, G. E. (2015). Prevalence of comorbid substance use, anxiety and mood disorders in epidemiological surveys, 1990–2014: A systematic review and meta-analysis. *Drug and Alcohol Dependence*, 154, 1–13. https://doi.org/10.1016/j.drugalcdep.2015.05.03.

Lee, D. C., Crosier, B. S., Borodovsky, J. T., Sargent, J. D., & Budney, A. J. (2016). Online survey characterizing vaporizer use among cannabis users. *Drug and Alcohol Dependence*, 159, 227–233. https://doi.org/10.1016/j.drugalcdep.2015.12.020.

Morral, A. R., McCaffrey, D. F., & Paddock, S. M. (2002). Reassessing the marijuana gateway effect. *Addiction*, 97(12), 1493–1504. https://doi.org/10.1046/j.1360-0443.2002.00280.x.

NIDA. (2015). *The Biology and Potential Therapeutic Effects of Cannabidiol*. https://archives.nida.nih.gov/about-nida/legislative-activities/testimony-to-congress/2015/the-biology-and-potential-therapeutic-effects-of-cannabidiol (accesse 15 February 2024).

NIDA. (2023a). *What Are Marijuana's Long-Term Effects o the Brain?* https://nida.nih.gov/publications/research-reports/marijuana/what-are-marijuanas-long-term-effects-brai (accessed 4 March 2024).

NIDA. (2023b). *Is Marijuana a Gateway Drug?* https://nidc nih.gov/publications/research-reports/marijuana/mariju na-gateway-drug (accessed 4 March 2024).

Nkansah-Amankra, S., & Minelli, M. (2016). "Gateway hypot esis" and early drug use: Additional findings from trackin a population-based sample of adolescents to adulthooc *Preventive Medicine Reports*, 4, 134–141. https://do org/10.1016/j.pmedr.2016.05.003.

Pacher, P., Steffens, S., Haskó, G., Schindler, T. H., & Kuno G. (2018). Cardiovascular effects of marijuana and sy thetic cannabinoids: The good, the bad, and the ugl *Nature Reviews. Cardiology*, 15(3), 151–166. https://do org/10.1038/nrcardio.2017.130.

Pagano, C., Navarra, G., Coppola, L., Avilia, G., Bifulco, M & Laezza, C. (2022). Cannabinoids: Therapeutic use in cli ical practice. *International Journal of Molecular Science* 23(6), 3344. https://doi.org/10.3390/ijms23063344.

Radhakrishnan, R., Wilkinson, S. T., & D'Souza, D. C. (2014 Gone to pot – a review of the association between cannab and psychosis. *Frontiers in Psychiatry*, 5, 54. https://do org/10.3389/fpsyt.2014.00054.

Secades-Villa, R., Garcia-Rodríguez, O., Jin, C. J., Wang, S., Blanco, C. (2015). Probability and predictors of the cannab gateway effect: A national study. *The International Journal c Drug Policy*, 26(2), 135–142. https://doi.org/10.1016/drugpo.2014.07.011.

Seely, K. A., Lapoint, J., Moran, J. H., & Fattore, L. (2012 Spice drugs are more than harmless herbal blends: A revie of the pharmacology and toxicology of synthetic cannak noids. *Progress in Neuro-Psychopharmacology & Biologic Psychiatry*, 39(2), 234–243. https://doi.org/10.1016/pnpbp.2012.04.017.

Serrano, A. (2013). *Weed All About It: The Origins of th Word "Marijuana"*. http://america.aljazeera.com/ar cles/2013/12/14/weed-all-about-ittheoriginsofthewordan arijuanaaintheus.html (accessed 15 February 2024).

Tournebize, J., Gibaja, V., & Kahn, J. P. (2017). Acute effec of synthetic cannabinoids: Update 2015. *Substance Abus* 38(3), 344–366. https://doi.org/10.1080/08897077.2 16.1219438.

Troup, L. J., Andrzejewski, J. A., Braunwalder, J. T., & Torrenc R. D. (2016). The relationship between cannabis use ar measures of anxiety and depression in a sample of cc lege campus cannabis users and non-users post state legc ization in Colorado. *Peer Journal*, 4, e2782. https://do org/10.7717/peerj.2782.

UNDOC. (2022). *World Drug Report, 2022*. Vienna: Unite Nations Office on Drugs and Crime, United Natio Publication.

Van Gundy, K., & Rebellon, C. J. (2010). A life-course perspecti on the "gateway hypothesis". *Journal of Health and Soci Behavior*, 51(3), 244–259. https://doi.org/10.1177/0022 46510378238.

Chapter 10

Stimulants

Amphetamines, cocaine, and khat

Learning outcomes

- Discuss the therapeutic and non-therapeutic uses of amphetamine.
- Briefly describe the mechanism of action of stimulants.
- Describe amphetamine effects on the different modes of administration.
- Discuss the sought-after effects of stimulants.
- Discuss the psychological and physical effects of amphetamines and cocaine.
- List the withdrawal symptoms of amphetamine.
- List the withdrawal symptoms of cocaine.
- Discuss the phases in cocaine withdrawal.
- Discuss the physiological and psychological effects of khat.
- Discuss the effects of synthetic cathinones.
- Discuss the effects of synthetic stimulants

INTRODUCTION

Stimulants encompass a range of psychoactive substances known for increasing activity within various parts of the central nervous system or directly enhancing muscle activity. Commonly referred to as "uppers," stimulants are available in various forms, including legal and illegal varieties. They go by various street names, such as bennies, black beauties, coke, crystal, and speed. Available in synthetic powders, tablets, and capsules, stimulants can be legal or illegal. Legal stimulants such as caffeine, found in tea, coffee, and chocolate, are relatively mild and cause stimulation of the central nervous system, promoting alertness while reducing drowsiness. Nicotine, present in tobacco products, is another legal stimulant. In the past, amphetamines were widely prescribed in the 1950s and 1960s for depression symptoms and as appetite suppressants. They have also been used therapeutically for conditions like obesity, asthma, and attention-deficit hyperactivity disorder (ADHD). Prescription medications for ADHD often contain stimulants like methylphenidate, which help alleviate hyperactivity and fidgeting while enhancing alertness and physical activity. However, many stimulants, including nicotine and cocaine, are addictive and harmful. Illicit stimulants like amphetamines, cocaine, and crack are widely used despite their associated risks. Other substances, such as Ritalin (methylphenidate) and diethylpropion (tenuate, Apisate), offer similar effects to amphetamines, but with less potency. Illegally produced stimulants include substances like methamphetamine (including crystal meth) and methcathinone. These substances are part of the group known as amphetamine-type stimulants (ATS). They are synthetic stimulants that are commonly abused for their stimulating effects on the central nervous system.

Improper use of stimulants, beyond medical prescription, can lead to adverse effects, such as hostility, paranoia, and even psychotic symptoms. Additionally, unsafe elevation of body temperature, irregular heartbeat, heart failure, and seizures may result from improper stimulant consumption. Due to their potential for misuse and addiction, medical use of stimulants has decreased, with prescriptions now limited to conditions like ADHD, narcolepsy, and occasionally, treatment-resistant depression. Stimulant drugs are administered orally, inhaled,

DOI: 10.4324/9781003456674-12

smoked, or injected, with rapid development of tolerance and psychological dependence, particularly with potent stimulants such as amphetamine, methylphenidate, methamphetamine, cocaine, and methcathinone. This chapter sheds light on the usage and effects of amphetamine, cocaine, and khat.

LEGAL STATUS

Many stimulants have a legitimate medical use for the treatment of conditions such as obesity, narcolepsy, ADHD, and depression. Most countries regulate these substances as "prescription-only" drugs, requiring users to obtain a valid doctor's prescription for their use. However, despite their medical utility, stimulants, particularly amphetamines, are frequently abused in many countries, leading to various health complications and addiction issues. Cocaine, another potent stimulant, has limited commercial use and is strictly controlled in terms of sale and possession. In jurisdictions where medical use is permitted, prescribing cocaine is exceptionally rare, requiring specialised licensing from authorities. Additionally, certain stimulant ingredients like ephedrine and pseudoephedrine, found in over-the-counter allergy and cold medications, are regulated due to their stimulant properties, with restrictions imposed to prevent misuse and abuse. However, there are exceptions and variations in legal frameworks worldwide.

AMPHETAMINES

The term "amphetamine" derives from its chemical designation, alpha-methylphenethylamine, reflecting the similar chemical properties and actions of synthetic amphetamine, dextroamphetamine, and methamphetamine. These psychoactive substances collectively belong to the class of drugs known as amphetamines. Amphetamine was first synthesised in 1887 by Lazar Edeleanu at the University of Berlin and was first marketed in the 1930s as Benzedrine in an over-the-counter inhaler to treat nasal congestion. During World War II, amphetamine was widely used to combat fatigue and increase alertness in soldiers. Methamphetamine hydrochloride, commonly referred to as crystal amphetamine, is the crystalline form of methamphetamine and is typically smoked after being heated. Smokable methamphetamine, often called "ice," is a powder ranging in colour from off-white to grey or pinkish, primarily smoked using glass pipe. Methamphetamine, known by various street names, including meth, crystal, chalk, and ice, exists as a white, odourless, bitter-tasting crystalline powder, sharing chemical similarities with amphetamine. Amphetamines, recognised as speed, whizz, sulph, uppers, crystal, among other names, are consumed through ingestion, insufflation, smoking, or injection, with tablets being crushed for injection purposes.

During the past decades, amphetamine became popular as a recreational drug and performance enhancer amongst young people. Amphetamines are often manufactured in homemade laboratories in a matter of hours, with pseudoephedrine (a cold remedy) as the main ingredient and mixing a cocktail of about 15 chemicals. This process is highly toxic and dangerous. Compared to cocaine, amphetamine is cheaper and has a longer-lasting effect. Most "street stimulants" are made with illicitly manufactured amphetamine sulphate powder. Illicit amphetamine heavily diluted with adulterants is easily available. According to UK drug situation (2023), the average amphetamine sulphate powder purity at user level has ranged between 5% and 12% over the past decade. An occasional user may take a few weeks to consume half a gram, while a heavy user might consume up to 6 grams per day of relatively impure substance.

Mechanism of action

Amphetamines, structurally similar to dopamine and noradrenaline, induce the release of dopamine from nerve terminals, particularly elevating dopamine levels associated with pleasurable experiences. Dopamine, a primary neurotransmitter affected by stimulants, plays a pivotal role in the heightened energy and pleasure induced by amphetamine. The drug's impact intensifies with higher doses and varied routes of administration. At low doses, amphetamine enhances attention and reduces impulsivity, whereas higher doses suppress appetite and lead to weight loss. Orally ingested amphetamines boost wakefulness and physical activity while reducing appetite, whereas smoking or injection yields an immediate, albeit fleeting, rush of intense pleasure known as a "flash." Prolonged use of stimulants can diminish dopamine levels, impairing the user's capacity for pleasure and fostering tolerance over time.

Sought-after effects

The psychological effects of amphetamines vary based on dosage, individual personality, and the context of use. Amphetamines induce arousal and mimic the effects of adrenaline, accelerating heart and respiratory rates, dilating pupils, and suppressing appetite. Users often experience heightened energy, increased wakefulness, concentration, confidence, and cheerfulness, potentially leading to psychological dependence. As the drug's effects decline, feelings of anxiety, irritability, and restlessness may arise. Snorting or oral ingestion of amphetamines produces euphoric effects but lacks the intense rush of rapid-onset methods. The duration of amphetamine effects varies based on dosage but can last up to 12 hours. In contrast, cocaine is processed more rapidly by the body, with a significant portion eliminated within the first hour after consumption.

Therapeutic uses

Amphetamines have several therapeutic uses, including the treatment of attention-deficit hyperactivity disorder (ADHD). Amphetamines, such as Adderall and Ritalin, are commonly prescribed to manage symptoms of ADHD in children and adults. They help increase attention span, focus, and impulse control in individuals with ADHD. Amphetamines are also used to treat narcolepsy, a sleep disorder characterised by excessive daytime sleepiness and sudden episodes of falling asleep. They help promote wakefulness and reduce episodes of uncontrollable sleepiness. In some cases, amphetamines may be prescribed for short-term weight loss management in individuals who are obese. They work by suppressing appetite and increasing metabolism, leading to reduced food intake and weight loss. In certain rare cases where other treatments have been ineffective, doctors may prescribe low doses of amphetamines off-label (off-label use of amphetamines refers to the practice of prescribing these medications for conditions or purposes other than those approved by regulatory agencies) to help alleviate symptoms of depression. However, this use is less common and carefully monitored due to the potential for abuse and dependence.

Adverse effects

Short-term physiological effects of amphetamines vary based on dosage and administration method. Long-term use may lead to violent behaviour, anxiety, confusion, and insomnia. Heavy users may experience psychotic features like paranoia, auditory hallucinations, mood disturbances, and delusions (Farnia & Golshani, 2016), known as amphetamine psychosis, potentially resulting in homicidal or suicidal thoughts. These effects typically diminish upon discontinuation of the drug. Prolonged heavy use also heightens the risk of cardiovascular issues, especially among individuals with hypertension or those engaging in strenuous exercise. Amphetamine use may cause rapid heart rate, irregular heartbeat, stroke, high blood pressure, shortness of breath, nausea, vomiting, diarrhoea, and physical collapse. Methamphetamines share similar physical effects with amphetamines, including increased wakefulness, physical activity, decreased appetite, elevated respiration, rapid heart rate, irregular heartbeat, heightened blood pressure, and increased body temperature.

Psychologically, long-term methamphetamine use can cause dental problems ("meth mouth"), anxiety, confusion, insomnia, paranoia, hallucinations, mood disturbances, and even psychosis. Users may experience delusions and violent behaviour, which can pose risks to themselves and others. Additionally, long-term methamphetamine use can lead to cognitive deficits, including problems with memory, attention, decision-making, and addiction (NIDA, 2022). Overall, long-term methamphetamine use can have devastating effects on both physical and mental health, leading to significant impairments in daily functioning and quality of life. In addition, methamphetamine misuse can increase the risk of contracting or transmitting HIV and hepatitis B and C. This risk applies not only to individuals who inject the drug but also to those who use it through non-injecting methods, such as snorting or smoking (NIDA, 2021). A list of physical and psychological effects is presented in Table 10.1.

Amphetamines can induce rapid effects, depending on the method of intake, such as snorting or injecting, which can lead to near-instantaneous responses, or swallowing, which may take up to 30 minutes to manifest. The duration of a single dose's

Table 10.1
Physical and psychological effects of amphetamine

Physical effects: short-term	Psychological effects: short-term
• Decreased appetite	• Alertness
• Increased stamina	• Euphoria
• Increased sexual drive	• Increased concentration
• In some cases, decreased sexual drive	• Rapid talking
• Teeth-griding	• Increased confidence
• Hyperactivity	• Increased social awareness
• Agitation	• Hallucinations
• Nausea	• Loss of REM sleep
• Itchiness	• Insomnia
• Greasy skin	
• Tachycardia	
• Irregular heart rate	
• Hypertension	
• Headaches	
• Fatigue	
• Nystagmus	
Physical effects: long-term	**Psychological effects: long-term**
• Tolerance	• Irritability
• Deterioration of the lining of the nostrils	• Anxiety
• Difficulty in breathing	• Depression
• Tremor	• Aggressiveness
• Restlessness	• Obsessive behaviours
• Fatigue	• Delusions
• Changes in sleep patterns	• Paranoia
• Poor skin condition	• Dependence
• Twitching	• Withdrawal symptoms
• Gastric fluctuations and/or pain	
• Cardiovascular problems	
• Stroke	
• Damage to lung, kidney, and liver	
• Erectile dysfunction	

effects typically spans four to eight hours, with lasting after-effects that can persist for days. Chronic users often escalate to snorting or injecting to amplify the drug's potency, heightening the risk of infections, vein damage, and overdose. Excessive amphetamine use tends to foster rapid tolerance, with some experiencing "reverse tolerance" or heightened sensitivity to certain psychological effects over time.

Withdrawal from amphetamines, while not typ cally life-threatening, can be uncomfortable an protracted, with symptom severity correlated t the level of abuse. This process often perpetuat a perilous cycle of increased drug consumption an may involve the use of other substances to allevia withdrawal symptoms. Key withdrawal sympton of amphetamines are presented in Table 10.2.

Table 10.2
Withdrawal symptoms of amphetamine

- Cravings
- Nausea
- Irritability
- Depression
- Loss of energy
- Sweats
- Fatigue
- Decreased libido
- Decreased self-confidence
- Hyperventilation
- Convulsions
- Irregular heartbeat
- Insomnia
- Depression
- Long periods of sleep
- Paranoia
- Delusions

Activity 10.1

Please choose one correct answer for the following multiple-choice questions.

1. Which of the following is a therapeutic use of amphetamine?
   a. Enhancing memory recall
   b. Managing symptoms of depression
   c. Promoting weight loss
   d. Inducing sleep
   e. None of the above
2. What is the primary mechanism of action of stimulants like amphetamine?
   a. Increasing levels of serotonin in the brain
   b. Blocking the reuptake of dopamine and norepinephrine
   c. Inhibiting the release of GABA neurotransmitters
   d. Activating opioid receptors in the central nervous system
   e. None of the above
3. How do the effects of amphetamines differ when administered orally versus intravenously?
   a. Intravenous administration results in slower onset of effects.
   b. Oral administration produces a more intense high.
   c. Intravenous administration leads to longer duration of effects.
   d. Oral administration has a quicker onset of effects.
   e. Both routes produce similar effects.
4. What are some sought-after effects of stimulants like amphetamines?
   a. Sedation and relaxation.
   b. Increased energy and alertness.
   c. Enhanced sensory perception.
   d. Euphoria and pain relief.
   e. None of the above.
5. Which of the following is a psychological effect commonly associated with amphetamine use?
   a. Increased risk of heart attack
   b. Hallucinations and paranoia
   c. Slowed breathing and respiratory depression

d. Dilated pupils and blurred vision
e. Decreased appetite and weight loss

6. What are common withdrawal symptoms of amphetamine use?
   a. Extreme fatigue and depression
   b. Intense craving for the drug
   c. Increased heart rate and blood pressure
   d. Nausea, vomiting, and diarrhoea
   e. All of the above

Combining amphetamines

Combining amphetamines with other substances poses significant risks, particularly due to heightened strain on the cardiovascular system. The effects of mixing amphetamines with various drugs, including alcohol, cocaine, ecstasy, heroin, cannabis, hallucinogenic mushrooms, prescription medications, and over-the-counter medicines, can be unpredictable. When amphetamines are combined with other stimulants like cocaine or ecstasy, the stimulant effects intensify, leading to increased energy and euphoria, but also escalating toxicity and strain on the heart, potentially resulting in stroke. Similarly, mixing amphetamines with depressants like alcohol can mask alcohol's effects, potentially leading to over-consumption, impaired judgement, blackouts, loss of consciousness, and even fatal outcomes. Thus, combining amphetamines with other substances requires caution due to the potential for severe and harmful effects on health. It is difficult for people to gauge their level of intoxication, which can result in over-consumption, for example, significant impairment of coordination and judgement, blacking out, passing out, and potential death (University Health Service, 2017).

COCAINE

Cocaine, derived from the coca plant, is a highly addictive stimulant derived from the leaves of the coca shrub. Initially praised for its medicinal benefits, cocaine was widely used in tonics and as a local anaesthetic by surgeons, especially in ophthalmology. However, research has revealed its highly addictive nature and its ability to alter brain function with repeated use (NIDA, 2022a). It comes in various forms, including fine powder, crystal powder, paste, and solidified rock-like substances known as "crack cocaine." Street names for cocaine includ coke, Charlie, C, white, Percy, snow, rock, crac and toot. There are three main forms of cocain cocaine hydrochloride, freebase, and crack cocain In Europe and North America, the most commo form of cocaine is a white crystalline powder. User typically ingest cocaine by sniffing it through th nose or rubbing it onto the gums. It can also b dissolved in water and injected intravenously. Free basing consists of smoking cocaine base (or crack Crack cocaine (rocks, ready wash, ice, base, freebas stones) is whitish in colour and looks like irregul lumps of sugar. Crack is made by heating cocain hydrochloride with baking soda or ammonia i water. Smoking cocaine base is a more potent wa of administration than snorting and produces "rush" similar to the experience of injecting cocain

In recent times, there has been growing concer about the increasing use of cocaine in recreation settings, such as clubs and among young peo ple. Cocaine powder is generally used by social integrated recreational users, while crack cocain remains very rare, being mainly consumed by mor marginalised groups (for example, homeless, se workers). In many cases, cocaine users are polydru users, often consuming cocaine with alcohol an tobacco, with other illicit drugs such as other stim ulants and cannabis, or with heroin. When cocain is consumed alongside ethanol (alcohol), it form a psychoactive metabolite known as cocaethylen This compound shares similar properties wit cocaine but may pose greater cardiotoxicity. Coca ethylene has a longer half-life compared to cocain leading individuals who use both substances t experience extended and heightened psychoactiv effects due to the prolonged presence of cocaet ylene in the body (Pergolizzi et al., 2022). Man cocaine and crack users also take other drugs, inclu ing heroin and ecstasy. A highly dangerous practic is injecting a mixture of heroin and soluble cocaine (known as snowballing or speedballing). This combination increases the risk of adverse health effects and highlights the potential dangers associated with concurrent use of these psychoactive substances.

Therapeutic uses

In July 1884, Sigmund Freud, the father of psychoanalysis, published *Über Coca*, a paper in which he enthusiastically reported on the therapeutic uses of coca and its alkaloid, cocaine. Freud expected that cocaine would be used as a substitution therapy for morphine addiction and as a euphoriant in cases of melancholia (depression). Cocaine had been used as a local anaesthetic in ophthalmology, nasal surgery, dentistry, and as a diagnostic tool. Cocaine was also used in the treatment of asthma, cramps, mountain sickness, seasickness, and vomiting in pregnancy. Today, most of the therapeutic uses of cocaine are now obsolete due to its highly addictive nature and severe side effects of the drug. Consequently, safer and more effective alternatives have largely replaced cocaine in medical practice for most applications.

Mechanism of action

Cocaine exerts its effects by altering the action of dopamine in the brain's reward pathways, preventing the reabsorption of dopamine after its release from nerve cells. This leads to a buildup of dopamine in the synapse, resulting in intense feelings of euphoria and a "high" sensation. When cocaine use is discontinued, dopamine levels return to normal, but withdrawal symptoms, including strong cravings, occur due to the desire to restore dopamine levels. Additionally, cocaine blocks the reuptake of norepinephrine, leading to increased stimulation of the sympathetic nervous system. This manifests in symptoms such as tachycardia, hypertension, sweating, dilated pupils, and tremors. At high doses, cocaine can induce depression, disrupted sleep patterns, hallucinations, delusions, and paranoia. These effects underscore the potent and potentially harmful nature of cocaine use, highlighting its significant impact on both the brain and the body.

Cocaine's effects vary in intensity and duration based on the method of administration. Chewing coca leaves mixed with an alkaline substance is a traditional method that involves forming a bolus in the mouth, allowing the alkaloids to be absorbed through the stomach. Orally ingested cocaine takes around 30 minutes to enter the bloodstream, with effects peaking approximately 60 minutes after administration and lasting about 60 minutes thereafter. Snorting cocaine leads to maximum physiological effects within 40 minutes, with an activation period of 5 to 10 minutes, similar to oral ingestion, but with a faster onset due to quicker absorption. Smoking freebase cocaine results in immediate absorption into the blood, reaching the brain in about 5 seconds, producing a powerful rush that peaks rapidly and lasts for 5 to 10 minutes. Coca ethylene is produced when alcohol and cocaine are consumed together. Active in the brain, cocaethylene mimics the effects of cocaine. However, the subjective experience of the cocaine "high" and its impact on the heart do not escalate; instead, they diminish in intensity.

Sought-after effects

The sought-after effects of cocaine are:

- A rapid feeling of intense high
- Increased alertness and energy
- A feeling of well-being
- Delayed hunger and fatigue
- Increased confidence
- Stimulated sex drive
- Feelings of euphoria
- Elevated mood

Adverse effects

Repeated doses of cocaine can cause extreme agitation, panic attacks, restlessness, irritability, and anxiety. Chronic cocaine use can result in ongoing rhinitis (runny nose) and damage to the nasal septum, often accompanied by a burning sensation in the nostrils after the drug's anaesthetic effects wear off. Cocaine's effects on blood vessel constriction can lead to inadequate blood supply, contributing to nasal issues. Furthermore, cocaine users may experience paranoia, auditory hallucinations, or full-blown cocaine psychosis, which may take several months to fully recover from. Long-term cocaine use can lead to debilitation due to sleep and appetite disturbances, resulting in lowered resistance to illness. Hyperthermia (elevated body temperature) and convulsions occur with cocaine overdoses and, if not treated immediately, can result in death. Excessive doses, whether snorted, injected, or smoked, can lead to overdose, which can lead to sudden death from respiratory or heart failure. Cocaine-related deaths are often a result of cardiac arrest or seizures followed by respiratory arrest. The physical symptoms of cocaine overdose may include chest pain, nausea, blurred vision, fever, muscle spasms, convulsions, and coma. Some of the physical and psychological effects of low to moderate dose, excessive dose, and chronic use of cocaine are presented i Table 10.3.

Some polydrug users mix cocaine with othe psychoactive substances. The long-term use of th combination of alcohol and cocaine can result i cardiac diseases, such as cardiomyopathy, pathc logical arrhythmias, and even myocardial infarctio (heart attack). The effects of mixing cocaine wit alcohol, MDMA, heroin, and cannabis are presente in Table 10.4.

Table 10.3
Physical and psychological effects of cocaine

Dose	Physical effects	Psychological effects
Low to moderate dose	Loss of appetite	Euphoria
	Dry mouth	Sense of well-being
	Tachycardia	Impaired reaction time
	Raised heart rate	Increased self-confidence
	Hypertension	Suspiciousness
	Sweating	Increased sensory awareness
	Dilated pupils	Sense of superiority
	Reduced appetite	
	Reduced need for sleep	
	Impaired motor skills	
	Reduced lung function	
	Erratic or violent behaviour	
	Increased desire for sex	
Excessive dose	Convulsions	Anxiety
	Heart failure	Irritability
	Stroke	Insomnia
	Cerebral haemorrhage	Depression
	Respiratory arrest	Paranoia
	Exhaustion	Aggressiveness
		Delusions
		Disorientation
		Indifference
		Reduced psychomotor function
Chronic use	Destruction of nasal septum (snorting)	Tolerance
	Nasal eczema (snorting)	Psychological dependence
	Chest pains	Cocaine psychosis
	Muscle spasm	
	Respiratory problems (smoking)	
	Contraction of infection (injected cocaine)	
	Abscesses (injected cocaine)	
	Weight loss	
	Malnutrition	
	Sexual impotence	

Table 10.4 Effect of mixing cocaine with other psychoactive substances

Psychoactive substance with cocaine use	Effects
Alcohol[1]	Chest pain
	Heart palpitations
	Confusion
	Stroke
	Seizures
	Coma
	Nausea and vomiting
	Irritability
	HIV or hepatitis
	Malnutrition
	Traumatic injuries due to violence
Heroin[2]	Renal disease
	Breakdown of muscle tissue
	Nosebleeds
	Problems swallowing
	Nasal septum perforation
	Contraction of hepatitis or HIV
	Abscesses
	Track lines
	Collapsed veins
	Anxieties
	Irritability
	Paranoia
	Depressed breathing
	Severe itching
	Coma
	Drowsiness
	Dizziness
Ecstasy (MDMA)[3]	Increased blood pressure
	Increased heart rate
	Increased body temperature
	Severe organ damage
	Death (in some cases)
Cannabis[4]	Increased blood pressure
	Cardiovascular effects

Source:

[1]*APA (2013).*

[2]*APA (2013), NIDA (2022b), Jaffe and Kimmel (2006).*

[3]*Mental Health.Net (2016).*

[4]*Foltin and Fischman (1990).*

Withdrawal syndrome

Cocaine users develop tolerance to its euphoric effects quickly, necessitating increased doses for the same high. Conversely, regular users may experience a "reverse tolerance," intensifying adverse effects. Both physical and psychological dependence develop, with severity influenced by the administration route. Psychological dependence outweighs physical symptoms, especially with injection or smoking. Withdrawal involves strong cravings and drug-seeking behaviour, with symptoms diminishing over time, as observed in outpatient studies. Coffey et al. (2000) found milder craving during cocaine withdrawal compared to other drugs, with symptoms decreasing steadily. In contrast to earlier inpatient studies, outpatient research provides valuable insights into cocaine withdrawal dynamics. Cocaine withdrawal symptoms encompass a range of physical and psychological manifestations: these symptoms reflect the challenging experience of discontinuing cocaine use, highlighting both the physical and mental implications of withdrawal.

Stages in cocaine withdrawal

Cocaine withdrawal generally occurs in three phases: the "crash," the "withdrawal," and the "extinction." Not all cocaine users may go through the three distinct phases, as this may be influenced by the level of cocaine consumption, the set, and the setting.

The crash

The crash occurs in the first few days when a person who has used cocaine for an extended period suddenly stops using cocaine. Even first-time users of cocaine can experience the crash, depending on dosage and length of use. The withdrawal symptoms experienced can last between nine hours and four days. The withdrawal symptoms can include:

- Agitation
- Depression
- Anxiety
- Anorexia
- Intense craving for cocaine
- Uncontrollable appetite
- Insomnia or prolonged, but disturbed, sleep
- Extreme fatigue and exhaustion

Withdrawal

The withdrawal phase may last up to ten weeks from the end of the crash. During this early stage of this phase, there is a gradual return to normal sleep and mood, often accompanied by a low level of cocaine craving and low level of anxiety. This may last from one to ten weeks. In the middle phase of the withdrawal, severe cravings for cocaine are experienced. This may be reinforced by cues, such as cocaine paraphernalia or other environmental cues, which may lead to intense craving. This may induce physiological responses, such as runny nose, taste sensations, and fidgetiness. Other withdrawal symptoms during this phase include:

- Low energy
- Anhedonia (inability to feel pleasure)
- Anxiety
- Angry outbursts

Extinction

The final phase of cocaine withdrawal is called the extinction phase. This may, for some cocaine users, last for a least six months, and for others indefinitely. Some cocaine users may experience cravings when faced with strong cues. This is in response to people, places, or objects that are conditioned cues and provoke memories of taking the drug. These cravings may surface months or years after cocaine use has stopped. The person returns to a normal mood but still feels an occasional craving for cocaine. The risk of relapse is high because of continued cravings.

KHAT

Khat, also known as quat, qat, or kat, serves as a social stimulant in predominantly Muslim countries, notably Yemen, Ethiopia, and Somalia, with cultural significance. It originates from the evergreen shrub *Catha edulis*, found in parts of East Africa and the Middle East. Khat use for medical purposes is documented in *Kitab al-Saidana fi al-Tibb*, the oldest

Activity 10.2

There is only one correct answer to the following multiple-choice questions.

1. Which of the following is a common withdrawal symptom of cocaine use?
   a. Insomnia and vivid dreams
   b. Muscle aches and tremors
   c. Bradycardia and hypotension
   d. Increased appetite and weight gain
   e. None of the above
2. What are the phases in cocaine withdrawal?
   a. Tolerance, withdrawal, addiction
   b. Crash, withdrawal, recovery
   c. Intoxication, hangover, withdrawal
   d. Acute withdrawal, protracted withdrawal, extinction
   e. None of the above
3. The traditional method of coca consumption to alleviate altitude sickness:
   a. Ingesting
   b. Drug injecting
   c. Smoking
   d. Mate de coca
   e. Snorting
4. Forms of cocaine include:
   a. Crack and cocaine hydrochloride
   b. Cannabis and crack
   c. Heroin and cocaine
   d. Sulphate and freebase
   e. Cocaine and alcohol
5. The therapeutic use of cocaine was:
   a. Anaesthetic
   b. Stimulant
   c. Appetite suppressant
   d. Depressant
   e. Hallucinogen
6. The popularity of crack cocaine is known as the:
   a. Cocaine epidemic
   b. Crack epidemic
   c. Speedball endemic
   d. Drug epidemic
   e. None of the above
7. What is the route of administration of cocaine?
   a. Injecting
   b. Snorting
   c. Smoking
   d. All of the above
   e. None of the above
8. Snorting cocaine produces effects:
   a. Within 3 to 5 minutes
   b. Within 5 to 10 minutes

c. Within 20 to 25 minutes
d. Within 20 to 30 minutes
e. Within 30 to 45 minutes

9. Crack is:
a. A form of cocaine
b. Chemically altered cocaine
c. Deadlier than other forms of cocaine
d. All of the above
e. None of the above

10. Which is a long-term effect of cocaine?
a. Seizures
b. Increased heart rate
c. Blood vessel constriction
d. Insomnia
e. Addiction

11. A "speedball" is a combination of which two drugs?
a. LSD and heroin
b. Alcohol and cocaine
c. Cocaine and heroin
d. Amphetamines and alcohol
e. Ecstasy and cocaine

12. Which is a long-term effect of crack?
a. Cardiac arrest
b. Hallucinations
c. Seizures
d. Paranoia
e. None of the above

13. Freebasing is:
a. The sale price of the drug
b. A method of cutting the drug
c. A method of taking cocaine or crack
d. Mixing cocaine and crack
e. None of the above

14. What are some of the effects of cocaine?
a. Euphoria
b. Arousal
c. Anxiety
d. All of the above
e. Only a and b

15. Cocaine's mechanism of action works by:
a. Blocking the chemical in the brain
b. Blocking the reuptake of dopamine
c. Breaking down the blood–brain barrier
d. None of the above
e. All of the above

16. The immediate effect of crack has an influence on:
a. Respiratory system
b. Circulatory system

c. Excretory system
d. Central nervous system
e. Cardiovascular system

17. One of the effects of crack cocaine is the feeling of euphoria. How long does this effect last?
   a. 15 minutes
   b. 30 minutes
   c. 60 minutes
   d. 180 minutes
   e. 200 minutes

Activity 10.3

Questions

- Briefly describe the mechanism of action of cocaine.
- What are the adverse effects of cocaine?
- What are the features of the withdrawal syndrome of cocaine?
- Describe the stages in cocaine withdrawal.
- What are the dangers of mixing cocaine with other psychoactive substances?

Activity 10.4

State whether the statements are true or false.

Statements	True	False
Khat is a depressant.		
The main active substances in khat are cathine and cathinone.		
Effects start about a quarter of an hour into chewing and finish up to two hours after stopping.		
The khat plant is illegal in many countries.		
Khat generally produces talkativeness, mild euphoria, and hallucinations.		
The onset of the effect of khat is immediate.		

known (11th century) pharmaceutical and medical description of khat (Al-Biruni, 1973). The primary psychoactive compounds in khat leaves are cathinone, cathine, and norephedrine. While cathinone and cathine are stimulant drugs with effects similar to amphetamine, they are less potent. Due to the highly unstable nature of cathinone, khat leaves have a short shelf life and decompose within 72 hours of harvesting. To maintain freshness, khat plants are often wrapped in materials like plastic bags, banana leaves, or newspapers and regularly moistened. Within the European Union, khat use is confined to immigrants from the sub-Saharan countries and surrounding the Horn of Africa. In the United States, Khat is used by the Somali, Ethiopian, and Yemeni communities. It has been reported that "most regular khat chewers acquired their habit before coming to Europe. In second generation immigrants, khat use is less common" (EMCDDA, 2011).

Consumption of khat usually takes place in "mafrish" cafés, private apartments, and other private venues. Khat users usually chew about 100 to 300 grams of leaves or stems during three to six hours, swallowing the juice. Dryness of the mouth is caused by the juice, so large amounts of liquid are also drunk. Effects start about a quarter of an hour into chewing and finish up to two hours after stopping. The prevalence data on the use of khat range from 34% to 67% of the Somali community, who identify themselves as current users of khat (ACMD, 2005). Khat users appear to have very low levels of other drug or alcohol use. There is no evidence that khat use is a gateway to the use of other stimulant drugs, although there is, however, a significant prevalence of tobacco use within this population (Kassim et al., 2015).

Mechanism of action

Chewing khat leaves results in the release of cathinone, a potent stimulant that induces feelings of euphoria. As cathinone is metabolised in the body, it breaks down into various chemicals, including cathine and norephedrine. These compounds possess structural similarities to amphetamine and adrenaline (epinephrine), contributing to their stimulant effects. However, it is important to note that the effects of khat consumption can vary depending on factors such as dosage, frequency of use, individual tolerance, and the presence of other substances.

Legal status

Khat leaves are not under the International Convention of Psychotropic Drugs (1971). However, cathinone and cathine and some of their synthetically produced derivates (e.g. methcathinone) are controlled substances under this treaty. In the United States, Canada, and most of Europe, khat is a controlled substance, often placed in the same category as cocaine.

Sought-after effects

Khat generally produces talkativeness, mild euphoria, and hallucinations. In many countries, it has social and cultural significance, and it is mostly used as a social stimulant on festive occasions.

Adverse effects

Effects start after approximately 30 minutes with stimulation and talkativeness. This is followed by a relaxed and introspective state that can last up to five hours, often with insomnia. This is then followed by periods of lethargy, irritability, and general hangover. Dependence can develop, and heavy use can be problematic. Nausea, vomiting, mouth ulcers, abdominal pain, headache, palpitations, increased aggression, and hallucinations can occur. Continued use can lead to cycles of sleeplessness and irritability and can, in the longer-term, lead to psychiatric problems, such as paranoia and possibly psychosis. Digestive problems, such as constipation and stomach ulcers, have been reported frequently to affect regular users. Khat is also often used with tobacco and hypno-sedatives, such as benzodiazepines, which bring additional associated risks. Long-term khat use is linked to notable cognitive impairments across various domains. Human studies indicate deficits in learning, motor speed, coordination, set-shifting, response inhibition functions, cognitive flexibility, short-term and working memory, as well as conflict resolution abilities (Ahmed et al., 2021). These findings highlight the adverse cognitive effects associated with prolonged khat consumption.

The physical and psychological risks associated with khat are presented in Table 10.5.

Although numerous somatic and psychological health problems have been reported with khat use, there is little robust information on the subject and limited evidence to permit conclusive statements of causality (EMCDDA, 2011). The chronic use of khat is linked to severe complications across multiple bodily systems, including cardiac, neurological, psychological, and gastrointestinal issues. Psychological dependence and withdrawal symptoms contribute to the prolonged use of khat, highlighting the challenges associated with discontinuing its consumption (Silva et al., 2022). Khat typically induces moderate psychological dependence, without evident physical dependence. However, along with psychological reliance, withdrawal symptoms contribute to its continued use (Abede, 2018; Odenwald & al'Absi, 2017). Depressive disorder, sedation, and hypotension are sometimes seen after withdrawal of khat (Cox & Rampes, 2003). Khat consumption is associated with anecdotal reports of social harms in various UK cities, including unemployment, criminal behaviour, minor antisocial actions like public spitting, and potential links to violent behaviour. However, empirical evidence establishing direct causal connections between khat

Table 10.5
Khat: risks to physical, psychological, and social harms

Risks to physical health	Risks to psychological health	Social harms
Increase in blood pressure	Insomnia	No evidence shows a causal relationship between
Risk factor for oral cancer	Anorexia	khat and various social harms for which its consumption is supposedly responsible*
Risk factor for myocardial infarction	Low mood	
Affects reproductive health	Depression	
Delivery of low-birth-weight babies	Manic and delusional behaviour	
Lower sperm motility	Violence	
Increased libido	Suicidal depression hallucinations	
Decreased libido (chronic use)	Paranoia	
Residual pesticides	Khat-induced psychosis	
Gingivitis and loose teeth	Exacerbated pre-existing mental health problems	
Incidence of oesophageal cancer		
Gastric disorders		
Liver damage		

*Sources: Adapted from Silva et al. (2022). *Anderson and Carrier (2011).*

use and these issues is lacking (Anderson & Carrier, 2011). While heavy and frequent khat use may impact employment prospects, the literature does not clearly demonstrate a causal relationship with unemployment or criminality. Limited evidence suggests associations with minor antisocial behaviour and violence, but clear causal connections remain elusive (Anderson & Carrier, 2011).

SYNTHETIC CATHINONES

Synthetic cathinones, often referred to as "bath salts" or "research chemicals," are a class of synthetic drugs designed to mimic the effects of cathinone, the primary psychoactive component found in the khat plant. Synthetic cathinones are included "new psychoactive substances" that can be much stronger than the natural product and, in some cases, very dangerous. These substances are chemically similar to amphetamines and can produce stimulant effects, such as increased energy, alertness, and euphoria. Synthetic cathinones gained popularity as recreational drugs and were sold under various names like "Flakka," "mephedrone," "MDPV," and others. They are typically consumed orally, nasally (snorting), or by injection. The synthetic cathinones include mephedrone and methylone and are used as a recreational drug and can be addictive. The synthetic drugs are in the form of a white or brown crystal-like powder and are sold in small plastic or foil packages. The products sold as "molly" (MDMA) often contain synthetic cathinones. These psychoactive substances are marketed "not for human consumption" as plant food or household cleaners. Most users tend to snort (insufflate) mephedrone, but most of the cathinones are ingested. These psychoactive substances are sometimes injected because they are soluble in water. Mephedrone or substituted cathinone drugs can be smoked, but it is not a "cost-effective" way of consuming them. Some synthetic cathinones, including bupropion, have medical approval for treating specific conditions or are under investigation as potential treatments for substance use disorders (NIDA, 2024). Some of the effects of synthetic cathinones are presented in Table 10.6.

In addition, there are other health effects. The psychoactive substances are associated with cravings and severe withdrawal symptoms. The withdrawal symptoms may include depression, anxiety, tremors, insomnia, and paranoia. Research shows illicit synthetic cathinone use can be life-threatening and cause other serious health and safety problems. People who use synthetic cathinones regularly may develop stimulant use disorder (NIDA, 2024). These drugs are often produced clandestinely in illegal laboratories, making their composition and potency unpredictable and potentially dangerous.

Table 10.6
Effects of synthetic cathinones

Physical effects	Psychological effects
• Rapid heartbeat	• Euphoria
• Hypertension	• Alertness
• Hyperthermia	• Confusion
• Prolonged dilation of the pupil of the eye	• Acute psychosis
• Breakdown of muscle fibres	• Agitation
• Teeth grinding	• Combativeness
• Sweating	• Aggressiveness
• Headaches	• Violence
• Palpitations	• Self-destructive behaviour
• Seizures	• Paranoia
	• Hallucinations
	• Delusions

Source: Department of Justice/Drug Enforcement Administration (2022).

Activity 10.5

There is only one correct answer to the following multiple-choice questions.

1. What is a common name for the stimulant plant *Catha edulis*?
   a. Cocaine
   b. Khat
   c. Cannabis
   d. Opium
   e. LSD
2. Which psychoactive compound found in khat leaves produces feelings of euphoria and alertness?
   a. Nicotine
   b. Cathinone
   c. Caffeine
   d. THC
   e. Psilocybin
3. What are some psychological effects commonly associated with khat use?
   a. Increased sociability and euphoria
   b. Depression and anxiety
   c. Paranoia and hallucinations
   d. Enhanced cognitive function and memory
   e. None of the above
4. What is a potential consequence of chronic khat use on the body?
   a. Reduced heart rate
   b. Weight gain
   c. Hypotension
   d. Dental problems
   e. Decreased appetite

5. Which of the following is NOT a reported psychological effect of khat consumption?
   a. Paranoia
   b. Hallucinations
   c. Euphoria
   d. Memory enhancement
   e. Confusion

6. How do individuals typically consume khat leaves?
   a. Smoking
   b. Inhalation
   c. Chewing
   d. Injection
   e. Vaporisation

7. What is one of the social implications associated with chronic khat consumption?
   a. Increased social integration
   b. Improved cognitive function
   c. Reduced stress levels
   d. Family conflicts
   e. Enhanced academic performance

8. Which neurotransmitter system does khat primarily affect in the brain?
   a. Serotonin
   b. Dopamine
   c. GABA
   d. Glutamate
   e. Endorphins

9. Which of the following statements about synthetic cathinones is true?
   a. They are derived from the opium poppy.
   b. They primarily act as depressants on the central nervous system.
   c. They are synthetic stimulants similar to amphetamines.
   d. They have no effect on mood or perception.
   e. None of the above is correct.

10. What are some effects commonly associated with synthetic stimulants?
    a. Sedation and relaxation
    b. Enhanced sensory perception
    c. Decreased heart rate and blood pressure
    d. Altered perception and hallucinations
    e. None of the above

11. For what are synthetic cathinones primarily known?
    a. Acting as sedatives
    b. Mimicking the effects of opioids
    c. Producing hallucinogenic effects
    d. Acting as synthetic stimulants
    e. None of the above

12. How do synthetic cathinones affect the central nervous system?
    a. By increasing GABA activity
    b. By blocking the reuptake of serotonin
    c. By inhibiting the release of dopamine
    d. By mimicking the effects of endorphins
    e. None of the above

13. What are some common street names for synthetic cathinones?
    a. Ice and crank
    b. Ecstasy and MDMA
    c. Bath salts and flakka
    d. Heroin and opium
    e. None of the above

Activity 10.6

Questions

- List the physical risk associated with khat
- List the psychological risk associated with khat

KEY POINTS

- Amphetamine, dextroamphetamine, and methamphetamine are collectively referred to as amphetamines.
- The increase of dopamine is the primary mechanism for its behavioural-stimulant effects, with intense pleasure and increased energy.
- Chronic users of amphetamines typically snort or resort to drug injection to experience the full-intensity effects of the drug.
- Injecting cocaine has the added risks of infection, vein damage, and higher risk of overdose.
- Many amphetamine users will repeat the amphetamine cycle by taking more of the drug during the withdrawal.
- Smoking cocaine base is a more potent way of administration than snorting and produces a "rush" similar to the experience of injecting cocaine.
- Many cocaine and crack users also take other drugs, including heroin. Alcohol is often mixed with cocaine to produce coca-ethylene, which is highly toxic.
- Cocaine users are polydrug users, often consuming cocaine with alcohol and tobacco, with other illicit drugs, such as other stimulants and cannabis, or with heroin.
- During the withdrawal symptoms of cocaine, such as craving, the user experiences a very strong need for the drug to get the level of dopamine back up.
- The intensity and the duration of the effects of cocaine are influenced by the route of administration.
- Cocaine users may also experience paranoia, auditory hallucinations, or full-blown cocaine psychosis.
- Withdrawal leads to strong craving and drug-seeking behaviour, followed by a withdrawal syndrome.
- The long-term use of the combination of alcohol and cocaine can result in cardiac diseases, such as cardiomyopathy, pathological arrhythmias, and even myocardial infarction (heart attack).
- Cocaine withdrawal generally occurs in three phases the "crash," the "withdrawal," and the "extinction."
- Khat is an evergreen shrub (*Catha edulis*) native to East Africa and the Arabian Peninsula.
- The leaves of the khat plant contain psychoactive compounds, like cathinone, cathine, and norephedrine.
- Chewing khat leaves releases cathinone, producing stimulant effects, such as euphoria and increased alertness.
- Khat is traditionally consumed in social settings for its stimulant effects, particularly in East African and Middle Eastern cultures.
- Chronic use of khat is associated with various health issues, including cardiovascular problems, psychological dependence, and gastrointestinal complications.
- While khat is legal in some countries where it is traditionally used, it is classified as a controlled substance in others due to its psychoactive properties and potential for abuse.
- Synthetic cathinones are a class of psychoactive substances designed to mimic the effects of cathinone found in the khat plant.
- They are commonly known as "bath salts" or "research chemicals" and are often abused for their stimulant effects.
- Synthetic cathinones can produce euphoria, increased energy, alertness, and heightened sociability.
- Adverse effects of synthetic cathinones include rapid heartbeat, hypertension, hyperthermia, paranoia, hallucinations, and agitation.

- Long-term abuse of synthetic cathinones can lead to addiction, cardiovascular problems, and psychological issues.
- Synthetic cathinones are often produced clandestinely in illegal laboratories, leading to variability in potency and composition.
- Due to their potential for abuse and adverse effects, synthetic cathinones are classified as illicit substances in many countries.
- Some synthetic cathinones, like bupropion, have medical applications and are used to treat depression and aid in smoking cessation.

References

Abebe, W. (2018). Khat: A substance of growing abuse with adverse drug interaction risks. *Journal of the National Medical Association,* 110(6), 624–634. https://doi.org/10.1016/j.jnma.2018.04.001.

Ahmed, A., Ruiz, M. J., Cohen Kadosh, K., Patton, R., & Resurrección, D. M. (2021). Khat and neurobehavioral functions: A systematic review. *PLOS One,* 16(6), e0252900. https://doi.org/10.1371/journal.pone.0252900.

Al-Biruni, A. R. M. A. (1973). *Kitab-al-Saydanah fi Al-Tibb*. Volumes 1–2 of Pakistan series of Central Asian studies. Karachi, Pakistan: Hamdard National Foundation.

American Psychiatric Association. (2013). *Diagnostic and Statistical Manual of Mental Disorders: DSM-5* (5th ed.). Washington, DC: American Psychiatric Publishing.

Anderson, D. M., & Carrier, N. C. M. (2011). *Khat: Social Harms and Legislation: A Literature Review* (Occasional Paper 95). University of Oxford. https://assets.publishing.service.gov.uk/media/5a7ab058ed915d670dd7de76/occ95.pdf (accessed 5 March 2024).

Coffey, S. F., Dansky, B. S., Carrigan, M. H., & Brady, K. T. (2000). Acute and protracted cocaine abstinence in an outpatient population: A prospective study of mood, sleep and withdrawal symptoms. *Drug and Alcohol Dependence,* 59(3), 277–286. https://doi.org/10.1016/S0376-8716(99)00126-X.

Cox, G. & Rampes, H. (2003). Adverse effects of khat: A review. *Advances in Psychiatric Treatment,* 9(6), 456–463. https://doi.org/10.1192/apt.9.6.456.

Department of Justice, Drug Enforcement Agency. (2022). *Drug Fact Sheet: Bath Salts*. https://www.dea.gov/sites/default/files/2023-03/Bath%20Salts%202022%20Drug%20Fact%20Sheet%20NEW.pdf (accessed 5 March 2024).

EMCDDA. (2011). *Khat Use in Europe: Implications for European Policy* (Drugs in Focus No. 21). Lisbon: European Monitoring Centre for Drugs and Drug Addiction.

Farnia, V., & Golshani, S. (2016). Chapter 26 – amphetamine-induced psychosis. In V. R. Preedy (Ed.), *Neuropathology of Drug Addictions and Substance Misuse*. Cambridge, MA: Academic Press, pp. 269–280.

Foltin, R. W., & Fischman, M. W. (1990). The effects of combinations of intranasal cocaine, smoked marijuana, and task performance on heart rate and blood pressure. *Pharmacology, Biochemistry, and Behavior,* 36(2), 311–315. https://doi.org/10.1016/0091-3057(90)90409-b.

Jaffe, J. A., & Kimmel, P. L. (2006). Chronic nephropathies of cocaine and heroin abuse: A critical review. *Clinical Journal of the American Society of Nephrology: CJASN,* 1(4), 655–667. https://doi.org/10.2215/CJN.00300106.

Kassim, S., Jawad, M., Croucher, R., & Akl, E. A. (2015). The epidemiology of tobacco use among Khat users: A systematic review. *Biomed Research International,* 2015, 313692. https://doi.org/10.1155/2015/313692.

Mental Health.Net. (2016). *Effects of Mixing Cocaine & Ecstasy*. https://www.mentalhelp.net/substance-abuse/cocaine/mixing-with-ecstasy/ (accessed 4 March 2024).

NIDA. (2021). *Are People Who Misuse Methamphetamine at Risk for Contracting HIV/AIDS and Hepatitis B and C?* https://nida.nih.gov/publications/research-reports/methamphetamine/are-people-who-misuse-methamphetamine-risk-contracting-hivaids-hepatitis-b-c (accessed 4 March 2024).

NIDA. (2022a). *What Are the Long-Term Effects of Methamphetamine Misuse?* https://nida.nih.gov/publications/research-reports/methamphetamine/what-are-long-term-effects-methamphetamine-misuse (accessed 4 March 2024).

NIDA. (2022b). *What Is Cocaine?* https://nida.nih.gov/publications/research-reports/cocaine/what-cocaine (accessed on 4 March 2024).

NIDA. (2024). *Synthetic Cathinones ("Bath Salts")*. https://nida.nih.gov/research-topics/synthetic-cathinones-bath-salts (accessed 5 March 2024).

Odenwald, M., & al'Absi, M. (2017). Khat use and related addiction, mental health and physical disorders: The need to address a growing risk. *Eastern Mediterranean Health Journal = La Revue De Sante De La Mediterranee Orientale = Al-Majallah Al-Sihhiyah Li-Sharq Al-Mutawassit,* 23(3), 236–244. https://doi.org/10.26719/2017.23.3.236.

Pergolizzi, J., Breve, F., Magnusson, P., LeQuang, J. A. K., & Varrassi, G. (2022). Cocaethylene: When cocaine and alcohol are taken together. *Cureus,* 14(2), e22498. https://doi.org/10.7759/cureus.22498.

Silva, B., Soares, J., Rocha-Pereira, C., Mladěnka, P., Remião, F., & On Behalf of the Oemonom Researchers (2022). Khat, a cultural chewing drug: A toxicokinetic and toxicodynamic summary. *Toxins,* 14(2), 71. https://doi.org/10.3390/toxins14020071.

United Kingdom Drug Situation. (2023). *Focal Point Annual Report*. https://www.gov.uk/government/publications/united-kingdom-drug-situation-focal-point-annual-report/united-kingdom-drug-situation-focal-point-annual-report-2019 (accessed 4 March 2024).

University Health Service. (2017). *The Effects of Combining Alcohol with Other Drugs*. University of Michigan. https://uhs.umich.edu/effects-combining-alcohol-other-drugs (accessed 4 March 2024).

Chapter 11

Psychedelics

A journey into hallucinogenic drugs

Learning outcomes

- State the meaning of *hallucinogens*.
- Understand the legal aspects of hallucinogens.
- Describe the physiological effects of LSD, MDMA, GHB, ketamine, psilocybin, and PCP.
- Describe the psychological effects of LSD, MDMA, GHB, ketamine, psilocybin, and PCP.
- List the withdrawal symptoms of MDMA and GHB.
- Describe the risk factors in using MDMA.
- List the effects ayahuasca, *Salvia divinorum*, and 2C-B.

Activity 11.1

Please choose one answer for the following multiple-choice questions. There is only one correct answer.

1. *Hallucinogens* refer to:
   a. A group of drugs causing hyperactivity
   b. A group of drugs causing hallucinogenic experiences
   c. A group of synthetic drugs
   d. A group of natural drugs
2. The following drugs are hallucinogens:
   a. LSD, alcohol, cannabis, PCP
   b. LSD, alcohol, PCP, GHB
   c. LSD, PCP, GHB, ecstasy
   d. LSD, PCP, heroin, cocaine
   e. LSD, PCP, GHB, ecstasy, ayahuasca, *Salvia divinorum*, and 2C-B
3. Most hallucinogenic drugs:
   a. Cause hallucinations
   b. Do not cause hallucinations
   c. Cause changes in mood or thought
   d. Do not change mood or thought
   e. None of the above
4. The effects of LSD start:
   a. About 10 minutes after taking it
   b. About 20 minutes after taking it

DOI: 10.4324/9781003456674-13

c. About 30 minutes after taking it
d. Immediately
e. None of the above

5. Acid, microdots, dots, tabs, or trips are slang names for:
   a. PCP
   b. GHB
   c. Ecstasy
   d. LSD
   e. Ayahuasca
6. LSD is associated with:
   a. Physical dependence
   b. Withdrawal symptoms
   c. Dependence
   d. Tolerance
   e. None of the above
7. *Ecstasy* refers to which of the following drugs?
   a. Alcohol
   b. Cocaine
   c. MDMA
   d. Steroids
   e. *Salvia divinorum*
8. Ecstasy tablets contain:
   a. MDMA
   b. Amphetamine
   c. Caffeine
   d. Heroin
   e. Cannabinoids
9. The effects of ecstasy start:
   a. About 10 minutes after taking it
   b. About 20 minutes after taking it
   c. About 30 minutes after taking it
   d. Immediately
   e. None of the above
10. Which of the following are considered "club drugs"?
    a. Ecstasy
    b. Rohypnol
    c. Ketamine
    d. All of the above
    e. Only a is correct
11. The effects of ecstasy may cause:
    a. Physical dependence
    b. Psychological dependence
    c. No dependence
    d. Both physical and psychological dependence
    e. None of the above
12. The effects of GHB start:
    a. Anywhere from 10 to 30 minutes
    b. Anywhere from 10 to 60 minutes

c. Anywhere from 30 to 60 minutes
d. Immediately
e. None of the above

13. In terms of physical and social harms, GHB:
a. Is more dangerous than alcohol
b. Is less dangerous than alcohol
c. Has the same danger as alcohol
d. Does not have any harm
e. Only has physical harm

14. Regular use of GHB can cause:
a. Physical dependence
b. Psychological dependence
c. No dependence
d. Both physical and psychological dependence
e. None of the above

15. Special K is known as
a. GHB
b. PCP
c. Ketamine
d. Cannabis
e. 2C-B

16. The effects of injecting ketamine start:
a. Anywhere from 10 to 15 minutes
b. Anywhere from 30 to 60 minutes
c. Anywhere from 30 to 40 minutes
d. Immediately
e. None of the above

17. Psilocybin is known as:
a. Angel dust
b. PCP
c. Magic mushrooms
d. Special K
e. Ketamine

18. The effects of injecting psilocybin start:
a. Anywhere from 10 to 20 minutes
b. Anywhere from 30 to 50 minutes
c. Anywhere from 50 to 60 minutes
d. Immediately
e. None of the above

19. Phencyclidine (PCP) is known as:
a. Angel dust
b. PCP
c. Magic mushrooms
d. Special K
e. MDMA

20. Regular use of PCP can cause:
a. Physical dependence
b. Psychological dependence

c. No dependence
d. Both physical and psychological dependence
e. None of the above

21. Which indigenous tribes traditionally use ayahuasca for spiritual and healing purposes?
a. Native Americans
b. Aborigines of Australia
c. Indigenous people of the Amazon basin
d. Maori of New Zealand
e. Inuit of the Arctic

22. What is the primary hallucinogenic compound in *Salvia divinorum*?
a. DMT
b. Mescaline
c. Psilocybin
d. Salvinorin A
e. MDMA

23. Which of the following best describes the typical method of consuming *Salvia divinorum*?
a. Smoking
b. Ingesting as a tea
c. Snorting
d. Injecting
e. Chewing

24. 2C-B belongs to which class of hallucinogens?
a. Phenethylamines
b. Tryptamines
c. Dissociative
d. Deliriants
e. Antidepressants

INTRODUCTION

The chapter discusses hallucinogens, a group of substances capable of inducing alterations in perception, thought, emotion, and consciousness. Hallucinogens encompass a diverse range of drugs, both natural and synthetic. The widespread experimentation with substances like LSD during the 1960s counterculture movement resurfaced in the late 1980s, coinciding with the emergence of the rave scene and club drugs. This resurgence led to renewed interest and experimentation with hallucinogens in recent times, particularly within specific subcultures.

Hallucinogens encompass both naturally occurring substances found in trees, vines, seeds, fungi, and leaves and as well as synthetic compounds manufactured in laboratories. Examples of hallucinogens include lysergic acid diethylamide (LSD), derived from the alkaloid ergot, and psilocybin from liberty cap mushrooms. Other natural hallucinogens include *Amanita muscaria* mushrooms, morning glory seeds, mescaline from peyote cactus, and ayahuasca tea containing DMT (dimethyltryptamine). Synthetic hallucinogens include phencyclidine (PCP), ketamine (surgery anaesthetic), ecstasy (MDMA and related drugs, in high doses), dextromethorphan (DXM) (cough suppressant), *Salvia divinorum* (salvia), and cannabis (in high quantities). Among these, 2C-B stands out as a synthetic hallucinogen belonging to the phenethylamine class of drugs.

Hallucinogens constitute a diverse array of substances with varying chemical compositions, mechanisms of action, and adverse effects. Unlike other psychoactive drugs, they induce subjective experiences that markedly differ from normal consciousness. While most hallucinogens do not consistently produce hallucinations, they often lead to alterations in perception, mood, and thought, rather than outright hallucinations. However, certain substances like dimethyltryptamine (DMT) and atropine may indeed induce true hallucinations. Additionally, some hallucinogens such as dextromethorphan (DXM), ketamine, phencyclidine (PCP), and *Salvia divinorum* (salvia) may provoke feelings of being out of control or experiencing "out of body" sensations. PCP is known for inducing hallucinations, delusions, and distorted perceptions of reality. Its effects are unpredictable and may lead to agitation, aggression, and violence. Ayahuasca induces intense hallucinogenic experiences, often accompanied by profound insights and emotional catharsis. *Salvia divinorum* produces short-lived but intense psychedelic effects, including altered perception, dissociation, and visual distortions. 2C-B produces visual hallucinations, changes in sensory perception, and altered mood. Limited research indicates that psychedelic drugs like psilocybin and LSD are not typically associated with addiction (Nichols, 2016; Nichols & Grob, 2018). Researchers speculate that one reason psychedelic drugs like psilocybin and LSD are not typically associated with addiction is the common occurrence of unpleasant side effects, such as headaches and nausea, which diminishes the desire to use them again (Johnson et al., 2012).

MECHANISM OF ACTION

The exact mechanism of action of hallucinogens remains unclear, but there is some evidence that hallucinogens bind with one type of serotonin receptor (5-HT2) in the brain. Studies indicate that psychedelic drugs like psilocybin, LSD, and DMT primarily target 5-HT2A receptors in the brain, which are typically activated by the neurotransmitter serotonin (Vollenweider & Smallridge, 2022). These substances control neurotransmitter activity, resulting in changes in perception, mood, and cognition. The exact mechanisms vary depending on the specific hallucinogen but often entail the disruption of typical neurotransmission patterns, leading to the distinctive hallucinatory experiences associated with these drugs. Furthermore, certain hallucinogens may influence other neurotransmitter systems, such as serotonin and glutamate, contributing to their varied effects on perception and consciousness. Serotonin has been linked to the occurrence of hallucinations, as in certain hallucinogenic drugs like LSD, mescaline, psilocybin, and ecstasy. Glutamate may also play a role in hallucinations, as evidenced by the fact that glutamate antagonists like phen cyclidine and ketamine can induce hallucinatio (Kumar et al., 2009).

LSD (LYSERGIC ACID DIETHYLAMIDE)

Lysergic acid diethylamide, known as LSD, is derive from an alkaloid (ergot, a fungus that grows on ry and other grains). It was first synthesised by Swi chemist Albert Hofmann in 1938. LSD becan popular in the 1960s counterculture movement ar has since been studied for its potential therapeut effects as well. LSD is also known as acid, microdo dots, tabs, or trips. In pure state, LSD is an odourle colourless, and tasteless powder. LSD usually com in the form of liquid, tablets or capsules, squar of gelatine, or blotter paper. The blotter paper divided into small decorated squares, with eac square representing one dose. LSD can be swa lowed, sniffed, injected, or smoked. LSD is take by mouth in extremely small doses (50–150 micr grams), which are usually on small paper squar LSD is a powerful hallucinogenic drug known for i profound effects on perception, mood, and though The effects of LSD can vary widely depending factors such as dosage, set (mindset of the use setting (environment), and individual differenc While some users report positive and profou spiritual experiences, others may experience anx ety, paranoia, or even psychotic reactions, especial at higher doses. The effects tend to start about ha an hour after taking it and last up to 12 hours, sometimes even longer, depending on the dosage.

Legal status

LSD is a controlled drug, and the United Natio Convention on Psychotropic Substances (adopte in 1971) requires the signing parties to prohib LSD. This means it is illegal to manufacture, bu possess, or distribute (sell, trade, or give) LS However, medical and scientific research with LS in humans is permitted.

Therapeutic use

In ancient cultures, various plants and extrac were utilised in religious rituals, witchcraft, ar medicinal practices as intoxicants. Hallucinogens, including LSD, have been explored for their potential therapeutic benefits in treating various disorders, such as depression, obsessive-compulsive disorder, alcohol dependence, and opiate addiction. In the 1960s, LSD was used in the treatment of anxiety, depression, psychosomatic diseases, and addiction (Abramson, 1966). In recent times, there has been a renewed interest in researching the therapeutic potential of LSD, particularly in the context of psychotherapy. Studies, such as the one conducted by Gasser et al. (2014), have shown promising results. Participants in LSD-assisted psychotherapy sessions reported reductions in anxiety and improvements in quality of life. They also experienced insightful, cathartic, and interpersonal experiences during the sessions. Research into psychedelic-assisted psychotherapy, including the use of LSD, has shown promising results for various mental illnesses, particularly depression, anxiety, post-traumatic stress disorder (PTSD), and addiction (Belouin & Henningfield, 2018; Reiff et al., 2020). LSD has emerged as a potential therapeutic agent in addiction psychiatry, with growing evidence supporting its use, particularly in the treatment of alcohol use disorder. Research findings suggest that LSD-assisted therapy may offer significant benefits in addressing alcohol addiction (Fuentes et al., 2020). This resurgence of research interest suggests that LSD-assisted psychotherapy could be a valuable approach in addressing certain mental health disorders. However, further research and clinical trials are necessary to fully understand the effectiveness, safety, and potential long-term effects of using LSD in therapeutic settings.

Sought-after effects

The effects of the drug are dependent on the user's prior experience, mood, expectations, and setting. It is much stronger in effect than psychedelic mushrooms or mescaline. A moderate dose will produce profound alteration in mood, sensation, and consciousness, intensified sensory experiences, and perceptual distortions. Some users report an experience of intense enlightenment. Confusion of time, space, body image, and boundaries can occur with what have been called the blending of sight and sound. The user may "see" sounds and "hear" colours. Mushrooms are similar to LSD, but the trip is often milder and shorter.

Adverse effects

LSD, while potentially therapeutic in controlled settings, can induce a range of adverse effects and risks when used recreationally or improperly. Users may experience panic, confusion, impulsive behaviour, and unpleasant illusions during a "bad trip." Strong feelings of anxiety, paranoia, and fear can emerge, along with hallucinations, such as feeling insects crawling on the skin. Users may feel a lack of control, leading to panic. LSD trips can last 12 to 36 hours, causing physical and psychological exhaustion. Users often underestimate the duration, leading to surprise and discomfort. Physiological effects include elevated heart rate, increased blood pressure, dilated pupils, higher body temperature, sweating, loss of appetite, sleeplessness, dry mouth, and tremors. Users may experience synaesthesia, hearing colours and seeing sounds. Large doses can induce delusions and visual hallucinations. Panic, paranoia, and fear may lead to risky behaviour, potentially causing injury or accidents. While accidental deaths due to impaired judgement are rare, they can occur. Negative effects are more likely in negative moods or situations, or when mixed with other drugs or alcohol. LSD poses a significant risk of relapse in individuals susceptible to schizophrenia or psychotic disorders. Evidence suggests that psychedelic drugs may potentially trigger schizophrenia-like illness in individuals with predisposing factors. However, there is limited evidence indicating that they cause long-term psychiatric problems for the majority of users (NIDA, 2024a). In summary, while LSD may have therapeutic potential, its recreational use carries substantial risks, including psychological distress, physiological discomfort, and the potential for dangerous behaviour. It is crucial to approach LSD with caution, especially in individuals with pre-existing mental health conditions or in situations where negative mood or environment prevails. Table 11.1 presents the physical and psychological effects of LSD.

Tolerance, dependence, and withdrawal

As a recreational drug, LSD differs from substances like opioids, cocaine, cannabis, and methamphetamine in several key ways: LSD does not lead to physical dependence or withdrawal syndrome, unlike many other substances. Tolerance may

Table 11.1
The physical and psychological effects of LSD

	Physical effects	Psychological effects
Short-term effects	• Blurred vision • Dizziness • Chills • Sweating • Dry mouth • Dilated pupils • Nausea • Weakness • Palpitations • Elevated body temperature • Tremors • Rapid heartbeat	• Visual and auditory hallucinations • Distorted sense of time and body perception • Sensitivity to sounds, smells, and other sensations • Blending of the senses (synaesthesia) • Heightened sense of understanding and identity • Mystical or religious experiences
Long-term effects	• Altered vision • Change in appetite • Altered levels of neurotransmitters (brain chemicals: serotonin and dopamine) • Significant changes in blood pressure and heart rate • Loss of coordination	• Tolerance • Flashbacks • Increased risk of mental illness • Anxiety, depression, or panic attacks • Suicidal thoughts and feelings • Persistent psychosis • Hallucinogen persisting perception disorder

Activity 11.2 LSD.

- What is LSD (lysergic acid diethylamide)?
- List the sought-after effects of LSD.
- List the physiological effects of LSD.
- List the psychological effects of LSD.

develop with frequent or long-term use, but emotional, physical, and mental stability typically return quickly after a single dose (Bogenschutz & Johnson, 2016). There is no physical dependence or withdrawal symptoms associated with recreational use of LSD. LSD is not considered an addictive drug since it does not produce compulsive drug-seeking behaviour, for example, the experiences of cravings associated with physical addiction. LSD can also cause cross-tolerance to other psychedelic drugs that may last from a few days to a week. Recent assessments suggest that LSD is one of the safest psychoactive recreational substances available (Nutt et al., 2010; van Amsterdam et al., 2013, 2015). LSD stands out among recreational substances due to its lack of physical dependence, low physiological toxicity, and perceived safety compared to other psychoactive drugs.

MDMA (ECSTASY)

3,4-methylenedioxymethamphetamine (MDMA), commonly known as ecstasy or Molly, is a synthetic psychoactive drug with hallucinogenic and amphetamine-like properties. It shares some similarities with LSD and is often categorised as a hallucinogen. MDMA is typically manufactured from the components of methylamphetamine and safrole, a derivative of nutmeg. It is available in various forms, including tablets, powder, and capsules, with different shapes and colours. The most common route of administration is swallowing, but MDMA tablets can also be crushed and snorted or injected as a liquid. MDMA has primarily been used as a drug within the dance or rave culture. In the early 1990s, it garnered significant media attention, highlighting the perceived dangers associated with its use. This period coincided with the emergence of a vibrant youth culture centred on MDMA, house music, and all-night raves. However, due to its production in unregulated black market laboratories, the strength and contents of MDMA tablets sold on the street cannot be accurately known. MDMA, also known as Molly (slang for "molecular"), is sometimes mixed with other substances, such as amphetamines, caffeine, or fillers. The term "Molly" typically refers to the purportedly "pure" crystalline powder form of MDMA, commonly sold in capsules (NIDA, 2022).

Pills sold as "MDMA" may not contain MDMA but could be composed of amphetamine ("speed") base or synthetic cathinones ("bath salts"). Currently, MDMA is used by a broader demographic due to its positive effects experienced within an hour after a single dose. The effects typically begin in about half an hour and last between three and six hours, followed by a gradual comedown. Less than 1% of MDMA remains in the body after 48 hours, making it undetectable in blood or urine samples. However, MDMA users may test positive for amphetamines in standard drug tests. Some individuals combine MDMA with other substances such as alcohol or cannabis.

Ecstasy (MDMA) and the brain

MDMA affects the brain by altering the activity of neurotransmitters such as serotonin, dopamine, and norepinephrine (Liechti & Vollenweider, 2001). MDMA (ecstasy) causes the brain to release large amounts of serotonin, which likely contributes to the mood-elevating effects experienced by users. However, this excess release of serotonin leads to significant depletion of this neurotransmitter in the brain. Consequently, individuals may experience negative psychological after-effects for several days following MDMA use (Bolla et al., 1998; Kish et al., 2000). There is extensive evidence for chronic pharmacodynamic tolerance to recreational MDMA, but the underlying mechanisms are currently unclear (Ricaurte & McCann, 2005), and long-term physiological and psychological changes occurring in human recreational users (Green et al., 2003). There is evidence to suggest that compared to the non-users, heavy MDMA users had significant impairments in visual and verbal memory (Mathias, 1999). The findings of clinical studies suggest that MDMA may increase the risk of long-term, perhaps permanent, problems with memory and learning and that "heavy MDMA users experience long lasting confusion, depression, and selective impairment of working memory and attention processes" (Kish, 2002; Verkes et al., 2001).

Legal status

MDMA is a controlled drug and is generally illegal in most countries under the UN Convention on Psychotropic Substances and other international agreements. In general, the unlicensed use, sale, or manufacture of MDMA are all criminal offences.

Therapeutic use

MDMA was first manufactured in Germany in 1914 as an appetite suppressant, although it was never actually marketed for this purpose. It has been used in a limited way as an adjunct to various types of psychotherapy in order to facilitate the therapeutic process. In addition, the drug has also been used to some extent with terminally ill patients in order to help them come to terms with their situation and to communicate or ventilate their feelings more easily.

The evidence regarding MDMA's therapeutic effects is currently limited, although ongoing research is being conducted in this area. Advocates of MDMA-assisted therapy suggest its use exclusively for reactive disorders, like post-traumatic stress disorder (PTSD) (Mithoefer, 2015), as it may exacerbate certain psychiatric conditions (Parrott, 2014).

Sought-after effects

The effects start about 20 to 60 minutes after use and can last several hours. Users describe MDMA as making them empathic, producing a temporary state of openness with an enhanced perception of colours and sound. The user experiences euphoric feelings and feelings of empathy, relaxation, and meaningfulness. Tactile sensations are enhanced for some users, making physical contact with others more pleasurable. The user experiences euphoria which plateaus for two to three hours before wearing off. MDMA can also cause mild hallucinogenic effects.

Effects of MDMA

The effects of MDMA/ecstasy are multifaceted and influenced by a range of factors, including dosage, individual characteristics, past experiences, concurrent drug use, and the composition of the drug itself. MDMA use typically involves three phases: the "coming up" phase, characterised by an amphetamine-like rush and mild nausea; followed by a plateau of intoxication, where users feel happy and relaxed; and finally, the "coming down" phase, where users may feel physically exhausted, depressed, and irritable. Effects usually begin within 20 minutes and can last up to six hours. MDMA induces euphoria, increased energy, and empathy, along with physical effects, like dilated pupils, jaw clenching, and heightened senses. Large doses or potent batches may lead to perceptual changes, irrational behaviour, anxiety, and aggression. Both physical and psychological effects vary based on factors such as dosage, individual characteristics, and drug composition. Psychological effects can encompass intense euphoria, accompanied by heightened extroversion and a sense of floating. Perceptual changes, such as vivid visual and auditory hallucinations, may also occur. However, MDMA use can lead to out-of-character irrational behaviour, as well as feelings of anxiety, irritability, paranoia, and even aggression in some cases. Paradoxically, MDMA can also evoke emotional warmth, fostering empathy towards others and a willingness to engage in discussions about emotionally charged memories. The physiological and psychological effects of MDMA are presented in Table 11.2.

Adverse effects

Long-term use of MDMA or ecstasy can lead to a range of adverse health effects, including depression, tolerance, and dependence. Users may also experience memory and concentration problems, along with financial, work, and social difficulties. Chronic use increases the risk of serious medical conditions, such as stroke, liver and kidney failure, lung dysfunction, and weight loss. Furthermore, MDMA use can result in dehydration, malnutrition, and exhaustion, while also suppressing the immune system and increasing the risk of infection. Cardiovascular health is also compromised, with acute risks of heart attack and premature heart disease, along with conditions like coronary artery disease, heart enlargement, and cardiomyopathy associated with psychostimulant use. These long-term effects underline the importance of understanding the risks associated with MDMA and ecstasy consumption. Among recreational ecstasy/MDMA users, polydrug use is a phenomenon whose common purpose is to experience the synergistic effect of the combined drugs, moderate MDMA effects, prevent potential toxicity, enhance a high or come down from a high from other drugs, or simply to treat existing medical conditions.

Overdose

The characteristics of psychostimulant toxicity or overdose, particularly with MDMA, are not clearly defined, and there is no specific dose–response relationship that reliably triggers toxicity. Toxic reactions can occur unpredictably regardless of the drug's form, method of administration, or apparent purity. Most cases of toxicity and overdose stem from interactions with other drugs, including unknown substances within MDMA, or from the use of other illicit (such as opioids or methamphetamine) or prescribed (such as antidepressant) medications. It is noteworthy that overdose can result from MDMA or ecstasy use alone (Darke et al., 2019).

Overdosing on MDMA can lead to severe symptoms, such as high body temperature, elevated blood pressure, hallucinations, and rapid heartbeat, posing significant risks to individuals with underlying health conditions or psychological disorders. Sudden death from overheating, dehydration, or complications from excessive water or alcohol intake is possible. Drinking excessive water, in attempt to mitigate risks, can result in dilutional hyponatremia, causing brain swelling and fatal outcomes. Harm reduction strategies, like wearing light clothing, staying hydrated with non-alcoholic fluids, and resting when fatigued, are advised. MDMA contamination with substances like bath salts or amphetamines underscores the need for caution. While MDMA-related deaths are comparatively low, vigilance is crucial.

Table 11.2
Immediate and adverse effects of ecstasy

	Physiological	Psychological
Immediate effects	Dilated pupils	Euphoria
	Jaw clenching and teeth grinding	Increased extroversion
	Heightened senses (sight, hearing, and touch)	Floating sensations
	Increased heart rate	Perceptual changes, such as visual and auditory hallucinations
	Dehydration	Out-of-character irrational behaviour
	High blood pressure	Anxiety
	Faintness	Irritability, paranoia, and aggression
	Panic attacks	Emotional warmth
	Loss of consciousness	Empathy towards others
	Seizures	Willingness to discuss emotionally charged memories
	Risky sexual behaviours	
	Fatal overdoses on MDMA rare	
Adverse effects	Increased risk of stroke	Feeling energetic and confident
	Liver failure	Depression
	Kidney failure	Tolerance
	Lung dysfunction	Dependence
	Weight loss, dehydration, malnutrition, exhaustion	Memory and concentration problems
	Immunosuppression increasing risk of infection	Mild detachment from oneself (depersonalisation)
	Rise in body temperature	Illogical or disorganised thoughts
	Lack of appetite	Impulsivity
	Restless legs	Concentration difficulties
	Nausea	Decreased cognitive function
	Hot flashes or chills	
	Headache	
	Sweating	
	Muscle or joint stiffness	
	Sleep disturbances	
	Lack of appetite	
	Heart disease	
	Motor delays in the offspring up to 2 years after birth (use in pregnancy)	
	Congenital abnormalities (particularly heart defects) in infants exposed to it during pregnancy	

Source: Adapted from NIDA (2021a); NIDA (2024a); NDARC (2021).

Tolerance, dependence, and withdrawal symptoms

Some individuals may develop tolerance to the effects of MDMA, and psychological dependence on MDMA can occur, making it challenging for individuals to reduce or cease their use. The existence of MDMA dependence has been debated but is now well-demonstrated, with a recognised psychostimulant withdrawal syndrome. Some individuals who use MDMA report symptoms of addiction, indicating continued use despite experiencing negative physical or psychological consequences (NIDA, 2021b). These consequences may include health issues or social and interpersonal problems. Additionally, tolerance to MDMA's effects can develop, requiring users to consume larger doses to achieve the desired effects. Withdrawal symptoms,

Activity 11.3 Ecstasy

- What is *ecstasy* (MDMA)?
- List the sought-after effects of ecstasy.
- List the physiological effects of ecstasy.
- List the psychological effects of ecstasy.
- What are the risks associated with ecstasy?

such as dysphoria, agitation, anxiety, fatigue, and insomnia, may also occur when individuals attempt to reduce or stop their MDMA use. Moreover, users may experience strong cravings for MDMA (NIDA, 2021b), which can further contribute to difficulties in quitting or reducing use.

GHB

GHB (gamma-hydroxybutyrate) is a central nervous system depressant known by various names, such as liquid ecstasy, GBL, BDO, and GBH. It is often referred to as a "club drug" or "date-rape" drug due to its psychoactive effects. GHB is a colourless liquid with a slightly salty taste and can be found in small quantities in certain beers and wines. Like MDMA, GHB is popular among teenagers and young adults in recreational and club settings, offering an alcohol-like high with potent positive sexual effects. It is typically sold in small plastic containers and consumed in capfuls, often mixed with alcoholic drinks. Despite being sometimes referred to as "liquid MDMA," GHB is distinct from MDMA in terms of its chemical composition and effects. GHB can take anywhere from ten minutes to an hour to take effect, with effects lasting from one and a half to three hours or longer. It induces intoxication resembling alcohol or ketamine intoxication and can lead to respiratory depression and death, particularly when combined with alcohol.

GHB has gained notoriety as a date-rape drug due to its colourless and odourless nature, making it easy to add to drinks without detection. Its sedative properties can render individuals comatose and unable to give consent, increasing the risk of sexual assault. This risk is high regardless of whether the individual knowingly or unknowingly ingests the substance. Additionally, GHB is abused by bodybuilders and athletes. National surveys show low rates of GHB use, with high-risk populations identified among men who have sex with men and polysubstance users. GHB is among the three most commonly used drugs in "chemsex" (Tay et al., 2022), where it is frequently co-ingested with other psychoactive substances, increasing the risk of adverse effects and complications. GHB is difficult to trace because they quickly leave the body and may be difficult to detect.

Mechanism of action

GHB has a similar structure to gamma aminobutyric acid (GABA). GHB acts on at least two sites in the brain: the GABA-B receptor and a specific GHB binding site (NIDA, 2010). Pharmacologically, GHB acts as a central nervous system depressant by interacting with and binding to receptors for the major inhibitory neurotransmitter γ-aminobutyric acid (GABA) (Busardò & Jones, 2015). Both alcohol and GHB act on GABA-B receptors in the brain. Their action at these receptor sites results in central nervous system (CNS) depressant effects, as well as stimulant and psychomotor impairment effects of GHB (Drugs.com, 2017). This shared mechanism of action contributes to the similar physiological and behavioural effects observed with both substances, including sedation, relaxation, and impaired coordination.

Legal status

GHB, or gamma-hydroxybutyrate, is a controlled substance and is highly regulated. In some European countries, GHB is an approved drug available by prescription.

Therapeutic use

Gamma-hydroxybutyrate (GHB) has a complex history of use, including both therapeutic and non-therapeutic applications. Initially, GHB was utilised as an anaesthetic due to its sedative properties. However, its use in anaesthesia has declined due to its narrow therapeutic window and potential for respiratory depression and other side effects. It has also been used as a hypnotic for insomnia, and as a treatment for depression. Additionally, it has been suggested to improve athletic performance. Sodium oxybate, another name for GHB, under the brand name Xyrem, has been approved by the FDA for the treatment of cataplexy or excessive daytime sleepiness (EDS) treatment in patients with narcolepsy who are 7 years of age and older (Dominguez et al., 2023). In Italy and Austria, sodium oxybate is utilised in the management of alcohol withdrawal and for preventing relapse in individuals with alcohol dependence (Skala et al., 2014). Additionally, beyond alcohol withdrawal management, pharmaceutical gamma-hydroxybutyrate has shown promise in treating GHB withdrawal. This treatment approach has been investigated and is now commonly used for GHB withdrawal in the Netherlands (Beurmanjer et al., 2020).

Sought-after effects

Gamma-hydroxybutyrate (GHB) affects dopamine release in the brain, inducing effects from relaxation to sleep at low doses. Even a small amount can lead to feelings of uninhibitedness, euphoria, and relaxation, which can be appealing to individuals seeking stress relief or recreational enjoyment. Users often report increased sociability, enhanced social interactions, perceived heightened sensory experiences, including intensified tactile sensations, and altered perception of colours and sounds. GHB has been associated with increased libido and enhanced sexual experiences in some individuals, contributing to its popularity as a party or club drug. GHB has been explored for its potential to improve sleep quality and duration, making it appealing to individuals seeking relief from sleep disturbances or insomnia. Determining a safe dose is challenging due to varying liquid concentrations.

Adverse effects

It is important to note that while GHB may offer desirable effects to some users, it also poses significant risks, including addiction, overdose, respiratory depression, and coma. Use of GHB can lead to severe health complications and even death. Toxicity of GHB is dose-dependent, with higher doses causing adverse effects, like headache, dizziness, nausea, vomiting, speech impairment, and anterograde amnesia (Andresen et al., 2011). Severe toxicity or poisoning can manifest as respiratory depression, bradycardia, seizures, and reduced consciousness, leading to deep coma. Death may result from respiratory compromise, aspiration, asphyxia, pulmonary oedema, or traumatic injury due to sudden loss of consciousness (Tay et al., 2022). Users experience loss of body control similar to alcohol intoxication, lasting several hours, accompanied by grogginess and potential audiovisual hallucinations. Combining GHB with sedatives, especially alcohol, is extremely hazardous and can result in emergencies, such as convulsions, necessitating intensive care admission and prolonging hospital stays (Galicia et al., 2019). Driving or operating machinery under GHB influence heightens the risk of accidents or injuries to oneself and others. Table 11.3 presents the effects of GHB related to dosage.

Table 11.3
Doses and effects of GHB

Doses	Effects
Recreational	Euphoria
	Increased enjoyment of movement and music
	Increased libido
	Increased sociability
	Intoxication
Higher	Nausea
	Vomiting
	Desire to sleep
	Giddiness
	Slurred speech
	Dizziness
	Respiratory depression
	Drowsiness
	Agitation
	Visual disturbances
	Depressed breathing
	Amnesia
	Convulsions
	Unconsciousness
	Death

Dependence and withdrawal

Although gamma-hydroxybutyrate use disorder is not officially recognised in *DSM-V*, chronic recreational use of GHB can lead to the development of tolerance, dependence, and withdrawal syndrome (Tay et al., 2022). Regular use of GHB can lead to physical dependence, and withdrawal symptoms may vary in severity and progression. The symptoms may include tremor, anxiety, agitation, sleep disturbances, diaphoresis, and autonomic instability. Severe withdrawal may lead to acute delirium, visual or auditory hallucinations, and seizures, necessitating intensive care management to prevent fatal outcomes. The most severe withdrawal symptoms typically resolve within two weeks. However, insomnia, mood disruption, and anxiety may persist beyond the acute phase, similar to other sedative-hypnotic withdrawals (Tay et al., 2022). Withdrawal onset may occur within one to two hours after the last dose, with symptoms subsiding within 2 to 21 days based on dosage and frequency of use. GHB withdrawal resembles acute withdrawal from alcohol or barbiturates (delirium tremens), potentially leading to convulsions, paranoia, and hallucinations. Ceasing GHB use abruptly or attempting self-detoxification is strongly discouraged.

Overdose

Overdose presentations are generally associated with recreational use. Accidental overdose on GHB is common due to the narrow margin between the desired effect and toxicity. Signs of overdose include confusion, vomiting, dizziness, seizures, lowered body temperature, agitation, hallucinations, difficulty breathing, and coma. Individuals with respiratory or low blood pressure disorders, including asthmatics, should avoid GHB. Most fatalities occur when GHB is combined with alcohol or other drugs, intensifying its effects and the risk of toxic outcomes. Combining GHB with substances like ketamine, prescription tablets, cocaine, MDMA, mephedrone, or crystal meth amplifies the danger of overdose and toxic effects. The risk of choking on vomit while sleeping increases, and taking higher-than-normal doses elevates the likelihood of an unexpected overdose.

KETAMINE

Ketamine is a dissociative anaesthetic that is commonly used for medical and veterinary purposes. Ketamine, also known as "special K," "green," "super K," or "vitamin K," is a substance that comes in powdered or liquid form and resembles pharmaceutical cocaine. It can act as both a depressant and a hallucinogen. The World Health Organization (WHO, 2006) conducted a critical review of ketamine due to concerns about its increasing recreational use in Europe, Asia, and North America, as well as its misuse by medical personnel in some countries. The conclusions of the report, in line with recommendations from the European Union (EMCDDA, 2002), suggest that while there is evidence of Ketamine abuse, it does not constitute a significant public health and social problem when compared to other drugs in the cyclidine class. Ketamine has become a significant player in the recreational drug market, appealing to a broader group of partygoers due to its effects and availability. Ketamine is typically inhaled, injected, or mixed into drinks, with effects appearing within 10 to 15 minutes and lasting about an hour. It can also be smoked when mixed with cannabis and tobacco. The drug is often combined with other psychoactive substances like cocaine and MDMA to enhance their potency. Ketamine's onset is immediate when injected, reaching peak effects within minutes. Snorting ketamine leads to effects within 5 to 10 minutes, while ingestion may take up to 20 minutes. Ketamine is odourless and tasteless, making it easy to add to beverages without detection, and it can induce amnesia.

Activity 11.4 GHB

- What is GHB?
- List the sought-after effects of GHB.
- List the adverse effects of GHB.
- What are the risks associated with GHB?
- List the withdrawal effects of GHB

Legal status

Ketamine is one of the essential medicines in the WHO's Essential Drugs List (WHO, 2023). In most countries, ketamine is a classified as a controlled drug.

Therapeutic use

Ketamine, initially recognised as an anaesthetic for inhibiting painful sensations in human anaesthesia and veterinary medicine, has gathered attention for its therapeutic potential. A growing body of scientific research strongly supports the rapid antidepressant and anti-suicidal effects of ketamine in treating treatment-resistant depression (TRD) and bipolar depression (Yavi et al., 2022). However, ketamine has been used in the treatment of resistant depression with immediate improvements in mood (Diamond et al., 2014), including the reduction of suicidal thoughts (Ballard et al., 2014).

Ongoing research, such as the Ketamine for Reduction of Alcoholic Relapse (KARE) trial funded by the Medical Research Council in the UK, investigates whether ketamine injections combined with psychological therapy can prevent relapse in abstinent alcoholics (University of Exeter). Systematic reviews and meta-analyses have consistently demonstrated robust, rapid, and transient antidepressant and anti-suicidal effects of ketamine. These findings have been notable in various clinical settings, including treatment-resistant depression and acute suicidal ideation (Walsh et al., 2021). However, it is important to note that the long-term efficacy, safety, and optimal dosing strategies of ketamine for individuals with TRD, bipolar depression, and suicidal ideation are still areas of ongoing research and clinical investigation. Ketamine-based psychotherapy has also been explored. A study (Dore et al., 2019) involving 235 participants with various diagnoses examined ketamine-assisted psychotherapy across three private practices. The average ketamine dose administered was 200–250 mg sublingually or 80–90 mg intramuscularly. The findings showed that patients reported clinically significant improvements in depressive and anxiety symptoms. However, the study lacked a control group, and the diversity of settings and methods used limits the generalizability of the results.

Sought-after effects

Ketamine users often report experiencing sensations of dissociation, which can range from a pleasant feeling of floating to a sense of being separated from their bodies. At lower doses, users may feel a giddy euphoria, but this can be followed by bursts of anxiety or mood swings. Some individuals may also experience a terrifying sense of almost complete sensory detachment, which is referred to as the "K-hole." This experience, akin to a "bad trip" on LSD, can be deeply unsettling. These sought-after effects are strongly dose-related and may persist for up to two hours.

Adverse effects

At higher doses, ketamine induces a withdrawn state known as dissociation. At even higher doses, dissociation can become severe, resulting in what is termed a "K-hole," characterised by ataxia, dysarthria, muscular hypertonicity, and myoclonic jerks. Very high doses may lead to coma and severe hypertension, although deaths are rare. The acute effects of ketamine typically diminish after about 30 minutes. Ketamine use may impair memory and exacerbate existing psychosis, anxiety, or depression. Prolonged use can result in disorientation and a gradual detachment from reality. While ketamine does induce mild respiratory depression, it generally does not significantly affect cardiovascular status. Furthermore, ketamine possesses analgesic and amnesic properties and is associated with less confusion, irrationality, and violent behaviour compared to phencyclidine (PCP), another dissociative drug. Large or repeated doses of ketamine can induce hallucinations, including experiences such as a loss of sense of time, feeling disconnected from the body, and near-death experiences. In extreme cases, large doses of ketamine can lead to loss of consciousness. Some of the long-term effects include memory impairment and deficits in executive functioning (Strous et al., 2022). A summary of the physiological and psychological effects of ketamine is shown in Table 11.4.

Withdrawal and overdose

Excessive use of ketamine can lead to psychological dependence and subsequent withdrawal symptoms upon discontinuation, which may exacerbate cravings and prompt further abuse. Common withdrawal symptoms include agitation, confusion, depression with suicidal risk, psychosis, loss of motor skills, double vision, hearing loss, increased heart rate, rapid breathing, loss of coordination, insomnia, shakes, fatigue, and cognitive impairment. Acute withdrawal symptoms typically manifest within 24 hours of cessation and may persist for up to two weeks, with duration influenced by factors such as drug quantity, tolerance level, duration of use, and co-administration with other substances. A ketamine overdose may result from a high dose, adverse reaction, or combination with other drugs and alcohol. Complications include loss of consciousness, airway obstruction leading to breathing difficulties, coma, nausea, vomiting, and hallucinations. Respiratory failure poses the most significant risk of death in ketamine overdose. Combining ketamine with other depressants like alcohol, Valium, or GHB can result in delirium, amnesia, "K-hole" experiences, loss of coordination, and depression, with potential suicidal risk. A few deaths have occurred due to ketamine overdose, often involving complications such as heart or respiratory failure. The underlying cause

Table 11.4
The physiological and psychological effects of ketamine

Dose	Physiological effects	Psychological effects
Low	Vertigo	Euphoria
	Ataxia	
	Slurred speech	
	Slow reaction time	
Higher	Analgesia	Amnesia
	Movement difficulty	Dissociation (K-hole)
	Muscular hypertonicity	Disorganised thinking
	Hypertension	Unintelligible speech
	Mild respiratory depression	Altered body image
	Coma	Feeling of unreality
		Visual hallucinations

Activity 11.5 Ketamine

- What is *ketamine*?
- List the sought-after effects of ketamine.
- List the adverse effects of ketamine.
- Evaluate the therapeutic use of ketamine.

of death with ketamine is accidental poisoning and impaired judgement (Corkery et al., 2021).

PSILOCYBIN

Psilocybin is a hallucinogenic compound found in over 180 species of mushrooms, commonly known as magic mushrooms. It belongs to the tryptamine class of psychedelics and is structurally similar to serotonin, a neurotransmitter in the brain. Psilocybin has a long history of traditional and ceremonial use in various cultures, particularly in Central and South America. It is widely available as dried mushrooms or in various forms derived from mushrooms. Similar to LSD, psilocybin induces hallucinogenic effects and can be consumed fresh, cooked, or brewed into a tea. A typical hallucinogenic experience requires ingestion of about 30 to 50 mushrooms and lasts up to six hours. Other hallucinogens include *Amanita muscaria* (fly agaric mushrooms), mescaline from the peyote cactus, and psilocybin found in liberty cap mushrooms.

The physical effects of psilocybin manifest within 20 minutes of ingestion. When ingested, psilocybin is metabolised into psilocin, which is responsible for its psychoactive effects. These effects can include alterations in perception, mood, thought patterns, and consciousness. Users may experience vivid hallucinations, changes in sensory perception, euphoria, introspection, and altered sense of time. In modern times, it has gained attention for its potential therapeutic applications, particularly in the treatment of depression, anxiety, PTSD, and other mental health conditions.

Legal status

Psilocybin and psilocybin-containing mushrooms are listed as Schedule I drugs under the United Nations 1971 Convention on Psychotropic Substances, indicating that they are considered to have a high potential for abuse and no recognised medical uses. However, the legal status of psilocybin mushrooms varies widely worldwide, and there is often ambiguity in legislation regarding their possession, sale, transport, and cultivation.

Therapeutic use

Studies investigating the therapeutic advantages of psilocybin have yielded promising findings, yet regulatory challenges persist across many regions. Nevertheless, there is a burgeoning interest in its potential therapeutic applications. Psilocybin has shown therapeutic promise, particularly in treating cancer-related depression, treatment-resistant depression, and potentially OCD, cluster headaches, migraines, and AIDS-related demoralisation (MacCallum et al., 2022). Preliminary research indicates positive outcomes in these areas. Ongoing clinical trials are investigating psilocybin's efficacy in addressing addiction, anorexia, bipolar disorder, chronic pain, major depressive disorder, and OCD (MacCallum et al., 2022), reflecting growing interest in its diverse therapeutic applications.

Sought-after effects

The sought-after effects are similar to LSD's, but the hallucinogenic trip is often milder and shorter.

Adverse effects

Psilocybin, when consumed in small quantities, induces relaxation and mild mood changes.

Physically, it may cause an increase in blood pressure and heart rate, headaches, nausea, fatigue, migraines, vomiting, and physical discomfort. Psilocybin typically raises blood pressure and heart rate, which may be dangerous for people with heart conditions. Psychologically, it can induce anxiety, confusion, strong or extreme fear, paranoia, psychotic-like symptoms, and psychological discomfort. Some people who take magic mushrooms have extreme fear, anxiety, panic, or paranoia as they experience its hallucinogenic effects, which is known as a "bad trip" (NIDA, 2024b). Hallucinogen persisting perception disorder, commonly known as flashbacks, refers to the reoccurrence of sensory disturbances or perceptual abnormalities experienced after the use of hallucinogenic substances. These disturbances may involve visual, auditory, or other sensory perceptions that resemble those experienced during intoxication. Flashbacks can occur briefly or persistently over time, even years after the initial substance use. However, research indicates that flashback episodes are relatively rare, and they are not always negative experiences (NIDA, 2024b). However, when they do occur, they can significantly impact an individual's daily functioning and quality of life. Research conducted thus far suggests that the use of psilocybin, the psychoactive compound found in certain mushrooms, does not typically lead to addiction. While psilocybin itself may not be addictive, it is essential to recognise that individual responses to any substance can vary, and misuse or overuse of psilocybin can still lead to negative consequences.

Activity 11.6 Psilocybin

- What is *psilocybin*?
- List the sought-after effects of psilocybin.
- List the adverse effects of psilocybin.
- Explain hallucinogen persisting perception disorder.

Accidental poisoning from ingesting poisonous mushrooms is a potential risk for some psilocybin users. Symptoms of mushroom poisoning may include muscle spasms, confusion, and delirium, indicating the need for immediate medical attention. Given the prevalence of hallucinogenic and poisonous mushrooms in various environments, it is essential to regularly remove all mushrooms from areas accessible to children to prevent accidental consumption. While most cases of accidental mushroom ingestion result in minor gastrointestinal illness, severe instances may necessitate medical attention.

PCP

PCP (phencyclidine), commonly known as "angel dust," is a pure white crystalline powder that can be found in various forms, such as crystal, capsules, tablets, and liquid. Phencyclidine (PCP) is a dissociative drug initially developed in the 1950s as a surgical aesthetic. It was later discontinued for human use due to its severe side effects, including hallucinations, delusions, and agitation. PCP can be ingested orally, smoked, snorted, or injected. PCP is sometimes combined with cannabis, MDMA, or other drugs, and it has been sold under various names, including mescaline or THC. PCP continues to be detected in PCP-laced marijuana cigarettes, known as "whacko tobacco," and has been found in up to 24% of street marijuana samples (Bey & Patel, 2007). When PCP is swallowed, its effects are delayed for about 30 to 60 minutes, and depending on the dose, they may last from 4 to 48 hours.

Legal status

PCP is a controlled substance in most countries because there is a possibility that the user may become physically or psychologically dependent.

Sought-after effects

- PCP usage causes alterations in thought, mood, sensory perception, and body awareness. However, its effects on mood states are unpredictable. In small amounts, PCP can act as either a stimulant or a depressant, varying among users. A drug-taking episode may induce feelings of well-being, euphoria, numbness, and relaxation, or it may trigger panic, fear, and detachment from reality. Common experiences include distortions of space, time, and body image. Additionally, episodes may lead to odd, erratic, or unexpected behaviours, hallucinations, and catatonic posturing, highlighting the diverse and often unpredictable nature of PCP's effects on users.

Adverse effects

PCP intoxication leads to a spectrum of effects, including unpredictable behaviour, drunkenness, euphoria, disorientation, combativeness, rage, and obscenity. Users may experience alternating periods of lethargy and fearful agitation, with sympton waxing and waning. PCP use may result in decrease but intact pain perception, midpoint pupils, nysta mus, and ataxia, distinguishing it from stimula intoxication. PCP reactions vary based on dosage. A doses between 5 and 25 milligrams, individuals m show signs of stupor, mild coma, intact response deep pain, muscle contractions, and bizarre posture However, doses exceeding 25 milligrams can lead coma with no response to deep pain, hypertherm convulsions, and potentially fatal outcomes (Bey Patel, 2007). This underlines the severe risks assoc ated with PCP use, emphasising the importance understanding its dosage-related effects.

Dependence and withdrawal

PCP is highly addictive, and repeated use will oft lead to psychological dependence, cravings, and co pulsive drug-seeking behaviour (Bey & Patel, 2007 Cravings for PCP can persist even after months abstinence. Withdrawal symptoms include fe

Table 11.5
Physiological and psychological effects of PCP

Dose	Physiological Effects	Psychological Effects
Low to moderate	Shallow rapid breathing	Decreased awareness
	Increased blood pressure	Detached, distant, and estranged from surroundings
	Elevated heart rate	
	Increased temperature	
	Sweating	
	Nausea	
	Blurred vision	
	Dizziness	
	Numbness of extremities	
	Loss of muscular coordination	
High	Decreased blood pressure	Disordered thinking
	Decreased pulse rate	Disordered speech
	Decreased respiration	Delusions
	Nystagmus	Delirium
	Drooling	Suicide
	Loss of balance	Violent behaviour
	Dizziness	Hallucinations
	Convulsions	Paranoia
	Hyperthermia	Catatonia
	Coma	
	Death	

Activity 11.7 PCP.

- What is *PCP?*
- List the sought-after effects of PCP.
- List the adverse effects of PCP.

agitation, anxiety, irritability, sweating, headache, muscle twitching, hallucinations, seizures, and elevated body temperature, typically occurring within eight hours of abstinence. Long-term withdrawal effects can include depression, suicidal thoughts, memory loss, weight loss, speech impairment, impaired cognitive function, sleep disturbances, and mood disorders. Withdrawal symptoms may last several months to a year after detoxification. The physiological and psychological effects of PCP are presented in Table 11.5.

AYAHUASCA, *SALVIA DIVINORUM*, AND 2C-B

Ayahuasca is a traditional Amazonian brew made from the *Banisteriopsis caapi* vine and the *Psychotria viridis* bush, containing beta-carboline alkaloids and N,N-dimethyltryptamine (DMT), respectively. It has been used for centuries by indigenous shamans for spiritual communication, healing practices, and religious rituals in South America. Some Brazilian churches routinely use ayahuasca for spiritual experiences. In contemporary times, it has been used for recreational experiences. Ayahuasca induces various psychological effects, including altered perception, ego dissolution (a dissolution of the sense of self, leading to feelings of unity with others, nature, or the universe), introspection, emotional release, spiritual experiences, healing, and catharsis. Users often report deep introspection, encounters with spiritual entities, and therapeutic benefits, such as resolving psychological conflicts. These effects are highly subjective and influenced by factors like dosage and individual psychology. The ayahuasca experience typically begins around 40 minutes after ingestion, reaching its peak between 60 and 120 minutes, and fading within approximately four hours (Hamill et al., 2019). Users of ayahuasca experience shifts in consciousness without complete loss, often gaining profound self-assurance, fresh insights into internal conflicts, intimate truths unveiled, and the possibility of aiding psychotherapeutic processes (Mabit, 2007).

The primary physical side effects of ayahuasca include nausea, vomiting, and diarrhoea. However, in traditional settings, these effects are regarded as integral to the ayahuasca healing process, often seen as a form of spiritual cleansing rather than mere side effects (Fotiou & Gearin, 2019). Despite the prevalence of adverse physical and psychological effects associated with ayahuasca usage, they are typically not severe (Bouso et al., 2022). As a therapeutic substance, ayahuasca is found to bring about lasting enhancements in mood and cognitive patterns (Uthaug et al., 2018) and significant reductions in depression and psychopathology, self-transcendence, and improved quality of life (Jiménez-Garrido et al., 2020).

Salvia divinorum, native to Mexico, has been utilised spiritually and medicinally by Mazatec tribes for centuries. It is a potent natural hallucinogen known for inducing intense psychedelic experiences. While gaining popularity in the West for recreational purposes, it is also being explored for potential therapeutic applications. *Salvia divinorum* induces intense but short-lived hallucinogenic experiences, often characterised by distortions in perception, paranoia, mood changes, detachment from one's body, altered visual perceptions, slurred speech, sweating, and dizziness. The effects of *Salvia divinorum* can be unpredictable and sometimes unsettling, leading to a unique set of experiences compared to other hallucinogens. Therapeutically, the traditional preparations of *Salvia divinorum* have been employed in treatments addressing illnesses associated with inflammatory conditions and pain (Coffeen & Pellicer, 2019).

2C-B is a synthetic hallucinogen belonging to the phenethylamine class of compounds. It produces psychedelic effects similar to those of LSD and mescaline but is often considered to have a more manageable and gentle experience by some users. Acute effects include elevated blood pressure and heart rate, euphoria, hallucinatory effects, experienced alterations in perceptions, such as distances, colours, shapes, and lights, as well as changes in body sensations and surroundings (Papaseit et al., 2018). However, like with other hallucinogens, the effects of 2C-B can vary widely depending on the dose, individual characteristics, and environmental factors.

KEY POINTS

- Hallucinogens are a diverse group of substances that have different chemical structures, mechanisms of action, and adverse effects.
- Ketamine is an odourless, colourless, and tasteless powder that can be swallowed, sniffed, injected, or smoked.
- The effects of LSD may cause panic, confusion, impulsive behaviour and unpleasant illusions (bad trip), and flashbacks and may precipitate psychotic reactions.
- In MDMA, the user experiences euphoric feelings and feelings of empathy, relaxation, and meaningfulness.
- The adverse effects of MDMA include tiredness, confusion, anxiety, and depression.
- Some people may develop tolerance to the effects of MDMA; using larger amounts will increase the severity of undesirable effects rather than increase the pleasurable effects.
- GHB causes intoxication resembling alcohol or ketamine intoxication and can lead to respiratory depression and death, especially when combined with alcohol.
- GHB, at high doses, can cause convulsions, coma, and respiratory collapse.
- Most deaths have occurred when GHB was taken with alcohol or other drugs.
- Withdrawal from GHB may cause symptoms similar to acute withdrawal from alcohol or barbiturates (delirium tremens) and can cause convulsions, paranoia, and hallucinations.
- Some ketamine users' experiences involve a terrifying feeling of almost-complete sensory detachment that is likened to a near-deat experience.
- With very high doses, coma and severe hyperten sion may occur; deaths are unusual.
- Psilocybin usually takes about 30 to 50 mush rooms to produce a hallucinogenic experienc similar to that experienced with LSD.
- Higher doses cause perceptual changes, distor tion of body image, and hallucinations.
- Some people eat poisonous mushrooms thinkin they are mushrooms containing psilocybin.
- High doses of PCP can cause convulsions, coma hyperthermia, and death.
- Long-term PCP users report memory loss, difficulties with speech and thinking, depression, an weight loss.
- Recent research suggests that repeated or prolonged use of PCP can cause withdrawal syndrome when drug use is stopped.
- Ayahuasca induces various psychological effects including altered perception, ego dissolution introspection, emotional release, spiritual experiences, healing, and catharsis.
- Despite the prevalence of adverse physical and psychological effects associated with ayahuasca usage, they are typically not severe.
- *Salvia divinorum* induces intense but short-lived hallucinogenic experiences, often characterised by distortions in perception, paranoia, mood changes, detachment from one's body, altered visual perceptions, slurred speech, sweating, and dizziness.
- *Salvia divinorum* has been employed in treatments addressing illnesses associated with inflammatory conditions and pain.

References

Abramson, H. A. (1966). LSD in psychotherapy and alcoholism. *American Journal of Psychotherapy*, 20(3), 415–438. https://doi.org/10.1176/appi.psychotherapy.1966.20.3.415.

Andresen, H., Aydin, B. E., Mueller, A., & Iwersen-Bergmann, S. (2011). An overview of gamma-hydroxybutyric acid: Pharmacodynamics, pharmacokinetics, toxic effects, addiction, analytical methods, and interpretation of results. *Drug Testing and Analysis*, 3(9), 560–568. https://doi.org/10.1002/dta.254.

Ballard, E. D., Ionescu, D. F., Vande Voort, J. L., Niciu, M. J., Richards, E. M., Luckenbaugh, D. A., Brutsché, N. E., Ameli, R., Furey, M. L., & Zarate, C. A., Jr (2014). Improvement in suicidal ideation after ketamine infusion: Relationship to reductions in depression and anxiety. *Journal of Psychiatric Research*, 58, 161–166. https://doi.org/10.1016/j.jpsychires.2014.07.027.

Belouin, S. J., & Henningfield, J. E. (2018). Psychedelics: Where we are now, why we got here, what we must do. *Neuropharmacology*, 142, 7–19. https://doi.org/10.1016/j.neuropharm.2018.02.018.

Beurmanjer, H., Luykx, J. J., De Wilde, B., van Rompaey, K., Buwalda, V. J. A., De Jong, C. A. J., Dijkstra, B. A. G., & Schellekens, A. F. A. (2020). Tapering with pharmaceutical GHB or benzodiazepines for detoxification in GHB -dependent patients: A matched-subject observational study of treatment-as-usual in Belgium and The Netherlands.

CNS Drugs, 34(6), 651–659. https://doi.org/10.1007/s40263-020-00730-8.

Bey, T., & Patel, A. (2007). Phencyclidine intoxication and adverse effects: A clinical and pharmacological review of an illicit drug. *The California Journal of Emergency Medicine,* 8(1), 9–14.

Bogenschutz, M. P., & Johnson, M. W. (2016). Classic hallucinogens in the treatment of addictions. *Progress in Neuro-Psychopharmacology & Biological Psychiatry,* 64, 250–258. https://doi.org/10.1016/j.pnpbp.2015.03.002.

Bolla, K. I., McCann, U. D., & Ricaurte, G. A. (1998). Memory impairment in abstinent MDMA ("ecstasy") users. *Neurology,* 51(6), 1532–1537. https://doi.org/10.1212/wnl.51.6.1532.

Bouso, J. C., Andión, Ó., Sarris, J. J., Scheidegger, M., Tófoli, L. F., Opaleye, E. S., Schubert, V., & Perkins, D. (2022). Adverse effects of ayahuasca: Results from the global ayahuasca survey. *PLOS Global Public Health,* 2(11), e0000438. https://doi.org/10.1371/journal.pgph.0000438.

Busardò, F. P., & Jones, A. W. (2015). GHB pharmacology and toxicology: Acute intoxication, concentrations in blood and urine in forensic cases and treatment of the withdrawal syndrome. *Current Neuropharmacology,* 13(1), 47–70. https://doi.org/10.2174/1570159X13666141210215423.

Coffeen, U., & Pellicer, F. (2019). *Salvia divinorum:* From recreational hallucinogenic use to analgesic and anti-inflammatory action. *Journal of Pain Research,* 12, 1069–1076. https://doi.org/10.2147/JPR.S188619.

Corkery, J. M., Hung, W. C., Claridge, H., Goodair, C., Copeland, C. S., & Schifano, F. (2021). Recreational ketamine-related deaths notified to the national programme on substance abuse deaths, England, 1997–2019. *Journal of Psychopharmacology,* 35(11), 1324–1348. https://doi.org/10.1177/02698811211021588.

Darke, S., Lappin, J., & Farrell, M. (2019). *The Clinician's Guide to Illicit Drugs and Health.* Great Britain: Silverback Publishing.

Diamond, P. R., Farmery, A. D., Atkinson, S., Haldar, J., Williams, N., Cowen, P. J., Geddes, J. R., & McShane, R. (2014). Ketamine infusions for treatment resistant depression: A series of 28 patients treated weekly or twice weekly in an ECT clinic. *Journal of Psychopharmacology,* 28(6), 536–544. https://doi.org/10.1177/0269881114527361.

Dominguez, A., Soca Gallego, L., & Parmar, M. (2023). Sodium oxybate. In *StatPearls* [Internet]. Treasure Island, FL: StatPearls Publishing. https://www.ncbi.nlm.nih.gov/books/NBK562283/ (accessed 6 March 2024).

Dore, J., Turnipseed, B., Dwyer, S., Turnipseed, A., Andries, J., Ascani, G., Monnette, C., Huidekoper, A., Strauss, N., & Wolfson, P. (2019). Ketamine assisted psychotherapy (KAP): Patient demographics, clinical data and outcomes in three large practices administering ketamine with psychotherapy. *Journal of Psychoactive Drugs,* 51(2), 189–198. https://doi.org/10.1080/02791072.2019.1587556.

Drugs.com. (2017). *GHB or Gamma-Hydroxybutyrate.* www.drugs.com/illicit/ghb.html (accessed 24 June 2024).

EMCDDA. (2002). *Report on the Risk Assessment of Ketamine in the Framework of the Joint Action on New Synthetic Drugs.* Luxembourg: European Monitoring Centre for Drugs and Drug Addiction.

Fotiou, E., & Gearin, A. K. (2019). Purging and the body in the therapeutic use of ayahuasca. *Social Science & Medicine (1982),* 239, 112532. https://doi.org/10.1016/j.socscimed.2019.112532.

Fuentes, J. J., Fonseca, F., Elices, M., Farré, M., & Torrens, M. (2020). Therapeutic use of LSD in psychiatry: A systematic review of randomized-controlled clinical trials. *Frontiers in Psychiatry,* 10, 943. https://doi.org/10.3389/fpsyt.2019.00943.

Galicia, M., Dargan, P. I., Dines, A. M., Yates, C., Heyerdahl, F., Hovda, K. E., Giraudon, I., Euro-DEN Plus Research Group, Wood, D. M., Miró, Ò., & Euro-DEN Plus Research Group (2019). Clinical relevance of ethanol coingestion in patients with GHB/GBL intoxication. *Toxicology Letters,* 314, 37–42. https://doi.org/10.1016/j.toxlet.2019.07.001.

Gasser, P., Holstein, D., Michel, Y., Doblin, R., Yazar-Klosinski, B., Passie, T., & Brenneisen, R. (2014). Safety and efficacy of lysergicacid diethylamide-assisted psychotherapy for anxiety associated with life-threatening diseases. *Journal of Nervous and Mental Disease,* 202(7), 513–520. https://doi.org/10.1097/NMD.0000000000000113.

Green, A. R., Mechan, A. O., Elliott, J. M., O'Shea, E., & Colado, M. I. (2003). The pharmacology and clinical pharmacology of 3,4-methylenedioxymethamphetamine (MDMA, "ecstasy"). *Pharmacological Reviews,* 55(3), 463–508. https://doi.org/10.1124/pr.55.3.3.

Hamill, J., Hallak, J., Dursun, S. M., & Baker, G. (2019). Ayahuasca: Psychological and physiologic effects, pharmacology and potential uses in addiction and mental illness. *Current Neuropharmacology,* 17(2), 108–128. https://doi.org/10.2174/1570159X16666180125095902.

Jiménez-Garrido, D. F., Gómez-Sousa, M., Ona, G., Dos Santos, R. G., Hallak, J. E. C., Alcázar-Córcoles, M. Á., & Bouso, J. C. (2020). Effects of ayahuasca on mental health and quality of life in naïve users: A longitudinal and cross-sectional study combination. *Scientific Reports,* 10(1), 4075. https://doi.org/10.1038/s41598-020-61169-x.

Johnson, M. W., Sewell, R. A., & Griffiths, R. R. (2012). Psilocybin dose-dependently causes delayed, transient headaches in healthy volunteers. *Drug and Alcohol Dependence,* 123(1–3), 132–140. https://doi.org/10.1016/j.drugalcdep.2011.10.029.

Kish, S. J. (2002). How strong is the evidence that brain serotonin neurons are damaged in human users of ecstasy? *Pharmacology, Biochemistry, and Behavior,* 71(4), 845–855. https://doi.org/10.1016/s0091-3057(01)00708-0.

Kish, S. J., Furukawa, Y., Ang, L., Vorce, S. P., & Kalasinsky, K. S. (2000). Striatal serotonin is depleted in brain of a human MDMA (Ecstasy) user. *Neurology,* 55(2), 294–296. https://doi.org/10.1212/wnl.55.2.294.

Kumar, S., Soren, S., & Chaudhury, S. (2009). Hallucinations: Etiology and clinical implications. *Industrial Psychiatry Journal,* 18(2), 119–126. https://doi.org/10.4103/0972-6748.62273.

Liechti, M. E., & Vollenweider, F. X. (2001). Which neuroreceptors mediate the subjective effects of MDMA in humans? A summary of mechanistic studies. *Human Psychopharmacology,* 16(8), 589–598. https://doi.org/10.1002/hup.348.

Mabit, J. (2007). Ayahuasca in the treatment of addictions. *Psychedelic Medicine: New Evidence for Hallucinogenic Substances as Treatments,* 2, 87–105.

MacCallum, C. A., Lo, L. A., Pistawka, C. A., & Deol, J. K. (2022). Therapeutic use of psilocybin: Practical considerations for dosing and administration. *Frontiers in Psychiatry,* 13, 1040217. https://doi.org/10.3389/fpsyt.2022.1040217.

Mathias, R. (1999). *Ecstasy-Damages the Brain and Impairs Memory in Humans* (Vol. 14, No. 4). The National Institute on Drug Abuse, NIDA Notes. https://www.ehd.org/pdf/ecstasy5.pdf (accessed 6 March 2024).

Mithoefer, M. C. (2015). *A Manual for MDMA-Assisted Psychotherapy in the Treatment of Posttraumatic Stress Disorder*. Santa Cruz, CA: MAPS. https://maps.org/research-archive/mdma/MDMA-Assisted-Psychotherapy-Treatment-Manual-Version7-19Aug15-FINAL.pdf (accessed 6 March 2024).

National Drug and Alcohol Research Centre (NDARC). (2021). *MDMA/Ecstasy*. Fact Sheets. https://ndarc.med.unsw.edu.au/sites/default/files/ndarc/resources/NDARC%20Fact%20Sheet_MDMA_Ecstasy.pdf (accessed 6 March 2024).

Nichols, D. E. (2016). Psychedelics. *Pharmacological Reviews*, 68(2), 264–355. https://doi.org/10.1124/pr.115.011478.

Nichols, D. E., & Grob, C. S. (2018). Is LSD toxic? *Forensic Science International*, 284, 141–145. https://doi.org/10.1016/j.forsciint.2018.01.006.

NIDA. (2010). *Drug Infofacts: Club Drugs (GHB, Ketamine, and Rohypnol)*. National Institute of Drug Abuse, National Institutes of Health; U.S. Department of Health and Human Services. www.drugabuse.gov/sites/default/files/clubdrugs10.pdf (accessed 24 June 2024).

NIDA. (2021a). *What Are the Effects of MDMA?* https://nida.nih.gov/publications/research-reports/mdma-ecstasy-abuse/what-are-effects-mdma (accessed 6 March 2024).

NIDA. (2021b). *Is MDMA Addictive?* https://nida.nih.gov/publications/research-reports/mdma-ecstasy-abuse/mdma-addictive (accessed 6 March 2024).

NIDA. (2022). *What Is MDMA?* https://nida.nih.gov/publications/research-reports/mdma-ecstasy-abuse/what-mdma (accessed 6 March 2024).

NIDA. (2024a). *Psychedelic and Dissociative Drugs*. https://nida.nih.gov/research-topics/psychedelic-dissociative-drugs (accessed 5 March 2024).

NIDA. (2024b). *Psilocybin (Magic Mushrooms)*. https://nida.nih.gov/research-topics/psilocybin-magic-mushrooms (accessed 8 March 2024).

Nutt, D. J., King, L. A., Phillips, L. D., & Independent Scientific Committee on Drugs. (2010). Drug harms in the UK: A multi-criteria decision analysis. *Lancet*, 376(9752), 1558–1565. https://doi.org/10.1016/S0140-6736(10)61462-6.

Papaseit, E., Farré, M., Pérez-Mañá, C., Torrens, M., Ventura, M., Pujadas, M., de la Torre, R., & González, D. (2018). Acute pharmacological effects of 2C-B in humans: An observational study. *Frontiers in Pharmacology*, 9, 206. https://doi.org/10.3389/fphar.2018.00206.

Parrott, A. C. (2014). The potential dangers of using MDMA for psychotherapy. *Journal of Psychoactive Drugs*, 46(1), 37–43. https://doi.org/10.1080/02791072.2014.873690.

Reiff, C. M., Richman, E. E., Nemeroff, C. B., Carpenter, L. L., Widge, A. S., Rodriguez, C. I., Kalin, N. H., McDonald, W. M., & The Work Group on Biomarkers and Novel Treatments, a Division of the American Psychiatric Association Council of Research. (2020). Psychedelics and psychedelic-assisted psychotherapy. *The American Journal of Psychiatry*, 177(5), 391–410. https://doi.org/10.1176/appi.ajp.2019.19010035.

Ricaurte, G. A., & McCann, U. D. (2005). Recognition and management of complications of new recreational drug use. *Lancet*, 365(9477), 2137–2145. https://doi.org/10.1016/S0140-6736(05)66737-2.

Skala, K., Caputo, F., Mirijello, A., Vassallo, G., Antonel Ferrulli, A., Walter, H., Lesch, O., & Addolorato, G. (2 Sodium oxybate in the treatment of alcohol dependence: the alcohol withdrawal syndrome to the alcohol relaps vention. *Expert Opinion on Pharmacotherapy*, 15(2), 257. https://doi.org/10.1517/14656566.2014.863

Strous, J. F. M., Weeland, C. J., van der Draai, F. A., Daa G., Denys, D., Lok, A., Schoevers, R. A., & Figee, M. (2 Brain changes associated with long-term ketamine abu systematic review. *Frontiers in Neuroanatomy*, 16, 795 https://doi.org/10.3389/fnana.2022.795231.

Tay, E., Lo, W. K. W., & Murnion, B. (2022). Current in on the impact of gamma-hydroxybutyrate (GHB) Abuse *stance Abuse and Rehabilitation*, 13, 13–23. https:/ org/10.2147/SAR.S315720.

University of Exeter. *Ketamine for reduction of Alcoholic Re (KARE)*. https://www.exeter.ac.uk/research/projects chology/kare/ (accessed 7 March 2024).

Uthaug, M. V., van Oorsouw, K., Kuypers, K. P. C., van tel, M., Broers, N. J., Mason, N. L., Toennes, S. W., J., & Ramaekers, J. G. (2018). Sub-acute and long effects of ayahuasca on affect and cognitive thinking and their association with ego dissolution. *Psychopha cology*, 235(10), 2979–2989. https://doi.org/10.1C s00213-018-4988-3.

van Amsterdam, J., Nutt, D., Phillips, L., & van den B W. (2015). European rating of drug harms. *Journa Psychopharmacology*, 29(6), 655–660. https:/ org/10.1177/0269881115581980.

van Amsterdam, J., Pennings, E., Brunt, T., & van den Brink (2013). Physical harm due to chronic substance use. *ulatory Toxicology and Pharmacology: RTP*, 66(1), 83 https://doi.org/10.1016/j.yrtph.2013.03.007.

Verkes, R. J., Gijsman, H. J., Pieters, M. S., Schoemaker, R de Visser, S., Kuijpers, M., Pennings, E. J., de Bruin, D., de Wijngaart, G., Van Gerven, J. M., & Cohen, A. F. (20 Cognitive performance and serotonergic function in use ecstasy. *Psychopharmacology*, 153(2), 196–202. http doi.org/10.1007/s002130000563.

Vollenweider, F. X., & Smallridge, J. W. (2022). Classic psyche drugs: Update on biological mechanisms. *Pharmacopsychi* 55(3), 121–138. https://doi.org/10.1055/a-1721-2914

Walsh, Z., Mollaahmetoglu, O. M., Rootman, J., Golsof, Keeler, J., Marsh, B., Nutt, D. J., & Morgan, C. J. A. (20 Ketamine for the treatment of mental health and substance disorders: Comprehensive systematic review. *BJPsych Op* 8(1), e19. https://doi.org/10.1192/bjo.2021.1061.

WHO. (2006). *Critical Review of KETAMINE*. Geneva: W Health Organization. ECDD 2006/4.3. www.who. medicines/areas/quality_safety/4.3KetamineCritReview (accessed 24 June 2024).

WHO. (2023). Web Annex A. World Health Organiza model list of essential medicines 23rd list, 2023. In *Selection and Use of Essential Medicines 2023: Execu Summary of the Report of the 24th WHO Expert Commi on the Selection and Use of Essential Medicines*. Gene World Health Organization, 24–28 April.

Yavi, M., Lee, H., Henter, I. D., Park, L. T., & Zarate, C. A., (2022). Ketamine treatment for depression: A review. *cover Mental Health*, 2(1), 9. https://doi.org/10.10C s44192-022-00012-3.

Chapter 12

Anabolic steroids, amyl and butyl nitrite, hypno-sedatives, volatile substances, over-the-counter drugs, smart and eco drugs

Learning outcomes

- Describe the therapeutic and adverse effects of anabolic steroids.
- Describe the therapeutic and adverse effects of amyl nitrite.
- Describe the therapeutic and adverse effects of hypno-sedatives.
- Describe the short-term and long-term effects of volatile substances.
- Identify the use and misuse of over-the-counter drugs.
- Identify the risk of using smart and eco drugs.

Activity 12.1

Please choose one correct answer to the following multiple-choice questions.

1. Which of the following statements about steroids is true?
   a. Steroids are only used for medical purposes.
   b. Steroids are not addictive.
   c. Steroids are primarily used to treat bacterial infections.
   d. Steroids can have adverse effects on physical and mental health.
   e. Steroids are harmless when used without a prescription.
2. Which of the following is a common reason athletes and bodybuilders misuse steroids?
   a. To reduce inflammation
   b. To enhance physical performance and muscle mass
   c. To promote relaxation and stress relief
   d. To improve concentration and focus
   e. To prevent allergic reactions
3. Which of the following statements accurately describes the use of steroids?
   a. Steroids are typically used to treat diabetes.
   b. Steroids are not associated with any adverse effects on health.
   c. Steroids are often misused by athletes and bodybuilders to enhance muscle growth.
   d. Steroids are primarily used as painkillers.
   e. Steroids have no impact on reproductive system development.

DOI: 10.4324/9781003456674-14

4. Steroids are synthetic versions of:
   a. Bacteria
   b. Testosterone
   c. Oestrogen
   d. Hormone
   e. None of the above
5. Steroids are hormones that occur naturally in the body:
   a. To control the digestive system
   b. To control the respiratory system
   c. None of the above
   d. To control the reproductive system
   e. To control the circulatory system
6. Steroids are typically used:
   a. To stimulate muscle growth
   b. To increase intelligence
   c. To decrease performance
   d. To increase confidence
   e. None of the above
7. Steroids are hormones that occur naturally in the body
   a. To control the digestive system
   b. To control the respiratory system
   c. None of the above
   d. To control the reproductive system
   e. To control the circulatory system
8. Steroids are typically used:
   a. To stimulate muscle growth
   b. To increase intelligence
   c. To decrease performance
   d. To increase confidence
   e. None of the above
9. Which organ is the first to be affected with heavy use of steroids?
   a. Kidneys
   b. Liver
   c. Heart
   d. Brain
   e. None of the above
10. Steroid abuse can cause
    a. Brain tumours
    b. Heart tumours
    c. Liver tumours
    d. Kidney tumours
    e. None of the above
11. Steroids cannot do which of the following?
    a. Increase muscle mass
    b. Improve visual acuity
    c. Increase stamina
    d. Increase strength
    e. None of the above

12. Female steroid misusers become more masculine. Among other things, their voice:
    a. Deepens
    b. Gets lower
    c. Gets higher
    d. Gets hoarse
    e. None of the above
13. Male steroid misusers may suffer from
    a. A decrease in sperm production
    b. An increase in testes size
    c. An increase in sperm production
    d. All of the above
    e. None of the above

Activity 12.2

State whether the statements are true or false.

Statements	True	False
Anabolic steroids are classified as a controlled drug.		
Anabolic steroids are available on prescription only.		
Anabolic steroids can be taken orally, injected, or with skin patches.		
The sought-after effects of steroids are to enhance physical appearance/body image.		
Steroids can cause hair loss, acne, breast development, and low sperm production.		
Physical dependence is common in steroid users.		

ANABOLIC STEROIDS

Steroids, naturally occurring hormones in the body, regulate reproductive system development and function. Anabolic steroids, synthetic versions of testosterone, enhance muscle growth and are commonly used by athletes and bodybuilders to boost performance and physique. They are administered orally or via injection in cycles, often at higher doses than medically prescribed. Commonly known as roids, juice, gear, and stackers, anabolic steroids are used to build muscle mass, reduce fatigue, and enhance self-confidence. Synthetic testosterone derivatives dominate the market, available in various forms, including creams, gels, and patches. Anabolic steroids come in various forms: oral, injectable, and topical gels or creams. Users often start with oral steroids, progressing to injectable forms due to reduced liver damage. However, oral steroids clear from the body faster, preferred by those wary of drug testing. Misusers take doses 10 to 100 times higher than medically prescribed (NIDA, 2018). Steroid misuse commonly involves cycling, where doses are taken over a set period, followed by breaks and restarts. Users often stack multiple steroids, including oral, injectable, and veterinary types, believing in enhanced muscle effects, though scientifically unproven. Pyramiding is another method, tapering doses up and down in cycles of 6–12 weeks, followed by drug-free intervals for hormonal recovery. Plateauing, a technique to avoid tolerance, involves staggering or substituting steroids yet lacks scientific validation (NIDA, 2018). These practices reflect users' beliefs in optimising muscle gains but remain unverified by scientific research.

Legal status

Most of the developed countries have very strict laws when it comes to the sale, possession, purchase, and use of anabolic steroids. That is, using or possessing any anabolic steroid without a prescription is illegal. However, some countries have very different views when it comes to the sale and possession of anabolic steroids.

Therapeutic use

Anabolic steroids are used therapeutically to address hormonal deficiencies, muscle wasting diseases, delayed puberty, osteoporosis, and chronic illnesses. They help supplement hormone levels, promote muscle growth, stimulate puberty, improve bone density, and counteract muscle weakness. Anabolic steroids are prescribed to treat body wasting in patients with AIDS and other conditions causing loss of lean muscle mass. They are also used when patients fail to gain or maintain normal weight due to unexplained medical reasons. Additionally, anabolic steroids are employed in the treatment of certain types of anaemia, breast cancer in women, blood clotting diseases, growth failure, Turner's syndrome, and hereditary angioedema. Medical supervision is crucial to ensure safe and effective use, with adherence to prescribed dosages and monitoring for potential side effects.

Sought-after effects

The desired effects of steroids include enhancing muscle size, increasing body strength, and improving performance, driven by the desire for a favourable physical appearance and body image. Anabolic steroids facilitate nitrogen retention in the body, promoting muscle growth. They also stimulate the production of red blood cells, leading to the misconception that they may enhance endurance, although empirical evidence does not support this notion.

Adverse effects

Anabolic steroids, while sought for their muscle-building and strength-enhancing effects, entail a host of adverse consequences for both physical and mental health. These include cardiovascular complications, hormonal imbalances, liver damage, musculoskeletal issues, psychological disturbances, skin and hair problems, as well as disruptions to the endocrine system. Such adverse effects highlight the necessity for informed and supervised use, emphasising caution to prevent misuse and safeguard individual well-being. In addition, there are some gender-specific side effects. Table 12.1 presents the potential adverse effects of anabolic steroids.

Table 12.1
Potential adverse effects of anabolic steroids

Effects	
Cardiovascular effects	Elevated blood pressure
	Increased risk of heart attack and stroke
	Adverse changes in cholesterol levels
	Artery damage
	Predisposing individuals to cardiovascular diseases
Hormonal imbalances	Disrupt the body's natural hormone balance, leading to infertility
	Decreased libido and impotence in men
	Decreased sperm production
	Enlarged breasts (men)
	Decreased breast size (women)
	Menstrual irregularities and infertility in women

Table 12.1 (*Continued*)

Effects	
Liver damage	Liver damage
	Jaundice
	Liver tumours or cancer
Musculoskeletal problems	Tendon ruptures
	Ligament injuries
	Musculoskeletal pain (weightlifters and bodybuilders)
Skin and hair issues	Acne
	Oily skin
	Accelerated hair loss or baldness (if genetically predisposed)
Endocrine disruptions	Disrupt the normal functioning of the endocrine system
	Hormonal imbalances
	Potential long-term health consequences
Infection	HIV/AIDS
	Hepatitis
Development of secondary sexual characteristics	Anabolic steroid
	In men: development of breast tissue (gynecomastia)
	In women: masculinisation, including deepening of the voice and excessive facial and body hair growth
Psychological effects	Mood swings
	Aggression
	Irritability
	Delusions
	Mania
	Depression and anxiety
	Steroid dependence and addiction

Anabolic steroids are seldom associated with overdose, but acute overdose of corticosteroids can manifest in various symptoms, including burning/itchy skin, agitation or psychosis, convulsions, high blood pressure, muscle and bone weakness, nausea or vomiting, extreme sleepiness, worsening health conditions, nervousness, depression, and swelling in the legs (National Library of Medicine, 2023). These symptoms may occur due to intentional or accidental excessive doses of corticosteroids. Withdrawal from anabolic steroids occurs in individuals who develop dependence, with approximately 32% of users becoming dependent. Symptoms include tolerance, needing higher doses for the same effects, and withdrawal upon cessation, marked by fatigue, restlessness, loss of appetite, insomnia, reduced sex drive, and cravings. Notably, depression, a dangerous symptom, may escalate to suicide attempts (NIDA, 2018).

AMYL AND BUTYL NITRITE

Amyl and butyl nitrites, collectively known as alkyl nitrites, are stimulants commonly referred to as "poppers," "TNT," "liquid gold," and "rush." Chemically related to nitrous oxide, they are clear, yellow, volatile, and inflammable liquids with a sweet smell when fresh but develop a foul odour when stale, often described as "smelly socks." Users inhale the vapours through the nose or mouth from small bottles or tubes. Sold in sex shops, pubs, bars, and clubs in some countries, these drugs come in small bottles with screw or plug tops. Amyl nitrite, classified as an inhalant, is typically snorted from an open bottle, while some individuals inhale it through a cigarette dipped in the liquid. It acts as a vasodilator, dilating blood vessels upon inhalation.

Activity 12.3

- What are the physical effects of anabolic steroids?
- What are the psychological effects of anabolic steroids?

Activity 12.4

Please choose one correct answer for the following multiple-choice questions.

1. What are the common effects of amyl and butyl nitrites?
   a. Sedation and drowsiness
   b. Increased heart rate and blood pressure
   c. Euphoria and enhanced sensory perception
   d. Decreased respiratory rate and muscle relaxation
   e. None of the above
2. Which term is commonly used to refer to amyl and butyl nitrites?
   a. Roids
   b. Juice
   c. Gear
   d. Poppers
   e. None of the above
3. What is a potential risk associated with the misuse of amyl and butyl nitrites?
   a. Liver damage
   b. Kidney failure
   c. Cardiovascular complications
   d. Respiratory depression
   e. None of the above
4. How are amyl and butyl nitrites typically consumed?
   a. Orally
   b. Injected intramuscularly
   c. Inhaled
   d. Applied topically
   e. None of the above
5. Which of the following is a common slang term for amyl and butyl nitrites?
   a. TNT
   b. Gear
   c. Stackers
   d. Roids
   e. None of the above
6. What is a potential side effect of using amyl and butyl nitrites?
   a. Increased alertness
   b. Enhanced memory
   c. Headaches
   d. Improved concentration
   e. None of the above
7. How do amyl and butyl nitrites affect blood vessels?
   a. They cause vasoconstriction
   b. They cause vasodilation

c. They have no effect on blood vessels
d. They decrease blood pressure
e. None of the above

8. What is a potential danger of combining amyl and butyl nitrites with other drugs?
   a. Increased effectiveness of both drugs
   b. Decreased risk of side effects
   c. Heightened euphoric effects
   d. Increased risk of adverse reactions and complications
   e. None of the above
9. The therapeutic use of amyl nitrite is for
   a. The treatment of angina
   b. The treatment of cancer
   c. No therapeutic medical uses
   d. The treatment of liver disease
   e. None of the above
10. Tolerance to the drug develops:
   a. Within two to three weeks of regular use
   b. After a few days of abstinence
   c. Within four to five weeks of regular use
   d. Within two days of occasional use
   e. None of the above

Legal status

The legal status of amyl and butyl nitrites varies from country to country and jurisdiction. In many places, they are legally sold as industrial chemicals or room odorises, but their recreational use as inhalants is often prohibited or restricted. In many countries, poppers are sold in nightclubs, bars, sex shops, drug paraphernalia head shops, over the internet, and in markets. These substances are sold as odourises or DVD or leather cleaner. In some countries, possession, sale, or distribution of poppers for recreational purposes may be illegal or subject to regulations due to their potential health risks and abuse. However, they may be legally available for certain industrial or commercial purposes.

Therapeutic use

Amyl nitrite has historically been used medically to treat angina and as an antidote to cyanide poisoning. It was first produced in 1857 specifically for angina treatment. Amyl nitrite evaporates at room temperature, and its vapor causes veins and arteries to dilate, leading to faster blood flow through the heart and brain. Recreationally, users report intense sensations when inhaling amyl nitrite. On the dance floor, it is described as feeling like a percussive thunderbolt, while during sex, users may feel like their sexual organs have grown significantly. These effects are short-lived, typically lasting only a few moments, with some individuals experiencing light-headedness afterward. However, reactions to amyl nitrite can vary. Some users may suffer from pounding headaches, dizziness, flushed face, or sensations. Unlike amyl nitrite, butyl nitrite lacks therapeutic medical uses.

Sought-after effects

Amyl and butyl nitrite are potent drugs that induce a rapid burst of dizzy energy lasting two to five minutes upon inhalation. They cause immediate dilation of blood vessels, increased heart rate, and a rush of blood to the brain. Users, especially those seeking enhanced sexual pleasure, report a slowed sense of time, prolonged sensation of orgasm, and prevention of premature ejaculation. Additionally, alkyl nitrites are utilised for relaxing the anal sphincter, facilitating anal intercourse.

Adverse effects

Nitrites induce various effects, including dizziness, muscle relaxation, increased heart rate, low blood pressure, flushing, blurred vision, headaches, vomiting, burning sensations in the mouth and nose, and in severe cases, death, particularly among individuals with existing heart problems or low blood pressure. People with cardiovascular issues, glaucoma, and anaemia should refrain from using nitrites. While the drug is rapidly excreted from the body in healthy individuals, there are concerns regarding its potential to suppress the immune system. Individuals with anaemia, high blood pressure, a history of cerebral haemorrhaging, or pregnancy should also avoid nitrite use. Combining nitrites with alcohol, cannabis, or cocaine can exacerbate adverse effects. Concurrent use of Viagra or other drugs for sexual dysfunction with nitrites may lead to hypotension, fainting, stroke, or heart attack. The immediate and long-term effects of nitrites are presented in Table 12.2.

Table 12.2
Immediate and long-term effects of amyl nitrites

Dizziness	Reduced resistance to infections
Relaxation of muscles	Suppressed immune system
Increased heart rate	Skin lesions
Low blood pressure	Dermatological problems, particularly around the nose, mouth, lips, and face
Feeling flushed	Increased intraocular pressure (risky for people with underlying glaucoma)
Blurred vision	
Headaches	
Vomiting	
Burning feeling (mouth and nose)	
Death (due to existing heart problems or low blood pressure)	

Activity 12.5

Questions

- Describe the immediate effects of nitrites.

Activity 12.6

Please choose one correct answer for the following multiple-choice questions.

1. Which class of drugs includes both hypnotics and minor tranquillisers?
   a. Opioids
   b. Stimulants
   c. Hypno-sedatives
   d. Hallucinogens
   e. Sedatives
2. Barbiturates are known for their:
   a. Stimulating effects
   b. Sedative-hypnotic effects
   c. Analgesic effects
   d. Anxiolytic effects
   e. Mood-enhancing effects

3. Benzodiazepines are commonly used as:
   a. Analgesics
   b. Antidepressants
   c. Minor tranquillisers
   d. Hallucinogens
   e. Stimulants
4. Which of the following is NOT a barbiturate?
   a. Tuinal
   b. Valium
   c. Sodium amytal
   d. Phenobarbitone
   e. Seconal
5. What are street names for hypno-sedative drugs?
   a. Uppers
   b. Downers
   c. Speed
   d. Euphorics
   e. Trippers
6. How are benzodiazepines typically administered?
   a. Injection
   b. Inhalation
   c. Oral ingestion
   d. Transdermal patch
   e. Rectal suppository
7. Which drug is NOT a benzodiazepine?
   a. Librium
   b. Ativan
   c. Temazepam
   d. Heminevrin
   e. Xanax
8. What term is used to describe the combined effects of hypno-sedative drugs?
   a. Hallucinations
   b. Delirium
   c. Euphoria
   d. Sedation
   e. Analgesia

Activity 12.7

State whether the statements are true or false.

Statements	True	False
The hypno-sedatives include both hypnotics and major tranquillisers.		
Benzodiazepines cannot be injected.		

Statements	True	False
Benzodiazepines and barbiturates are not controlled drugs.		
Withdrawal of barbiturates can be dangerous .		
Hypno-sedatives, such as barbiturates and minor tranquillisers, induce effects similar to alcohol intoxication.		
Mixing hypno-sedatives with alcohol or other drugs can lead to respiratory failure and death.		
Injecting hypno-sedatives increases the risk of overdose, gangrene, and abscesses.		
Tolerance, physical dependence, and psychological dependence on hypno-sedatives develop slowly with prolonged use.		
The therapeutic dose and lethal dose margin of hypno-sedatives widen as tolerance develops.		
Withdrawal from hypno-sedatives can be dangerous and should be supervised medically due to potential symptoms, like anxiety and headaches.		
Hypno-sedatives are not addictive.		

HYPNO-SEDATIVES

Hypno-sedatives encompass both hypnotics and minor tranquillisers, with barbiturates and benzodiazepines being the primary classes. Barbiturates, introduced in 1903, include Tuinal, Nembutal, sodium amytal, and phenobarbitone, known for their sedative-hypnotic effects. Benzodiazepines, such as Valium (diazepam), Librium, Ativan, and Mogadon, are also widely used as minor tranquillisers. Other drugs like heminevrin and chloral hydrate are also part of this category. Commonly referred to as downers, barbs, and tranx on the street, hypno-sedatives are misused not only among illicit drug users but also in the general population. While benzodiazepines are typically taken orally, they can also be ground up and injected, as seen with temazepam.

Legal status

Benzodiazepines and barbiturates are prescription-only medicines and are controlled drugs, respectively. In most countries, it is illegal to supply these psychoactive substances.

Therapeutic use

Barbiturates have been used medically in anaesthesia and in the treatment of epilepsy and, rarely nowadays, insomnia. Minor tranquillisers are often prescribed for the relief of anxiety and stress.

Adverse effects

Barbiturates and minor tranquillisers are depressant drugs that induce effects akin to alcohol intoxication, including slurred speech, confusion, reduced inhibition, and impaired judgement. Minor tranquillisers commonly lead to fatigue, drowsiness, and ataxia, along with various other adverse effects, such as constipation, urinary retention, and blurred vision. Overdosing, especially in combination with alcohol or other drugs, can result in respiratory failure and even death. Injection of these drugs heightens the risk of overdose, gangrene, and abscesses. They are highly addictive, and tolerance, physical dependence, and psychological dependence can develop rapidly with prolonged use. The therapeutic dose and lethal dose margin narrows as tolerance develops. Withdrawal from barbiturates can

Activity 12.7

Questions

- What are the effects of hypno-sedative drugs?

Activity 12.8

State whether the statements are true or false.

Statements	True	False
Volatile substances produce effects similar to alcohol or anaesthetics.		
Volatile substance misuse is the deliberate inhalation of a volatile substance to achieve a change in mental state.		
Sniffers of volatile substances heighten the desired effect by decreasing the concentration of the vapour and including air.		
The pattern of use includes children from all lower social classes.		
The peak age of experimentation is approximately 17–18 years.		
There are more deaths from volatile substances compared to other illicit psychoactive substances.		
Volatile substances are more common in women than men.		
Anyone can buy solvents in the local shop.		
After inhalation of volatile substances, effects are experienced within a matter of minutes.		
The experiences of taking volatile substances are like being drunk on alcohol.		
Tolerance does not develop with volatile substances.		
Psychological dependence may develop.		

Activity 12.9

Please choose one correct answer for the following multiple-choice questions.

1. What is the legal status of volatile substances in many jurisdictions?
   a. Regulated
   b. Unrestricted
   c. Prohibited
   d. Controlled
   e. Limited
2. Which of the following is NOT a common volatile substance?
   a. Glue
   b. Aerosols

c. Paint thinners
d. Water
e. Butane

3. What legal measures are often enacted to prevent the misuse of volatile substances among young people?
a. Age restrictions
b. Mandatory education programmes
c. Public awareness campaigns
d. Community service requirements
e. None of the above

4. What is the primary purpose of legal regulations regarding volatile substances?
a. Economic control
b. Environmental protection
c. Preventing misuse and harm
d. Promoting recreational use
e. None of the above

5. Which of the following is a potential consequence of misusing volatile substances?
a. Increased intelligence
b. Improved memory
c. Respiratory failure
d. Enhanced physical health
e. Mental clarity

6. What is the primary mode of intake for volatile substance abuse?
a. Injection
b. Ingestion
c. Inhalation
d. Transdermal absorption
e. Oral administration

7. Which organ is most affected by chronic solvent abuse?
a. Heart
b. Liver
c. Lungs
d. Brain
e. Kidneys

8. Which of the following is a short-term effect of inhaling volatile substances?
a. Increased appetite
b. Heightened concentration
c. Euphoria
d. Decreased heart rate
e. Improved memory

9. What is the long-term consequence of repeated solvent abuse?
a. Enhanced cognitive abilities
b. Improved respiratory function
c. Liver damage
d. Reduced risk of mental illness
e. Increased lifespan

10. Which of the following is NOT a common volatile substance abused by inhalation?
    a. Paint thinner
    b. Glue
    c. Acetaminophen
    d. Gasoline
    e. Aerosol sprays

be perilous, necessitating medical supervision due to symptoms like anxiety, headaches, abdominal cramps, limb pain, and potentially epileptic fits.

VOLATILE SUBSTANCES

Volatile substance misuse involves inhaling organic-based substances like glues, aerosols, and cleaning fluids to induce effects akin to alcohol or anaesthetics. Deliberate inhalation is required to alter mental states, often intensified by increasing vapor concentration. Solvent misuse occurs predominantly in localised areas and among young people, leading to accidents and serious health risks. Around one in ten secondary school children experiment with sniffing, with some progressing to heavy use. Both genders and various social classes are affected, with inner-city areas experiencing higher prevalence. The peak age for experimentation is around 13 to 14 years old, and chronic dependence is rare, making volatile substance misuse a transient phenomenon. The extent of young children's involvement in volatile substance abuse surpasses that typically observed with other forms of substance misuse (Flanagan et al., 1997).

Legal status

The legal status of volatile substances varies depending on the country and specific regulations in place. In many jurisdictions, volatile substances are legally available for certain purposes, such as industrial use, cleaning, or medical applications. However, their sale and distribution may be regulated to prevent misuse, especially among young people. In some regions, there are laws and regulations specifically targeting the sale, possession, and use of volatile substances for recreational purposes. For example, certain jurisdictions may have age restrictions on purchasing volatile substances, and some products may be classified as controlled substances, making their possession and distribution illegal without proper authorisation. Additionally, there may be laws addressing the sale of volatile substances to minors or prohibiting the sale of certain types of products known to be misused, such as certain types of glue, aerosols, or solvents.

Sought-after effects

After inhalation of volatile substances, effects are experienced within a matter of minutes. Users typically experience a sensation similar to taking alcohol – being giggly and disoriented, possibly being uncoordinated and feeling dizzy. Nausea is not uncommon.

Short- and long-term use

Inhalation of solvent vapours leads to rapid absorption through the lungs, affecting the brain and reducing oxygen intake. This results in depressed respiratory and heart rates, potentially leading to disorientation, loss of control, and unconsciousness, akin to being drunk. Sniffers seek a dream-like state, but effects typically dissipate within 45 minutes post-inhalation, sometimes leaving a headache and poor concentration for up to a day. Accidental injury or death risk is high, particularly in hazardous environments, and suffocation may occur during vomiting or if a plastic bag is used for inhalation. Certain substances sensitise the heart, increasing the risk of heart failure, while direct inhalation into the mouth can cause suffocation. Particularly, inhaling from small bags poses fewer risks than using bags over the head with gases like butane.

Table 12.3
Volatile substances: short- and long-term effects

Short-term effects	Long-term effects
• Depressed respiration rate	• Damage to brain, kidneys, and liver
• Depressed heart rate	• Exhaustion
• Loss of coordination	• Amnesia
• Disorientation	• Loss of concentration
• Loss of consciousness	• Weight loss
• Drowsiness	• Depression
• Hangover	
• Accidental death	
• Heart failure	

Activity 12.10

- What are the short-term effects of volatile substances?
- What are the long-term effects of volatile substance?

Activity 12.11

State whether the statements are true or false

Statements	True	False
Over-the-counter drugs (OTC) are medications that can be purchased without a prescription.		
Codeine linctus, Collis Browne's mixture, Gee's Linctus, and kaolin and morphine are stimulants.		
Over-the-counter drugs are always safe for consumption without any risk of side effects.		
Over-the-counter drugs may interact with prescription medications and cause adverse effects.		
Over-the-counter drugs are often used for the treatment of minor ailments and symptoms.		
Some travel sickness tablets contain hallucinogenic compounds.		
Antihistamines may be used for their sedative and/or mixed with methadone or heroin.		
Amphetamine derivatives in decongestants may be used as a depressant.		
Over-the-counter drugs are typically regulated by health authorities to ensure their safety and efficacy.		

Statements	True	False
Smart drugs are reported to enhance sexual behaviour, physical endurance, muscle power, and emotional intelligence.		
Eco drugs are pharmaceuticals that have been developed to minimise environmental impact.		
Eco drugs are only concerned with minimising environmental impact during the disposal phase.		
Eco drugs are not widely available and are mainly experimental in nature.		
Eco drugs such as kava kava and yohimbe are vegetable substances that can produce a psychotropic or physical effect.		

Activity 12.12

Please choose one correct answer for the following multiple-choice questions.

1. Which of the following best defines over-the-counter (OTC) drugs?
   a. Medications that require a prescription from a doctor
   b. Drugs that are available only in hospitals
   c. Medications that can be purchased without a prescription
   d. Drugs that are illegal to sell
   e. Medications that can only be obtained from online pharmacies
2. Over-the-counter drugs are medications that can be obtained:
   a. Only with a prescription
   b. Without a prescription
   c. From specialised pharmacies only
   d. Only through online pharmacies
   e. Only with a doctor's recommendation
3. The main purpose of over-the-counter drugs is to:
   a. Be affordable
   b. Require minimal dosage
   c. Treat serious diseases
   d. Provide quick relief for minor health issues
   e. Be accessible without professional advice
4. Over-the-counter drugs can be purchased from:
   a. Hospitals only
   b. Licensed pharmacies and stores without a prescription
   c. Online marketplaces exclusively
   d. Specialty medical clinics
   e. Government dispensaries
5. Over-the-counter drugs are typically used for:
   a. Serious medical conditions
   b. Chronic illnesses only
   c. Minor ailments and symptoms
   d. Hospital treatments only
   e. Mental health disorders

6. What is the primary advantage of over-the-counter drugs?
   a. They are cheaper than prescription drugs.
   b. They are more potent than prescription drugs.
   c. They can be purchased without a prescription.
   d. They have fewer side effects.
   e. They are available in larger quantities.
7. Which of the following is NOT typically considered an over-the-counter drug?
   a. Aspirin
   b. Ibuprofen
   c. Penicillin
   d. Antihistamines
   e. Acetaminophen
8. Which statement about over-the-counter drugs is true?
   a. They always require a prescription from a doctor.
   b. They can be sold only in certain countries.
   c. They are available without a doctor's recommendation.
   d. They are typically stronger than prescription drugs.
   e. They are only used for chronic diseases.
9. Which statement about over-the-counter drugs is false?
   a. They are accessible without professional advice.
   b. They can be purchased in limited quantities.
   c. They are regulated to ensure safety and efficacy.
   d. They are primarily used for serious medical conditions.
   e. They provide quick relief for minor health issues.
10. Smart drugs are often used to:
    a. Treat bacterial infections
    b. Enhance memory and concentration
    c. Reduce inflammation
    d. Induce relaxation
    e. Lower blood pressure
11. Smart drugs are designed to:
    a. Be addictive
    b. Improve physical endurance only
    c. Enhance cognitive abilities
    d. Induce hallucinations
    e. Treat chronic pain
12. Smart drugs, also known as nootropics, are substances that:
    a. Cause immediate euphoria
    b. Improve cognitive function
    c. Induce deep sleep
    d. Increase heart rate
    e. Enhance physical strength
13. Smart drugs may include substances like:
    a. Antibiotics
    b. Painkillers
    c. Stimulants
    d. Sedatives
    e. Antacids

Long-term heavy solvent abuse results in enduring impairment of brain function, particularly affecting movement control. Chronic misuse of aerosols and cleaning fluids can damage the kidneys and liver. Sniffing leaded petrol can lead to lead poisoning. Chronic misuse manifests in general performance decline, weight loss, depression, and tremors, which typically dissipate upon cessation of sniffing. While tolerance may develop, physical dependence is not prevalent. Psychological dependence is more common in susceptible individuals with family or personality issues, often leading to solitary sniffing instead of group behaviour. The short-term and long-term effects are presented in Table 12.3.

OVER-THE-COUNTER DRUGS

The misuse of over-the-counter (OTC) drugs is a concerning issue, with individuals often seeking non-medical therapeutic effects or attempting to alleviate withdrawal symptoms from other substances. Dextromethorphan (DXM), a cough suppressant found in many OTC cough and cold medications, is commonly misused for its hallucinogenic and dissociative effects, leading to addiction and severe health consequences, including hallucinations and seizures. Pseudoephedrine, ephedrine, diphenhydramine, loperamide, and caffeine are other OTC drugs frequently misused. Pseudoephedrine is sought for its stimulant effects and is a key ingredient in illegal methamphetamine production. Ephedrine is misused for its stimulant effects but poses risks like high blood pressure and stroke. Diphenhydramine, an antihistamine, is abused for sedative effects and hallucinations. Loperamide is misused to alleviate opioid withdrawal symptoms but can lead to cardiac complications. Excessive caffeine consumption from OTC medications and beverages can result in caffeine intoxication, manifesting symptoms like rapid heartbeat and insomnia.

Legal status

No prescriptions are required to purchase those substances.

Therapeutic use

Some medical preparations, particularly over-the-counter medications, are utilised for pain relief, cough suppression, treating the common cold, diarrhoea management, and respiratory conditions. However, some individuals misuse these substances by taking them in large doses or combining them with other drugs to achieve specific effects. Antihistamines, for instance, may be used for their sedative properties and may be mixed with substances like methadone or heroin. Decongestants containing amphetamine derivatives can be misused as stimulants, while cough syrups and diarrhoea medications with opiate content may also be abused.

SMART AND ECO DRUGS

Smart drugs, also known as nootropics or cognitive enhancers, are substances that are purported to improve cognitive function, memory, creativity, or motivation in healthy individuals. These drugs may include prescription medications, like modafinil and methylphenidate, as well as over-the-counter supplements, such as caffeine and omega-3 fatty acids. Marketed as mind enhancers or boosters, they claim to improve intelligence, emotional intelligence, physical endurance, and even sexual behaviour. While some have therapeutic uses for neurological or mental disorders, healthy individuals increasingly use them in hopes of cognitive enhancement. Smart drugs, smart products (herbal mixtures), and smart drinks are promoted as safe alternatives to illicit drugs, offering cognitive enhancement and various other benefits. However, concerns persist regarding their safety, efficacy, and potential for misuse, especially among healthy individuals seeking cognitive improvement.

Eco drugs include herbs, plants, and mixtures, some of which may induce hallucinogenic or euphoric effects. Energising drinks with high caffeine content, often including guarana and taurine, are also prevalent. The effects of these substances can vary significantly, ranging from highly stimulating to inducing mild excitement or euphoria. Vegetable substances like hallucinogenic mushrooms, kava kava, and yohimbe fall under eco drugs and can elicit psychotropic or physical effects. These substances are derived from natural sources, namely, plants and fungi, and are often used for their psychoactive or physiological effects. Kava kava is a plant native to the Pacific Islands, where its root is traditionally used to prepare a ceremonial beverage with sedative and anxiolytic properties. It has been used to promote relaxation and alleviate stress and anxiety. Yohimbe comes from the bark of a tree native to West Africa and contains yohimbine, a compound that has been used for its stimulant and aphrodisiac effects. It is sometimes used as a dietary supplement to enhance sexual performance. There is limited evidence regarding their effects and associated risks.

KEY POINTS

- Anabolic steroids can be taken orally, injected, or with skin patches.
- The sought-after effects of steroids are to build up muscle size and body strength to enhance performance.
- Abuse of anabolic steroids can lead to serious health problems, some irreversible.
- Amyl and butyl nitrites are stimulant and are known collectively as alkyl nitrites.
- The effects of using nitrites may lead to sudden death if the individual has existing low blood pressure or heart conditions.
- Hypno-sedatives are drugs of misuse not only among the illicit drug population but also in the population in general.
- Benzodiazepines and barbiturates are prescription-only medicines and are class C and B controlled drugs, respectively.
- Barbiturates are depressant drugs, and their effects are similar to alcohol intoxication.
- Some organic-based substances produce effects similar to alcohol or anaesthetics when their vapours are inhaled.
- After inhalation of volatile substances, effects are experienced within a matter of minutes.
- Over-the-counter drugs are taken in large doses and often combined with other drugs to obtain the desired effects.
- The amphetamine derivatives in decongestants may be used as a stimulant; cough linctus and diarrhoea drugs treatment may be used for their opiate content.
- Smart drugs are referred to as substances taken with the purpose of enhancing cognitive functions and may have stimulating, sedating, or hallucinogenic effects.

References

Flanagan, R. J., Streete, P. J., & Ramsey, J. D. (1997). *Volatile Substance Abuse: Practical Guidelines for Analytical Investigation of Suspected Cases and Interpretation of Results.* Vienna: UN International Drug Control Programme.

National Library of Medicine. (2023). *Corticosteroids Overdose.* MedlinePlus [Internet]. Bethesda, MD: National Library of Medicine (US). https://medlineplus.gov/ency/article/002582.htm (accessed 9 March 2024).

NIDA. (2018). *Steroids and Other Appearance and Performance Enhancing Drugs (APEDs).* National Institute on Drug Abuse. https://www.drugabuse.gov.

Chapter 13

Nicotine addiction, electronic nicotine delivery systems, and shisha smoking

Learning outcomes

- Have an awareness of the global tobacco strategy.
- Examine the advantages and limitations of the global tobacco strategy.
- Give a definition of an *e-cigarette*.
- Describe the features of electronic cigarettes or e-cigarettes.
- Understand the mechanism of action of tobacco smoking.
- Describe briefly the harmful constituents of tobacco smoke.
- List the medical effects of nicotine addiction.
- List the psychological effects of nicotine addiction.
- Examine the relationship between tobacco smoking and type 2 diabetes.
- Discuss the issues regarding the safety of using e-cigarettes.
- Discuss the harms caused by shisha smoking.
- Describe the withdrawal symptoms associated with nicotine addiction.

Activity 13.1

There is only one correct answer to the following multiple-choice questions.

1. What is the primary psychoactive component found in tobacco products?
   a. Caffeine
   b. Nicotine
   c. THC
   d. Alcohol
   e. Benzene
2. Nicotine addiction primarily affects which system in the human body?
   a. Cardiovascular system
   b. Respiratory system
   c. Nervous system
   d. Endocrine system
   e. Digestive system
3. Which of the following is NOT a common method of nicotine delivery?
   a. Smoking cigarettes
   b. Chewing tobacco

DOI: 10.4324/9781003456674-15

c. Vaping
d. Drinking nicotine-infused beverages
e. Snorting nicotine powder

4. Which neurotransmitter is primarily affected by nicotine in the brain?
a. Serotonin
b. Dopamine
c. GABA
d. Acetylcholine
e. Norepinephrine

5. What is the addictive potential of nicotine compared to heroin or cocaine?
a. Less addictive
b. Equally addictive
c. More addictive
d. Nicotine is not addictive
e. Depends on the individual

6. Chronic exposure to nicotine can lead to which of the following health conditions?
a. Hypertension
b. Lung cancer
c. Heart disease
d. All of the above
e. None of the above

7. Which of the following is a common withdrawal symptom experienced by individuals trying to quit smoking?
a. Increased appetite
b. Increased energy levels
c. Decreased irritability
d. Decreased cravings
e. Improved mood

8. How does nicotine addiction affect the brain's reward system?
a. It decreases dopamine levels.
b. It increases GABA production.
c. It sensitises nicotinic receptors.
d. It has no effect on the brain's reward system.
e. It increases serotonin release.

9. Second-hand smoke exposure has been linked to an increased risk of:
a. Lung cancer
b. Cardiovascular disease
c. Respiratory infections
d. All of the above
e. None of the above

10. Which of the following medications is commonly used to aid in smoking cessation by reducing cravings and withdrawal symptoms?
a. Nicotine replacement therapy (NRT)
b. Ibuprofen
c. Vitamin C
d. Antibiotics
e. Antidepressants

11. Which of these gynaecological disorders is especially common among women who smoke?
    a. Endometriosis
    b. Polycystic ovary syndrome (PCOS)
    c. Pelvic inflammatory disease (PID)
    d. Premenstrual syndrome (PMS)
    e. Vaginal yeast infection
12. How do electronic cigarettes deliver nicotine to users?
    a. Through combustion
    b. Through vaporisation
    c. Through injection
    d. Through absorption in the skin
    e. Through ingestion
13. What is the primary psychoactive component found in electronic cigarettes (e-cigarettes) and shisha?
    a. Caffeine
    b. Nicotine
    c. THC
    d. Alcohol
    e. Benzene
14. Which of the following is a common flavouring agent used in electronic cigarettes?
    a. Mint
    b. Chocolate
    c. Fruit
    d. All of the above
    e. None of the above
15. Which of the following statements about second-hand vapor from e-cigarettes is true?
    a. It contains only water vapor.
    b. It contains harmful chemicals and nicotine.
    c. It is completely harmless.
    d. It smells pleasant.
    e. It is less harmful than second-hand smoke from traditional cigarettes.
16. What is the primary reason for the popularity of e-cigarettes among young people?
    a. Health benefits
    b. Flavour variety
    c. Cost-effectiveness
    d. Social acceptance
    e. Availability in vending machines
17. Which of the following is a potential health risk associated with e-cigarette use?
    a. Increased risk of lung cancer
    b. Nicotine addiction
    c. Decreased risk of heart disease
    d. Improved lung function
    e. Decreased risk of respiratory infections
18. What is the primary concern regarding the long-term effects of e-cigarette use?
    a. Cardiovascular disease
    b. Respiratory infections
    c. Nicotine addiction

d. Tooth decay
e. All of the above

19. What is the term commonly used to describe the act of smoking shisha?
    a. Vaping
    b. Dripping
    c. Hookahing
    d. Juuling
    e. Blowing smoke

20. Shisha smoking involves the use of which apparatus?
    a. Vaporiser
    b. Hookah
    c. Nicotine patch
    d. Inhaler
    e. E-cigarette

21. True or false: Shisha smoking is considered less harmful than cigarette smoking.
    a. True
    b. False
    c. Depends on the frequency of use
    d. Depends on the type of shisha
    e. Depends on the flavouring agent

22. In a single session, shisha smokers inhale up to:
    a. 200 times more smoke than from a cigarette
    b. 300 times more smoke than from a cigarette
    c. 400 times more smoke than from a cigarette
    d. 500 times more smoke than from a cigarette
    e. None of the above

Activity 13.2

State whether the following statements are true or false. Give reasons for your answers.

Statements	True	False
Tobacco is not an addictive substance.		
Smoking can hamper the sexual function of both men and women.		
Smoking causes stomach ulcers.		
Smoking helps reduce a person's stress level.		
Chewing tobacco does not have health risks because it is smoke-free.		
Switching to light- or low-tar cigarettes will save me.		
Smoking a cigar is better for you than smoking a cigarette.		
Some people gain weight when they quit smoking.		
Chewing tobacco does not have the same adverse effects as smoking tobacco.		

Even when a smoker inhales, two-thirds of the smoke from the cigarette goes into the environment.		
Children who breathe second-hand smoke are more likely to develop asthma.		
When one person smokes in a room, everyone smokes, because they are inhaling second-hand smoke.		
Second-hand smoke is more dangerous for children than adults because children breathe faster and their lungs are not as developed.		
Water pipe tobacco smokers generally believe that it is less harmful than cigarette smoking.		
People exposed to second-hand smoke from water pipe smoking are at risk for the same kinds of diseases as are caused by cigarette smoking.		
The longer the hookah session, the less nicotine and toxins one takes in.		

INTRODUCTION

Tobacco smoking is highly addictive and contains toxic and carcinogenic substances, making it the leading cause of preventable illness and premature death worldwide. Cigarettes are the most common form of tobacco, though products such as electronic nicotine delivery systems (e.g. e-cigarettes, vape pens) are gaining in popularity and provide nicotine, the psychoactive and addictive component in tobacco. Smoking is associated with various cancers, chronic lung diseases, heart disease, pregnancy complications, and other serious health issues. Smokeless tobacco, such as snuffing and chewing tobacco, also poses increased risks of cancers of the mouth, oesophagus, and pancreas. Exposure to environmental tobacco smoke, or second-hand smoke, increases the risk of cancer and causes DNA damage, especially in non-smokers and children. Tobacco use exacerbates social inequalities in health and contributes to poverty among disadvantaged smokers. The smoke from cigarettes, cigars, and pipes contains thousands of chemicals, including nicotine, tar, carbon monoxide, acetaldehyde, and nitrosamines. Nicotine, found in chewing tobacco as well, is the primary addictive component of tobacco.

The declining prevalence of cigarette smoking globally, however, is not reflected in patients with mental illnesses. In particular, people with mental illness and substance use disorders are disproportionately affected with high smoking prevalence (Prochaska et al., 2017). Smoking rates among adults with common mental disorders, such as depression, anxiety, schizophrenia, or bipolar disorder, are significantly higher compared to mentally well adults. Specifically, individuals with depression and anxiety are almost twice as likely to smoke, while those with schizophrenia or bipolar disorder are three times more likely to smoke (Robson & Potts, 2014). This highlights a concerning association between mental health conditions and tobacco use, indicating the need for targeted smoking cessation interventions and mental health support for individuals with mental disorders.

The World Health Organization (WHO, 2008) has introduced the MPOWER strategy, comprising six evidence-based measures to combat the morbidity and mortality associated with tobacco use. These measures include monitoring tobacco use, protecting individuals from second-hand smoke, assisting with tobacco cessation, educating about tobacco hazards, enforcing bans on tobacco advertising, and increasing tobacco taxes. Despite global acceptance, significant gaps remain in implementing effective tobacco control measures. Progress has been made, with more countries adopting MPOWER measures and increased public awareness through mass media campaigns. Continuous efforts are required to improve the efficacy and reach of tobacco control initiatives globally. One limitation of the global strategy and the WHO Framework Convention on Tobacco Control is the lack of anticipation for emerging nicotine delivery systems like electronic cigarettes (e-cigarettes). These non-tobacco nicotine delivery systems have the potential to undermine global tobacco strategies and policies, including taxation, marketing regulations, and product control (Yach, 2014). Major transnational tobacco companies are investing more in smokeless tobacco and e-cigarette production, presenting new challenges to tobacco control efforts. However, there is a positive aspect to the reduction in the global tobacco epidemic through a unified approach to preventing non-communicable diseases (NCDs), such as cancer, cardiovascular disease, chronic obstructive pulmonary disease, and diabetes. Tobacco use is a significant risk factor for these diseases, and addressing it is crucial for NCD prevention efforts. Nonetheless, new challenges in public health policy regarding the supply and demand of tobacco products are expected to arise, especially as transnational tobacco companies seek opportunities to market their products in developing countries in South America, Asia, and Africa.

ELECTRONIC CIGARETTES OR E-CIGARETTES

There is a trend in the use of electronic cigarettes, also called e-cigarettes or electronic nicotine delivery systems, and they are popular with smokers. Currently, there is a great deal of marketing of electronic cigarettes, e-liquids, and next-generation vaping devices, with an array of high-quality e-cigarette accessories available to smokers to join the global vape community. Vaping devices are battery-operated devices that people use to inhale an aerosol, which typically contains nicotine (though not always), flavourings, and other chemicals (NIDA, 2020). E-cigarettes come in various designs, resembling traditional tobacco cigarettes, cigars, pipes, or everyday items like pens or USB memory sticks. Despite their appearance, these devices generally operate similarly and share common components. With over 460 different brands available, e-cigarettes deliver nicotine through an inhalable aerosol by heating a solution containing nicotine, propylene glycol and/or glycerol, and flavours (McEwen & McRobbie, 2016). The aerosol produced is known as vapour, and the act of using an e-cigarette is commonly referred to as vaping.

More than 600 different e-cigarette brands are currently on the market, which means less time filling. The use of e-cigarette is to simulate the act of tobacco smoking without combustion (smokeless) by producing a flavoured aerosol that looks like tobacco smoke. It delivers nicotine, but with less of the toxic chemicals, such as tar and carbon monoxide, produced by burning tobacco.

Are e-cigarettes safe or harmful?

While e-cigarettes are often promoted as safer alternatives to traditional cigarettes, whether e-cigarettes are safer than conventional cigarettes or not is debatable. There is limited information about the health risks of these products. However, it is reported that "e-cigarettes are considerably safer than smoking cigarettes, are popular with smokers and that they have a role to play in reducing smoking rates" (McEwen & McRobbie, 2016, p. 4). However, evidence suggests that vaping may act as a gateway for preteens and teens, leading them to use other nicotine products, such as cigarettes, known to cause disease and premature death (NIDA, 2020). Studies indicate that students who use e-cigarettes are more likely to start smoking cigarettes and other tobacco products within a year (Leventhal et al., 2015). High school students who use e-cigarettes are significantly more likely to report smoking cigarettes approximately six months later compared to non-users (Bold et al., 2017). There is an association between vaping and progression to smoking actual cigarettes, indicating that vaping nicotine may encourage cigarette smoking in adolescents (Chaffee et al., 2018). Among adult smokers in Europe, those who vaped nicotine were less likely to have quit smoking and tended to smoke more cigarettes (Kulik et al., 2018). A study of individuals using e-cigarettes to quit traditional smoking found that only 9% had successfully quit after a year (Weaver et al., 2018). The Office of the Surgeon General's (2016) report highlights concerns regarding e-cigarettes, stating that they can expose users to various potentially harmful chemicals, including nicotine, carbonyl compounds, and volatile organic compounds. Despite these findings, there is a lack of safety data and precise information regarding the specific chemicals, flavourings, and colourings contained in e-cigarettes. Additionally, the report emphasises the absence of comprehensive understanding regarding the short-term and long-term effects of e-cigarette use on human health.

In contrast with some of the aforementioned findings, the Report from Public Health England (2015) provides evidence suggesting that e-cigarettes pose minimal risks compared to traditional smoking. According to the report, e-cigarettes do not pose a risk of nicotine poisoning when used as intended, and they contain fewer harmful chemicals associated with smoking-related diseases. It is estimated that e-cigarettes are approximately 95% safer than traditional smoking. Regarding second-hand exposure, evidence suggests that e-cigarettes release negligible amounts of nicotine into the environment, posing no identified health risks to bystanders. Additionally, there is good-quality evidence supporting the potential of e-cigarettes as a low-cost and effective intervention for smoking cessation. However, further research is needed to determine if experimenting with e-cigarettes leads to regular use of tobacco products.

Legal status

E-cigarettes are subject to varying legal statuses worldwide. In the United States, regulations are set by the FDA, while the European Union regulates them under the Tobacco Products Directive. In the UK, they fall under tobacco-related regulations, and in Canada, they are governed by the Tobacco and Vaping Products Act. Australia treats them as prescription-only medicine, while Japan requires approval from health authorities. China has minimal regulation, while India has a national ban on their sale and use. These regulations encompass advertising, packaging, nicotine concentration, and prescription requirements. The global landscape reflects a range of approaches, from strict controls to more permissive policies.

NICOTINE: MECHANISM OF ACTION

Nicotine, a harmful component of tobacco smoke, is rapidly absorbed by the body, reaching the brain within seconds and having a half-life of 10 to 20 minutes. While cigarettes deliver nicotine quickly, chewing tobacco and snuff result in slower absorption. Nicotine activates brain reward pathways, leading to pleasurable sensations similar to other addictive drugs. Specifically, nicotine increases dopamine levels, affecting brain circuits associated with reward and pleasure. This dopamine release in the midbrain is thought to contribute to the addictive nature of nicotine and the pleasurable feelings experienced by smokers.

Nicotine addiction

Indeed, there is substantial evidence to support the assertion that tobacco smoking is addictive. Nicotine, the primary psychoactive ingredient in tobacco, is highly addictive (NIDA, 2021). Smoking is widely recognised as a behaviour driven by dependence on the addictive substance nicotine rather than a choice made by free will (Roh, 2018). The addictive nature of nicotine leads individuals to repeat smoking behaviour despite awareness of its harmful effects. This understanding underscores the importance of addressing nicotine addiction through effective cessation interventions and public health policies aimed at reducing tobacco use. The WHO International Classification of Diseases (ICD)-10 (WHO, 1992) and the *Diagnostic and Statistical Manual of Mental Disorders* (*DSM-V*) (American Psychiatric Association, 2013) offer frameworks for understanding nicotine addiction, now termed *tobacco use disorder* in *DSM-V*. *Tobacco* in ICD-10 is replaced by *nicotine* in ICD-11, reflecting the increasing use of alternate forms of nicotine, such as through vaporisers (Poznyak et al., 2018). Key features of nicotine addiction include:

- Higher priority given to drug use
- Craving or strong desire to use tobacco
- Continued use despite harmful consequences
- Tolerance to the effects of nicotine
- Withdrawal symptoms upon cessation

These criteria help clinicians and researchers diagnose and assess the severity of nicotine addiction, highlighting the compulsive and addictive nature of tobacco use. The addictive nature of tobacco smoking has been shown in research studies to (1) indicate the role of nicotine to activate the reward pathways – the brain circuitry that regulates feelings of pleasure – and (2) nicotine increases levels of dopamine in the reward circuits. This reaction is similar to that seen with other drugs of abuse and is thought to underlie the pleasurable sensations experienced by many smokers (NIDA, 2021). This indicates that nicotine affects the brain's reward pathways, leading to the release of neurotransmitters such as dopamine, which produce pleasurable sensations. Over time, individuals develop a tolerance to nicotine, requiring increased amounts to achieve the same effects. Additionally, withdrawal symptoms such as irritability, anxiety, and cravings occur when nicotine levels drop, reinforcing the addictive cycle.

Sought-after effects

Tobacco, like many psychoactive substances, is subjectively pleasurable, and the effects often produce rewarding effects in the relief of stress and in enhancing mood and performance. The rapid absorption of nicotine from cigarette smoking and the high arterial levels which reach the brain as a result allow for rapid behavioural reinforcement from smoking. For e-cigarettes, smokers have an electronic fix for numerous reasons, including reducing appetite, boosting mood, or increasing their heart rate, alertness, and endurance.

HARMFUL CONSTITUENTS OF TOBACCO SMOKE

The burning of tobacco or cigarettes produces different gases and chemicals, and the main components include tar, nicotine, and carbon dioxide. Nicotine, a highly addictive toxic component of cigarette smoking, typically yields 8 milligrams to 20 milligrams per cigarette and up to 40 milligrams per cigar, with only around 1 milligram being absorbed. While nicotine is poisonous, its slow absorption rate when inhaled makes it unlikely to be fatal. In the body, nicotine is metabolised into cotinine, which has a 24-hour half-life, allowing for cotinine screening in urine to detect recent smoking. Nicotine acts on the nervous system, increasing heart rate and blood pressure, and can make blood platelets stickier, potentially triggering arrhythmias in patients with coronary heart disease.

Tar in cigarette smoke is composed of approximately 4,000 different organic chemicals, including carcinogens, which remain in the lungs upon exhalation, causing irritation and damage. As cigarettes burn down, the tar content increases, with the end of a cigarette potentially containing twice as much tar as the initial puffs. Despite the belief that low-tar cigarettes deliver less tar to the lungs, smokers tend to modify their behaviour to ensure they inhale enough smoke for a satisfactory nicotine hit, inadvertently increasing their tar intake from cigarettes (Jarvis & Bates, 1999). The components of tar ar[e] cancer-initiating and cancer-accelerating, contribut[-]ing to lung diseases like emphysema, bronchitis, an[d] lung cancer.

Carbon monoxide, a colourless and odourles[s] gas present in tobacco smoke, swiftly enters th[e] bloodstream. Its toxicity arises from its bindin[g] to haemoglobin, forming carboxyhaemoglobin[.] Consequently, habitual smokers exhibit reduce[d] haemoglobin levels and an elevated red blood cel[l] count. This reduction in the blood's oxygen-carrying capacity among smokers can lead to advers[e] health effects, particularly in diseases of the peripheral circulation.

Medical effects of tobacco smoking

The chronic effects of nicotine use are of significant concern due to its addictive nature, contributing to various toxic and adverse outcomes associated with high morbidity and mortality rates. Smoking, driven by nicotine addiction, stands as the most crucial modifiable risk factor for coronary heart disease across all age groups. The heightened risk of heart attacks among smokers, irrespective of age, gender, or ethnicity, has been well-established for decades. Moreover, passive smoking, or exposure to second-hand smoke, also leads to similar adverse health effects. Chronic nicotine use can result in a spectrum of acute effects, including headache, dizziness, insomnia, abnormal dreams, nervousness, gastrointestinal distress, dry mouth, nausea, vomiting, dyspepsia, diarrhoea, and musculoskeletal symptoms. Table 13.1 depicts the medical effects of tobacco smoking.

Nicotine withdrawal symptoms

These withdrawal symptoms of nicotine dependence happen with the sudden stopping or reduction of smoking or other tobacco use. The extent of withdrawal symptoms of nicotine is dependent on the duration of smoking and number of cigarettes smoked. These symptoms may begin within a few hours after the last cigarette, quickly driving people back to tobacco use. Symptoms peak within the first few days of smoking cessation and may subside within a few weeks. For some people, however, symptoms may persist for months. While

Table 13.1
Effects of tobacco smoking

Diseases	Examples
Cardiovascular diseases	Coronary heart disease: common in female smokers
	Nicotine and carbon monoxide: precipitate angina attacks
	Risk factor for stroke: especially with high blood pressure
	Effects: increased blood cholesterol, hypertension, arteriosclerosis
Respiratory diseases	Deaths: majority from chronic obstructive lung disease
	Relationship: smoking linked to chronic cough, mucus hypersecretion
	Patients: chronic bronchitis, pulmonary emphysema, bronchial asthma – mostly smokers
Cancer	Deaths: 84% lung cancer
	Risk: 20 times higher for 20+ cigarettes/day
	Increased risks: mouth, pharynx, larynx, bladder, pancreas, kidney, stomach cancers, cervical cancer
	Leading cause: mouth, oesophageal cancers; combined with alcohol, causing 90% of cases
Sexual health	Impaired fertility, delayed conception, early menopause, increased risk, cardiovascular disease, oral contraceptives
Effects of maternal smoking during pregnancy	Increased foetal and perinatal mortality, low birth weight, hindered blood flow, reduced nutrients, second-hand smoke, complications, miscarriage, stillbirth, ectopic pregnancy, cot death, growth retarding, delayed development, increased risk, miscarriages, adverse long-term growth, behavioural, educational
Psychological effects	Acts as a mood regulator, increasing pleasure; provides relief during highly stressful situations and strong emotional periods; reduces aggression and irritability; enhances performance and concentration on minor tasks; helps with anxiety disorders and depression

Table 13.2
Effects of nicotine withdrawal

Physiological	Dryness of the mouth
	Nausea
	Sore throat
	Drowsiness
	Cough problems
	Headache
	Tiredness
	Postnasal drip
	Bleeding in the gums
	Stomach pain
	Constipation
	Hunger pangs
	Increased appetite
	Increased weight gain
	Insomnia
	Tightness/stiffness in the chest
Psychological	Craving
	Restlessness
	Feeling of loneliness
	Inability to concentrate
	Anger
	Irritability
	Anxiety
	Depression

withdrawal is related to the pharmacological effects of nicotine, many behavioural factors can also affect the severity of withdrawal symptoms. For some people, the times, places, or situations associated with the pleasurable effects of smoking can make withdrawal or cravings worse. The physiological and psychological effects of nicotine withdrawal are presented in Table 13.2. A milder form of nicotine withdrawal, involving some of or all these symptoms, can occur when a smoker switches from regular to low-nicotine cigarettes or significantly cuts down on the number of cigarettes smoked. The symptoms of nicotine withdrawal can mimic, disguise, or aggravate the symptoms of other psychological problems. Depressed smokers appear to experience more withdrawal symptoms upon quitting, are less likely to be successful at quitting, and are more likely to relapse.

Smoking and type 2 diabetes

There is a relationship between tobacco smoking and type 2 diabetes. Smoking has been linked to an increased risk of type 2 diabetes. Several studies have demonstrated that while smoking itself may not directly cause diabetes, a growing evidence suggests that regular smokers are at risk of developing incident diabetes (Campagna et al., 2019). The exact mechanisms underlying this association are not fully understood, but smoking is thought to contribute to insulin resistance, impaired glucose metabolism, and inflammation, all of which are key factors in the development of type 2 diabetes. Additionally, smoking is often associated with other unhealthy behaviours, such as poor diet and lack of physical activity, which further exacerbate the risk of diabetes.

SHISHA SMOKING

The popularity of shisha smoking, particularly among younger generations, has surged in Western countries, often associated with the trendy café culture. Shisha use is most prevalent among individuals aged 18 to 25 but declines with age. For many, shisha smoking represents a leisurely activity akin to enjoying a glass of wine or a cigarette to unwind. Shisha consists of a glass-bottomed water pipe, with fruit-flavoured tobacco heated with charcoal and inhaled deeply and slowly through a water chamber. Enthusiasts find the experience smooth and sweet-smelling, masking the natural odours of tobacco tar and nicotine. However, due to the concerning increase in young people smoking shisha, many countries have initiated educational campaigns to raise awareness about its health risks.

Despite misconceptions surrounding shisha smoking, there is evidence refuting claims that it is less harmful than cigarette smoking. While some believe that shisha smoking, particularly in the Middle East, has no health consequences, research suggests otherwise. Shisha smoking involves the inhalation of nicotine, carcinogens, and toxins to a similar extent as other forms of tobacco use. In fact, shisha smoke contains carcinogens at levels comparable to ordinary tobacco smoke, but with significantly higher levels of carbon monoxide due to the way the tobacco is burned. Carbon monoxide testing has been used to demonstrate the effects of shisha smoking on the body, leading some individuals to reconsider their consumption habits.

Harms of shisha smoking

The World Health Organization (WHO) advises against shisha smoking due to its harmful health effects. In a report, WHO (2005) highlights the risks associated with shisha smoking, emphasising that it exposes individuals to significant levels of nicotine, carcinogens, and toxins. Water pipe smoking shares similar health risks with cigarette smoking and is associated with comparable diseases (El-Hakim & Uthman, 1999). Despite popular misconceptions about shisha being less harmful than cigarette smoking, the WHO's stance highlights the dangers inherent in shisha use. The organisation recommends raising awareness about the health risks of shisha smoking and implementing policies to regulate its use to protect public health. Shisha smoking poses significant health risks comparable to or even exceeding those of cigarette smoking. In a single shisha session lasting 20–80 minutes, a smoker can inhale the equivalent amount of smoke as consuming over 100 cigarettes (British Heart Foundation, 2024). This exposes individuals to toxins that increase the risk of heart and circulatory diseases, cancers, nicotine addiction, and respiratory infections and conditions. Hookah smoking appears to be associated with lung cancer, respiratory disease, and low birth weight in babies (Patil et al., 2022).

Shisha smoking exposes individuals to significantly higher levels of aldehyde compounds, carbon monoxide, and tar compared to cigarette smoking, ranging from 4 to 30 times higher in a single session (Patil et al., 2022). These substances are known human carcinogens and lead to stress on our bodies. Additionally, they can make us sick from inhaling too much carbon monoxide, resulting in carbon monoxide poisoning. Shisha smoke also contains heavy metals that can lead to carcinogenesis. Evidence suggests that shisha smoking is a risk factor for various cancers, including lung, oral, oesophageal, stomach, bladder, colorectal, and nasopharyngeal cancers (Patil et al., 2022). Exposure to tobacco juices during hookah smoking increases the risk of oral cancers more than pipe or cigar smoking due to its frequent and prolonged practice (El-Hakim & Uthman, 1999; WHO, 2005). Exposure to second-hand smoke from water pipe smoking poses risks for diseases similar to those caused by cigarette smoking, including cancer, heart disease, respiratory disease, and adverse effects during pregnancy (Nuwayhid et al., 1998). Despite evidence indicating that water pipe smoking carries health risks comparable to cigarette smoking, there are widespread misconceptions about its health impact, with many people believing it to be less harmful (Knishkowy & Amitai, 2005). Sharing a hookah can transmit infectious diseases (Akl et al., 2010). Additionally, babies

Table 13.3
Harmful effects of shisha smoking

Substance–disease	Harmful effects
Nicotine	Acute and chronic cardiovascular effects and increased heart rate
Blood chromium and nickel	Chronic obstructive pulmonary disorder, bronchitis, and nasal congestion
Heavy metals and tar	Carcinogens
Risk factor	Lung, oral, oesophageal, stomach, bladder, colorectal, and nasopharyngeal cancer
Sharing of the shisha's mouthpiece	High risk of transmission of communicable diseases, including hepatitis A and tuberculosis
Cardiovascular disease and metabolic syndrome	Hypertriglyceridemia, hyperglycaemia, hypertension, and abnormal obesity
Respiratory effects	Carbon monoxide poisoning: carboxyhaemoglobin, leading to cell hypoxia and impaired cell respiration; nausea, vomiting, headache, and muscle lethargy
Periodontal disease (gum disease)	*Periodontal health* – condition of the tissues that surround and support the teeth, including the gums, periodontal ligament, and alveolar bone
Pregnancy and infertility	Low-birth-weight babies and increased pulmonary problems for the new-born; harmful impacts of second-hand smoke on the mother and the foetus; male infertility associated with shisha

Source: Adapted from Patil et al. (2022).

born to women who smoked one or more water pipes daily during pregnancy tend to have lower birth weights, at least three and a half ounces less, compared to babies born to non-smokers. These infants also face an increased risk for respiratory diseases (U.S. Department of Health & Human Services, 2021; Patil et al., 2022). Table 13.3 presents the harmful effects of shisha smoking.

Shisha: the facts

- Hookah smoke contains harmful components, like nicotine, tar, and heavy metals, similar to those found in cigarette smoke.
- Water pipe smoking delivers nicotine, the highly addictive substance found in other tobacco products.
- During a typical 1-hour hookah session, users may inhale 100–200 times the amount of smoke they would inhale from a single cigarette, along with up to 9 times the carbon monoxide and 1.7 times the nicotine.
- In a single session, shisha smokers inhale up to 200 times more smoke than from a cigarette.
- The longer the hookah session, the more nicotine and toxins one takes in.
- Despite passing through water, the smoke from a hookah retains high levels of these toxic agents.
- The tobacco in hookahs is exposed to high heat from burning charcoal, making the smoke at least as toxic as cigarette smoke, including carbon monoxide, posing additional risks to users.
- Tobacco juices from hookahs can irritate the mouth, raising the risk of developing oral cancers.
- Hookah smokers face risks for similar diseases as cigarette smokers, including oral, lung, stomach, and oesophageal cancers, as well as reduced lung function and decreased fertility.
- Hookah tobacco and smoke contain numerous toxic agents that can contribute to clogged arteries and heart disease.
- Babies born to individuals who smoked water pipes daily during pregnancy tend to have lower birth weights, at least 3 1/2 ounces less, compared to babies born to non-smokers.
- Babies born to individuals who use hookah are also at an elevated risk for respiratory diseases.
- Hookah users may absorb more toxic substances than cigarette smokers due to the way hookahs are used.
- Second-hand smoke from hookahs poses a health risk for non-smokers as it contains smoke from both the tobacco and the heat source, such as charcoal.

adapted from the US Department of Health and Human Services (2021)

KEY POINTS

- Smoking is the single greatest cause of preventable illness and premature death in the world.

- Tobacco smoking is highly addictive, and the contents of cigarette contain the most toxic and carcinogenic substances.
- There are multiple impacts on non-smokers and children exposed to tobacco smoke.
- The declining prevalence of cigarette smoking globally, however, is not reflected in patients with mental illnesses.
- The WHO has identified six evidence-based tobacco control measures that are the most effective in reducing tobacco use.
- There is a trend in the use of electronic cigarettes, also called e-cigarettes or electronic nicotine delivery systems, and they are popular with smokers.
- E-cigarettes often look like cigarettes, cigars, or pipes or can be manufactured to resemble pens or USB memory sticks, and some with refillable tanks look different.
- Many countries ban the importation, distribution, commercialisation, and advertising of e-cigarettes and accessories.
- Smokers could be forgiven for believing that low-tar cigarettes deliver less tar to the smoker's lung.
- Nicotine, a main toxic component of cigarette smoking, is highly addictive.
- The health and risk factors associated with active cigarette smoking include cancer, cardiovascular disease, respiratory diseases, sexual health, and maternal health.
- There is an increased risk of type 2 diabetes for those who smoked at least 20 cigarettes a day.
- Whether e-cigarettes are safe or pose many health risks remains controversial.
- The Report from Public Health England indicates that e-cigarettes pose no risk of nicotine poisoning, and the chemicals which are present pose limited danger.
- Using a water pipe to smoke tobacco poses a serious potential health hazard to smokers and others exposed to the smoke emitted.
- Water pipe use may increase exposure to carcinogens by smokers and those exposed to second-hand smoke from water pipe smoking.
- Tuberculosis outbreaks in Middle Eastern countries were linked to shisha.
- Carbon monoxide (from the coal) is 30 times harder to dissolve in water than oxygen.
- In a single session, shisha smokers inhale up to 200 times more smoke than from a cigarette.
- Nicotine withdrawal symptoms happen with the sudden stopping or reduction of smoking or other tobacco use.
- The extent of withdrawal symptoms of nicotine is dependent on the duration of smoking and number of cigarettes smoked.

Activity 13.3

Questions

- Why is tobacco considered an addictive psychoactive substance?
- List the medical effects of tobacco smoking.
- List the psychological effects of tobacco smoking.
- Describe the effects of withdrawal symptoms of nicotine addiction.
- Describe the harmful effects of shisha smoking.

References

Akl, E. A., Gaddam, S., Gunukula, S. K., Honeine, R., Jaoude, P. A., & Irani, J. (2010). The effects of waterpipe tobacco smoking on health outcomes: A systematic review. *International Journal of Epidemiology,* 39(3), 834–857. https://doi.org/10.1093/ije/dyq002.

American Psychiatric Association. (2013). *Diagnostic and Statistical Manual of Mental Disorders* (5th ed.). Washington, DC: American Psychiatric Association.

Bold, K. W., Kong, G., Camenga, D. R., Simon, P., Cavallo, D. A., Morean, M. E., & Krishnan-Sarin, S. (2018). Trajectories of e-cigarette and conventional cigarette use among youth. *Pediatrics,* 141(1), e20171832. https://doi.org/10.1542/peds.2017-1832.

British Heart Foundation. (2024). *Shisha.* https://www.bhf.org.uk/informationsupport/risk-factors/smoking/shisha (accessed 10 March 2024).

Campagna, D., Alamo, A., Di Pino, A., Russo, C., Calogero, A. E., Purrello, F., & Polosa, R. (2019). Smoking and diabetes: Dangerous liaisons and confusing relationships. *Diabetology & Metabolic Syndrome,* 11, 85. https://doi.org/10.1186/s13098-019-0482-2.

Chaffee, B. W., Watkins, S. L., & Glantz, S. A. (2018). Electronic cigarette use and progression from experimentation to established smoking. *Pediatrics,* 141(4), e20173594; 142(3), e20181885. https://doi.org/10.1542/peds.2018-1885.

El-Hakim, I. E., & Uthman, M. A. (1999). Squamous cell carcinoma and keratoacanthoma of the lower lip associated with "goza" and "shisha" smoking. *International Journal of Dermatology,* 38(2), 108–110. https://doi.org/10.1046/j.1365-4362.1999.00448.x.

Jarvis, M., & Bates, C. (1999). *Why Low Tar Cigarettes Don't Work and How the Tobacco Industry Has Fooled the Smoking Public* (1999 ed.). https://ash.org.uk/uploads/ASH_780.pdf?v=1648215029 (accessed 10 March 2024).

Knishkowy, B., & Amitai, Y. (2005). Water-pipe (narghile) smoking: An emerging health risk behavior. *Pediatrics,* 116(1), e113–e119. https://doi.org/10.1542/peds.2004-2173.

Kulik, M. C., Lisha, N. E., & Glantz, S. A. (2018). E-cigarettes associated with depressed smoking cessation: A cross-sectional study of 28 European Union countries. *American Journal of Preventive Medicine,* 54(4), 603–609. https://doi.org/10.1016/j.amepre.2017.12.017.

Leventhal, A. M., Strong, D. R., Kirkpatrick, M. G., Unger, J. B., Sussman, S., Riggs, N. R., Stone, M. D., Khoddam, R., Samet, J. M., & Audrain-McGovern, J. (2015). Association of electronic cigarette use with initiation of combustible tobacco product smoking in early adolescence. *JAMA,* 314(7), 700–707. https://doi.org/10.1001/jama.2015.8950.

McEwen, A., & McRobbie, H. (2016). *Electronic Cigarettes: A Briefing for Stop Smoking Services.* National Centre for Smoking Cessation and Training. https://cloudfront.ncsct.co.uk/pdfs/Electronic_cigarettes._A_briefing_for_stop_smoking_services.pdf (accessed 10 March 2024).

Nuwayhid, I. A., Yamout, B., Azar, G., & Kambris, M. A. (1998). Narghile (hubble-bubble) smoking, low birth weight, and other pregnancy outcomes. *American Journal of Epidemiology,* 148(4), 375–383. https://doi.org/10.1093/oxfordjournals.aje.a009656.

NIDA. (2020). *Vaping Devices (Electronic Cigarettes) Drug Facts.* https://nida.nih.gov/publications/drugfacts/vaping-devices-electronic-cigarettes (accessed 10 March 2024).

NIDA. (2021). *Is Nicotine Addictive?* https://nida.nih.gov/publications/research-reports/tobacco-nicotine-e-cigarettes/nicotine-addictive (accessed 10 March 2024).

Office of the Surgeon General. (2016). *E-Cigarette Use Among Youth and Young Adults: A Report of the Surgeon General.* Washington, DC: U.S. Department of Health and Human Services, Centers for Disease Control and Prevention. https://www.cdc.gov/tobacco/data_statistics/sgr/ecigarettes/pdfs/2016_sgr_entire_report_508.pdf (accessed 10 March 2024).

Patil, S., Mahuli, A. V., & Warnakulasuriya, S. (2022). Effects of smoking shisha, cancer risk, and strategies for prevention of shisha habit. *Journal of Oral Biology and Craniofacial Research,* 12(4), 439–443. https://doi.org/10.1016/j.jobcr.2022.05.008.

Poznyak, V., Reed, G. M., & Medina-Mora, M. E. (2018). Aligning the ICD-11 classification of disorders due to substance use with global service needs. *Epidemiology and Psychiatric Sciences,* 27(3), 212–218. https://doi.org/10.1017/S2045796017000622.

Prochaska, J. J., Das, S., & Young-Wolff, K. C. (2017). Smoking, mental illness, and public health. *Annual Review of Public Health,* 38, 165–185. https://doi.org/10.1146/annurev-publhealth-031816-044618.

Public Health England. (2015). *E-Cigarettes: An Evidence Update.* A report commissioned by Public Health England. London: Public Health England. https://www.gov.uk/government/publications/e-cigarettes-an-evidence-update (accessed 10 March 2024).

Robson, D., & Potts, J. (2014). *Smoking Cessation and Mental Health.* Dorchester: National Centre for Smoking Cessation and Training (NCSCT). https://www.ncsct.co.uk/library/view/pdf/mental%20health%20briefing%20A4.pdf.

Roh, S. (2018). Scientific evidence for the addictiveness of tobacco and smoking cessation in tobacco litigation. *Journal of Preventive Medicine and Public Health = Yebang Uihakhoe chi,* 51(1), 1–5. https://doi.org/10.3961/jpmph.16.088.

U.S. Department of Health & Human Services. (2021). *Hookahs.* Centers for Disease Control and Prevention. https://www.cdc.gov/tobacco/data_statistics/fact_sheets/tobacco_industry/hookahs/index.htm (accessed 11 March 2024).

Weaver, S. R., Huang, J., Pechacek, T. F., Heath, J. W., Ashley, D. L., & Eriksen, M. P. (2018). Are electronic nicotine delivery systems helping cigarette smokers quit? Evidence from a prospective cohort study of U.S. adult smokers, 2015–2016. *PLOS One,* 13(7), e0198047. https://doi.org/10.1371/journal.pone.0198047.

WHO. (1992). *International Statistical Classification of Diseases and Related Health Problems* (10th rev. ed.). Geneva: World Health Organization.

WHO. (2005). *Advisory Note: Waterpipe Tobacco Smoking: Health Effects, Research Needs, and Recommended Action by Regulators.* WHO Study Group on Tobacco Product Regulation (TobReg). Geneva: WHO.

WHO. (2008). WHO Report on the Global Tobacco Epidemic, 2008: The MPOWER Package. Geneva: WHO.

Yach, D. (2014). The origins, development, effects, and future of the WHO framework convention on tobacco control: A personal perspective. *Lancet,* 383(9930), 1771–1779. https://doi.org/10.1016/S0140-6736(13)62155-8.

Part 3

Special issues and populations

Chapter 14

Blood-borne infections

Learning outcomes

- Relate to practice the impact of stigma and discrimination towards people with blood-borne viruses.
- Define terminology used in relation to HIV, hepatitis C, and hepatitis B.
- Describe current trends in HIV, hepatitis C, and hepatitis B infection.
- Identify the transmission routes of HIV, hepatitis C, and hepatitis B to risk behaviours.
- Discuss the risks of injecting drug use to the transmission of blood-borne viruses.
- Describe the process of HIV pre-discussion and post-test counselling.
- Examine effective prevention measures to reduce blood-borne virus infection.
- Identify current treatment and vaccinations available for viral infections.

Activity 14.1

Please choose one correct answer to the following multiple-choice questions.

1. Which virus causes HIV/AIDS?
   a. Hepatitis A
   b. Hepatitis B
   c. Hepatitis C
   d. Human papillomavirus
   e. Human immunodeficiency virus
2. Which of the following bodily fluids can transmit HIV?
   a. Sweat
   b. Tears
   c. Urine
   d. Saliva
   e. Semen
3. What is the primary mode of transmission for HIV?
   a. Contaminated food and water
   b. Sexual contact
   c. Blood-borne transmission
   d. Respiratory droplets
   e. Vector-borne transmission

DOI: 10.4324/9781003456674-17

4. What type of virus is HIV?
   a. Bacterium
   b. Fungus
   c. Retrovirus
   d. Protozoan
   e. Prion
5. Which cells does HIV primarily target in the human body?
   a. White blood cells
   b. Red blood cells
   c. Platelets
   d. Liver cells
   e. Nerve cells
6. What is the main function of HIV?
   a. Attacking the liver
   b. Attacking the nervous system
   c. Attacking the immune system
   d. Attacking the digestive system
   e. Attacking the respiratory system
7. Which of the following is NOT a common symptom of HIV infection?
   a. Fever
   b. Weight loss
   c. Persistent cough
   d. Swollen lymph nodes
   e. High blood pressure
8. How does HIV weaken the immune system?
   a. By increasing white blood cell count
   b. By suppressing the production of antibodies
   c. By destroying red blood cells
   d. By increasing platelet count
   e. By promoting inflammation
9. What is the most effective way to prevent HIV transmission?
   a. Eating a healthy diet
   b. Using condoms during sexual intercourse
   c. Getting vaccinated
   d. Avoiding sharing needles
   e. Wearing gloves
10. Which of the following is a common symptom of acute HIV infection?
    a. Persistent cough
    b. Skin rash
    c. Fatigue
    d. Joint pain
    e. Visual disturbances
11. Which population is at the highest risk for HIV infection?
    a. Children under 5 years old
    b. Elderly individuals over 65 years old
    c. Young adults aged 18–35 years old
    d. Pregnant women
    e. Healthcare workers

12. What is the primary method of preventing vertical transmission of HIV from mother to child?
    a. Vaccination
    b. Antiretroviral therapy during pregnancy
    c. Avoiding breastfeeding
    d. Caesarean section delivery
    e. Abstaining from sexual activity
13. What is the window period for HIV testing?
    a. 1 day
    b. 1 week
    c. 1 month
    d. 3 months
    e. 6 months
14. What is the difference between HIV and AIDS?
    a. HIV is a virus, while AIDS is a syndrome.
    b. HIV is a syndrome, while AIDS is a virus.
    c. HIV is caused by a weakened immune system, while AIDS attacks the immune system.
    d. HIV is the later stage of AIDS.
    e. HIV and AIDS are interchangeable terms.
15. You can find out if you have HIV by getting:
    a. A blood test
    b. Skin lesions checked
    c. An eye examination
    d. Symptoms
    e. None of the above
16. The standard, most common HIV test:
    a. Predicts how fast you will develop AIDS
    b. Measures the amount of virus in your blood
    c. Detects antibodies to the virus
    d. None of the above
    e. All of the above
17. If you have another sexually transmitted infection, your chance of getting HIV/AIDS through having sex:
    a. Is safe
    b. Stays the same
    c. Is higher
    d. Is lower
    e. None of the above
18. Sharing a needle and syringe to inject drugs is safe when . . .
    a. You only share with your partner.
    b. You only inject crack cocaine.
    c. It is never safe.
    d. You only inject heroin.
    e. None of the above is correct.
19. Which protects you most against HIV infection?
    a. Contraceptive pills
    b. Spermicide jelly
    c. Condoms
    d. Condoms and spermicide jelly
    e. None of the above

20. HIV affects the immune system; this increases:
    a. The likelihood of people acquiring TB infection
    b. The likelihood of people not acquiring TB infection
    c. The likelihood of people acquiring sexually transmitted disease
    d. The likelihood of people not acquiring sexually transmitted disease
    e. None of the above
21. Which type of hepatitis can lead to chronic liver disease and liver cancer?
    a. Hepatitis A
    b. Hepatitis B
    c. Hepatitis C
    d. Hepatitis D
    e. Hepatitis E
22. Which type of hepatitis is primarily transmitted through blood-borne contact, such as sharing needles?
    a. Hepatitis A
    b. Hepatitis B
    c. Hepatitis C
    d. Hepatitis D
    e. Hepatitis E
23. Which of the following is a characteristic of chronic hepatitis B infection?
    a. Jaundice
    b. Abdominal pain
    c. Joint stiffness
    d. Fatigue
    e. Rash
24. Which type of hepatitis can cause liver failure and death in severe cases?
    a. Hepatitis A
    b. Hepatitis B
    c. Hepatitis C
    d. Hepatitis D
    e. Hepatitis E
25. Which type of hepatitis can be prevented through vaccination?
    a. Hepatitis A
    b. Hepatitis B
    c. Hepatitis C
    d. Hepatitis D
    e. Hepatitis E
26. What is the recommended treatment for chronic hepatitis C infection?
    a. Antibiotics
    b. Antifungal medication
    c. Antiretroviral therapy
    d. Interferon and ribavirin
    e. Hepatitis B vaccine
27. Which type of hepatitis is primarily transmitted through sexual contact and sharing needles?
    a. Hepatitis A
    b. Hepatitis B
    c. Hepatitis C
    d. Hepatitis D
    e. Hepatitis E

28. What is the main route of transmission for hepatitis C?
    a. Contaminated food and water
    b. Sexual contact
    c. Blood-borne transmission
    d. Respiratory droplets
    e. Vertical transmission (from mother to child)
29. The increased likelihood of progression to severe liver complications may be caused by
    a. Alcohol consumption and co-infection with HIV
    b. Drug consumption and co-infection
    c. Alcohol and drug consumption
    d. Tobacco consumption
    e. None of the above
30. Many people with chronic hepatitis B:
    a. Are aware that they are infected
    b. Remain well but become chronic carriers
    c. Cannot pass on the virus to others
    d. Do not remain infectious
    e. None of the above

BLOOD-BORNE VIRUSES

Blood-borne viruses (BBVs) are pathogens primarily found in blood or bodily fluids. Transmission of BBVs occurs when infected blood or body fluids come into contact with an open lesion on the skin or through injury with a sharp object contaminated with infected blood. The risk of BBV transmission varies based on factors such as the frequency and scale of contact with blood and body fluids, behaviours of individuals involved, and the infectiousness of the person or material. Among BBVs, HIV and hepatitis viruses B and C (HBV, HCV) are particularly significant due to their potential health risks, especially for individuals engaging in illicit drug injection. This heightened risk stems from the transfer of blood through the sharing of contaminated injecting equipment or environmental contamination in injecting settings. The main BBVs include HIV, hepatitis B, and hepatitis C, which pose significant health risks, particularly among individuals who inject illicit drugs, due to the sharing of contaminated equipment and environmental factors in injecting settings.

GLOBAL HEALTH STRATEGY

The global health sector strategies on, respectively, HIV, viral hepatitis, and sexually transmitted infections for the period 2022–2030 (WHO, 2022) highlight the importance of the health sector in leading efforts to end epidemics like HIV, viral hepatitis, and STIs (sexually transmitted infections). The report advocates for a comprehensive approach that addresses systemic barriers, targets affected populations, promotes universal health coverage, and contributes to the broader goals of sustainable development and health equity. These new strategies take into account shifts in epidemiology, advancements in technology, and changes in contextual factors observed in recent years. By fostering cross-learning across various disease areas, including HIV, viral hepatitis, and STI, the strategies aim to capitalise on innovations and emerging knowledge to enhance responses to these health challenges.

The strategies call for renewed investments in primary prevention interventions for HIV, with a focus on comprehensive education, correct and consistent condom use, addressing substance use, implementing evidence-based strategies, and promoting sexual and reproductive health within a holistic framework of well-being. They advocate for the implementation of a comprehensive package of accessible harm reduction and treatment services as part of broader interventions aimed at preventing, treating, and caring for HIV among people who inject drugs and individuals who use stimulant drugs. In addition, the strategies aim to advance the triple elimination of vertical (mother-to-child) transmission of HIV, syphilis, and hepatitis B virus by implementing comprehensive and accessible prevention, testing, treatment, and follow-up services for women, children, and their families.

The strategies outline a comprehensive approach to prevent new infections among children, address the needs of affected children and adolescents, ensure infection prevention in healthcare settings, integrate testing for various diseases, implement partner notification services, and eliminate stigma and discrimination in healthcare settings. The strategies emphasise the importance of addressing tuberculosis in the context of HIV and viral hepatitis, promoting integrated services and access to sexual and reproductive health services, addressing mental health needs, ensuring disability-inclusive programming, and preventing and responding to gender-based violence to improve health outcomes and well-being for affected populations. Finally, the strategies emphasise the integration of gender equality promotion across all actions, addressing underlying gender inequalities, empowering female health workers, and recognising and supporting women's unpaid care work within the community. These efforts aim to create a more equitable and inclusive environment in the health sector and society as a whole.

WHAT IS HIV?

HIV, or human immunodeficiency virus, is a retrovirus that attacks CD4 host cell receptors, particularly certain lymphocytes, known as T4 helper cells, as well as macrophages and microglial cells. HIV replicates within these cells, ultimately leading to their destruction. As the immune system loses too many CD4 cells and becomes impaired, the infected person becomes vulnerable to opportunistic infections and tumours. AIDS, or acquired immunodeficiency syndrome, is the advanced stage of HIV infection, characterised by a weakened immune system. It is diagnosed when an individual has less than 200 CD4 cells and/or one of 21 AIDS-defining opportunistic infections. AIDS comprises a collection of rare infections and cancers that people with HIV can develop. WHO now defines *advanced HIV disease* (AHD) as CD4 cell count less than 200 cells/mm^3 or WHO stage 3 or 4 in adults and adolescents. All children with HIV younger than 5 years of age are considered to have advanced HIV disease. Some of the opportunistic infections and tumours associated with late-stage AIDS are presented in Table 14.1.

HIV transmission

Blood, blood products, semen, vaginal secretions, donor organs and tissues, and breast milk have been implicated in the transmission of infection. There is good evidence from studies of household contacts of infected people that HIV is not spread by close social contact. Most HIV transmission occurs through:

- Unprotected vaginal or anal intercourse
- Sharing contaminated needles and syringes
- Transfusion of contaminated blood and blood products
- From mother to baby in utero, at birth, or via breastfeeding

Nature and extent of HIV infection

AIDS is among the leading causes of death globally and remains the primary cause of death in Africa (WHO, 2022). While the expansion of antiretroviral therapy has significantly reduced HIV-related deaths, mortality rates remain unacceptably high, with over 1.5 million new HIV infections annually. Key populations, including men who have sex with men, people who inject drugs, sex workers, transgender

Table 14.1
Opportunistic infections and tumours in late stage of AIDS

Bacterial	Viral	Fungal	Protozoal	Tumours
Mycobacterial tuberculosis	Papovaviruses	*Candida*	*Pneumocystis carrini*	Kaposi's sarcoma
Mycobacterium avium complex	Cytomegalovirus	*Cryptococcus*	Toxoplasmosis	Non-Hodgkin's lymphoma
Salmonella	Herpes (*simplex* and *zoster*)	*Aspergillus*	*Cryptosporidium isospora*	Cervical cancer
Shigella				

people, and those in prisons, face significant barriers to accessing services, contributing to the persistence of HIV transmission. Similarly, although the viral hepatitis response has gained momentum, funding remains insufficient to meet global goals. While progress has been made in reducing hepatitis B incidence and increasing treatment for chronic hepatitis C, a large proportion of cases remains undiagnosed, and access to affordable treatments remains a challenge. The response to sexually transmitted infections has lagged severely, with a lack of visibility, funding, and implementation support leading to high disease burden and a significant number of undiagnosed and untreated cases, contributing to long-term health complications and adverse outcomes (WHO, 2022).

Testing for HIV

To determine HIV infection, individuals undergo an HIV antibody test, which detects antibodies in their blood. The presence of HIV antibodies indicates HIV infection, except for cases like an HIV-negative baby born to an HIV-positive mother. Babies may retain maternal antibodies for up to 18 months, potentially yielding positive results despite being HIV-negative. Typically, most individuals develop detectable HIV antibodies within 6 to 12 weeks post-infection, although it may take up to six months in rare cases. Testing earlier than three months may yield unclear results, as antibodies might not have developed yet. The HIV antibody test, commonly known as the HIV test, is used to determine HIV infection by detecting antibodies in an individual's blood.

HIV testing is conducted across various settings, including genitourinary clinics, emergency rooms, primary care services, same-day test clinics, drug units, antenatal clinics, TB clinics, and acute hospitals. Individuals seek testing for various reasons, including potential exposure to HIV, presence of symptoms related to immunodeficiency, and as part of antenatal care. Antenatal clinics routinely offer HIV testing to women to allow for early detection, counselling, and decision-making regarding conception, pregnancy management, and breastfeeding. Moreover, individuals who test positive for HIV receive counselling and health information to prevent further transmission, including practicing safe sex and informing past sexual partners. Overall, HIV testing plays a crucial role in early detection, prevention, and management of HIV infection for individuals across diverse healthcare settings. Encouraging couples to test together for HIV infection and mutually disclose their HIV status offers numerous benefits. Joint testing allows couples to make informed decisions regarding HIV prevention and reproductive health, including contraception and conception. Couples testing together are more likely to adopt behaviours that protect each other from HIV transmission. Providing antiretroviral treatment (ART) to the positive partner significantly reduces the risk of transmission to the negative partner, while pre-exposure prophylaxis (PrEP) for the negative partner can prevent HIV acquisition. Moreover, couples can support each other in accessing and adhering to ART and interventions to prevent mother-to-child transmission of HIV if one or both partners are HIV-positive.

Pre-test discussion and post-test counselling

In HIV counselling, healthcare professionals must adhere to strict principles of confidentiality when notifying clients of their HIV status. Confidentiality is crucial as it fosters trust between doctors and patients, enabling patients to share necessary information for quality care without fear. Patients have the right to know their HIV status, and research indicates that individuals who are aware of their HIV status are more likely to adopt preventive behaviours compared to those who are unaware. Therefore, maintaining confidentiality while informing patients of their HIV status not only respects their rights but also facilitates better health outcomes through informed decision-making and behaviour change. The notification of a test result (if positive) should be given directly to the patient and not via any third party because of confidentiality clause. This clause may be waived if the patient has specifically agreed to the test result being given to a significant partner or relatives. The notification of a test result needs to be comprehensive and include examination of high-risk behaviours, knowledge of the HIV virus and AIDS, and resources, unsafe sex, unborn babies, and the exploration of the patient's concerns. It is important for the health professional in the role of counsellor to be aware of the following (Canadian Aboriginal AIDS Network, 2012):

- Never make assumptions about the client's level of knowledge, concerns, values, and possible reactions.
- Ensure that the objectives are small, limited, and attainable.

- Draw on own assessment skills. Intuition is important when trying to understand a client's needs, their level of understanding, and the pace of information provided.
- Help the client view their health challenges differently.
- Where appropriate, help reduce a client's anxiety.
- Take less control over trying to solve the client's situation.
- Denial by a client can be a way of coping that protects the client from anxiety, depression, and possibly suicide.
- Feelings of being overwhelmed could happen to healthcare professionals who are in frequent contact with HIV-positive clients, and in this depressing situation, they may resort to falsely reassuring clients.

The primary purpose of pre-test discussion is to establish informed consent for HIV testing. However, some patients, because of anxieties and health concerns, may need to have a pre-test HIV counselling. Guidelines on pre-test discussion and post-test counselling are available from health and social care services. Key components of the pre-test discussion are presented in Table 14.2.

Post-test counselling should be available for both those diagnosed as HIV-negative and those diagnosed positive. The main features of post-test counselling are outlined in Table 14.3. The contents and the timing of the discussion will depend on the patients' reactions to their positive result.

Stigma and discrimination

Fear, negative attitudes, prejudice, and abuse towards people living with HIV and AIDS persist as persistent issues across societies. HIV-related stigma and discrimination profoundly affect the health, lives, and overall well-being of individuals living with or at risk of HIV infection, particularly among

Table 14.2
Pre-test discussion

Pre-test contents	Discussion
Nature of HIV	Modes of transmission
	Difference between HIV and AIDS
	Methods to reduce transmission
	Provision of materials of risk reduction strategies
Risk activities/need for test	Unsafe sexual practices
	History of drug use
	Injecting behaviour
	History of exposure to blood/blood products
	Tattooing
	Occupational risk
	Overseas travel with exposure to high-risk activity
Advantages of testing	Allows individual to form strategies to protect sexual partners
	Allows interventions to reduce vertical transmission (pregnant women)
	Allows for appropriate medical care
	Allows effective prophylactic care
	Allows decisions for future plan
	Reduction of needless anxiety about HIV infection
Disadvantages of testing	Psychological complications
	Possible adverse impact on relationships (family, partners, work)
	Possible restrictions, such as travelling abroad
Test procedure and result giving	Positive, negative, and indeterminate results
Obtaining informed consent	Written note

Source: Adapted from Expert Advisory Group on AIDS (2002). Department of Health.

Table 14.3
Post-test counselling

Aims	If HIV positive
• Address immediate concerns. • Provide support for those who are positive. • Provide information on prevention of HIV transmission.	• Address patient's immediate reactions. • Refer for specialist management and treatment. • Give details of support service. • Offer follow-up appointments. • Ongoing support (legal issues, support for carers and partners, etc.).

key populations, such as men who have sex with men, injecting drug users, and sex workers. HIV-related stigma and discrimination have wide-ranging implications, including hindering disclosure of HIV status, social rejection, limited access to services, impede access to HIV testing and treatment, loss of income, marriage, and childbearing options, poor healthcare, withdrawal of caregiving, loss of hope, worthlessness, and damage to reputation. Addressing stigma and discrimination is crucial for ensuring rights, access to care, and dignity for individuals living with HIV.

Discriminatory laws, regulations, and policies pertaining to HIV in a country can exacerbate stigma and exclusion, alienating individuals living with HIV and perpetuating societal stigma surrounding HIV and AIDS. Such legal frameworks contribute to further marginalisation and hinder efforts to combat HIV-related stigma and discrimination effectively.

> HIV-related discrimination-and stigma, where it leads to rights violations-is a human rights issue. People have a right to protection from discrimination and to a life of dignity where stigmatising attitudes do not impede the enjoyment of their other rights, including the rights to education, health care, work, access to justice, privacy, family, bodily autonomy and other rights.
>
> (UNAIDS, 2021, p. 1)

The recognition of HIV-related discrimination and stigma as a human rights issue is crucial in promoting equality, dignity, and justice for all individuals, including those living with HIV. Stigmatising attitudes and discriminatory practices not only violate the fundamental rights of individuals but also hinder their access to essential services and opportunities. People living with HIV have the right to protection from discrimination and deserve to lead lives of dignity where their rights to education, healthcare, work, access to justice, privacy, family, bodily autonomy, and other rights are respected and upheld.

Efforts to address HIV-related discrimination and stigma must be grounded in human rights principles, including the principles of equality, non-discrimination, and dignity. Laws, policies, and practices should be enacted and enforced to prevent and address discrimination based on HIV status and to ensure that individuals living with HIV are treated with respect and provided with the necessary support and resources to live fulfilling lives. Additionally, education, awareness-raising, and advocacy efforts are essential to challenge stigma and discrimination associated with HIV and to promote a culture of inclusivity, empathy, and understanding. By promoting human rights and combating discrimination and stigma, we can create a more equitable and supportive environment for all individuals affected by HIV.

HIV prevention and harm reduction

Public health policies, such as HIV prevention and harm reduction programmes, aim to decrease the transmission of HIV by considering various socio-cultural, economic, political, legal, and contextual factors, as highlighted by UNAIDS (2010). Harm reduction encompasses policies, programmes, and practices designed to minimise the adverse health, social, and legal consequences associated with drug use, drug policies, and drug laws. Rooted in the principles of justice and human rights, harm reduction emphasises positive change and collaboration with individuals without judgement, coercion, discrimination, or the precondition of cessation of drug use for support. Its focus lies in reducing the negative impacts of drug use while respecting the dignity and autonomy of individuals involved (Harm Reduction International, 2022).

HIV transmission occurs primarily through sexual contact, exposure to contaminated blood, and mother-to-child transmission. Key determinants of HIV transmission include sexual behaviours and needle/syringe use, with HIV being transmissible through specific body fluids like blood, semen, pre-seminal fluid, rectal fluids, vaginal fluids, and breast milk. Transmission occurs when these fluids come into contact with mucous membranes or damaged tissue, or through contaminated needle/syringe use during injecting drug use. Harm reduction approaches have been widely implemented as a public health response to the HIV epidemic, particularly among people who inject drugs. Evidence suggests that these approaches have effectively reduced the number of new HIV infections among this population, as highlighted by Harm Reduction International (2022). Professionals across various sectors, including health, education, social care, and voluntary services, play a crucial role in HIV prevention and harm reduction efforts. By combining prevention and harm reduction approaches, these professionals can make significant contributions to mitigating the spread of HIV and minimising the negative health, social, and legal impacts associated with drug use.

To prevent HIV transmission, various strategies are available, including:

- Promotion of safe sexual practices, including condom use and reducing the number of sexual partners
- Providing access to HIV testing and counselling services for early detection and prevention
- Needle and syringe programmes (NSPs)
- Opioid substitution therapy (OST) and other drug dependence treatment
- HIV testing and counselling (HTC)
- Offering antiretroviral therapy (ART) for individuals living with HIV to suppress the virus and reduce the risk of transmission
- Promoting voluntary medical male circumcision to reduce the risk of HIV acquisition in heterosexual men
- Offering pre-exposure prophylaxis (PrEP) to individuals at high risk of HIV infection
- Prevention and treatment of sexually transmitted infections (STIs)
- Condom programmes for people who inject drugs and their sexual partners
- Targeted information, education, and communication for people who inject drugs and their sexual partners
- Vaccination, diagnosis, and treatment of viral hepatitis
- Prevention, diagnosis, and treatment of tuberculosis (TB)

These prevention strategies play a crucial role in reducing the transmission of HIV and promoting public health.

Preventive measures for HIV and STIs include undergoing HIV testing for oneself and one's partner and being aware of each other's HIV status before engaging in sexual activity. The prevention of poor sexual health relies on individuals that have access to information, skills, and services necessary for making informed choices. Targeting high-risk groups is crucial for effective HIV and STI prevention efforts. These groups, often deemed as "higher risk," include young people (both in and out of care), individuals from Black and minority ethnic backgrounds, gay and bisexual men, people who inject drugs, individuals living with HIV (both adults and children), sex workers, and individuals in prisons and youth offending establishments. Tailored prevention initiatives and support services are necessary to address the specific vulnerabilities and needs of these groups and to promote sexual health and well-being.

In the realm of sexual health information and prevention of HIV and STIs, the emphasis is on engaging in less-risky sexual behaviours. Anal and vaginal sex pose the highest risk for HIV transmission, whereas oral sex is considered less risky. To mitigate HIV transmission, it is important to limit the number of sexual partners and consistently use condoms during sexual activity. Additionally, avoiding the sharing of needles and syringes among injecting drug users is essential. Utilising sterile drug injection equipment and refraining from sharing injecting equipment can significantly reduce the risk of HIV transmission. Having an STI increases the likelihood of acquiring or transmitting HIV; thus, it is imperative to get tested and seek treatment for STIs, including sexual partners. Overall, these preventive measures play a critical role in promoting sexual health and reducing the spread of HIV and STIs within communities. Furthermore, pharmacological interventions are utilised to prevent mother-to-child transmission of HIV. Pregnant women living with HIV can take HIV medications during pregnancy and childbirth to decrease the likelihood of transmitting the virus to their babies. Moreover, newborn babies born to HIV-infected mothers are administered HIV medications for six weeks post-birth to further reduce the risk of transmission. These measures form integral components of comprehensive HIV prevention strategies, aiming to reduce HIV transmission rates and improve health outcomes for both affected individuals and their offspring.

UNAIDS (2010) advocates for combination prevention programmes in the fight against HIV/AIDS. These programmes emphasise the simultaneous use of complementary behavioural, biomedical, and structural prevention strategies, rather than relying solely on single interventions like condom distribution. The approach targets individual, community, and population levels, particularly in high-prevalence regions or "hot spots" and among high-risk groups. An example of combination prevention includes integrating pre-exposure prophylaxis with HIV testing, needle and syringe programmes, antiretroviral treatment, and opioid substitution therapy (UNAIDS, 2024). This comprehensive strategy aims to address the multifaceted aspects of HIV prevention and control.

Treatment of HIV

The goal of HIV treatment is to reduce the viral load to undetectable levels and bolster the immune system to prevent HIV-related illnesses (HIVinfo, 2024). Treatment typically begins when CD4+ lymphocyte cell counts fall towards 350 or below, even if the individual remains asymptomatic. Antiretroviral treatment consists of drugs that slow down HIV replication in the body. Treatment options have significantly improved the lives of people with HIV by reducing AIDS-related illnesses, hospital admissions, and death rates. These treatments offer individuals the opportunity to maintain their health for extended periods.

Antiretroviral treatment (ART) has enabled many individuals with HIV to return to full-time employment by effectively controlling the virus. Typically, ART involves combinations of three or more antiretroviral drugs, known as combination therapy or highly active antiretroviral therapy (HAART). HAART has proven effective in controlling HIV and delaying the onset of AIDS for numerous individuals. However, it is important to note that not everyone responds positively to ART, and some may experience adverse effects or develop drug resistance. In cases of drug resistance, alternative combination therapies may be necessary, althoug HIV may still persist in the body. Some individual with HIV may also integrate complementary therapies, such as vitamin supplements, herbal remedie meditation, massage, and acupuncture, either alon or alongside their antiretroviral treatment. Despit the effectiveness of ART, individuals undergoin treatment should still refrain from unprotected se or sharing needles or injecting equipment, as ART does not eliminate the risk of transmitting the virus It is crucial for individuals with HIV to continu practicing safe behaviours to prevent the spread o the virus to others.

TUBERCULOSIS

Tuberculosis (TB) is a contagious and airborne disease and ranks as the second leading infectious killer globally, following COVID-19, and is the 13th leading cause of death worldwide (WHO, 2021). It was also the primary cause of death among individuals with HIV and a significant contributor to deaths associated with antimicrobial resistance. Tuberculosis is caused by the bacterium *Mycobacterium tuberculosis* and primarily affects the lungs, though it can impact any part of the body. Transmission occurs through the coughing of infectious droplets and usually requires prolonged close contact with an infected individual. TB is curable with a combination of specific antibiotics, but treatment must continue for at least six months. Common symptoms include chronic cough, fatigue, lack of appetite, weight loss, night sweats, and fever.

The burden of HIV-associated TB is highest in the WHO African Region (WHO, 2021). HIV/AIDS and TB are closely intertwined, often described as a "co-epidemic" or "dual epidemic." HIV weakens the immune system, making individuals more susceptible to TB infection. TB tends to occur earlier in the course of HIV infection and is a significant risk factor for converting latent TB into active disease. On the contrary, TB bacteria accelerate the progression of AIDS in HIV-infected individuals. The two diseases together pose a formidable threat, with TB being more challenging to diagnose and progressing faster in HIV-infected individuals. Without proper treatment, approximately 90% of those living with HIV die within months of contracting TB. Treatment involves a six-month course of four antimicrobial drugs and should be supported by healthcare professionals to ensure adherence to the treatment regimen.

HEPATITIS

Hepatitis refers to liver inflammation, which can result from various factors, including alcohol, drugs, immune disorders, and infections. The primary cause of hepatitis is through blood-borne viruses. There are six main types of viral hepatitis: A, B, C, D, E, and G. Hepatitis A and E are transmitted via the faecal–oral route, while the others are spread through blood and body fluids. In the context of drug misuse, hepatitis C, B, and A are particularly concerning. In England, the most common route of infection currently is through the sharing of contaminated needles or injecting equipment among injecting drug users.

Hepatitis C

Hepatitis C is increasingly recognised as a significant public health concern, often remaining undetected for years or even decades due to the delayed onset of symptoms. Its prevalence remains high among injecting drug users, primarily transmitted through the sharing of contaminated needles and syringes, along with other equipment used for drug injection. While transmission from mother to baby is uncommon, caution is advised against breastfeeding. Sexual transmission of hepatitis C is possible but rare. Transmission may also occur through sharing personal items contaminated with blood, such as toothbrushes or razors, and during medical procedures abroad where infection control is lacking. Risks from tattooing, piercing, and acupuncture with unsterile equipment are also documented. Health and social care workers face occupational hazards, including needle stick injuries, that put them at risk of hepatitis infection.

Hepatitis C infection often goes unnoticed in its early stages, as it typically presents no signs or symptoms. However, some individuals may experience mild symptoms, such as muscle aches, fatigue, nausea, and loss of appetite. In more severe cases, symptoms may include jaundice, liver discomfort, dark urine or "tea-coloured" urine. Progression of hepatitis C can lead to severe liver complications, particularly in cases of alcohol consumption or co-infection with HIV or hepatitis B. The infection's long latency period, spanning decades in some cases, complicates its recognition and diagnosis. The signs and symptoms of the early stage and later stage of hepatitis are presented in Table 14.4. Alcohol consumption and co-infection with HIV or hepatitis B are strongly associated with increased likelihood of progression to severe liver complications.

Table 14.4
Signs and symptoms of hepatitis C

Early stage	Later stage
• Slight fatigue	• Fatigue
• Nausea	• Lack of appetite
• Poor appetite	• Nausea
• Muscle and joint pains	• Vomiting
• Tenderness (area of the liver)	• Jaundice (yellow skin and eyes)
	• High temperature
	• Weight loss
	• Poor memory
	• Anxiety
	• Depression
	• Alcohol intolerance

Testing for hepatitis C

Like HIV testing, there are clear guidelines on testing and counselling in hepatitis C infection, similar to those for HIV. There is the need for coordinated discussions before and after testing to address the serious implications of hepatitis C infection. Health professionals must be knowledgeable about transmission routes, prevention measures, and treatment options to effectively counsel clients. Prevention and harm reduction strategies include education, safe injection practices, blood safety measures, safer sex practices, harm reduction programmes, screening, treatment access, and supportive services. These measures aim to reduce transmission and mitigate the impact of hepatitis C on individuals and communities.

Prevention and harm reduction of hepatitis C

The absence of a hepatitis C vaccine highlights the importance of prevention strategies aimed at reducing both acute and chronic infections. These efforts focus on educating healthcare professionals and the general public about the risks associated with hepatitis C. Specifically targeting high-risk groups, such as injecting drug users, requires comprehensive approaches, including health information dissemination, harm reduction initiatives, and counselling services. Various prevention and promotion strategies can be implemented at primary, secondary, and tertiary levels to minimise the risk of virus exposure in vulnerable populations. Table 14.5 offers examples of primary, secondary, and tertiary prevention interventions.

Preventive measures would not be effective unless there is a range of service provisions for the reduction or minimisation of hepatitis C infections. These include:

- *Needle and syringe exchange services*. Providing access to sterile injecting equipment helps prevent the transmission of hepatitis C among injecting drug users.
- *Safe disposal of needles and syringes*. Ensuring the proper disposal of used needles and syringes reduces the risk of accidental needle stick injuries and potential transmission of the virus.
- *Outreach and peer education services*. Engaging with communities through outreach and peer education helps disseminate information about hepatitis C risks and prevention measures effectively.
- *Specialist addiction treatment services*. Offering specialised addiction treatment services supports individuals in overcoming substance abuse issues, thereby reducing the likelihood of hepatitis C transmission through injecting drug use.
- *Health education and promotion*. Increasing awareness about hepatitis C and other blood-borne viruses through health education campaigns helps individuals understand the risks associated with injecting drugs and encourage safer practices.
- *Disinfecting tablets in prisons*. Providing disinfecting tablets throughout prison facilities helps inmates maintain hygienic conditions, reducing the risk of hepatitis C transmission within correctional settings.

On an individual level of prevention, there is a need to discuss some of the issues and problems associated with hepatitis C. The harm reduction strategies that patients should adopt in order to minimise the transmission of hepatitis C include:

- Take the test.
- Become abstinent or reduce alcohol consumption.
- Carry an organ donor card.
- Do not donate blood.
- Never share any injecting equipment.
- Use condoms.
- Do not share razors or toothbrushes or any toiletry equipment contaminated with blood.
- Avoid body piercing.

Treatment of hepatitis C

Currently, there is no vaccination available for hepatitis C. Individuals who test positive for hepatitis C

Table 14.5
Primary, secondary, and tertiary prevention interventions for hepatitis C

Primary prevention	Secondary and tertiary prevention
Hand hygiene: including surgical hand preparation, handwashing, and use of gloves	Education and counselling on options for care and treatment
Safe and appropriate use of healthcare injections	Immunisation with the hepatitis A and B vaccines to prevent coinfection from these hepatitis viruses and to protect the liver
Safe handling and disposal of sharps and waste	Early and appropriate medical management, including antiviral therapy, if appropriate
Provision of comprehensive harm reduction services to people who inject drugs, including sterile injecting equipment	Regular monitoring for early diagnosis of chronic liver disease
Testing of donated blood for hepatitis B and C (as well as HIV and syphilis)	
Training of health personnel	
Promotion of correct and consistent use of condoms	

Source: Adapted WHO (2023a).

should undergo regular liver function tests to monitor for any signs of liver damage. They are advised to reduce or stop alcohol intake to minimise further liver damage. In cases where liver function deteriorates, a liver biopsy may be conducted to assess the extent of liver changes. Testing and diagnosis involve serological tests for anti-HCV antibodies and nucleic acid tests for HCV RNA to confirm chronic infection and determine treatment necessity. Early detection prevents health complications and transmission. WHO (2023a) recommends testing high-risk groups and implementing blood donor screening in regions with high HCV prevalence.

Treatment options for hepatitis C have seen significant advancements. With the introduction of direct-acting antiviral medications, the treatment landscape for hepatitis C has improved considerably. Antiviral medications, particularly direct-acting antivirals (DAAs) like sofosbuvir and daclatasvir, can cure over 95% of hepatitis C cases (WHO, 2023a). Treatment typically lasts 12 to 24 weeks, depending on cirrhosis status. Lifestyle changes such as avoiding alcohol and maintaining a healthy weight complement treatment efforts. WHO (2023a) recommends pan-genotypic DAAs for all adults, adolescents, and children over 3 years old with chronic hepatitis C. These medications offer higher cure rates with shorter treatment durations compared to older regimens. As a result, individuals diagnosed with hepatitis C have better prospects for successful treatment outcomes and improved long-term liver health.

The findings from a meta-analysis of prospective studies on the combination treatment of chronic hepatitis C in illicit drug users showed that using antiviral combinations to treat chronic hepatitis C was effective and well tolerated in illicit drug users, as in the general population (Zanini et al., 2010). Despite highly effective therapy, eliminating hepatitis C remains challenging due to gaps in diagnosis and access to care. Pangenotypic treatment options and ongoing vaccine research offer hope for improved outcomes (Alshuwaykh & Kwo, 2021). While successful elimination efforts have been reported, sustained innovation and collaboration are essential for achieving global hepatitis C eradication.

Hepatitis B

Hepatitis B is a viral infection that attacks the liver and can cause both acute and chronic disease. Hepatitis B is primarily transmitted through contact with infected bodily fluids, such as blood, semen, and vaginal fluids. Transmission commonly occurs through unprotected sexual intercourse, sharing contaminated needles among drug users, receipt of infected blood or blood products, and from infected mothers to their babies during childbirth. Additionally, transmission can occur through household contact among children and via tattooing and body piercing practices. The virus can cause acute infection, which may present with symptoms like sore throat, fatigue, joint pains, nausea, vomiting, and loss of appetite. Severe cases may involve abdominal discomfort and jaundice. After acute infection, some individuals, particularly babies, may develop chronic hepatitis B, where the virus persists in the body. Many carriers of chronic hepatitis B remain asymptomatic but can still transmit the virus to others, posing a risk of developing serious complications such as cirrhosis and primary liver cancer. In severe cases, acute hepatitis B can progress to liver failure, leading to death. Chronic hepatitis B infection affects millions globally and poses significant health risks, including liver cirrhosis and hepatocellular carcinoma (liver cancer) (WHO, 2023b).

Early detection and intervention are crucial in managing hepatitis B and preventing its transmission. However, the infection can be prevented through vaccination, which is highly effective and safe. Vaccination strategies typically involve administering the hepatitis B vaccine to newborns shortly after birth, followed by additional doses, to establish long-term immunity. Booster vaccines are generally not required for individuals who have completed the recommended vaccination series. Prevention strategies for hepatitis B also include practicing safe sex, using condoms, and reducing the number of sexual partners to minimise the risk of transmission. Individuals should also avoid sharing needles or any equipment used for injecting drugs, piercing, or tattooing. Proper hand hygiene, including thorough handwashing with soap and water after contact with blood, body fluids, or contaminated surfaces, is crucial in preventing the spread of the virus.

Diagnosis and monitoring of hepatitis B infection involve various blood tests, physical examinations, and imaging techniques to assess liver health and disease progression. Regular monitoring is essential to detect any changes in liver function and adjust treatment accordingly. Additionally, screening of all blood donations for hepatitis B helps ensure blood safety and prevent accidental transmission of the virus. Treatment options for chronic hepatitis B include oral antiviral medications, such as tenofovir or entecavir (WHO, 2023b). These drugs can slow disease progression, reduce the risk of liver complications, and improve long-term survival. However, most individuals with chronic hepatitis B require lifelong treatment to manage the infection effectively. Furthermore, antiviral medications can be administered during pregnancy to prevent mother-to-child transmission of hepatitis B (WHO, 2023b). These comprehensive prevention and intervention measures are essential in controlling the spread of hepatitis B and reducing the burden of liver disease and mortality associated with the infection.

KEY POINTS

- Blood-borne viruses (BBVs) are mainly found in blood or bodily fluids.
- BBVs, especially the human immunodeficiency virus (HIV) and hepatitis B and C viruses (HBV, HCV), pose major risks to the health of people who inject illicit drugs.
- HIV stands for human immunodeficiency virus. HIV is the virus that causes AIDS (acquired immunodeficiency syndrome).
- Most HIV transmission occurs from: Unprotected vaginal or anal intercourse. Sharing contaminated needles and syringes. Transfusion of contaminated blood and blood products. From mother to baby in utero, at birth, or via breastfeeding. Transfusion of contaminated blood and blood products.
- It is important to encourage couples to test together for HIV infection and to mutually disclose their HIV status.
- In the context of HIV counselling, the approac of a counsellor is required when healthcare pro fessionals notify a client of their HIV status.
- The primary purpose of pre-test discussion is t establish informed consent for HIV testing.
- Post-test counselling should be available for botl those diagnosed as HIV-negative and those diag nosed positive.
- Public health policies such as HIV preventio and harm reduction programmes are aimed a reducing the transmission of HIV.
- Fear and prejudice regarding HIV infection act a a barrier to prevention, treatment, and care ser vices for people with, or at risk from, HIV.
- Those people who are in the high-risk group but do not have HIV have the choice of having pre-exposure prophylaxis (PrEP) treatment.
- Antiretroviral treatment has had a huge impact on the lives of people with HIV.
- The antiretroviral drugs are usually prescribed in combinations of three or more. This is called combination therapy or highly active antiretroviral therapy (HAART).
- There is evidence to suggest that harm reduction approaches have reduced the number of new HIV infections among people who inject drugs.
- TB is common in people with AIDS and is one of the leading causes of death in HIV-infected people.
- Hepatitis means inflammation of the liver. The main cause of hepatitis is through blood-borne viruses.
- Many people with chronic hepatitis B remain well but become chronic carriers.

Activity 14.2

Questions

- Describe current trends in HIV infection.
- List the transmission routes of HIV.
- Describe the process of HIV pre-discussion and post-test counselling.
- Discuss the prevention of HIV.
- Discuss the risks of injecting drug use to the transmission of blood-borne viruses.
- Outline the global health sector strategies on, respectively, HIV, viral hepatitis, and sexually transmitted infections.

Activity 14.3

Questions

- Describe current trends in hepatitis C and B infections.
- List the transmission routes of hepatitis C and B infections.
- Describe the effective prevention measures to hepatitis C and B infections.
- What current treatment and vaccinations are available for viral infections?

References

Alshuwaykh, O., & Kwo, P. Y. (2021). Current and future strategies for the treatment of chronic hepatitis C. *Clinical and Molecular Hepatology,* 27(2), 246–256. https://doi.org/10.3350/cmh.2020.0230.

Canadian Aboriginal Aids Network. (2012). *Pre and Post HIV Test Counselling Guide.* http://caan.ca/wp-content/uploads/2012/05/get-tested-guide.pdf (accessed 11 March 2024).

Harm Reduction International. (2022). *What Is Harm Reduction?* London: Harm Reduction International. https://hri.global/what-is-harm-reduction/ (accessed 11 March 2024).

HIVinfo. (2024). *HIV Prevention.* https://hivinfo.nih.gov/understanding-hiv/fact-sheets/basics-hiv-prevention (accessed 11 March 2024).

UNAIDS. (2010). *Combination HIV Prevention: Tailoring and Coordinating Biomedical, Behavioural and Structural Strategies to Reduce New HIV Infections.* https://www.unaids.org/en/resources/documents/2010/20101006_JC2007_Combination_Prevention_paper (accessed 11 March 2024).

UNAIDS. (2021). *HIV and Stigma and Discrimination* (Human Rights Fact Sheet Series #7). https://www.unaids.org/sites/default/files/media_asset/07-hiv-human-rights-factsheet-stigma-discrmination_en.pdf (accessed 11 March 2024).

UNAIDS. (2024). *HIV Treatment.* https://www.unaids.org/en/topic/treatment (accessed 11 March 2024).

WHO. (2021). *Global Tuberculosis Report 2021.* https://cdn.who.int/media/docs/default-source/hq-tuberculosis/tb-report-2021/factsheet-global-tb-report-2021.pdf?sfvrsn=86011b1e_5&download=true (accessed 11 March 2024).

WHO. (2022). *Global Health Sector Strategies on, Respectively, HIV, Viral Hepatitis and Sexually Transmitted Infections for the Period 2022–2030.* Geneva: World Health Organization.

WHO. (2023a). *Hepatitis C: Key Facts.* https://www.who.int/news-room/fact-sheets/detail/hepatitis-c (accessed 11 March 2024).

WHO. (2023b). *Hepatitis B: Key Facts.* https://www.who.int/news-room/fact-sheets/detail/hepatitis-b (accessed 12 March 2024).

Zanini, B., Covolo, L., Donato, F., & Lanzini, A. (2010). Effectiveness and tolerability of combination treatment of chronic hepatitis C in illicit drug users: Meta-analysis of prospective studies. *Clinical Therapeutics,* 32(113), 2139–2215.

Chapter 15

Alcohol and drug use in women

Learning outcomes

- Describe the prevalence of alcohol and substance use disorder with women.
- Discuss the psychosocial and environmental issues related to alcohol and substance use disorder.
- List the features of foetal alcohol spectrum disorders.
- Discuss the problems associated with illegal drug use in pregnancy.
- Discuss the issues of blood-borne viruses in pregnancy.
- Discuss the barriers in preventing women from accessing treatment services.
- Discuss the special treatment needs of women with alcohol and/or substance use disorder.

Activity 15.1

There is only one correct answer to the following multiple-choice questions.

1. Which of the following factors may contribute to the development of alcohol or substance use disorder in women?
   a. Genetic predisposition
   b. Socio-economic status
   c. Trauma history
   d. All of the above
   e. None of the above
2. Compared to men, women generally metabolise alcohol:
   a. Faster
   b. Slower
   c. At the same rate
   d. Depends on the individual's body weight
   e. None of the above
3. Women who misuse alcohol or drugs are at increased risk of:
   a. Cardiovascular diseases
   b. Liver damage
   c. Breast cancer
   d. All of the above
   e. None of the above

DOI: 10.4324/9781003456674-18

4. Pregnant women who use substances like alcohol or drugs may expose their foetus to:
   a. Developmental delays
   b. Birth defects
   c. Neonatal withdrawal symptoms
   d. All of the above
   e. None of the above
5. Which of the following is a common barrier for women seeking treatment for substance use disorder?
   a. Lack of childcare
   b. Stigma
   c. Limited access to specialised programmes
   d. All of the above
   e. None of the above
6. Women with substance use disorder may have higher rates of co-occurring:
   a. Depression
   b. Anxiety disorders
   c. Postpartum depression
   d. All of the above
   e. None of the above
7. The term "telescoping" refers to:
   a. Rapid progression from substance use to addiction in women
   b. Long-term recovery from substance use disorder
   c. Use of telescopic lenses in treatment programmes
   d. None of the above
   e. None of the above
8. Women are more likely to experience shame and guilt related to their substance use due to:
   a. Societal expectations
   b. Biological factors
   c. Genetic predisposition
   d. All of the above
   e. None of the above
9. In women, substance use disorder may manifest as:
   a. Increased risk-taking behaviour
   b. Physical health issues
   c. Mood swings
   d. All of the above
   e. None of the above
10. Which of the following is a potential consequence of substance use disorder in women?
    a. Financial instability
    b. Legal problems
    c. Relationship conflicts
    d. All of the above
    e. None of the above
11. Women with substance use disorder are at higher risk of:
    a. Intimate partner violence
    b. Employment stability
    c. Social acceptance
    d. All of the above
    e. None of the above

12. Which of the following is a common coping mechanism for women with substance use disorder?
    a. Social support
    b. Avoidance behaviour
    c. Seeking professional help
    d. All of the above
    e. None of the above
13. Women with substance use disorder may face unique challenges related to:
    a. Hormonal changes
    b. Menstrual cycles
    c. Menopause
    d. All of the above
    e. None of the above
14. Which of the following interventions may be particularly effective for women with substance use disorder?
    a. Trauma-informed care
    b. Pharmacotherapy
    c. Detoxification programmes
    d. All of the above
    e. None of the above
15. Co-occurring mental health disorders in women with substance use disorder:
    a. Often go undiagnosed
    a. Are easily treated with medication
    b. Do not impact the course of substance use disorder
    c. All of the above
    d. None of the above
16. Women with substance use disorder may benefit from treatment programmes that address:
    a. Trauma history
    b. Parenting skills
    c. Financial management
    d. All of the above
    e. None of the above
17. Which of the following is a common feature of substance use disorder treatment programmes for women?
    a. Gender-specific counselling
    b. Mandatory drug testing
    c. Isolation from family members
    d. All of the above
    e. None of the above
18. Which of the following strategies may help prevent substance use disorder in women?
    a. Education on the risks of substance misuse
    b. Access to affordable healthcare
    c. Strengthening social support networks
    d. All of the above
    e. None of the above

19. Which one of the following is not true?
    a. Although women are less likely than men to abuse alcohol, they are more likely to have alcohol-related health problems, such as liver disease.
    b. Women are less likely to have problems with prescribed medications compared to men.
    c. Alcohol and drug misuse in women increases the risk of developing other health problems, such as osteoporosis or depression.
    d. Women who misuse alcohol and drugs attempt suicide four times more frequently than non-users.
    e. None of the above is correct.
20. The only safe, sensible drinking regarding taking alcohol during pregnancy is:
    a. Women should avoid alcohol.
    b. Women should drink 3–4 units.
    c. Drinking 2–3 can enhance childbirth.
    d. Women should drink 3–5 units.
    e. None of the above is correct.
21. Which of the following is the most serious outcome of maternal drinking during pregnancy?
    a. Social, emotional, and cognitive development
    b. Learning deficits
    c. Growth retardation
    d. Foetal alcohol spectrum disorders
    e. None of the above
22. Tobacco smoking can cause reproductive problems, such as
    a. Fertility problems
    b. Premature babies
    c. Low-birth-weight babies
    d. All of the above
    e. None of the above
23. HIV can be transmitted from mother to baby
    a. Pre-natal
    b. Peri-natal
    c. Through breastfeeding
    d. All of the above
    e. None of the above

INTRODUCTION

Alcohol and substance use disorders among women represent a complex and often overlooked aspect of public health. Traditionally, societal norms and gender roles have shaped perceptions and expectations surrounding women's behaviour, including their relationship with alcohol and drugs. Historically, discussions surrounding addiction have predominantly focused on men, yet women's experiences with alcohol and substance use are distinct and multifaceted. Societal norms have favoured alcohol consumption among men, while women's drinking has been relatively less socially acceptable. However, there has been a shift toward greater acceptance of women consuming alcohol in both developed and developing countries. Despite this trend, women are less likely to engage in frequent or heavy drinking compared to men and are less likely to report alcohol-related problems (WHO, 2005).

Women's engagement with alcohol and psychoactive substances is influenced by a multitude of factors, including biological, psychological, social, and cultural determinants. Women often navigate a complex landscape of societal pressures, familial responsibilities, and cultural stigmas that can contribute to the development and continuation of substance use disorders. Moreover, women's experiences with addiction are intricately linked to broader issues, such as trauma, domestic violence, mental health disorders, and socio-economic inequalities. Women's drinking behaviour and drug use are often perceived differently than men's, characterised by stigmatisation, marginalisation, and labelling within society. Negative attitudes toward intoxicated women and those who struggle with substance misuse contribute to their social marginalisation. Interestingly, it has been observed that it is not merely intoxication that draws societal condemnation but rather the perceived deviation from traditional gender norms (Robbins & Martin, 1997). Women's behaviour while intoxicated, particularly if it is seen as aggressive or unruly, is often considered unfeminine and therefore attracts significant condemnation. These factors further complicate the prevention and management of alcohol and substance use disorders among women and underline the importance of holistic and gender-sensitive approaches to treatment and support.

ISSUES OF ALCOHOL AND DRUG USE

There is an increasing trend in the use of alcohol and drug amongst young women. Women, on average, have 10% more body fat and less body fluid than men, which leads to alcohol being more concentrated in their bodies and causing greater harm. Consequently, women face an elevated risk of various alcohol-related health issues compared to men, including alcohol hepatitis, heart disease, liver disease, ulcers, reproductive problems, osteoporosis, pancreatitis, brain damage, breast cancer, memory loss, and other illnesses stemming from alcohol and drug misuse.

In the context of women's health and alcohol use, understanding the influence of sex-related factors on pharmacokinetics and pharmacodynamics is important. *Pharmacokinetics* refers to how the body processes a substance, including absorption, distribution, metabolism, and elimination, while *pharmacodynamics* refers to how the substance affects the body. Research indicates that alcohol has sex-specific health effects, with females experiencing higher damage from lower alcohol amounts compared to males (Greaves et al., 2022). For example, evidence shows that pharmacokinetics and pharmacodynamics affect the processing of alcohol, including the absorption, distribution, metabolism, and elimination of drugs (Anderson, 2008; Beierle et al. 1999; Greenblatt & von Moltke, 2008). Sex-related factors such as hormonal differences, body composition, and enzyme activity can significantly impact how women metabolise and respond to alcohol compared to men. For example, women tend to have lower levels of the enzyme alcohol dehydrogenase, which is involved in metabolising alcohol, leading to slower alcohol metabolism and potentially higher blood alcohol concentrations compared to men consuming the same amount of alcohol. Moreover, hormonal fluctuations during the menstrual cycle and hormonal changes during pregnancy and menopause can further influence how women respond to alcohol. These factors contribute to variations in alcohol sensitivity, tolerance, and risk of alcohol-related health problems among women. Moreover, gender-related factors, such as increased susceptibility to sexual assault and intimate partner violence, along with negative gender norms and stereotypes about alcohol or substance use for women, further influence drinking behaviours.

However, women are just as likely as men to develop a substance use disorder. Women with substance use disorders often have shorter histories of using substances like cocaine, opioids, marijuana, or alcohol compared to men (NIDA, 2022). Research suggests that women with substance use issues are more likely than men to be younger, have partners with substance use problems, possess fewer resources, have dependent children, frequently reside with a partner who uses drugs, present more severe problems at treatment onset, have experienced trauma related to physical and sexual abuse, and have concurrent psychiatric disorders (UNDOC, 2004). Women may experience heightened cravings and relapse tendencies, crucial phases of addiction. Research indicates that women exhibit distinct patterns in drug use and responses and encounter specific barriers to treatment, such as childcare issues or receiving treatments not adequately tested on women (NIDA, 2022). However, when they seek treatment for substance use disorder, women tend to present with more severe medical, behavioural, psychological, and social issues. This is attributed to women's faster progression from initial substance use to developing dependence and addiction.

Women are disproportionately affected by misuse of central nervous system depressants, such as sedatives used for seizures, sleep disorders, and anxiety, as well as medications like antidepressants (NIDA, 2022). They are more likely to seek treatment for misuse and also face higher mortality rates from overdoses involving mental health medications. Women also visit emergency departments more frequently due to antidepressants and benzodiazepines. Given that women are at higher risk for anxiety and insomnia, they may receive more prescriptions for these drugs, leading to increased risk of misuse, substance use disorder, and overdose.

PROBLEMS RELATED TO ILLEGAL DRUG MISUSE DURING PREGNANCY

The use of tobacco, alcohol, and illicit drugs or the misuse of prescription drugs by pregnant women can have severe health consequences for infants. Drug and alcohol consumption during pregnancy poses significant risks to the developing foetus, with the first trimester being the most critical period for organ and limb formation. However, drugs can also interfere with functional development in later trimesters, leading to serious consequences for the central nervous system and organ systems. In the final 12 weeks of pregnancy, drug use increases the risk of stunting foetal growth and premature birth. All drugs taken during pregnancy reach the baby through the placenta, but individual responses vary depending on factors such as drug type, frequency of use, method of consumption, amount taken, polydrug use, and the baby's individual response. Mothers who use illegal drugs during pregnancy heighten their risk of various complications, including anaemia, blood and heart infections, skin infections, hepatitis, and other infectious diseases. Research indicates that smoking tobacco or marijuana, taking prescription pain relievers, or using illegal drugs during pregnancy doubles or triples the risk of stillbirth (Reddy, 2013). Approximately 5% of pregnant women use one or more addictive substances, according to estimates (Wendell, 2013).

The World Health Organization (WHO, 1997) states that there is reliable scientific evidence indicating that cannabis does not cause chromosomal or genetic damage. However, the findings from experimental studies showed that cannabinoids can cause widespread genetic damage in communities, affecting both the occurrence of birth defects and cancer rates at the chromosomal level (Reece & Hulse, 2021). Maternal cannabis use is linked to reduced birth weight and cognitive/memory deficits in offspring (Fergusson et al., 2002; Fried et al., 2003). Additionally, research suggests that chronic cannabis consumption by women of reproductive age may increase the risk of ectopic pregnancies (Wang et al., 2004). Furthermore, the use of heroin, cocaine, and other psychoactive substances during pregnancy can lead to newborn withdrawal symptoms and growth retardation in the unborn baby. It is essential for women to be cautious about recreational or pain-alleviating cannabis use during pregnancy.

Cocaine use during pregnancy can result in various adverse outcomes, including premature delivery, premature detachment of the placenta, haemorrhage, high blood pressure, and stillbirth. Babies exposed to cocaine in the womb are at higher risk of health problems during the newborn period, including behaviour issues, deficits in cognitive performance, information processing, sustained attention, language, and memory (Buckingham-Howes et al., 2013; Lester & Lagasse, 2010; Lambert & Bauer, 2012). Cocaine use during pregnancy can result in placental abruption, spontaneous abortion, or foetal neurologic damage if the infant survives. Babies born to addicted mothers often have low birth weight, reduced body length, smaller head circumference, and lower Apgar scores (Dysart, 2022). Cocaine exposure can cause cerebral infarcts and rare anomalies, such as limb amputations, genitourinary malformations, intestinal issues, attention/alertness deficits, lower IQ, and impaired motor skills (Dysart, 2022). Neonates exposed to cocaine do not typically experience withdrawal from cocaine, but they might display withdrawal symptoms if their mother used cocaine, heroin, methadone, alcohol, or other depressants before delivery. Cocaine-exposed babies may face feeding and sleep issues, hindering mother–child bonding. Research on the long-term impacts of pre-natal cocaine exposure is lacking.

In utero opioid exposure can result in neonatal withdrawal (narcotic abstinence syndrome) within 72 hours of birth, characterised by irritability, jitteriness, hypertonicity, vomiting, diarrhoea, sweating, seizures, and respiratory alkalosis. Infants may be monitored for up to five days for symptoms. Heroin use during pregnancy poses severe risks to both the mother and the unborn child. Women who use heroin during pregnancy significantly increase the likelihood of harming their babies and experiencing serious pregnancy complications. These risks include low birth weight, poor foetal growth, premature rupture of the membranes, premature delivery, and stillbirth. Babies born to heroin-dependent mothers often face numerous health challenges, such as being born premature, underdeveloped, and with respiratory issues and infections. They also have an increased risk of lifelong disabilities and sudden infant death syndrome (SIDS) (NICE, 2010a, 2021). SIDS has been noted to have associations with psychoactive substances. Research, including studies cited by Phillips et al. (2011), indicates that women addicted to various drugs, including alcohol, during pregnancy may have children who experience breathing difficulties and are at a heightened risk of SIDS compared to the general population. However, further evidence is required to fully understand the extent of this correlation and its underlying mechanisms. In utero opioid exposure can result in neonatal withdrawal (narcotic abstinence syndrome) within 72 hours of birth, including fever, high-pitched crying, excessive sucking, muscle spasms, sneezing, trembling, irritability, diarrhoea, vomiting, and occasionally, seizures. Infants may be monitored for up to five days for symptoms. The sudden cessation of heroin use by pregnant women can also harm the baby and lead to poor growth, miscarriage, or premature labour. Babies born to mothers taking methadone, a common treatment for heroin addiction, may also experience withdrawal symptoms. Additionally, injecting heroin increases the risk of acquiring HIV infection, which can be transmitted to the baby. Overall, heroin use during pregnancy presents significant dangers to both maternal and foetal health, with potential long-term consequences for the child's well-being.

Limited studies exist regarding the risks of "club drugs" like PCP, ketamine, LSD, and ecstasy during pregnancy. However, available evidence suggests potential dangers. Babies born to mothers who used PCP during pregnancy may experience withdrawal symptoms, while exposure to PCP or ketamine before birth could increase the risk of learning and behavioural problems (AGOG, 2021). Ecstasy use during pregnancy may be linked to congenital deformities, similar to other amphetamines. Methamphetamine use during pregnancy is associated with poor foetal growth, premature delivery, placental problems, and potential birth defects (Smith et al., 2006). Babies exposed to methamphetamine may exhibit withdrawal-like symptoms. The long-term effects of ecstasy and methamphetamines on babies are still unknown. The use of volatile substances during pregnancy increases the risk of miscarriage, slow foetal growth, preterm birth, and birth defects (AGOG, 2021). GHB use during pregnancy poses risks similar to alcohol. Additionally, LSD and other hallucinogens may increase the risk of miscarriage, birth complications, and a higher incidence of birth defects. Continued hallucinogen use while breastfeeding may expose the baby to adverse effects through breast milk. Overall, further research is needed to fully understand the risks associated with club drugs during pregnancy. In the case of barbiturates, prolonged maternal abuse of barbiturates can lead to neonatal drug withdrawal, presenting with agitation, irritability, and fussiness typically appearing 7 to 10 days after birth. Maternal cannabis use does not consistently increase congenital malformations or neurobehavioural issues in infants. However, it often accompanies alcohol and cigarette use, which can pose foetal risks (Dysart, 2022).

FOETAL ALCOHOL SPECTRUM DISORDERS

Maternal alcohol use during pregnancy is associated with a range of negative outcomes for the offspring, including social, emotional, and cognitive development issues. These may manifest as learning deficits, hyperactivity, and attention problems. The most severe consequence is the development of foetal alcohol spectrum disorders (FASD). FASD encompasses a spectrum of mental and physical features observed in babies exposed to alcohol before birth. The characteristics of FASD include distinctive facial anomalies, growth retardation, and significant learning and behavioural problems. These signs, symptoms, and long-term effects of FASD can have profound impacts on the affected individuals' quality of life and functioning, requiring specialised support and intervention strategies. The signs, symptoms, and long-term features of FASD are presented in Table 15.1.

Foetal alcohol spectrum disorders are lifelong conditions and are not always diagnosed at birth. Diagnosis may be made later, when the conditions can significantly impact on the life of the individual with learning and behavioural problems. The American Academy of Pediatrics (AAP) (2023) emphasises the necessity of universal screening for pre-natal alcohol exposure in all children. A diagnosis of foetal alcohol spectrum disorders involves various criteria, including evidence of central nervous system (CNS) problems, physical abnormalities such as growth deficits and specific facial anomalies, health issues, and documented pre-natal

Table 15.1
Foetal alcohol spectrum disorders

Signs at birth	Long-term effects
• Small body size and weight	• Learning difficulties
• Facial abnormalities	• Delays in normal development
• Small eyes	• Behavioural problems
• Small head circumference	• Memory problems
• Flattened face	• Attention-deficit hyperactivity disorder
• Flattened bridge of the nose	• Depression
• Sunken nasal bridge	• Psychosis
• Small jaw	• Increased risk of alcohol and drug use
• Opening in roof of mouth	
• Organ deformities	
• Heart defects	
• Genital malformations	
• Kidney and urinary defects	
• Mental retardation	
• Learning disabilities	
• Short attention span	
• Irritability in infancy	
• Hyperactivity in childhood	

alcohol exposure. The AAP recommends that initial assessment and diagnosis be conducted by the child's paediatrician. Referrals for further evaluation and treatment may be made to other healthcare professionals or, if available, to a specialised multidisciplinary team for comprehensive evaluation and care. Studies have indicated elevated rates of stillbirth among individuals who consume alcohol during pregnancy. Alcohol consumption during pregnancy also heightens the risk of preterm delivery (birth before 37 weeks of pregnancy) and can result in the baby being smaller than anticipated (Brentwood (TN), 2023). Additionally, alcohol use during pregnancy may lead to temporary symptoms in newborns shortly after birth, similar to withdrawal. These symptoms, often termed *withdrawal*, are more likely to occur if the baby has been exposed to alcohol close to delivery. Withdrawal symptoms may encompass involuntary shaking movements (tremors), heightened muscle tone, restlessness, and excessive crying.

The prevention of FASD requires a coordinated and multifaceted approach that incorporates universal prevention strategies in targeting the general population through public awareness campaigns and educational initiatives to raise awareness about the risks of alcohol consumption during pregnancy. Selective prevention strategies are aimed at women of childbearing age, especially those contemplating pregnancy. These strategies involve screening for maternal alcohol consumption to identify at-risk individuals early on. Specific prevention strategies are tailored for women at high risk of alcohol-exposed pregnancies. This involves referring them to specialised alcohol services for comprehensive support and intervention. Various approaches have been implemented to prevent foetal alcohol spectrum disorders (FASD) (Bazzo et al., 2017; WHO, 2016).

These approaches target different groups:

- *General public*. Initiatives include labelling drink containers, distributing posters and flyers, and media campaigns, such as International FASDay on 9 September annually.
- *Professionals*. Training sessions are provided for physicians and midwives to increase awareness and knowledge about FASD.
- *Women at risk or pregnant women*. Programmes range from brief interventions to intensive support during pregnancy, aiming to reduce alcohol consumption and prevent alcohol-exposed pregnancies.

Developing effective interventions for preventing FASD is a complex process. To address this challenge, programme developers can utilise pre-existing protocols and evidence-based strategies. One such approach is intervention mapping, which provides a systematic framework for designing, implementing, and evaluating interventions aimed at preventing FASD (Roozen et al., 2016). Overall, prevention strategies encompass a combination of public education, professional training, and targeted interventions to address FASD and reduce the incidence of alcohol consumption during pregnancy. There is no cure for foetal alcohol spectrum disorders (FASD), requiring comprehensive, multimodal approaches tailored to individual patient needs for management. Various approaches can help alleviate the symptoms of FASD and mitigate its impact on affected individuals and their families (NIAAA, 2023):

- *Education and behavioural interventions*. Target individuals with FASD and their caregivers, aiming to improve understanding and coping strategies.
- *Medications*. Offered to manage specific symptoms and behaviours associated with FASD.
- *Social support and case management*. Provide essential assistance and guidance for children and adults affected by FASD and their families.
- New interventions under development and evaluation include:

  1. Pre-natal and post-natal nutritional supplements for pregnant women and their children.
  2. Learning and behavioural interventions focusing on enhancing cognition, daily life skills, and managing impulsive behaviour.
  3. School-based approaches utilising specialised teaching strategies and computer-based games.
  4. Mobile health apps and other interventions to support families and caregivers in caring for children with FASD.

These interventions aim to improve the quality of life for individuals with FASD and their families, highlighting the ongoing efforts to develop effective treatments and support services in this field. Due to uncertainty about foetal risk and lack of clear guidelines, the safest approach is abstaining from alcohol during pregnancy. The World Health Organization strongly advises pregnant women to avoid alcohol consumption altogether.

SMOKING DURING PREGNANCY

Smoking during pregnancy is associated with numerous adverse outcomes for both the mother and the baby. These include preterm birth, low birth weight, intrauterine growth restriction, neonatal respiratory and gastrointestinal issues, prolonged admissions, intrauterine death, and neonatal infection (Tarasi et al., 2022). Smoking has detrimental effects on reproductive health, hindering conception and increasing the risk of pregnancy complications. Although fertility can improve after quitting smoking, continued smoking during pregnancy poses serious risks to both maternal and foetal health. Chemicals like nicotine and carbon monoxide are believed to contribute to adverse pregnancy outcomes. Babies born to smoking mothers are at a higher risk of low birth weight and preterm delivery. These infants face a greater likelihood of health issues in the newborn period; long-term disabilities, such as cerebral palsy and mental retardation; and even mortality. Women who smoke face increased challenges in conceiving and have a higher likelihood of never achieving pregnancy. Studies also indicate a connection between tobacco use and miscarriage. Furthermore, babies exposed to maternal smoking during pregnancy or second-hand smoke after birth tend to have weaker lungs, elevating their risk for various health complications (Centers for Disease Control and Prevention, 2020).

Smoking during pregnancy exacerbates health inequalities, disproportionately affecting women of lower socio-economic status and cultural capital. The findings of a study (Penn & Owen, 2002) reveal that pregnant women are more likely to smoke if they have lower education levels, reside in rented accommodations, belong to unskilled manual labour or unemployed groups, are single, or have partners who smoke. This underlines the significance of implementing tobacco control strategies that target the socio-economic status of pregnant women and address individual smoking behaviours, aiming to mitigate the adverse effects of smoking on maternal and foetal health, particularly within marginalised communities.

Quitting smoking is crucial for safeguarding the health of both mothers and their babies during pregnancy. These findings emphasise the critical importance of smoking cessation during pregnancy to protect maternal and foetal health. Promoting smoking cessation among pregnant women is deemed cost-effective (NICE, 2010a, 2010b). Additionally,

Table 15.2
Maternal, pre-natal, and post-natal effects of psychoactive substances

Maternal	Pre-natal (baby)	Post-natal (mother and baby)
• Insomnia	• Low birth weight	• Withdrawal symptoms
• Poor appetite	• Early delivery	• Sudden infant death syndrome
• Premature labour	• Miscarriage	• Cognitive dysfunction
• Cognitive functioning	• Mental retardation	• Difficulty in bonding with newborn
• Risk of infections (transmitted through sex)	• Death	• Meeting needs of newborn
• Water breaks early		• Depression
• Sudden haemorrhage		• Psychosis
• Inability to cope with normal changes in pregnancy		

a randomised controlled trial by Tappin et al. (2015) suggests the effectiveness of financial incentives in aiding smoking cessation during pregnancy. The maternal, pre-natal, and post-natal effects of psychoactive substances are presented in Table 15.2.

BLOOD-BORNE INFECTIONS

Early detection of blood-borne viruses, such as HIV, hepatitis B, and hepatitis C, during pregnancy is crucial for preventing transmission from mother to baby. HIV can be transmitted during pregnancy, childbirth, or breastfeeding, while hepatitis B transmission can be significantly reduced through timely vaccination and immunoglobulin administration to newborns. The risk of hepatitis C transmission to the unborn child is low, but pregnant women with potential exposure to the virus should undergo blood testing. Breastfeeding carries minimal risk of transmitting hepatitis B or C as long as the nipples are intact. Testing and vaccination during pregnancy can help mitigate the risk of transmission and protect the health of both mother and baby. Blood-borne viruses such as HIV, hepatitis B, and hepatitis C are transmitted from mother to baby. There is a high risk that an infected mother will transmit HIV on to her baby either during pregnancy, at birth, or while breastfeeding. Pregnant women who have hepatitis B should have their babies vaccinated with the hepatitis B vaccine and immunoglobulin soon after delivery. This greatly reduces the chance of their babies becoming infected. The risk of a mother passing the hepatitis C virus onto her unborn child during pregnancy and birth is low. Pregnant women should have a blood test if there is any chance they have been exposed to this virus. The risks of passing on hepatitis B or C through breastfeeding are very low, as long as the nipples are not cracked or bleeding. Early detection of the blood-borne viruses through testing or vaccinations is recommended.

Universal screening for the three major blood-borne viruses, namely, hepatitis B, hepatitis C, and human immunodeficiency virus (HIV), along with screening for sexually transmitted infections (STIs), is recommended during antenatal testing. Additionally, all pregnant women should be offered screening for rubella antibody. For pregnant women with hepatitis B, administering hepatitis B immune globulin (HBIG) can help protect the baby against the virus. Antenatal administration of HBIG may have a beneficial effect in preventing mother-to-child transmission of HBV, as evidenced by a higher proportion of treated babies showing protection compared to non-treated babies (Eke et al., 2017). Newborns should receive the first shot of the hepatitis B vaccine before leaving the hospital, ideally within the first 12 hours of life, for optimal effectiveness. Completing the full course of hepatitis B vaccination provides the best protection for the baby. Guidelines on hepatitis B immune globulin (HBIG) (what parents need to know) are provided by the Centers for Disease Control and Prevention (2018).

PARENTAL SUBSTANCE USE AND CHILDCARE ISSUES

Parental substance use disorders can significantly influence children's lives, impacting various aspects of their development. However, it is important to note that alcohol or substance use disorder does not automatically translate to poor parenting. There are instances where non-using parents may also exhibit inadequate parenting styles due to personal or relationship challenges. The impact of alcohol and drug use on parenting styles and responsibilities can lead to ineffective or inconsistent parenting. These may manifest in the following ways (Child Welfare Information Gateway, 2014):

- Physical or mental impairments resulting from alcohol or drug use
- Reduced ability to recognise and respond to a child's cues and needs
- Challenges in regulating emotions and managing anger and impulsivity
- Disruptions in forming healthy parent–child attachments
- Prioritising spending on alcohol or drugs over essential household needs like food
- Devoting time to seeking, using, or manufacturing alcohol or drugs
- Incarceration, leading to inadequate supervision of children
- Estrangement from family and other support networks

Parental substance use detrimentally impacts parenting by impairing judgement and decision-making, leading to inconsistent discipline practices, emotional instability, and an inability to provide a safe environment for children. Substance use compromises the ability of parents to make sound decisions, enforce rules consistently, regulate emotions, and create a secure environment, increasing the risk of accidents, exposure to danger, and neglect, ultimately impacting the well-being and development of children. Overall, parental substance use can impact parenting styles and responsibilities, potentially leading to ineffective or inconsistent caregiving, which can have adverse effects on children's well-being and development. Studies indicate that compared to non-drug-using parents, drug-dependent parents are more likely to neglect their children. Consequently, children in families grappling with addiction often find themselves compelled to take on parental duties and responsibilities, such as managing household affairs and caring for younger siblings (EMCDDA, 2012; Tedgård et al., 2019). However, these children are at risk of experiencing significant psychological and emotional challenges that can persist into adulthood (Tedgård et al., 2019).

Research has explored the relationship between alcohol use and child abuse, although definitive conclusions regarding parental alcohol abuse as a cause or consequence of child abuse remain elusive (Widom & Hiller-Sturmhöfel, 2001). The authors pointed out that multiple studies suggest that parental alcohol abuse may heighten a child's vulnerability to physical or sexual abuse, whether perpetrated by a family member or an external individual

Research studies also indicate that parental drug or alcohol abuse has been identified as a risk factor for child maltreatment, abuse, and neglect, and these children have limited engagement with their parents (EMCDDA, 2012; Committee on Child Maltreatment Research, Policy, and Practice for the Next Decade, 2014).

Pregnant women with alcohol or substance use disorder often hesitate to seek assistance from health and social care agencies due to concerns about potential child removal. However, there is a prevailing sentiment among these agencies emphasising the importance of preserving the family whenever feasible, as substance use disorder does not necessarily indicate a lack of parental commitment. In some nations, support services are available to help drug-dependent mothers stay with their children, while in others, extended family structures are utilised to provide appropriate childcare. Legislation regarding pregnant women with substance use disorder and children before birth varies globally. Some countries uphold the mother's right to self-determination, allowing voluntary treatment-seeking, while others employ coercive measures, such as mandatory referral to specialist services or pre-natal supervision orders after 24 weeks of pregnancy. This diversity reflects inherent conflicts between parental human rights and ensuring child safety and welfare. In certain nations, health and social care personnel are mandated by law to report concerns about child safety and welfare to specialised authorities when children are at risk of significant harm.

Risk assessment in families of drug users is complex but should be a routine part of child health and safety investigation and monitoring. A number of practical guidelines or checklists have been produced for health and care professionals working with drug-using parents for assessing risk to children. One of the checklists (Local Government Drug Forum and Standing Conference on Drug Abuse, 1997) focuses on seven key domains that can be used as part of risk assessment with parental drug use:

- The pattern of parental drug use
- Accommodation and home environment

- Provision of basic necessities
- Procurement of drugs
- Health risks
- Family's social network and support systems
- The parents' perception of the situation

When assessing families with parental alcohol and drug use, it is essential to consider specific domains outlined in checklists, but drug use alone does not always indicate child neglect or abuse. Automatic reporting to child protection agencies may discourage parents from seeking support, so professionals should only take action if there is genuine concern for child safety. Comprehensive assessments should evaluate the relationship between parental drug use and childcare on an individual basis, with interagency collaboration ensuring proper procedures and services are in place to address parental substance use and safeguard children's well-being.

BARRIERS TO TREATMENT AND TREATMENT SERVICES

Women with substance use disorder face tremendous barriers that impede them from accessing addiction service provision and delivery. Alcohol and drug treatment have been available to women, but the provision of services is seldom based on the special physical, psychological, and social needs of women. Most of the alcohol and drug treatment services are male-orientated. Despite the recognition of the need for women-sensitive services for alcohol and drug misusers, the provision of services is still scant.

In a review of the needs, barriers, and challenges of women suffering from drug addiction (Motyka et al., 2022), the findings indicate that women struggling with drug use disorder encounter a multitude of barriers when seeking help or treatment. These barriers include societal stigma and hostility towards women with drug use issues, lack of familial support, inadequate therapeutic programmes tailored to women's needs, low effectiveness of interventions, and limited understanding of women's needs by healthcare providers. Additionally, there is a lack of specialised rehabilitation centres for women, especially those serving prison sentences, and difficulties accessing comprehensive healthcare services. Practical obstacles such as transportation difficulties and lack of awareness of available support services further hinder women's ability to seek help. Emotional challenges, such as shame, guilt, loneliness, anxiety, and depression, also act as significant barriers to seeking treatment. The reluctance for women alcohol and drug misusers to seek treatment includes low self-esteem and guilt, social withdrawal, and fear of sexual harassment. Additional barriers include the lack of childcare, fear of stigma, lack of family or financial support, denial, and co-occurring disorders (Taylor, 2010).

In another review that explores the barriers and facilitators to substance use disorder treatment (Farhoudian et al., 2022), the findings reveal how individuals with substance use disorders face various obstacles to seeking treatment, including false beliefs about their ability to manage their addiction independently, denial of the severity of their problem, and reluctance to seek help. For example, many believe they can withdraw from substances on their own or view replacement medications like methadone as just another addictive substance. Loneliness often intensifies these issues, with a significant portion of individuals with alcohol problems underestimating the severity of their difficulties and feeling they can handle it alone. Moreover, motivations for seeking treatment may be driven by factors such as family disputes, mood disorders, or other mental health issues. Supportive connections with family, friends, and healthcare providers can significantly influence treatment-seeking behaviour, while unsupportive relationships can act as barriers. Motivation to seek treatment is influenced by both individual and social factors, with low motivation, denial, and resistance commonly observed in individuals with SUD.

At the service provider and policy level, barriers include financial concerns, inadequate treatment structures, legal constraints, and policy limitations, which can hinder access to and effectiveness of treatment services (Farhoudian et al., 2022). Research suggests that women with substance use problems face unique challenges compared to men. They are more likely to have partners with substance use issues, experience more severe problems at the start of treatment, and have a higher prevalence of trauma related to physical and sexual abuse, as well as concurrent psychiatric disorders (UNDOC, 2004). Additionally, women from large ethnic or culturally diverse communities, as well as Indigenous populations, may face barriers to engaging in treatment due to cultural and religious factors, as well as issues related to service availability, accessibility, and acceptability. These complex factors contribute to women's reluctance to access treatment programmes for substance use disorders.

In terms of provision of services to women, men and women are generally presented to services with different problems and characteristics. Research consistently shows that women suffer greater physical, psychological, and social consequences from drug and alcohol use Park et al., 2019). For instance, women who inject drugs have higher rates of associated infections, such as HIV and hepatitis C, compared to men (Degenhardt et al., 2017; El-Bassel & Strathdee, 2015). The severity of substance use disorder is more severe: they have more physical and mental health problems; have experienced emotional, physical, and sexual abuse; have depressive episodes, anxiety disorders, post-traumatic stress disorders (PTSD), and eating disorders and concerns about child-related issues (Ravndal, 2011).

Alcohol and drug treatment services often overlook the unique needs of women, failing to address issues like violence, sexual exploitation, and lack of childcare and pre-natal services. Implementing policy recommendations, such as providing day care and treatment services for women, could reduce barriers to seeking help. Key components for attracting and retaining women in treatment include female-oriented services, supportive environments, and non-coercive approaches. Health and social care professionals should enhance their understanding of gender issues related to substance use, and service provision should be more sensitive to women's needs. Overall, addressing these barriers is crucial to ensuring that women with drug abuse problems can access the support and treatment necessary for recovery.

KEY POINTS

- Gender-related and religio-social rules have defined what is considered appropriate behaviours for women, including the use of alcohol and drugs.
- Women's alcohol and drug misuse is considered to be deviant behaviour, and women are more stigmatised, marginalised, and labelled.
- Women's alcohol consumption, particularly in the younger and older women, has been increasing over the last few decades.
- The physical, psychological, and social effects of alcohol are more severe for women than for men.
- Women develop alcohol-related problems and alcohol dependence faster than men, and many die younger than men with similar drinking problems.
- The most serious outcome of maternal drinking during pregnancy is foetal alcohol spectrum disorders (FASD).
- Smoking during pregnancy not only harms a woman's health but can also lead to pregnancy complications and serious health problems in newborns.
- Premature and low-birth-weight babies face an increased risk of serious health problems during the newborn period, chronic lifelong disabilities, and even death.
- All drugs taken during pregnancy will reach the baby through the placenta.
- Tobacco smoking can cause reproductive problems before a woman even becomes pregnant, and women who smoke may have more trouble conceiving than nonsmokers.
- Alcohol and drug treatments have been available to women, but the provision of services is seldom based on the special physical, psychological, and social needs of women.
- Blood-borne viruses such as HIV and hepatitis B and C are transmitted from mother to baby.
- Pregnant women who have hepatitis B should have their babies vaccinated with the hepatitis B vaccine and immunoglobulin soon after delivery.
- All pregnant women should be offered antenatal screening for blood-borne viruses.
- The behaviours and lifestyles of parents with substance use disorders have a significant impact on the children.
- Drug use by parents does not automatically indicate child neglect or abuse.
- Risk assessment in families of drug users is complex but should be a routine part of child health and safety investigation and monitoring.
- Women who misuse alcohol or drugs face a variety of barriers, including barriers to treatment entry, to engagement in treatment, and to long-term rehabilitation.
- In terms of provision of services to women, men and women are generally presented to services with different problems and characteristics.
- The complex needs of women include the provision of comprehensive services, such as housing, transportation, education, and income support.
- Health and social care professionals need to increase their understanding of gender issues in relation to alcohol and drug use, and service provision should be more sensitive to women's needs.

Activity 15.2

Questions

- Describe the prevalence of alcohol and drug misuse with women.
- Discuss the psychosocial and environmental issues related to alcohol and drug misuse.
- List the features of foetal alcohol spectrum disorders.
- List the problems associated with the following drugs during pregnancy:
  a. Alcohol
  b. Heroin
  c. Cocaine
  d. Methamphetamine
  e. LSD
- Discuss the issues of blood-borne viruses in pregnancy.
- List the barriers in preventing women from accessing treatment services.
- Discuss the special treatment needs of women with alcohol and drug problems.

References

American Academy of Pediatrics. (2023). *Screening for Prenatal Alcohol Exposure*. https://www.aap.org/en/patient-care/fetal-alcohol-spectrum-disorders/screening-assessment/screening-for-prenatal-alcohol-exposure/ (accessed 13 March 2024).

American College of Obstetricians and Gynecologists (ACOG). (2021). *Your Pregnancy and Childbirth, Month to Month* (7th rev. ed.). Washington, DC: ACOG.

Anderson, G. D. (2008). Gender differences in pharmacological response. *International Review of Neurobiology*, 83, 1–10. https://doi.org/10.1016/S0074-7742(08)00001-9.

Bazzo, S., Black, D., Mitchell, K., Marini, F., Moino, G., Riscica, P., & Fattori, G. (2017). "Too young to drink": An international communication campaign to raise public awareness of fetal alcohol spectrum disorders. *Public Health*, 142, 111–115. https://doi.org/10.1016/j.puhe.2016.08.001.

Beierle, I., Meibohm, B., & Derendorf, H. (1999). Gender differences in pharmacokinetics and pharmacodynamics. *International Journal of Clinical Pharmacology and Therapeutics*, 37(11), 529–547.

Brentwood (TN): Organization of Teratology Information Specialists (OTIS). (2023). *Mother to Baby | Fact Sheets Alcohol*. https://www.ncbi.nlm.nih.gov/books/NBK582563/ (accessed 13 March 2024).

Buckingham-Howes, S., Berger, S. S., Scaletti, L. A., & Black, M. M. (2013). Systematic review of prenatal cocaine exposure and adolescent development. *Pediatrics*, 131, e1917–e1936.

Centers for Disease Control and Prevention. (2018). *Hepatitis B Immune Globulin (HBIG): What Parents Need to Know*. https://www.cdc.gov/vaccines/programs/perinatal-hepb/downloads/HBIGinfosheet-508.pdf (accessed 13 March 2024).

Centers for Disease Control and Prevention. (2020). *Smoking During Pregnancy*. https://www.cdc.gov/tobacco/basic_information/health_effects/pregnancy/index.htm (accessed 13 March 2024).

Child Welfare Information Gateway. (2014). *Parental Substance Use and the Child Welfare System*. Washington, DC: U.S. Department of Health and Human Services, Children's Bureau. www.childwelfare.gov/pubPDFs/parentalsubabuse.pdf (accessed 24 June 2024).

Committee on Child Maltreatment Research, Policy, and Practice for the Next Decade. (2014). Phase II; board on children, youth, and families. In Committee on Law and Justice, Institute of Medicine, National Research Council, A. C. Petersen, J. Joseph, & M. Feit (Eds.), *New Directions in Child Abuse and Neglect Research*. Washington, DC: National Academies Press.

Degenhardt, L., Peacock, A., Colledge, S., Leung, J., Grebely, J., Vickerman, P., Stone, J., Cunningham, E. B., Trickey, A., Dumchev, K., Lynskey, M., Griffiths, P., Mattick, R. P., Hickman, M., & Larney, S. (2017). Global prevalence of injecting drug use and sociodemographic characteristics and prevalence of HIV, HBV, and HCV in people who inject drugs: A multistage systematic review. *The Lancet: Global Health*, 5(12), e1192–e1207. https://doi.org/10.1016/S2214-109X(17)30375-3.

Dysart, K. C. (2022). *Prenatal Drug Exposure*. https://www.merckmanuals.com/en-pr/professional/pediatrics/metabolic-electrolyte-and-toxic-disorders-in-neonates/prenatal-drug-exposure (accessed 24 June 2024).

El-Bassel, N., & Strathdee, S. A. (2015). Women who use or inject drugs: An action agenda for women-specific, multilevel, and combination HIV prevention and research. *Journal of Acquired Immune Deficiency Syndromes (1999)*, 69(Suppl 2), S182–S190. https://doi.org/10.1097/QAI.0000000000000628.

Eke, A. C., Eleje, G. U., Eke, U. A., Xia, Y., & Liu, J. (2017). Hepatitis B immunoglobulin during pregnancy for prevention of mother-to-child transmission of hepatitis B virus. *Cochrane Database of Systematic Reviews*, 2017(2), Article ID CD008545. https://doi.org/10.1002/14651858.CD008545.pub2.

EMCDD. (2012). *Pregnancy, Childcare and the Family: Key Issues foe Europe's Response to Drugs*. European Monitoring Centre for Drugs and Drug Addiction. Luxembourg: Publications Office of the European Union. www.emcdda.europa.eu/attachements.cfm/att_190454_EN_TDSI12001ENC.PDF (accessed 13 March 2024).

Farhoudian, A., Razaghi, E., Hooshyari, Z., Noroozi, A., Pilevari, A., Mokri, A., Mohammadi, M. R., & Malekinejad, M. (2022). Barriers and facilitators to substance use disorder treatment: An overview of systematic reviews. *Substance Abuse: Research and Treatment*, 16. https://doi.org/10.1177/11782218221118462.

Fergusson, D. M., Horwood, L. J., Northstone, K., & ALSPAC Study Team. Avon Longitudinal Study of Pregnancy and Childhood. (2002). Maternal use of cannabis and pregnancy outcome. *BJOG: An International Journal of Obstetrics and Gynaecology*, 109(1), 21–27. https://doi.org/10.1111/j.1471-0528.2002.01020.x.

Fried, P. A., Watkinson, B., & Gray, R. (2003). Differential effects on cognitive functioning in 13- to 16-year-olds prenatally exposed to cigarettes and marihuana. *Neurotoxicology and Teratology*, 25(4), 427–436. https://doi.org/10.1016/s0892-0362(03)00029-1.

Greaves, L., Poole, N., & Brabete, A. C. (2022). Sex, gender, and alcohol use: Implications for women and low-risk drinking guidelines. *International Journal of Environmental Research and Public Health*, 19(8), 4523. https://doi.org/10.3390/ijerph19084523.

Greenblatt, D. J., & von Moltke, L. L. (2008). Gender has a small but statistically significant effect on clearance of CYP3A substrate drugs. *Journal of Clinical Pharmacology*, 48(11), 1350–1355. https://doi.org/10.1177/0091270008323754.

Lambert, B. L., & Bauer, C. R. (2012). Developmental and behavioral consequences of prenatal cocaine exposure: A review. *Journal of Perinatology: Official Journal of the California Perinatal Association*, 32(11), 819–828. https://doi.org/10.1038/jp.2012.90.

Lester, B. M., & Lagasse, L. L. (2010). Children of addicted women. *Journal of Addictive Diseases*, 29(2), 259–276. https://doi.org/10.1080/10550881003684921.

Local Government Drug Forum and Standing Conference on Drug Abuse. (1997). *Drug Using Parents: Policy Guidelines for Inter-agency Working*. London: London Government Association.

Motyka, M. A., Al-Imam, A., Haligowska, A., & Michalak, M. (2022). Helping women suffering from drug addiction: Needs, barriers, and challenges. *International Journal of Environmental Research and Public Health*, 19(21), 14039. https://doi.org/10.3390/ijerph192114039.

National Institute on Alcohol Abuse and Alcoholism (NIAAA). (2023). *Alcohol's Effects on Health: Research-Based Information on Drinking and Its Impact*. https://www.niaaa.nih.gov/publications/brochures-and-fact-sheets/understanding-fetal-alcohol-spectrum-disorders (accessed 13 March 2024).

NICE. (2010a). *Smoking: Stopping in Pregnancy and After Childbirth* (Public Health Guideline PH26). National Institute for Health and Care Excellence. www.nice.org.uk/guidance/ph26/chapter/appendix-c-the-evidence (accessed 13 March 2024).

NICE. (2010b). *Pregnancy and Complex Social Factors: A Model for Service Provision for Pregnant Women with Complex Social Factors* (Clinical Guideline CG110). www.nice.org.uk/guidance/cg110 (accessed 13 March 2024).

NICE. (2021). *Antenatal Care* (NICE Guideline (NG201)). https://www.nice.org.uk/guidance/ng201 (accessed 13 March 2024).

NIDA. (2022). *Sex and Gender Differences in Substance Use*. https://nida.nih.gov/publications/research-reports/substance-use-in-women/sex-gender-differences-in-substance-use (accessed 12 March 2024).

Park, J. N., Footer, K. H. A., Decker, M. R., Tomko, C., Allen, S. T., Galai, N., & Sherman, S. G. (2019). Interpersonal and structural factors associated with receptive syringe-sharing among a prospective cohort of female sex workers who inject drugs. *Addiction*, 114(7), 1204–1213. https://doi.org/10.1111/add.14567.

Penn, G., & Owen, L. (2002). Factors associated with continued smoking during pregnancy: Analysis of socio-demographic, pregnancy and smoking-related factors. *Drug Alcohol Review*, 2(1), 17–25.

Phillips, D. P., Brewer, K. M., & Wadensweiler, P. (2011). Alcohol as a risk factor for sudden infant death syndrome (SIDS). *Addiction*, 106(3), 516–525. https://doi.org/10.1111/j.1360-0443.2010.03199.x.

Ravndal, E. (2011). *Female Polydrug Abuse and Psychopathology: Gender Differences: An Overview* (SERAF Rapport nr 3/2011). https://www.med.uio.no/klinmed/forskning/sentre/seraf/publikasjoner/rapporter/2011/nedlastinger/seraf-rapport-3-2011-female-poly-drug-abuse-and-psychopathology-gender-differences.pdf (accessed 14 March 2024).

Reddy, U. M. (2013). *Tobacco, Drug Use in Pregnancy Can Double Risk of Stillbirth*. Eunice Kennedy Shriver National Institute of Child Health and Human Development. https://www.nichd.nih.gov/news/releases/Pages/121113-stillbirth-drug-use.aspx (accessed 12 March 2024).

Reece, A. S., & Hulse, G. K. (2021). Epidemiological overview of multidimensional chromosomal and genome toxicity of cannabis exposure in congenital anomalies and cancer development. *Scientific Reports*, 11(1), 13892. https://doi.org/10.1038/s41598-021-93411-5.

Robbins, C. A., & Martin, S. S. Cited in Thom, B. (1997). *Women and Alcohol. Issues for Prevention: A Literature Review*. London: Health Education Authority.

Roozen, S., Black, D., Peters, G. Y., Kok, G., Townend, D., Nijhuis, J. G., Koek, G. H., & Curfs, L. M. (2016). Fetal alcohol spectrum disorders (FASD): An approach to effective prevention. *Current Developmental Disorders Reports*, 3(4), 229–234. https://doi.org/10.1007/s40474-016-0101-y.

Smith, L. M., LaGasee, L. L., Derauf, C., Grant, P., Shah, R., Arria, A., Huestis, M., Haning, W., Strauss, A., Grotta, S. D., Liu, J., & Lester, B. M. (2006). The infant development, environment, and lifestyle study: Effects of prenatal methamphetamine exposure, polydrug exposure, and poverty on intrauterine growth. *Pediatrics*, 118(3),1149–1156.

Tappin, D., Bauld, L., Purves, D., Boyd, K., Sinclair, L., MacAskill, S., McKell, J., Friel, B., McConnachie, A., de Caestecker, L., Tannahill, C., Radley, A., & Coleman, T. (2015). Financial incentives for smoking cessation in pregnancy: Randomised controlled trial. *BMJ*, 350, h134.

Tarasi, B., Cornuz, J., Clair, C., & Baud, D. (2022). Cigarette smoking during pregnancy and adverse perinatal outcomes: A cross-sectional study over 10 years. *BMC Public Health*, 22, 2403. https://doi.org/10.1186/s12889-022-14881-4.

Taylor, O. D. (2010). Barriers to treatment for women with substance use disorders. *Journal of Human Behavior in the Social Environment*, 20(3), 393–409. https://doi.org/10.1080/10911351003673310.

Tedgård, E., Råstam, M., & Wirtberg, I. (2019). An upbringing with substance-abusing parents: Experiences of parentification and dysfunctional communication. *Nordisk Alkohol- & Narkotikatidskrift: NAT*, 36(3), 223–247. https://doi.org/10.1177/1455072518814308.

UNDOC. (2004). *Substance Abuse Treatment and Care for Women*. Vienna: United Nations Office on Drugs and Crime. www.UNDOC.org.

Wang, H., Guo, Y., Wang, D., Kingsley, P. J., Marnett, L. J., Das, S. K., DuBois, R. N., & Dey, S. K. (2004). Aberrant cannabinoid signaling impairs oviductal transport of embryos. *Nature Medicine*, 10, 1074–1080.

Wendell, A. D. (2013). Overview and epidemiology of substance abuse in pregnancy. *Clinical Obstetrics and Gynecology*, 56(1), 91–96. https://doi.org/10.1097/GRF.0b013e31827feeb9.

WHO. (1997). *Cannabis: A Health Perspective and Research Agenda*. Geneva: World Health Organization, Division of Mental Health and Prevention of Substance Abuse. https://iris.who.int/bitstream/handle/10665/63691/WHO_MSA_PSA_97.4.pdf?sequence=1http://apps.who.int/iris/bitstream/10665/63691/1/WHO_MSA_PSA_97.4.pdf (accessed 12 March 2024).

WHO. (2005). *Gender, Health and Alcohol Use*. World Health Organization, Pan American Health Organization. https://www.who.int/publications/m/item/gender-health-and-alcohol-use (accessed 12 March 2024).

WHO. (2016). *Prevention of Harm Caused by Alcohol Exposure in Pregnancy*. Copenhagen: World Health Organization.

Widom, C. S., & Hiller-Sturmhöfel, S. (2001). Alcohol abuse as a risk factor for and consequence of child abuse. *Alcohol Research & Health: The Journal of The National Institute on Alcohol Abuse and Alcoholism*, 25(1), 52–57.

Chapter 16

Mental health problems and substance use disorder

Co-occurring disorders

Learning outcomes

- Explain the meaning of the term *dual diagnosis* and *comorbidity*.
- Have an awareness of the prevalence rates nationally and internationally.
- List the associated consequences of having combined mental health and substance use problems.
- Examine the relationship of substance use disorder and mental health problems.
- Discuss some of the models of service delivery and treatment.
- Discuss some of the issues and problems relating to the management of patients with mental health problems and substance use disorder.

Activity 16.1

Before reading this chapter, reflect on the following statements.

Statements	**Agree**	**Disagree**
Substance use disorder (SUD) often co-occurs with mental health disorders.		
Substance use disorder can exacerbate existing mental health problems.		
Substance use disorder always leads to mental health problems.		
Ceasing drug use could lead to the alleviation of all symptoms associated with the mental disorder.		
Acknowledging one's addiction is essential for individuals with co-occurring disorder to derive benefits from treatment.		
Mental health problems can contribute to substance use disorder.		
Co-occurring disorder refers to the presence of both substance use disorder and a mental health disorder.		
Integrated treatment approaches are typically recommended for individuals with co-occurring disorders.		
Substance use disorder and mental health problems are completely independent of each other.		

DOI: 10.4324/9781003456674-19

Consuming a small quantity of cannabis is unlikely to have a significant impact on individuals with schizophrenia.		
Seeking help from a mental health professional is not necessary for treating substance use disorder.		
Alcohol consumption can exacerbate mental health problems.		
Alcohol use disorder can lead to an increased risk of developing depression and anxiety disorders.		
Alcohol consumption can worsen the symptoms of pre-existing mental health conditions, such as bipolar disorder or schizophrenia.		
Individuals with alcohol use disorder may experience mood swings, irritability, and difficulty concentrating as a result of their drinking.		
Chronic alcohol abuse can lead to cognitive impairment and memory problems, which may mimic symptoms of certain mental health disorders.		
Dual diagnosis involving alcohol use disorder and mental health issues requires specialised treatment that addresses both conditions simultaneously.		
Moderate alcohol consumption is safe for individuals with mental health disorders and does not exacerbate their symptoms.		
Seeking treatment for alcohol use disorder can improve overall mental health and functioning, even if no co-occurring mental health disorders are present.		
Alcohol use disorder is more prevalent among individuals with certain mental health disorders compared to the general population.		

Do you agree or disagree with the preceding statements? State the reasons that you either agree or disagree.

Activity 16.2

There is only one correct answer to the following multiple-choice questions.

1. What is meant by the term *co-occurring disorder*?
   a. Diagnosis of two unrelated medical conditions simultaneously
   b. Diagnosis of a mental health disorder and a substance use disorder simultaneously
   c. Diagnosis of a mental health disorder and a physical health disorder simultaneously
   d. Diagnosis of two mental health disorders simultaneously
   e. None of the above
2. Which of the following statements about the relationship between substance use disorder and mental health problems is true?
   a. Substance use disorder always precedes the onset of mental health problems.
   b. Mental health problems always precede the onset of substance use disorder.
   c. There is no relationship between substance use disorder and mental health problems.
   d. Substance use disorder and mental health problems often co-occur and influence each other.
   e. The Presence Of A Mental Health Disorder Eliminates The Risk Of Developing A Substance Use Disorder.

3. Which of the following is a consequence of co-occurring disorder?
   a. Improved social relationships
   b. Reduced risk of suicide
   c. Increased risk of homelessness
   d. Enhanced cognitive function
   e. None of the above
4. Which treatment model emphasises treating mental health and substance use disorders simultaneously and in the same setting?
   a. Sequential treatment model
   b. Parallel treatment model
   c. Integrated treatment model
   d. Dual-focused treatment model
   e. None of the above
5. What is a potential consequence of inadequate coordination between mental health and substance use disorder treatment providers?
   a. Improved treatment outcomes
   b. Enhanced patient satisfaction
   c. Suboptimal care and treatment efficacy
   d. Decreased risk of relapse
   e. None of the above
6. Which of the following is a consequence of co-occurring disorders?
   a. Improved social relationships
   b. Reduced risk of suicide
   c. Increased risk of homelessness
   d. Enhanced cognitive function
   e. None of the above
7. Which term describes the phenomenon where individuals with dual diagnosis often cycle between mental health services and substance use disorder treatment without achieving sustained improvement?
   a. Treatment success
   b. Relapse prevention
   c. Revolving door phenomenon
   d. Treatment adherence
   e. None of the above
8. Which model of service delivery involves treating mental health and substance use disorders separately, often in different settings?
   a. Sequential treatment model
   b. Parallel treatment model
   c. Integrated treatment model
   d. Stepped care model
   e. None of the above
9. What is one of the challenges associated with providing effective treatment for individuals with co-occurring disorders?
   a. Limited availability of specialised treatment programmes
   b. High success rates of treatment interventions
   c. Low prevalence of comorbid mental health and substance use disorders
   d. Minimal need for integrated care
   e. None of the above

10. What is the term used to describe the simultaneous presence of a mental health disorder and a substance use disorder?
    a. Co-occurrence
    b. Dual diagnosis
    c. Parallel disorder
    d. Concomitant disorder
    e. None of the above
11. What is a common challenge in the management of patients with co-occurring disorders?
    a. High success rates of treatment
    b. Low risk of relapse
    c. Limited availability of integrated treatment programmes
    d. Minimal need for specialised care
    e. None of the above
12. What is one of the consequences of untreated mental health problems in individuals with substance use disorder?
    a. Decreased risk of addiction
    b. Improved physical health outcomes
    c. Increased risk of substance abuse relapse
    d. Enhanced social functioning
    e. None of the above
13. What is a common challenge in the management of patients with co-occurring disorder?
    a. High success rates of treatment
    b. Low risk of relapse
    c. Limited availability of integrated treatment programmes
    d. Minimal need for specialised care
    e. None of the above
14. Which term describes the phenomenon where individuals with co-occurring disorder often cycle between mental health services and substance use disorder treatment without achieving sustained improvement?
    a. Treatment success
    b. Relapse prevention
    c. Revolving door phenomenon
    d. Treatment adherence
    e. None of the above

INTRODUCTION

Globally, there is broad recognition of the increase in the number of mentally ill patients who misuse psychoactive substances. Research provides strong evidence indicating a significantly higher prevalence of substance use disorder among individuals with mental illness compared to the general population. Within the severely mentally ill population, alcohol use and cannabis use are particularly common. Approximately 30–50% of individuals with substance use disorder also have a co-occurring mental health disorder, and vice versa. Among children and adolescents, the prevalence of dual diagnoses ranges from 18.3% to 54%, with boys being more likely to experience dual diagnoses and affective disorders being the most common psychiatric diagnoses (Tomáš & Lenka, 2023). However, prevalence rates can vary depending on factors such as the specific disorders studied and the population assessed.

The comorbidity of mental health problems and substance use disorder (SUD) represents a complex and multifaceted challenge within the realm of mental healthcare. Often occurring concurrently, these conditions significantly impact individuals' lives, presenting unique hurdles for treatment and recovery. *Co-occurring disorders* (COD) refer to the co-existence of two or more disorders or illnesses within the same individual, and the interaction between mental health problems and SUD typifies this phenomenon. The concepts of comorbidity, co-occurring disorders, and dual diagnosis will be used interchangeably. The combination of SUD and mental health problems is associated with a host of serious social, behavioural, psychological, and physical problems, resulting in increased demands on mainstream services. Dual diagnosis has gained prominence partly due to the closures of long-stay psychiatric institutions, which led to a greater focus on community-based mental health care and the identification of individuals with co-occurring substance use and mental health disorders in community settings (Rassool, 2002, 2006).

The comorbidity of mental health problems and SUD is not coincidental; instead, it often reflects a complex interplay of biological, psychological, and social factors. The easy availability of psychoactive substances has led individuals with mental health issues to become involved in the drug subculture. Some of these individuals resort to self-medication to manage their psychiatric symptoms, counteract the side effects of prescribed medications, or alleviate distress caused by chronic illnesses. Dual-diagnosis patients, according to Carey (1989), have separate and chronic psychiatric disorders as well as substance use issues. Despite being distinct, these conditions can influence each other, affecting their respective courses and characteristics. On the contrary, substance use can exacerbate existing mental health problems, leading to a vicious cycle of dependence and psychological distress. Patients with comorbid psychiatric disorders and substance misuse face significant challenges, including exclusion from mental health or addiction services, stigmatisation, and being labelled as "difficult patients." Health and social care professionals may hesitate to intervene due to a lack of expertise in substance use disorder or having negative attitudes towards individuals with SUD. Additionally, existing service provisions often fail to adequately address the complex needs of individuals with dual diagnosis or addiction problems. Addressing the comorbidity of mental health problems and SUD requires a comprehensive and integrated approach that acknowledges the interconnected nature of these disorders. Effective treatment strategies should involve collaboration between mental health professionals, addiction specialists, and other healthcare providers to provide holistic care tailored to individuals' unique needs.

CONCEPT AND CLASSIFICATION

The term "dual diagnosis" lacks a consensus or common understanding in the field, leading to confusion regarding its definition. It has been used to describe individuals with two co-existing disorders, such as physical illness and mental health problems, schizophrenia and SUD, or learning disability and mental health problems. Additionally, terms like *comorbidity, co-occurring illnesses, concurrent disorders,* and *comorbid disorders* are often used interchangeably with "dual diagnosis," further complicating the issue. The absence of a standardised definition hampers research comparisons and communication among practitioners, making it challenging to agree on appropriate treatment approaches for individuals with these complex needs (ECCAS, 2006; Hryb et al., 2007).

The term "dual diagnosis" encompasses the co-occurrence of a psychoactive substance use disorder and another psychiatric disorder within the same individual, according to the world health organization (WHO, 1994). Alternatively, it can refer to the co-occurrence of two psychiatric disorders not involving substance use, or even the co-occurrence of two diagnosable substance use disorders. This definition does not imply any specific association or etiological relationship between the conditions. Similarly, the european monitoring centre for drugs and drug addiction (Emcdda, 2004) defines *comorbidity* as the temporal co-existence of psychiatric or personality disorders, one of which involves problematic substance use. In the UK, co-occurring conditions include co-occurring mental health and alcohol and/or drug use conditions, including smoking (Public Health England, 2017). Another term commonly used in this context is "co-occurring disorders," which refers to the condition of having at least one mental disorder and at least one substance use disorder (Samhsa, 2021). Additionally, "comorbidity" describes two or more disorders or illnesses occurring in the same person. They can occur at the same time or one after the other. *Comorbidity* also implies interactions between the illnesses that can worsen the course of both (Nida, 2021a). All the terms describing the relationship between substance misuse and mental health problems cover a varied and complex range of issues. While all these terms denote a diagnostic entity, it is essential to recognise that "dual diagnosis" is not a diagnosis itself but rather describes the co-existence of mental health and substance misuse disorders (Banerjee et al., 2002). However, these terms serve as a generic index of complexity in understanding individuals' conditions (Rassool, 2002). Diagnosing and treating comorbid substance use disorders and mental illness present a complex challenge due to overlapping symptoms (Nida, 2024). This complexity highlights the need for comprehensive assessment and tailored treatment approaches to address the diverse needs of individuals experiencing both substance misuse and mental health issues.

The relationships between substance misuse and mental health problems can manifest themselves in the following ways, as shown in Table 16.1. There is no single type of co-occurring disorders, as there are many patterns of alcohol or drug misuse and different types of psychiatric disorders. In the "Dual Diagnosis Good Practice Guide" (Department of Health, 2002), a more manageable and clinically relevant interrelationship between psychiatric disorder and substance misuse has been described. The four possible relationships are:

- A primary psychiatric illness precipitating or leading to substance misuse
- Substance misuse worsening or altering the course of a psychiatric illness
- Intoxication and/or substance dependence leading to psychological symptoms
- Substance misuse and/or withdrawal leading to psychiatric symptoms or illnesses

Figure 16.1 presents the scope of co-existent psychiatric and substance misuse disorders (Department of Health, 2002). The horizontal axis represents the severity of mental illness, and the

Table 16.1
Substance use and psychiatric syndromes

- Substance use, even in small amounts, can result in psychiatric syndromes or symptoms.
- Harmful use of substances may give rise to psychiatric symptoms.
- Dependence on substances can lead to psychological symptoms.
- Intoxication from substances may induce psychological symptoms.
- Withdrawal from substances may trigger psychological symptoms.
- Withdrawal from substances may culminate in psychiatric syndromes.
- Substance use has the potential to worsen pre-existing psychiatric disorders.
- Psychological distress, even without meeting diagnostic criteria for a disorder, might prompt substance use.
- A primary psychiatric disorder could lead to the development of a substance use disorder.
- A primary psychiatric disorder might initiate a substance use disorder, subsequently leading to psychiatric syndromes.

Source: Based on Crome (1999).

For example, a dependent drinker with experiences increasing anxiety
For example, an individual with schizophrenia who misuses cannabis on a daily basis to compensate for social isolation
Low
High
For example, recreational misuser of 'dance drugs' who has begun to struggle with low mood after weekend use
For example, an individual with bi-polar disorder whose occasional binge drinking and experimental misuse of other substances de-stabilises their mental health

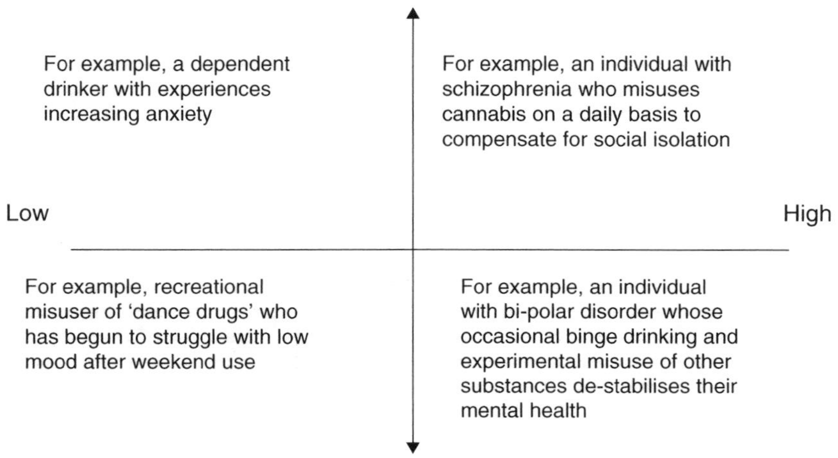

FIGURE 16.1 The scope of co-existent psychiatric and substance use disorders.
Source: Department of Health (2002).

vertical axis represents the severity of substance misuse. Intervention strategies would need to focus on those whose severity falls within the top right-hand and bottom right-hand quadrants.

AETIOLOGY OF CO-OCCURRING DISORDERS

The aetiology of dual diagnosis is unclear, and there is a wide consensus of opinions for the comorbidity to occur. There are a variety of theories that hypothesise why individuals with mental health problems are vulnerable in the misuse of alcohol and drugs. These include the self-medication hypothesis, the alleviation of dysphoria model, the multiple-risk-factor model, and the supersensitivity model. These theories or models are described in Rassool (2006, Chapter 1). The explanations of why substance use and psychiatric disorders occur are presented in Table 16.2.

MULTIPLE AND COMPLEX NEEDS

Individuals with co-occurring disorders, experiencing both substance use disorder and psychiatric disorders, represent a vulnerable group with complex needs. Various challenges arise from this dual diagnosis, including the potential for withdrawal from alcohol or drugs to mimic psychiatric disorders, masking of psychiatric symptoms by substance use, and the interplay between untreated substance use disorder and psychiatric symptoms. Additionally, untreated psychiatric disorders can contribute to substance use relapse, while individuals may face additional difficulties beyond medical or psychological issues, such as social, legal, housing, welfare, and lifestyle matters. This combination of problems often leads to a worse prognosis; increased service utilisation, including emergency clinic; and inpatient admissions (McCrone et al., 2000). In summary, the major problems associated with individuals with dual diagnosis are presented in Table 16.3.

Table 16.2
Why do substance misuse and psychiatric disorders commonly co-occur?

Factors	Explanations
Genetic vulnerabilities	There is evidence suggesting a shared genetic predisposition or neurobiological vulnerability underlying both substance misuse and psychiatric disorders. Certain genes and neurochemical pathways implicated in mental health conditions may also contribute to substance use disorders.
Environmental triggers	Stress, trauma (for example, physical or sexual abuse), and early exposure to drugs are common factors that can lead to addiction and to psychiatric disorders, particularly in those with underlying genetic vulnerabilities.
Involvement of similar brain regions	Some areas of the brain are affected by both drug misuse and psychiatric disorders. For example, brain circuits linked to reward processing as well as those implicated in the stress response are affected by abused substances and also show abnormalities in specific psychiatric disorders.
Developmental disorders	They often begin in adolescence or even childhood, periods when the brain is undergoing dramatic developmental changes. Early exposure to drugs of addiction can change the brain in ways that increase the risk for mental illness, just as early symptoms of a psychiatric disorder may increase vulnerability to alcohol and drug misuse.
Mental illnesses	Certain mental disorders serve as established risk factors for developing a substance use disorder, with individuals often using drugs as a form of self-medication, even in cases of mild or subclinical mental illness. While some drugs may temporarily alleviate symptoms, evidence suggests they can also exacerbate them, both acutely and over time. For instance, cocaine use has been linked to worsening symptoms of bipolar disorder and its progression.
Substance use and addiction	Substance use and addiction can contribute to the development of mental illness. Substance use can induce alterations in brain areas affected by various mental disorders, like schizophrenia, anxiety, mood, or impulse-control disorders. Preceding the onset of mental illness symptoms, drug use may lead to changes in brain structure and function, potentially triggering an underlying predisposition to develop the mental illness.
Comorbidity between mental illness and tobacco use	There exists a robust association between mental illness, particularly depression and schizophrenia, and tobacco product use. Individuals with schizophrenia exhibit the highest prevalence of smoking, with rates ranging from 70 to 80%, which can be up to five times higher than the general population.

Source: Adapted from NIDA (2021b).

Activity 16.2

Questions

Before reading the next section, try to answer the following questions:

- Why is there so much concern about patients with co-occurring disorders?
- Why do substance use disorder and psychiatric disorders commonly co-occur?
- List the problems associated with co-occurring disorders.
- List the common mental health problems associated with:
  - Alcohol
  - Stimulants
  - Hallucinogens
  - Opiates
- What are the problems and issues faced by healthcare professionals and service provision?
- Discuss some of the models of service delivery and treatment.

Table 16.3
Problems associated with co-occurring disorders

• Increased Likelihood Of Self-Harm	• Higher recidivism
• Increased Risk Of Hiv Infection	• Contact with the criminal justice system
• Increased Use Of Institutional Services	• Family problems
• Poor Compliance With Medication/Treatment	• Poor social outcomes, including impact on carers and family
• Homelessness	• Denial of substance use disorder
• Increased Risk Of Violence	• Negative attitudes of healthcare professionals
• Increased Risk Of Victimisation/Exploitation	• Social exclusion

Individuals from diverse ethnic or Indigenous backgrounds with co-occurring disorders encounter compounded challenges, such as stigma, prejudice, institutional racism, and ethnocentric intervention strategies. Addressing their complex needs necessitates a holistic approach spanning medical, psychological, social, spiritual, and legal domains, often involving multiple agencies or services. Managing and treating individuals with comorbid disorders is notably challenging due to these complexities and historical barriers to integrated treatment (Padwa et al., 2015). This vulnerable population also faces heightened risks of symptomatic relapses, hospitalisations, financial strain, social isolation, family discord, homelessness, victimisation, incarceration, and severe medical conditions (Psychology Today, 2021). Therapeutic interventions for individuals with comorbid disorders necessitate tailored care planning that matches various treatment and intervention strategies to each specific problem, ensuring comprehensive addressing of all complex needs within this client group. Gafoor and Rassool (1998) emphasise the importance of this approach, highlighting its significance not only in providing treatment but also in delivering the appropriate treatment for patients with comorbid disorders. Meeting this need calls for well-integrated health and social care services with clearly defined responsibilities and care pathways.

ALCOHOL AND MENTAL HEALTH PROBLEMS

Alcohol and mental health problems often co-exist and can have complex interactions. Excessive alcohol consumption can exacerbate existing mental health issues or even contribute to the development of new ones. Equally, individuals with mental health problems may be more prone to alcohol use disorder as a form of self-medication to alleviate symptoms or cope with distress. Having a dual diagnosis of alcohol use and mental disorders is prevalent, with approximately 86% of individuals receiving alcohol treatment services also experiencing co-occurring mental health difficulties. Similarly, about 44% of community mental health patients have reported substance use problems within the previous year (Public Health England, 2016a, 2017). The relationship between alcohol and mental health problems is bidirectional. Alcohol use can lead to symptoms of depression, anxiety, and other mental health disorders, especially when consumed in large quantities or over a prolonged period. On the contrary, individuals with pre-existing mental health conditions, such as depression or anxiety disorders, may be at higher risk of developing alcohol use disorder.

The most prevalent mental health conditions that frequently co-occur with alcohol use disorder include depressive disorders, anxiety disorders, bipolar disorder and antisocial personality disorder, trauma- and stress-related disorders, other substance use disorders, and sleep disorders (castillo-carniglia et al., 2019; De graaf et al., 2002; Koob & colrain, 2020; moeller & dougherty, 2001; public health england, 2016b). Additionally, psychotic disorders like schizophrenia commonly co-exist with aud and should be identified and treated concurrently during aud treatment (niaaa, 2024). It has been suggested that it is the psychiatric complaints that are often the first problems for which an alcoholic patient seeks help (anthenelli & schuckit, 1993). Alcohol use disorders can hinder the recovery process from psychiatric conditions, potentially delaying progress (greenfield, 2001). Additionally, alcohol use is linked to poorer outcomes among individuals receiving mental health services, with tragic consequences such as loss of life through suicide (public health england, 2016a). The links between alcohol and mental health can be extremely complex; however, there are four broad characteristics used in dual diagnosis to explain relationships (abdulrahim, 2001):

- Alcohol is used to medicate psychological distress/symptoms (self-medication).
- Alcohol use causes psychological distress/symptoms (side effect).
- Alcohol use has no causal or preventative mechanism for psychological distress or symptoms.
- Underlying trauma results in alcohol use and mood disorders.

RELATIONSHIP OF ALCOHOL AND ANXIETY DISORDERS

Anxiety disorders are prevalent, affecting approximately 10% of the population. According to the *Diagnostic and Statistical Manual of Mental Disorders (DSM-V)* (APA, 2013), substance/medication-induced anxiety disorder is diagnosed when persistent anxiety symptoms, including panic attacks, obsessions, and compulsions, occur in the absence of obsessive-compulsive disorders. These symptoms must develop during or within a month of substance use or intoxication, or within a month after withdrawal from a substance known to cause anxiety. Evidence suggests that individuals with high anxiety sensitivity may be prone to alcohol misuse (MacDonald et al., 2000). High anxiety sensitivity, characterised by symptoms like "butterflies," rapid breathing, or an increased heart rate in response to stress, may lead individuals to "soothe" their anxiety by drinking. Moreover, alcohol misuse may result from increased alcohol dosing, providing heightened relief from anxiety sensitivity. Researchers have identified a brain mechanism in rats that could play a pivotal role in regulating both anxiety and alcohol-drinking behaviours (Pandey et al., 2005), offering valuable insights into the neurobiology of alcohol consumption in humans.

Anxiety disorders can serve as a risk factor for the development of alcohol use disorder, with anxiety symptoms often present during chronic intoxication and withdrawal. While alcohol consumption may temporarily alleviate feelings of anxiety, prolonged alcohol misuse frequently exacerbates anxiety over time. Research suggests that alcohol can heighten clinical anxiety, particularly after extended periods of drinking and during withdrawal. Consequently, anxiety disorders such as panic disorder and generalised anxiety disorder may be linked more closely to these situations rather than serving as primary psychiatric disorders in affected individuals (Harrison & Abou-Saleh, 2001). This relationship may lead individuals with drinking problems into a harmful cycle, as they consume alcohol to self-medicate anxiety, inadvertently worsening their anxiety in the long run (Lingford-Hughes et al., 2002). Agoraphobia, social phobias, panic disorder, and generalised anxiety disorder are more frequently reported by heavy drinkers compared to the general population (Stockwell, 1995). The self-medication hypothesis has gained popularity, with many studies indicating that patients use alcohol to manage their phobic fears and anxiety (Bibb & Chambless, 1986). Gender differences may exist in the relationship between alcohol and anxiety. For instance, one study of hospitalised depressive patients found a robust association between anxiety and alcohol misuse among women, whereas the association was weaker among men (Fischer & Goethe, 1998).

Three distinct anxiety disorders commonly co-occur with alcohol use disorder (Smith & Randall, 2012):

- *Generalised anxiety disorder (GAD)*. Characterised by persistent and generalised worrying, individuals with GAD may experience symptoms such as poor sleep, fatigue, and difficulty relaxing.
- *Social anxiety disorder*. Marked by an extreme fear of situations involving the possibility of scrutiny by others or embarrassment, individuals with social anxiety disorder may avoid social situations or endure them with significant distress.
- *Panic Disorder*. Involves Recurrent "Panic Attacks" Characterised By Intense Fear Lasting Several Minutes To An Hour. These Panic Attacks Often Lead To Changes In Behaviour As Individuals May Attempt To Avoid Situations That Could Precipitate An Attack.

Research findings indicate that individuals with anxiety disorders, depression, and bulimia nervosa who consume alcohol are more prone to exceeding recommended limits. This heightened alcohol consumption raises the risk of developing more severe problems associated with alcohol use disorder (Palzes et al., 2020).

RELATIONSHIP OF ALCOHOL AND DEPRESSION

The relationship between alcohol and depression is complex and bidirectional. While alcohol consumption may initially provide temporary relief from depressive symptoms, excessive or prolonged alcohol use can exacerbate or contribute to the development of depression. This relationship can form a vicious cycle, as individuals with depression may turn to alcohol as a form of self-medication, which in turn can worsen their depressive symptoms and lead to further alcohol misuse. Depressive disorders are indeed the most prevalent psychiatric disorders among individuals with alcohol use disorder (Grant et al., 2004). The co-existence of these disorders is linked to increased severity and poorer prognosis compared to either disorder alone (Greenfield et al., 1998; Hasin et al., 2002). This includes a heightened risk for suicidal behaviour, highlighting the serious implications of comorbid depression and AUD (Conner et al., 2014).

Alcohol consumption can either be a cause or a consequence of depression. Evidence suggests a strong link between alcohol use disorders and depressive symptoms, with alcohol use disorder and depressive disorders co-occurring more frequently than expected by chance (Mental Health Foundation, 2006). Depressive symptoms are particularly prevalent among heavy drinkers or those engaging in hazardous alcohol use (Caldwell et al., 2002; Manninen et al., 2006). Gender differences exist among hazardous drinkers, with depressive symptoms correlated with frequency of intoxication, drinking to get drunk, and binge drinking (Bonin et al., 2000; Wang & Patten, 2001). However, it remains unclear whether depression precedes or leads to alcohol problems, or if alcohol consumption or alcohol problems cause depression. It is likely that alcohol problems and depression interact with various other factors, exacerbating or maintaining depressive symptoms. Risk factors for poor mental health may also contribute to alcohol misuse (Mental Health Foundation, 2006).

People may turn to alcohol use for various reasons, including experiencing moderate to high levels of shyness or fear, or to cope with social anxiety. A survey conducted by the Mental Health Foundation (2006) found that approximately one-third of participants reported that drinking made them feel less anxious (40%), less depressed (26%), and more capable of forgetting problems (30%). This aligns with the theory that individuals may use alcohol to self-medicate low levels of stress, anxiety, and depression. Self-medication has been proposed as an explanation for alcohol consumption in individuals with anxiety, and a similar self-perpetuating cycle may also apply to those with depression. Increased alcohol tolerance can lead to heightened drinking in an attempt to achieve the same desired effect. The pharmacological actions of alcohol can interact with an individual's pre-existing mood or personality, their beliefs and expectations about alcohol's effects, and the context in which it is consumed (Institute of Alcohol Studies, 2004). Alcohol can act as a reinforcing agent, exacerbating the cyclical pattern of increased alcohol consumption to alleviate feelings of depression. Moreover, there is evidence suggesting that abstaining from alcohol consumption can significantly reduce depressive symptoms in individuals who are alcohol-dependent within a short time frame (Schuckit & Monteiro, 1988).

Alcohol use disorder is closely associated with an increased risk of suicidal behaviour. the association between alcohol use and death by suicide is significant, with alcohol use being linked to a 94% increase in the risk of suicide (Isaacs et al., 2022). The findings of a study (Lange et al., 2022) suggest that that alcohol use preceding death by suicide is more prevalent among women compared to men. This indicates a gender difference in the relationship between alcohol use and suicide, with women showing a higher likelihood of alcohol use preceding suicide compared to men. The risk for attempted suicide is typically highest among adolescents and young adults in most countries. However, research suggests that alcohol-dependent middle-aged and older adults are at greater risk for suicide compared to alcohol-dependent young adults (Conner et al., 2003). This highlights the importance of recognising different demographic patterns in attempted suicide and suicide, with age playing a significant role in the risk profile. Additionally, studies have shown that alcohol intoxication is associated with violent methods of suicide and tends to decline markedly with age in both men and women (Kaplan et al., 2012). This underlines the complex interplay between alcohol use, age, and suicide risk, emphasising the need for targeted interventions and support strategies tailored to specific age groups within the population.

DRUGS AND MENTAL HEALTH

Individuals with substance use disorder may exhibit a range of psychiatric symptoms, including mania, psychosis, depression, anxiety, and personality disorder symptoms, which are influenced by factors such as the type of drug used, quantity consumed, and route of administration. These symptoms are common in drug-related problems and can complicate the diagnosis of dual diagnosis. For instance, regular cocaine users may experience euphoria, grandiosity, impulsiveness, impaired judgement, and marked psychomotor activity, resembling hypomania. Cocaine use can also lead to hallucinations, including visual, auditory, and tactile hallucinations, similar to those seen in schizophrenia. Prolonged or high-dose cocaine use may result in toxic psychosis, which can mimic acute psychosis of other causes but typically resolves within 24 hours (Harrison & Abou-Saleh, 2001).

In a study by Myrick and Brady (1997) examining the relationship between social phobia and cocaine dependence, a lifetime prevalence of social phobia was found to be 13.9% among cocaine-dependent individuals. These individuals with social phobia were also more likely to have additional psychopathology, use multiple psychoactive substances, and develop alcohol misuse at an earlier age. Similarly, amphetamines may produce toxic reactions, with psychosis lasting longer than that produced by cocaine but typically resolving within a few days (Connell, 1958). This condition, often observed in long-term users, manifests as disordered thinking, hallucinations, paranoid ideas, and repetitive behaviours, such as involuntary picking and scratching at the skin. The consumption of cannabis can lead to the development of anxiety and panic attacks, with symptoms typically brief in duration and including restlessness, depersonalisation, derealisation, paranoia, and transient mood disorders (Thomas, 1993). Additionally, acute toxic confusional states can result from high doses or prolonged cannabis consumption, resembling schizophrenia. However, it is challenging to differentiate whether these conditions represent relapses in previously psychotic patients, reactions precipitated in vulnerable individuals, or actual reactions produced by cannabis ingestion (Harrison & Abou-Saleh, 2001). Despite these associations, there is no conclusive evidence that cannabis can cause long-term psychiatric disorders or act as an independent risk factor for schizophrenia.

In a study examining the relationship between social phobia and cocaine dependence, Myrick and Brady (1997) found a lifetime prevalence of social phobia in these cocaine-dependant individuals to be 13.9%. They also found that the social phobic individuals were more likely to have additional psychopathology, use multiple psychoactive substances, and develop alcohol misuse at an earlier age. Amphetamines may produce similar toxic reactions; the psychosis may last longer than that produced by cocaine but will usually resolve within a few days (Connell, 1958). This condition usually occurs in long-term users but may start a day or two after use and consists of disordered thinking, hallucinations and paranoid ideas, and repetitive behaviour, such as involuntary picking and scratching at the skin. The consumption of cannabis can lead to the development of anxiety and panic attacks. Symptoms are usually brief in duration and may include restlessness, depersonalisation, derealisation, paranoia, and transient mood disorders (Thomas, 1993). Acute toxic confusional state can be developed as a result of high doses or prolonged consumption of cannabis and are indistinguishable from schizophrenia. It is difficult to differentiate whether these illnesses are, in fact, relapses in previously psychotic patients who use cannabis, precipitated in patients who are vulnerable or actual reactions produced by ingestion of cannabis (Harrison & Abou-Saleh, 2001). There is no conclusive evidence that cannabis can cause long-term psychiatric disorders or is an independent risk factor for schizophrenia. A summary of the negative effects of specific psychoactive substances is presented in Table 16.4.

RELATIONSHIP OF ALCOHOL, DRUGS, AND PERSONALITY DISORDERS

Personality disorders are associated with various serious outcomes, including impaired social functioning, difficulties in relationships, and decreased quality of life. They often co-occur with substance use disorders, such as alcohol use disorder, leading to more severe clinical presentations and poorer treatment outcomes (Helle et al., 2019). Individuals receiving treatment for alcohol dependence frequently have comorbid personality disorders. The prevalence of personality disorders varies across different populations, including community (nonclinical) samples, psychiatric outpatient samples, and clinical psychiatric samples. Epidemiological studies have shown prevalence rates ranging from 9% to 21% in community samples (Trull et al., 2010), indicating that a significant portion of the general population may meet criteria for at least one personality disorder. In psychiatric outpatient samples, the prevalence is higher, estimated to be approximately 31% (Zimmerman et al., 2005).

The European Monitoring Centre for Drugs and Drug Addiction (EMCDDA) (2016) suggests that individuals with a personality disorder tend to exhibit more problematic symptoms of substance use disorders compared to those without a personality disorder. Among illicit drug users, antisocial personality disorder (ASPD) and borderline personality disorder (BPD) are more frequently observed. It is important to note that many individuals in clinical settings may receive diagnoses of more than one personality disorder, further complicating the clinical picture. The study by Grant et al. (2004) found that associations between certain personality disorders and alcohol and drug use disorders varied between men and women. Specifically, obsessive-compulsive, histrionic, schizoid, and antisocial personality disorders were more strongly associated with specific alcohol and drug use disorders among women compared to men. In contrast, the association between personality disorders and drug dependence was significantly greater among men than women. These findings suggest that gender differences play a role in the relationship between personality disorders and substance use disorders, highlighting the importance of considering gender-specific factors in the assessment and treatment of these comorbid conditions.

Bernstein and Handelsman (1995) have proposed three mechanisms to try to explain the high levels of comorbidity:

- Substance misuse often takes place in the context of a deviant peer group and that antisocial behaviours are shaped and reinforced by social group norms.
- Psychoactive substances have the potential to alter behaviour through their effects as reinforcers or conditioning agents, linking environmental and internal cues to substance use.
- Chronic substance use may alter personality through its direct effects on brain chemistry.

Individuals with antisocial personality disorder exhibit increased susceptibility to alcohol's aggression-related effects compared to those without the disorder. Research, including studies by Moeller and Dougherty (2001), has shown that aggressive personality traits are correlated with heightened aggression following alcohol consumption. Moreover, personality disorders, including ASPD, have been linked to poor treatment response and outcomes in individuals with substance misuse and psychiatric issues. Such individuals are prone to engaging in risky behaviours, such as sharing injecting equipment and risky sexual practices, and they often face challenges in remaining compliant with treatment. Studies, such as those referenced by EMCDDA (2016) and Ball et al. (2006), suggest that impaired coping, social functioning, and low motivation or readiness to change contribute to higher attrition rates in treatment among individuals with personality disorders and substance use disorder.

Table 16.4
Psychoactive substance and psychiatric disorders

Category of substance	Type of substance	Common mental health problems
Depressant	Alcohol	Alcoholic hallucinosis (persecutory auditory hallucinations)
		Depression and suicidal ideation
		Social phobia
		Pathological jealousy
		Delirium tremens
		Wernicke's encephalopathy
		Korsakoff's "psychosis"
		Personality disorder
Stimulant	Amphetamine	Disordered thinking
		Hallucinations
		Paranoid ideas
		Production of random, pointless, repetitive behaviour (such as involuntary picking and scratching at the skin)
		Restlessness
		Sleep disturbances
Stimulant	Cocaine	Experience of hallucinations (visual, auditory, and tactile)
		Paranoid feelings
		Irritability
		Toxic psychosis with persecutory delusions and hallucinations
		Loss of insight (condition which usually subsides within 24 hours)
		Depression
		Sleep disturbances
Hallucinogen	Cannabis	Anxiety and panic attacks
		Restlessness
		Depersonalisation
		Derealisation
		Paranoia
		Transient mood disorders
		Acute toxic confusional state
Hallucinogen	LSD	Hallucinations
		Panic reactions
		Flashback (recurrence of symptoms)
Opiate	Heroin	Anxiety
		Depression
		Suicide
		Overdose
		Personality disorder
Synthetic cannabinoids	JWH-018	Depressive
	AM-2201	Anxiety
	AB-FUBINACA	Conduct disorder
	5F-ADB	Auditory hallucinations
	UR-144	Paranoia
	XLR-11.	Seizures
	CUMYL-PEGACLONE	Psychoses

Table 16.4 (*Continued*)

Category of substance	Type of substance	Common mental health problems
Synthetic stimulants	Bath salts (synthetic cathinones) Nootropics (smart drugs): modafinil, adrafinil, and phenylpiracetam Designer stimulants: α-PVP (alpha-Pyrrolidinopentiophenone) and 4-FA (4-Fluoroamphetamine)	Anxiety Agitation and aggression Panic attacks Mood disorders Cognitive impairment Psychosis
Synthetic opioids	Fentanyl and its analogues	Depressive symptoms Persistent sadness Loss of interest in activities Feelings of hopelessness Generalised anxiety disorder Panic disorder Social anxiety disorder Heightened feelings of fear Post-traumatic stress disorder Psychosis: hallucinations, delusions, and disorganised thinking Cognitive impairment Suicidal ideation and behaviour

RELATIONSHIP OF ALCOHOL, DRUGS, AND SCHIZOPHRENIA

Substance use disorders are highly prevalent co-occurring issues among individuals with schizophrenia, with lifetime rates reaching up to 80% in this population when tobacco use is included (Manseau & Bogenschutz, 2016). This comorbidity can result in challenges in diagnosis and treatment, as symptoms of substance misuse may overlap with those of schizophrenia, leading to misinterpretation. Additionally, substance use has the potential to worsen schizophrenic symptoms and even trigger psychotic symptoms independently. The impact of substance use on schizophrenia symptoms varies based on factors such as the type of drug used, quantity consumed, method of administration, and individual's state of use (Harrison & Abou-Saleh, 2001). Patients with schizophrenia often demonstrate a preference for activating drugs, including amphetamines, cocaine, cannabis, and hallucinogens (Ries et al., 2000). This preference may contribute to the heightened risk of substance use disorders within this population.

Schizophrenic patients who misuse alcohol may exhibit a higher likelihood of hostile behaviour, paranoid thoughts, and depression compared to non-alcohol-using patients (Harrison & Abou-Saleh, 2001). While drug misuse in schizophrenia is significantly correlated with both negative and positive symptoms, alcohol use is not associated with these symptoms unless it reaches the point of requiring alcohol treatment (Swofford et al., 2000). Substance misuse, including alcohol and drugs, can diminish the effectiveness of treatment for schizophrenia and increase the likelihood of non-compliance with treatment programmes. Nicotine addiction is the most common form of substance misuse among individuals with schizophrenia, and quitting smoking can be particularly challenging due to the exacerbation of psychotic symptoms during nicotine withdrawal.

PROBLEMS AND ISSUES FOR HEALTHCARE PROFESSIONALS

The term "co-occurring disorders" is frequently used to describe the co-existence of substance use disorders and mental health conditions. Individuals with co-occurring disorders tend to present more challenges in treatment and management due to higher rates of non-compliance, violence, homelessness, and suicide. The relationship between substance misuse and mental health problems is complex, as intoxication and withdrawal from drugs and alcohol can produce psychiatric symptoms, while individuals with certain psychiatric disorders like antisocial personality disorder and schizophrenia are more susceptible to substance misuse (Rassool, 2006). Four models of service provision have been identified for the treatment of co-occurring substance misuse and psychiatric disorders: the serial model, the parallel model, the integrated treatment model, and the joint liaison/collaborative approach (Rassool, 2002). Each model offers a different approach to addressing the complex needs of individuals with co-occurring disorders, highlighting the importance of tailored interventions to effectively manage and treat this population. The four models of service delivery and potential problems and difficulties of each model are presented in Table 16.5.

Integrated treatment, which addresses both schizophrenia and substance use disorders concurrently, has been shown to offer advantages over non-integrated treatment approaches in significantly improving psychiatric symptomatology among individuals with co-occurring disorders (Chetty et al., 2023). However, studies have not consistently found significant benefits of integrated treatment over non-integrated treatment, specifically regarding substance misuse and treatment retention. This suggests that while integrated treatment may effectively address psychiatric symptoms, additional interventions may be necessary to effectively target substance misuse and improve treatment retention rates in this population.

Assessing the needs of individuals with co-occurring disorders is challenging due to barriers such as their mental state, which may hinder their ability to understand or describe symptoms

Table 16.5
Models of treatment and potential difficulties

Model of treatment	Description		Problems/difficulties
Serial treatment	Treatment programmes provided consecutively by mental health and substance misuse services based on presenting problem.	An individual initially seeking treatment at a mental health clinic for symptoms of depression or anxiety. After some time, they may then be referred to a separate addiction services to address their alcohol or substance use disorder once their mental health symptoms have been stabilised or improved.	• Limited communication between the services. • Health problems treated as separate entities. • Patients are shunted between the two services.
Parallel treatment	Concurrent patient care by both services, facilitated by communication.	An individual attending therapy sessions at both a mental health clinic to address symptoms of depression or anxiety and simultaneously participating in a substance use treatment programme to manage their alcohol or substance use disorder.	• Patients are shunted between the two services. • Health problems are treated as separate entities. • Medical responsibility is not clearly defined.
Integrated treatment	Joint management of patient care by both services, possibly as a designated service.	An individual receiving comprehensive care within a single programme or facility that addresses both their mental health and substance use needs concurrently. For instance, they might participate in therapy sessions that incorporate techniques to address both their depression or anxiety symptoms and their substance use behaviours.	• Isolated from mainstream services. • Views dual diagnosis as a static condition. • Expensive service provision.
Joint liaison/ collaborative approach	Joint management of patient care by both services, possibly as a designated service.	An individual receiving coordinated care from both a mental health provider and addiction specialist working together as a team. For instance, the individual might have regular meetings where their mental health and substance use treatment providers discuss their progress, adjust treatment plans as needed, and ensure that both aspects of their care are effectively addressed.	• Joint working between mental health and substance misuse services. • Joint responsibility. • Ensures the skills and expertise of both spheres of healthcare are utilised.

Source: Adapted from NTA (2002).

accurately. The complexity is compounded by the use of multiple psychoactive substances, making it difficult to distinguish between substance-related symptoms and psychiatric symptoms. Failure to recognise and treat alcohol or substance use disorder early can lead to ineffective management and worsening symptoms. Additionally, individuals with co-occurring disorders often struggle to follow or comply with treatment regimens, further complicating their care. Compliance with taking prescribed medication has been shown to be poor in mentally ill clients with substance use disorders (Pristach & Smith, 1996). Co-occurring disorders, like substance use disorders, cannot be effectively addressed by a single discipline or specialist alone. A multidimensional approach is required, involving collaboration between various agencies and professionals. This collaboration is essential for collectively owning common goals aimed at meeting the complex physical/medical, social, psychological, and spiritual needs of individuals with co-occurring disorders.

KEY POINTS

- Co-occurring disorders, also known as dual diagnosis, refer to the simultaneous presence of mental health problems and alcohol or substance use disorders in an individual.
- Co-occurring disorders are common, with a high prevalence in both clinical and community populations.
- Mental health problems and substance use disorders often interact in complex ways, exacerbating each other's symptoms and making treatment more challenging.
- Individuals with co-occurring disorders may experience more severe symptoms, poorer treatment outcomes, and higher rates of relapse compared to those with either disorder alone.
- There is no single type of dual diagnosis as there are many patterns of alcohol or drug misuse and different types of psychiatric disorders.
- Substance use and/or withdrawal can lead to psychiatric symptoms or illnesses.
- There are a variety of theories that hypothesise why individuals with mental health problems are vulnerable in the misuse of alcohol and drugs.
- Individuals from ethnic or culturally and linguistically diverse communities and Indigenous populations with comorbidity face compounded pressure of stigma, prejudice, institutional racism, and ethnocentric intervention strategies.
- Most users of substance misuse services had affective disorders (depression) and anxiety disorders and psychosis.
- Individuals with alcohol or substance use disorders and psychiatric disorders are a vulnerable group of people with complex needs and problems.
- Self-medication has been proposed as an explanation for alcohol consumption in people with anxiety.
- Alcohol misusers had affective disorders (depression), anxiety disorders, and psychosis.
- Self-harm and suicides are much more common in people with alcohol problems.
- Evidence from research studies have shown substantial co-occurrence between anxiety disorders and alcohol problems.
- Drug misusers may show symptoms such as mania, psychosis, depression, anxiety, and personality disorder symptoms.
- Individuals receiving treatment for alcohol dependence are often also diagnosed with a personality disorder.
- The mental state of the patient may act as a barrier to recognition as some patients may not be able to understand the nature of the symptoms they experience or adequately describe them in a way that enables clinical staff to make an accurate assessment.
- The assessment is compounded by the fact that some patients are not able to understand or to describe the nature of the symptoms they experience.
- Integrated treatment approaches that address both mental health and substance use issues concurrently have been shown to be more effective than treating each disorder separately.
- Effective treatment for co-occurring disorders requires a comprehensive assessment of the individual's needs, including physical, psychological, social, and environmental factors.
- Coordinated care involving collaboration between mental health, substance abuse, and other healthcare providers is essential for ensuring holistic and effective treatment.
- Co-occurring disorders, similar to substance use disorders, require a multidimensional approach involving inter-agency collaboration.

References

Abdulrahim, D. (2001). *Substance Misuse and Mental Health Co-Morbidity (Dual Diagnosis)*. London: The Health Advisory Service.

American Psychiatric Association. (2013). *Diagnostic and Statistical Manual of Mental Disorders* (5th ed.). Washington, DC: APA Press.

Anthenelli, R. M., & Schuckit, M. A. (1993). Affective and anxiety disorders and alcohol and drug dependence: Diagnosis and treatment. *Journal of Addictive Diseases,* 12(3), 73–87. https://doi.org/10.1300/J069v12n03_07.

Ball, S. A., Carroll, K. M., Canning-Ball, M., & Rounsaville, B. J. (2006). Reasons for dropout from drug abuse treatment: Symptoms, personality, and motivation. *Addictive Behaviors,* 31(2), 320–330. https://doi.org/10.1016/j.addbeh.2005.05.013.

Banerjee, S., Clancy, C., & Crome, I. (2002). *Co-Existing Problems of Mental Disorder and Substance Misuse (Dual Diagnosis)*. London: The Royal College of Psychiatrists Research Unit.

Bernstein, D. P., & Handelsman, L. (1995). *The Neurobiology of Substance Abuse and Personality Disorders: Neuropsychiatry of Personality Disorders*. Oxford: Blackwell Science.

Bibb, J. L., & Chambless, D. L. (1986). Alcohol use and abuse among diagnosed agoraphobics. *Behaviour Research and Therapy,* 24(1), 49–58. https://doi.org/10.1016/0005-7967(86)90149-x.

Bonin, M. F., McCreary, D. R., & Sadava, S. W. (2000). Problem drinking behavior in two community-based samples of adults: Influence of gender, coping, loneliness, and depression. *Psychology of Addictive Behaviors: Journal of the Society of Psychologists in Addictive Behaviors,* 14(2), 151–161. https://doi.org/10.1037//0893-164x.14.2.151.

Caldwell, T. M., Rodgers, B., Jorm, A. F., Christensen, H., Jacomb, P. A., Korten, A. E., & Lynskey, M. T. (2002). Patterns of association between alcohol consumption and symptoms of depression and anxiety in young adults. *Addiction, 97,* 583–594.

Carey, K. B. (1989). Emerging treatment guidelines for mentally ill chemical abusers. *Hospital & Community Psychiatry,* 40(4), 341–342, 349.

Castillo-Carniglia, A., Keyes, K. M., Hasin, D. S., & Cerdá, M. (2019). Psychiatric comorbidities in alcohol use disorder. *The Lancet. Psychiatry,* 6(12), 1068–1080. https://doi.org/10.1016/S2215-0366(19)30222-6.

Chetty, A., Guse, T., & Malema, M. (2023). Integrated vs non-integrated treatment outcomes in dual diagnosis disorders: A systematic review. *Health SA = SA Gesondheid,* 28, 2094. https://doi.org/10.4102/hsag.v28i0.2094.

Connell, P. H. (1958). *Amphetamine Psychosis* (Maudsley Monograph No. 5). London: Oxford University Press.

Conner, K. R., Beautrais, A. L., & Conwell, Y. (2003). Moderators of the relationship between alcohol dependence and suicide and medically serious suicide attempts: Analyses of Canterbury suicide project data. *Alcoholism: Clinical Experimental Research,* 2(7), 156–1161.

Conner, K. R., Gamble, S. A., Bagge, C. L., He, H., Swogger, M. T., Watts, A., & Houston, R. J. (2014). Substance-induced depression and independent depression in proximal risk for suicidal behavior. *Journal of Studies on Alcohol and Drugs, 75*(4), 567–572. https://doi.org/10.15288/jsad.2014.75.567.

Crome, I. B. (1999). Substance misuse and psychiatric comorbidity: Towards improved service provision. *Drugs: Education, Prevention and Policy,* 6, 151–174.

de Graaf, R., Bijl, R. V., Smit, F., Vollebergh, W. A., & Spijker, J. (2002). Risk factors for 12-month comorbidity of mood, anxiety, and substance use disorders: Findings from the Netherlands mental health survey and incidence study. *The American Journal of Psychiatry,* 159(4), 620–629. https://doi.org/10.1176/appi.ajp.159.4.620.

Department of Health. (2002). *Dual Diagnosis Good Practice Guidance: Mental Health Policy Implementation Guide*. London: Department of Health.

EMCDDA. (2004). Selected issue 3: Co-morbidity. In *Annual Report 2004: The State of the Drugs Problem in the European Union and Norway*. European Monitoring Centre for Drugs and Drug Addiction. Luxembourg: Office for Official Publications of the European Communities, pp. 94–102.

EMCDDA. (2016). *Perspectives on Drugs: Comorbidity of Substance Use and Mental Health Disorders in Europe*. European Monitoring Centre for Drugs and Drug Addiction. Luxembourg: Publications Office of the European Union.

European Collaborating Centres in Addiction Studies (ECCAS). (2006). *Comorbidity* (ECCAS Monograph Series No. 4). London: European Collaborating Centres in Addiction Studies, International Centre for Drug Policy, St George's, University of London.

Fischer, E. H., & Goethe, J. W. (1998). Anxiety and alcohol abuse in patients in treatment for depression. *The American Journal of Drug and Alcohol Abuse,* 24(3), 453–463. https://doi.org/10.3109/00952999809016909.

Gafoor, M, & Rassool, G. H. (1998). The co-existence of psychiatric disorders and substance misuse: Working with dual diagnosis patients. *Journal of Advanced Nursing,* 27(3), 497–502.

Grant, B. F., Stinson, F. S., Dawson, D. A., Chou, S. P., Dufour, M. C., Compton, W., Pickering, R. P., & Kaplan, K. (2004). Prevalence and co-occurrence of substance use disorders and independent mood and anxiety disorders: Results from the national epidemiologic survey on alcohol and related conditions. *Archives of General Psychiatry,* 61(8), 807–816. https://doi.org/10.1001/archpsyc.61.8.807.

Greenfield, S. F., Weiss, R. D., Muenz, L. R., Vagge, L. M., Kelly, J. F., Bello, L. R., & Michael, J. (1998). The effect of depression on return to drinking: A prospective study. *Archives of General Psychiatry,* 55(3), 259–265. https://doi.org/10.1001/archpsyc.55.3.259.

Greenfield, T. K. (2001). Individual risk of alcohol-related disease and problems. Chapter 21 in N. Heather, T. J. Peter, & T. Stockwell (Eds.), *International Handbook Alcohol Dependence and Problems*. New York: John Wiley & Sons Ltd, pp. 413–439.

Harrison, C. A., & Abou Saleh, M. T. (2001). Psychiatric disorders and substance misuse: Psychopathology. In G. H.

Rassool (Ed.), *Dual Diagnosis: Substance Misuse and Psychiatric Disorders*. Oxford: Blackwell Publications.

Hasin, D., Liu, X., Nunes, E., McCloud, S., Samet, S., & Endicott, J. (2002). Effects of major depression on remission and relapse of substance dependence. *Archives of General Psychiatry, 59*(4), 375–380. https://doi.org/10.1001/archpsyc.59.4.375.

Helle, A. C., Watts, A. L., Trull, T. J., & Sher, K. J. (2019). Alcohol use disorder and antisocial and borderline personality disorders. *Alcohol Research: Current Reviews, 40*(1). https://doi.org/10.35946/arcr.v40.1.05.

Hryb, K., Kirkhart, R., & Talbert, R. (2007). A call for standardized definition of dual diagnosis. *Psychiatry, 4*(9), 15–16.

Institute of Alcohol Studies. (2004). *Alcohol and Mental Health*. St Ives, Cambridgeshire: Institute of Alcohol Studies.

Isaacs, J. Y., Smith, M. M., Sherry, S. B., Seno, M., Moore, M. L., & Stewart, S. H. (2022). Alcohol use and death by suicide: A meta-analysis of 33 studies. *Suicide & Life-Threatening Behavior, 52*(4), 600–614. https://doi.org/10.1111/sltb.12846.

Kaplan, M. S., McFarland, B. H., Huguet, N., Conner, K., Caetano, R., Giesbrecht, N., & Nolte, K. B. (2013). Acute alcohol intoxication and suicide: A gender-stratified analysis of the national violent death reporting system. *Injury Prevention: Journal of the International Society for Child and Adolescent Injury Prevention, 19*(1), 38–43. https://doi.org/10.1136/injuryprev-2012-040317.

Koob, G. F., & Colrain, I. M. (2020). Alcohol use disorder and sleep disturbances: A feed-forward allostatic framework. *Neuropsychopharmacology: Official Publication of the American College of Neuropsychopharmacology, 45*(1), 141–165. https://doi.org/10.1038/s41386-019-0446-0.

Lange, S., Kaplan, M. S., Tran, A., & Rehm, J. (2022). Growing alcohol use preceding death by suicide among women compared with men: Age-specific temporal trends, 2003–18. *Addiction, 117*(9), 2530–2536. https://doi.org/10.1111/add.15905.

Lingford-Hughes, A., Potokar, J., & Nutt, D. (2002). Treating anxiety complicated by substance misuse. *Advances in Psychiatric Treatment, 8*(2), 107–116. https://doi.org/10.1192/apt.8.2.107.

MacDonald, A. B., Baker, J. M., Stewart, S. H., & Skinner, M. (2000). Effects of alcohol on the response to hyperventilation of participants high and low in anxiety sensitivity. *Alcoholism: Clinical and Experimental Research, 24*(11), 1656–1665.

Manninen, L., Poikolainen, K., Vartiainen, E., & Laatikainen, T. (2006). Heavy drinking occasions and depression. *Alcohol and Alcoholism, 41*(3), 293–299. https://doi.org/10.1093/alcalc/agh246.

Manseau, M., & Bogenschutz, M. (2016). Substance use disorders and schizophrenia. *Focus, 14*(3), 333–342. https://doi.org/10.1176/appi.focus.20160008.

McCrone, P., Menezes, P. R., Johnson, S., Scott, H., Thornicroft, G., Marshall, J., Bebbington, P., & Kuipers, E. (2000). Service use and costs of people with dual diagnosis in South London. *Acta Psychiatrica Scandinavica, 101*(6), 464–472. https://doi.org/10.1034/j.1600-0447.2000.101006464.x.

Mental Health Foundation. (2006). *Cheers? Understanding the Relationship Between Alcohol and Mental Health*. London: Mental Health Foundation.

Moeller, F. G., & Dougherty, D. M. (2001). Antisocial personality disorder, alcohol, and aggression. *Alcohol Research & Health: The Journal of the National Institute on Alcohol Abuse and Alcoholism, 25*(1), 5–11.

Myrick, H., & Brady, K. T. (1997). Social phobia in cocaine-dependent individuals. *The American Journal on Addictions, 6*(2), 99–104.

NIAAA. (2024). *Mental Health Issues: Alcohol Use Disorder and Common Co-Occurring Conditions*. National Institute on Alcohol Abuse and Alcoholism. https://www.niaaa.nih.gov/health-professionals-communities/core-resource-on-alcohol/mental-health-issues-alcohol-use-disorder-and-common-co-occurring-conditions (accessed 21 March 2024).

NIDA. (2021a). Introduction. In *Common Comorbidities with Substance Use Disorders Research Report*. https://nida.nih.gov/publications/research-reports/common-comorbidities-substance-use-disorders/introduction (accessed 20 March 2024).

NIDA. (2021b). *Why Is There Comorbidity Between Substance Use Disorders and Mental Illnesses?* https://nida.nih.gov/publications/research-reports/common-comorbidities-substance-use-disorders/why-there-comorbidity-between-substance-use-disorders-mental-illnesses (accessed 20 March 2024).

NIDA. (2024). *What Are Some Approaches to Diagnosis?* https://nida.nih.gov/publications/research-reports/common-comorbidities-substance-use-disorders/what-are-some-approaches-to-diagnosis (accessed 20 March 2024).

NTA. (2002). *Models of Care for Treatment of Adult Drug Users*. London: National Treatment Agency.

Padwa, H., Guerrero, E. G., Braslow, J. T., & Fenwick, K. M. (2015). Barriers to serving clients with co-occurring disorders in a transformed mental health system. *Psychiatric Services, 66*(5), 547–550. https://doi.org/10.1176/appi.ps.201400190.

Palzes, V. A., Parthasarathy, S., Chi, F. W., Kline-Simon, A. H., Lu, Y., Weisner, C., Ross, T. B., Elson, J., & Sterling, S. A. (2020). Associations between psychiatric disorders and alcohol consumption levels in an adult primary care population. *Alcoholism, Clinical and Experimental Research, 44*(12), 2536–2544. https://doi.org/10.1111/acer.14477.

Pandey, S. C., Zhang, H., Roy, A., & Xu, T. (2005). Deficits in amygdaloid camp responsive element – binding protein signalling play a role in genetic predisposition to anxiety and alcoholism. *Journal of Clinical Investigations, 115*(10), 2762–2773. https://doi.org/10.1172/JCI24381.

Pristach, C. A., & Smith, C. M. (1996). Self-reported effects of alcohol use on symptoms of schizophrenia. *Psychiatric Services, 47*(4), 421–423. https://doi.org/10.1176/ps.47.4.421.

Psychology Today. (2021). *Co-Occurring Disorders*. https://www.psychologytoday.com/us/conditions/co-occurring-disorders#:~:text=People%20with%20co-occurring%20disorders%20are%20at%20high%20risk,and%20physical%20victimization%2C%20incarceration%2C%20and%20serious%20medical%20illnesses (accessed 21 March 2024).

Public Health England. (2016a). *Health Matters: Harmful Drinking and Alcohol Dependence*. London: Public Health England.

Public Health England. (2016b). *The Public Health Burden of Alcohol and the Effectiveness and Cost-Effectiveness of*

Alcohol Control Policies: An Evidence Review. London: Public Health England.

Public Health England. (2017). *Better Care for People with Co-Occurring Mental Health and Alcohol/Drug Use Conditions*. London: Public Health England.

Rassool, G. H. (Ed.). (2002). *Dual Diagnosis: Substance Misuse and Psychiatric Disorders*. Oxford: Blackwell Science Ltd.

Rassool, G. H. (2006). Understanding dual diagnosis: An overview. In G. H. Rassool (Ed.), *Dual Diagnosis Nursing*. Oxford: Blackwell Publishing.

Ries, R. K., Russo, J., Wingerson, D., Snowden, M., Comtois, K. A., Srebnik, D., & Roy-Byrne, P. (2000). Shorter hospital stays and more rapid improvement among patients with schizophrenia and substance use disorders. *Psychiatric Services*, 51(2), 210–215.

SAMHSA. (2021). *Substance Use Disorder Treatment for People with Co-Occurring Disorders, Advisory*. Rockville: The Substance Abuse and Mental Health Services Administration (SAMHSA). https://store.samhsa.gov/sites/default/files/pep20-06-04-006.pdf (accessed 20 March 2024).

Schuckit, M. A., & Monteiro, M. G. (1988). Alcoholism, anxiety and depression. *British Journal of Addiction*, 83(12), 1373–1380.

Smith, J. P., & Randall, C. L. (2012). Anxiety and alcohol use disorders: Comorbidity and treatment considerations. *Alcohol Research: Current Reviews*, 34(4), 414–431.

Stockwell, T. (1995). Anxiety and stress management. In R. K. Hester & W. R. Miller (Eds.), *Handbook of Alcoholism Treatment Approaches: Effective Alternatives* (2nd ed.). Needham Heights, MA: Allyn & Bacon, pp. 242–250.

Swofford, C. D., Scheller-Gilkey, G., Miller, A. H., Woolwine, B., & Mance, R. (2000). Double jeopardy: Schizophrenia and substance use. *The American Journal of Drug and Alcohol Abuse*, 26(3), 343–353. https://doi.org/10.1081/ada-100100248.

Thomas, H. (1993). Psychiatric symptoms in cannabis users. *The British Journal of Psychiatry: The Journal of Mental Science*, 163, 141–149. https://doi.org/10.1192/bjp.163.2.141.

Tomáš, J., & Lenka, Š. (2023). Prevalence of dual diagnoses among children and adolescents with mental health conditions. *Children*, 10(2), 293. https://doi.org/10.3390/children10020293.

Trull, T. J., Jahng, S., Tomko, R. L., Wood, P. K., & Sher, K. J. (2010). Revised NESARC personality disorder diagnoses: Gender, prevalence, and comorbidity with substance dependence disorders. *Journal of Personality Disorders*, 24(4), 412–426. https://doi.org/10.1521/pedi.2010.24.4.412.

Wang, J., & Patten, S. B. (2001). A prospective study of sex-specific effects of major depression on alcohol consumption. *The Canadian Journal of Psychiatry*, 46(5), 422–425. https://doi.org/10.1177/070674370104600507.

WHO. (1994). *Lexicon of Alcohol and Drug Terms*. Geneva, Switzerland: World Health Organisation. www.who.int/substance abuse/terminology/who lexicon/en/ (accessed 20 March 2024).

Zimmerman, M., Rothschild, L., & Chelminski, I. (2005). The prevalence of DSM-IV personality disorders in psychiatric outpatients. *The American Journal of Psychiatry*, 162(10), 1911–1918. https://doi.org/10.1176/appi.ajp.162.10.1911.

Chapter 17

Alcohol and drug use in culturally and linguistically diverse communities

Learning outcomes

- Understand the socio-political, economic, and health perspectives of multicultural societies in relation to alcohol and drug use.
- Recognise the heterogeneity of culturally and linguistically diverse communities and the influence of cultural and social factors on alcohol and substance use pattern.
- Identify the prevalence and impact of alcohol and drug use on physical, psychological, and social health within culturally and linguistically diverse communities.
- Evaluate the role of cultural values, attitudes, religious beliefs, and customs in shaping perceptions and behaviours related to alcohol and substance use.
- Examine the challenges and barriers faced by culturally and linguistically diverse communities in accessing culturally appropriate substance use interventions and services.
- Explore strategies for developing culturally sensitive and effective interventions for addressing alcohol and drug use issues in multicultural settings.
- Reflect on the ethical considerations and cultural competence required when working with individuals from diverse backgrounds affected by substance use.
- Identify potential interventions and prevention strategies tailored to the specific needs and contexts of culturally and linguistically diverse communities.
- Demonstrate an understanding of the intersectionality of factors such as race, ethnicity, language, and socio-economic status in shaping experiences of alcohol and substance use and access to care within diverse communities.

Activity 17.1 Alcohol and drug use in culturally and linguistically diverse communities.

State whether the statements are true or false.

Statements	True	False
The socio-political, economic, and health perspectives of a nation are intrinsically linked to the issues of race, culture, ethnicity, and substance misuse.		
Culturally and linguistically different communities have been the victims of negative stereotypes, social exclusions, health inequalities, etc.		
Culturally and linguistically different communities are a homogeneous group of people.		

DOI: 10.4324/9781003456674-20

The psychoactive substances misused by culturally and linguistically different communities are different from those used by the White population.		
Cultural and social factors have a significant influence role in the initiation, maintenance, and therapeutic intervention of substance misuse.		
Factors such as gender, age, and socio-economic status may be more important than cultural and religious factors.		
Some of the service provisions for those who are culturally and linguistically different are well-coordinated and ready to provide culturally appropriate care and interventions.		
Potential barriers occur at three different levels: patient level, provider level, and system level.		
There is a myriad of potential barriers that may inhibit culturally and linguistically different communities from utilisation of alcohol and drug services.		
There needs to be more explicit and overt organisational commitment to diversity and more resources dedicated to meeting the needs of people from ethnic and culturally diverse communities.		
The determinants of alcohol and drug misuse may differ between culturally and linguistically diverse communities because of the heterogeneity in the communities' structure, genetic differences, socio-economic differences, diversities in culture and religious beliefs, intergenerational and acculturation factors.		

Activity 17.2

Please choose one correct answer for the following multiple-choice questions.

1. In culturally diverse communities, substance abuse may be exacerbated by:
   a. Lack of community support
   b. Cultural celebrations
   c. Strict law enforcement
   d. Accessible addiction treatment
   e. Education programmes
2. Cultural beliefs and values may influence:
   a. Attitudes towards substance use
   b. Genetic make-up
   c. Access to rehabilitation centres
   d. Enforcement of drug laws
   e. Economic opportunities
3. Which of the following is a challenge in addressing alcohol and substance use disorder in culturally diverse communities?
   a. Homogeneous cultural beliefs
   b. Lack of language barriers
   c. Stigma associated with seeking help
   d. Equal access to treatment facilities
   e. High income levels

4. Effective intervention programmes should:
   a. Ignore cultural differences
   b. Be tailored to specific cultural contexts
   c. Focus solely on legal consequences
   d. Provide generic treatment plans
   e. Target affluent communities
5. The 1920sare associated with the popular myth that characterised the Chinese population as drug dealers and sexual deviants who preyed upon vulnerable young White women.
   a. "Birth of the British Drug Underground"
   b. "Birth of the European Drug Underground"
   c. "Birth of the American Drug Underground"
   d. Saw the "Birth of the British Drug Underground"
   e. None of the above
6. Which of the following is NOT a potential factor contributing to alcohol and drug use in culturally diverse communities?
   a. Social norms
   b. Economic status
   c. Language barriers
   d. Genetic predisposition
   e. Access to healthcare
7. Cultural competence training for healthcare providers may involve:
   a. Reinforcing stereotypes
   b. Ignoring cultural differences
   c. Understanding cultural norms and values
   d. Limiting communication channels
   e. Focusing solely on medical treatments
8. Alcohol and substance use prevention strategies should consider:
   a. One-size-fits-all approaches
   b. Cultural factors
   c. Criminalising substance users
   d. Ignoring community leaders
   e. Eliminating community involvement
9. Culturally sensitive interventions may include:
   a. Stereotyping individuals
   b. Providing culturally relevant resources
   c. Ignoring cultural differences
   d. Enforcing strict regulations
   e. Prioritising individual over community needs
10. The integration of traditional healing practices into alcohol and substance use treatment:
    a. May conflict with Western medical approaches
    b. Is unnecessary in diverse communities
    c. Can only be effective in affluent communities
    d. Should be discouraged
    e. Is culturally insensitive

11. Family dynamics in culturally diverse communities may:
    a. Play a minimal role in substance use
    b. Be irrelevant to treatment approaches
    c. Be central to understanding and addressing substance use
    d. Require no adjustments in intervention strategies
    e. Have no impact on cultural beliefs
12. Lack of access to culturally competent healthcare providers may result in:
    a. Increased stigma
    b. Improved treatment outcomes
    c. Greater community cohesion
    d. Reduced substance abuse rates
    e. Stronger social support networks
13. In addressing alcohol and substance use, it is important to:
    a. Overlook cultural differences
    b. Focus solely on individual responsibility
    c. Understand cultural contexts
    d. Disregard community input
    e. Ignore socio-economic factors
14. Culturally tailored prevention programmes may:
    a. Reinforce stereotypes
    b. Be less effective than generic programmes
    c. Increase community engagement
    d. Marginalise minority groups
    e. Prioritise legal consequences
15. Collaborative efforts between community leaders and healthcare providers can:
    a. Exacerbate cultural tensions
    b. Ignore community needs
    c. Improve treatment accessibility and effectiveness
    d. Undermine trust in healthcare systems
    e. Eliminate cultural diversity awareness
16. The low rates of presentation to alcohol and drug services by ethno-cultural groups may be due to a multitude of factors that include:
    a. Acculturation, acculturation stress, cultural values systems
    b. Cultural dissonance, education and literacy, previous experience of persecution
    c. Communication difficulties, religio-cultural prescriptions, discrimination, ethnicity of staff
    d. Religious values, stigma, and failure to meet their holistic needs
    e. All of the above

Activity 17.3

Questions

- List the potential barriers in the utilisation of services by culturally and linguistically different communities.

INTRODUCTION

Historically, drug laws and prohibitions of psychoactive substances have been intertwined with racism and prejudice, particularly in countries like Northern Europe, America, and Australasia, which boast multicultural societies. For instance, in the 1920s, the emergence of the British Drug Underground perpetuated myths portraying the Chinese population as drug dealers and sexual deviants preying on vulnerable White women (Kohn, 1992). Similarly, the "War on Drugs" in the United States originated in San Francisco due to fears of Chinese men luring White women into opium dens, reinforcing racist perceptions (Block, 2012, 2013). Cocaine was associated with African Americans, further perpetuating stereotypes of violence and antisocial behaviour (William, 1914), while Mexican Americans were linked to marijuana use and lawlessness (Block, 2013). Throughout history, addictive substances have been used to undermine non-European societies and advance White interests (Nunn, 2002). In Australia, the prohibition of opium was motivated by racism, with Anglo-Celtic Australians citing the use of opium by Chinese Australians as a threat to health and morality (Hamilton, 2001). Similarly, in Canada, negative stereotypes have been associated with Aboriginal peoples, including assumptions about alcoholism among Métis, Inuit, non-status, or First Nations individuals, although these beliefs are gradually changing. Alcohol has been used as a tool of exploitation and control by colonisers and oppressors against Indigenous peoples and minority groups. For example, European colonisers introduced alcohol to Indigenous communities in the Americas and other regions as a means of subjugation and exploitation. Alcohol has been associated with racial stereotypes and stigmatisation (Loersch et al., 2015). For instance, aggressive marketing of distilled drinks to African Americans has been encouraged, perpetuating racial stereotypes and potentially exacerbating alcohol-related harm within this community (Toner, 2020). Stereotypes have reduced opportunities for Asian Americans to seek help for drinking problems, highlighting the intersection of racial discrimination and access to healthcare (Caetano et al., 1998). Racially differentiated alcohol regulations in Australia, based on long-standing stereotypes about Indigenous drinking, have compounded rather than reduced alcohol-related harm, demonstrating the detrimental impact of racial bias on policy outcomes (D'Abbs, 2012). In the United States, the "drunken Indian" stereotype still influences attitudes of government officials involved in harm reduction programmes for Native Americans (Fish et al., 2017; Holmes & Antell, 2001). Overall, these examples illustrate how racial stereotypes perpetuate inequality and contribute to alcohol-related harm, highlighting the need for interventions that address both systemic racism and the specific needs of diverse communities in alcohol policy and harm reduction efforts.

CULTURE: ALCOHOL AND SUBSTANCE USE

Most culturally and linguistically diverse communities have used and misused alcohol, tobacco, and psychoactive substances throughout the ages for ceremonial, medicinal, or recreational purposes. These practices are often deeply rooted in cultural heritage and may play significant roles in social rituals and community bonding. Cultural and social factors have a significant influence role in the initiation, maintenance, and therapeutic intervention of substance misuse. It has been suggested that "different national cultures have their own ways of using intoxicants, with subcultures creating and renewing variations in use. All intoxicants are part of a cultural whole" (Seppälä & Salasuo, 2005, p. 1). Hoffman and Unger (2020) examined nine types of addictions – shopping, work, gambling, internet, substance use, exercise, food, sex, and love – which are intertwined with five aspects of role-of-culture information. They explore how these addictions are influenced by cultural factors, including ethnicity, nationality, gender, sexual orientation, and historical trends. These five key aspects of cultural influence are intertwined within the broader context of various addictive behaviours, emphasising that cultural influences shape perceptions, experiences, and responses to addiction.

The use of psychoactive substances among adolescents can stem from various factors, including rebellion against authority, the need for social inclusion, and differentiation from other peer groups. Alienation from one's social group and acculturation stress are significant determinants in the initiation of illicit drug use. Research suggests that adolescents who strongly identify with their communities and cultures are less susceptible to drug use risk factors and benefit more from protective factors (Zickler, 1999). Other influential factors in substance misuse include disengagement from education or employment, unsuccessful attempts to access education or employment, and familial or marital discord. While the types of psychoactive substances misused by ethnic communities may not differ significantly from those used by the White population, there are preferences for specific classes of substances and modes of consumption among different ethnic groups. These preferences are often linked to the historical and cultural characteristics of each ethnic group (Oyefeso et al., 2000).

Culturally and linguistically diverse communities encompass a broad spectrum of individuals with differing values, attitudes, religious beliefs, and customs, all of which influence patterns of alcohol and substance use. This diversity, characterised by variations in lifestyle, health behaviour, religion, and language, profoundly impacts how these communities perceive and recognise health problems and ill-health, particularly within the framework of Western medicine and the healthcare system (Rassool, 1995). While cultural and religious factors undoubtedly play a role in shaping health beliefs and behaviours, it is noted that factors such as gender, age, and socio-economic status may hold greater importance (Thom et al., 2010). Religious beliefs can significantly influence attitudes towards addiction and addiction treatment. There is evidence to suggest that over 84% of scientific studies demonstrate faith as a positive factor in addiction prevention or recovery (Grim & Grim, 2019). This suggests that incorporating spiritual beliefs and practices into addiction treatment and recovery programmes may be beneficial for many individuals. Additionally, it highlights the importance of recognising and respecting diverse spiritual beliefs and incorporating them into personalised treatment plans. Higher religiosity and adherence to religious/spiritual practices are related to the necessity and effectiveness of treatments for addiction, especially spiritually based treatments (Grant Weinandy & Grubbs, 2021). This implies that individuals with strong religious beliefs may place greater faith in interventions that incorporate spiritual elements as part of the recovery process.

ASSESSING HEALTH NEEDS

Health needs assessment, as defined by the National Institute for Health and Clinical Excellence (NICE, 2017), is a systematic process aimed at evaluating the health issues affecting a population. It involves identifying groups more susceptible to illness and uncovering any disparities in service provision ultimately leading to the establishment of priorities to enhance healthcare within a specific area. According to Rawaf (2002), a comprehensive health and social needs assessment serves as a vital foundation for developing intervention strategies, service improvements, and health promotion initiatives, particularly for culturally and linguistically diverse populations. The determinants of alcohol and drug use can vary among culturally and linguistically diverse communities due to differences in community structure, genetic make-up, socio-economic status, cultural and religious beliefs, as well as intergenerational and acculturation factors. It is essential for service provision to be informed by an understanding of the local ethnic population's composition, influencing not only service delivery but also the cultural competence training of the workforce. Rawaf and Marshall (1999) have outlined ten practical steps for conducting a health needs assessment for drug misusers, emphasising the importance of tailored and responsive services that address the diverse health needs of the population. These steps provide a framework for evaluating and addressing the unique challenges and requirements of culturally diverse communities in the provision of alcohol and drug services. Table 17.1 presents the ten steps in conducting a health needs assessment.

PREVENTION STRATEGIES

Tailored interventions and prevention strategies are essential for addressing substance misuse within culturally and linguistically diverse communities effectively. These strategies include culturally sensitive education and outreach programmes, community-based support networks, culturally competent counselling and treatment services, collaboration with faith leaders and community organisations and leaders, holistic approaches to health and well-being, promotion of cultural identity and pride, and prevention through education and empowerment. By implementing these strategies, stakeholders can better meet the unique needs of diverse communities and reduce disparities in substance misuse care. Table 17.2 depicts the prevention strategies

Table 17.1
Steps for assessing health needs of drug and alcohol users

Steps	Health needs assessment
Step 1	In looking at your population, you need to understand your population size, structure, dynamic segment, ethnic diversities, language diversities, etc.
Step 2	Identify the incidence and prevalence of the condition/problem. Use published local/national figures.
Step 3	Calculate the expected number of cases (total, age groups, gender, etc.). Apply step 2 to step 1.
Step 4	Measure service utilisation (health, social, housing, etc.) (self-help, primary care, secondary care, specialist service).
Step 5	Calculate unmet needs. Step 3 minus step 4.
Step 6	Assess effectiveness of intervention(s).
Step 7	Seek population's views (experience, expectations). Consult with local key stakeholders.
Step 8	Assess professionals' views (especially local) (clinical practice, feasibility, barriers, etc.). Their local views are therefore an essential step to define the services required.
Step 9	Define priorities (take into account current and new resources). Shifting resources from existing services, re-engineering services, and dis-investing in ineffective services should be considered as part of the defining priorities process.
Step 10	Advise on intervention(s)/healthcare programme(s)/strategy. Any emerging recommendations and plans need to be feasible, practical, and affordable.

Source: Adapted from Rawaf and Marshall (1999).

Table 17.2
Prevention strategies

Strategy	Activities
Holistic approach to health and well-being	Holistic approach to addressing alcohol and substance misuse. Addressing underlying social determinants of health, such as poverty, discrimination, and lack of access to healthcare. Provide resources and support for issues, such as housing, employment, and mental health, within culturally diverse communities.
Culturally tailored education and outreach programmes	Develop educational materials and outreach programmes that are culturally sensitive and linguistically appropriate. Translating materials into different languages, incorporating cultural symbols and references. Provide information on the risks and consequences of alcohol and substance misuse, as well as practical strategies for prevention and harm reduction.
Community-based support groups and peer networks	Establish support groups and peer networks. Groups can offer mutual support, encouragement, and understanding within a culturally relevant context.
Culturally competent counselling and treatment services	Train healthcare professionals and counsellors to be culturally competent. This includes understanding cultural beliefs about addiction, respecting cultural norms and values, and adapting treatment approaches to meet the needs of diverse populations.
Promotion of cultural identity and pride	Promote cultural identity and pride as protective factors against alcohol and substance use. Celebrate cultural traditions, customs, and heritage within communities to foster a sense of belonging and resilience.
Collaboration with community organisations and leaders	Partner with community organisations, religious leaders, and cultural institutions. These partnerships can help build trust, increase engagement, and ensure that services are culturally relevant and accessible.
Prevention through education and empowerment	Empower individuals within culturally diverse communities through education and skills-building initiatives.

SERVICE PROVISION AND BARRIERS TO SERVICE UTILISATION

Service provisions for culturally and linguistically different individuals often lack coordination and cultural appropriateness, presenting significant barriers to accessing alcohol and substance misuse services. Marginality, social exclusion, racial discrimination, and institutional racism further compound these challenges, impacting individuals' experiences and their ability to access care (Rassool, 2006). Barriers exist at three levels: the patient level, where cultural differences and stigma may deter individuals from seeking help; the provider level, where cultural competence and language barriers may hinder effective communication and care delivery; and the system level, where structural inequalities and inadequate resources may limit access to culturally appropriate services (Scheppers et al., 2006). Addressing these barriers is crucial for ensuring equitable access to substance misuse services for culturally and linguistically diverse communities.

- The barriers at patient level were related to the patient characteristics: demographic variables (age, gender, ethnicity), social structure variables, health beliefs and attitudes, personal enabling resources, community enabling resources, perceived illness, and personal health practices.
- The barriers at provider level were related to the provider characteristics: skills and attitudes.
- The barriers at system level were related to the system characteristics: the organisation of the healthcare system.

The low rates of engagement with alcohol and drug services among ethno-cultural groups can be attributed to various factors, including acculturation, acculturation stress, cultural values, cultural dissonance, education and literacy levels, past experiences of persecution, communication difficulties, religio-cultural beliefs, discrimination, ethnicity of staff, denial of substance misuse within Black and minority ethnic communities, and a lack of understanding of their culture (Rassool, 1995; Alcohol Concern, 2003). Ethnic minority groups often face barriers to accessing alcohol treatment services, including low awareness of health risks, difficulty navigating services, lack of recognition by professionals, stigma, and community shame (Institute of Alcohol Studies, 2020). Additionally, delayed help-seeking is common until serious health issues arise. These barriers highlight the need for increased awareness, culturally sensitive services, and improved trust in healthcare systems to address alcohol-related concerns among ethnic minorities effectively. Many service agencies tend to be mainstream and ethnocentric in their approach, leading to inadequate service delivery that fails to meet the health needs of culturally diverse communities (Rassool, 2006). Institutional racism and cultural dissonance have been found to marginalise South Asian service users from accessing quality and effective mental healthcare in the UK (Prajapati & Liebling, 2022). As a result, there are numerous potential barriers hindering these communities from accessing alcohol and drug services. These barriers must be addressed to ensure equitable access to care and support for all individuals, regardless of cultural background. Some of the barriers are presented in Table 17.3.

Table 17.3
Barriers to service utilisation

- Lack of awareness of local services
- Experience of racism
- Language barrier
- Lack of skills of staff
- Access to translated health information
- Access to trained interpreters
- Opiate focus of drug treatment
- Inadequate services
- Not meeting holistic needs
- Stigma
- Family honour
- Remoteness of services
- Immigration status and displacement
- Previous negative experiences
- Religious belief
- Islamophobia
- Microagression

SERVICE ACCESS: HOW TO ENCOURAGE CULTURALLY AND LINGUISTICALLY DIVERSE COMMUNITIES' UTILISATION OF ALCOHOL AND DRUG SERVICES

It is widely recognised that people from culturally and linguistically diverse communities often have limited knowledge of available support services. Many individuals with alcohol and drug problems are hesitant to seek help due to stigma, shame, adherence to family traditions, and religious beliefs. To address personal, provider, and organisational barriers, recommendations from the Black and Minority Ethnic Drug Misuse Needs Assessment Project (Bashford et al., 2003) are outlined in Table 17.3. These recommendations aim to improve access to and utilisation of support services among diverse communities. In Australia, the Network of Alcohol and Other Drug Agencies (NADA) has outlined strategies for addiction specialists to improve the accessibility, effectiveness, and appropriateness of services for culturally and linguistically diverse communities. These strategies include patient-centred communication, the use of trained interpreters, respect for cultural taboos, flexibility in intake and assessment procedures, and creating a welcoming environment through diverse signage and workforce recruitment. These efforts aim to address barriers and enhance the quality of care provided to diverse populations seeking addiction services.

In summary, addressing the needs of ethnic and culturally diverse communities requires a more explicit and committed organisational focus on diversity, along with increased resource allocation to meet their needs effectively. Research underlines several institutional failings, including a lack of equitable and accessible services, inadequate response to distinct patterns of misuse, failure to address cultural and diverse needs, and a lack of culturally competent services. To overcome these challenges, institutions must prioritise diversity, allocate resources accordingly, and enhance cultural competence among service providers to ensure equitable and effective support for diverse communities grappling with alcohol and substance use disorders.

KEY POINTS

- Culturally and linguistically different communities are a heterogeneous group.
- Historically, culturally and linguistically different communities have been the victims of negative stereotypes, social exclusions, health inequalities, disparate treatment, and racism.
- Cultural and social factors have a significant influence role in the initiation, maintenance, and therapeutic intervention of alcohol and substance use disorder.
- The psychoactive substances misused by culturally and linguistically different communities are not clearly different from those used by the White population, but there seem to be preferences for a certain class or classes of substances and mode of consumption.
- Tailored interventions and prevention strategies are essential for addressing substance misuse within culturally and linguistically diverse communities effectively.
- These prevention strategies include culturally sensitive education and outreach programmes, community-based support networks, culturally competent counselling and treatment services, collaboration with faith leaders and community organisations and leaders, holistic approaches to health and well-being, promotion of cultural identity and pride, and prevention through education and empowerment.
- Some of the service provisions for those who are culturally and linguistically different are sometimes patchy and uncoordinated and not ready to provide culturally appropriate care and interventions.
- Potential barriers occur at three different levels: patient level, provider level, and system level.
- There is a myriad of potential barriers that may inhibit culturally and linguistically different communities from utilisation of alcohol and drug services.
- There needs to be more explicit and overt organisational commitment to diversity and more resources dedicated to meeting the needs of people from ethnic and culturally diverse communities.

References

Alcohol Concern. (2003). *Alcohol Drinking Among Black and Minority Ethnic Communities (BME) in the United Kingdom*. London: Acquire.

Bashford, J., Buffin, J., & Patel, K. (2003). *The Department of Health's Black and Minority Ethnic Drug Misuse Needs Assessment Project. Part 2 The Findings*. The Centre for Ethnicity and Health, Faculty of Health, University of Central Lancashire. http://clok.uclan.ac.uk/2591/1/Buffi n_rep2comeng2.pdf (accessed 24 June 2024).

Block, F. (2012). *Disrobed: An Inside Look at the Life and Work of a Federal Trial Judge*. Minnesota: Thomson West.

Block, F. (2013). *Racism's Hidden History in the War on Drugs*. https://www.ungassondrugs.org/en/newsroom/latest-news/item/4249-racisms-hidden-history-in-the-war-on-drug-swww.huffingtonpost.com/judge-frederic-block/war-on-drugs_b_2384624.html (accessed 23 March 2024).

Caetano, R., Clark, C. L., & Tam, T. (1998). Alcohol consumption among racial/ethnic minorities: Theory and research. *Alcohol Health and Research World, 22*(4), 233–241.

D'Abbs, P. (2012). Problematizing alcohol through the eyes of the other: Alcohol policy and aboriginal drinking in the Northern Territory, Australia. *Contemporary Drug Problems, 39*(3), 371–396. https://doi.org/10.1177/009145091203900303.

Fish, J., Osberg, T. M., & Syed, M. (2017). "This is the way we were raised": Alcohol beliefs and acculturation in relation to alcohol consumption among Native Americans. *Journal of Ethnicity in Substance Abuse, 16*(2), 219–245. https://doi.org/10.1080/15332640.2015.1133362.

Grant Weinandy, J. T., & Grubbs, J. B. (2021). Religious and spiritual beliefs and attitudes towards addiction and addiction treatment: A scoping review. *Addictive Behaviors Reports, 14*, 100393. https://doi.org/10.1016/j.abrep.2021.100393.

Grim, B. J., & Grim, M. E. (2019). Belief, behavior, and belonging: How faith is indispensable in preventing and recovering from substance abuse. *Journal of Religion and Health, 58*, 1713–1750. https://doi.org/10.1007/s10943-019-00876-w.

Hamilton, M. (2001). Australia's drug policy – our own? In G. Jurg & E. L. Jensen (Eds.), *Drug War, American Style: The Internationalization of Failed Policy and Its Alternatives* (essay collection). New York: Taylor & Francis, pp. 97–120.

Hoffman, B. R., & Unger, J. B. (2020). The role of culture in addiction. In S. Sussman (Ed.), *The Cambridge Handbook of Substance and Behavioral Addictions*. Cambridge: Cambridge University Press, pp. 171–181.

Holmes, M. D., & Antell, J. A. (2001). The social construction of American Indian drinking: Perceptions of American Indian and white officials. *The Sociological Quarterly, 42*(2), 51–173.

Institute of Alcohol Studies. (2020). *Ethnic Minorities and Alcohol*. https://www.ias.org.uk/wp-content/uploads/2020/12/Ethnic-minorities-and-alcohol.pdf (accessed 23 March 2024).

Kohn, M. (1992). *Dope Girls: The Birth of the British Drug Underground*. London: Lawrence and Wishart.

Loersch, C., Bartholow, B. D., Manning, M., Calanchini, J., & Sherman, J. W. (2015). Intoxicated prejudice: The impact of alcohol consumption on implicitly and explicitly measured racial attitudes. *Group Processes & Intergroup Relations. GPIR, 18*(2), 256–268. https://doi.org/10.1177/1368430214561693.

NICE. (2017). *Glossary*. London: National Institute for Health and Care Excellence. www.nice.org.uk/glossary?letter=h (accessed 24 June 2024).

Nunn, K. B. (2002). *Race, Crime and the Pool of Surplus Criminality: Or Why the "War on Drugs" Was a "War on Blacks"*. https://www.semanticscholar.org/author/K.-Nunn/6153571s (accessed 23 March 2024).

Oyefeso, A., Ghodse, H., Keating, A., Annan, J., Phillips, T., Pollard, M., & Nash, P. (2000). *Drug Treatment Needs of Black and Minority Ethnic Residents of the London Borough of Merton* (Addictions Resource Agency for Commissioners (ARAC) Monograph Series on Ethnic Minority Issues). London: ARAC.

Prajapati, R., & Liebling, H. (2022). Accessing mental health services: A systematic review and meta-ethnography of the experiences of South Asian service users in the UK. *Journal of Racial and Ethnic Health Disparities, 9*(2), 598–619. https://doi.org/10.1007/s40615-021-00993-x.

Rassool, G. H. (1995). The health status and health care of ethno-cultural minorities in the United Kingdom: An agenda for action. *Journal of Advanced Nursing, 21*, 199–201.

Rassool, G. H. (2006). Black and ethnic minority communities: Substance misuse and mental health: Whose problem anyway? In G. H. Rassool (Ed.), *Dual Diagnosis Nursing*. Oxford: Blackwell Publications.

Rawaf, S. (2002). Assessing health and social needs and develop appropriate services: A public health perspective. In G. H. Rassool (Ed.), *Dual Diagnosis*. Oxford: Blackwell Publications.

Rawaf, S, & Marshall, F. (1999). Drug misuse: The ten steps for needs assessment. *Public Health Medicine, 1*, 21–26.

Scheppers, E., van Dongen, E., Dekker, J., Geertzen, J., & Dekker, J. (2006). Potential barriers to the use of health services among ethnic minorities: A review. *Family Practice, 23*(3), 325–348. https://doi.org/10.1093/fampra/cmi113.

Seppälä, P., & Salasuo, M. (2005). *Drug Use as Part of Culture*. www.paihdelinkki.fi/en/info-bank/articles/substance-use-and-society/drug-use-part-culture (accessed 24 March 2024).

Thom, B., Lloyd, C., Hurcombe, R., Bayley, M., Stone, K., Thickett, A., Watts, B., & Tiffany, C. (2010). *Black and Minority Ethnic Groups and Alcohol*. Report to the Department of Health. London: Department of Health.

Toner, D. (2020). *Why Is It Important to Understand the Development of Racial Stereotypes About Alcohol? Alcohol History: Alcohol, Race and Ethnicity: The United States, Mexico and the Wider World, 1845–1940*. https://alcoholhistory.le.ac.uk/?p=37 (accessed 23 March 2024).

William, E. (1914). Negro cocaine fiends are a New Southern Menace, 8 February 1914. *New York Times.com*. https://www.nytimes.com/1914/02/08/archives/negro-cocaine-fiends-are-a-new-southern-menace-murder-and-insanity.htm.

Zickler, P. (1999). Ethnic identification and cultural ties may help prevent drug use. *NIDA Notes, 14*, 7–9.

Chapter 18

Vulnerable people

The elderly and homeless and alcohol and drug use

INTRODUCTION

This chapter has two sections. Section I focuses on the use of alcohol and drugs among the elderly. Section II provides an overview of alcohol and drug misuse in homelessness.

Learning outcomes

- Describe the prevalence and pattern of alcohol and substance misuse amongst the elderly.
- List the signs and symptoms associated with alcohol misuse in the elderly.
- Identify the type of illicit and prescribed psychoactive substances used.
- Discuss the risk factors and effects of substance misuse in the elderly.
- Describe the nature and pattern of substance misuse among the homeless.
- List the factors which contribute to becoming homeless.
- Discuss the relationship between homelessness and substance misuse.

Activity 18.1

There is only one correct answer to the following multiple-choice questions.

1. What is a common but often overlooked problem among the elderly, leading to significant negative impacts on their health and quality of life?
   a. Obesity
   b. Substance misuse
   c. Hypertension
   d. Diabetes
   e. Arthritis
2. Which substance is most commonly used among older individuals?
   a. Cocaine
   b. Marijuana
   c. Heroin
   d. Tobacco
   e. Methamphetamine

DOI: 10.4324/9781003456674-21

3. What is a common form of substance misuse observed among the elderly?
   a. Daily marijuana use
   b. Weekly heroin injections
   c. Binge drinking
   d. Intravenous cocaine use
   e. Ecstasy consumption
4. Which of the following statements regarding tobacco use among the elderly is true?
   a. Elderly individuals are less likely to have ever smoked compared to younger individuals.
   b. Elderly individuals are more likely to have ever smoked compared to younger individuals.
   c. Elderly individuals have the same likelihood of smoking as younger individuals.
   d. Smoking rates among the elderly have declined to zero.
   e. Smoking rates among the elderly have increased dramatically.
5. What is a significant risk factor contributing to homelessness among the elderly population?
   a. Lack of education
   b. Family support
   c. History of problematic substance misuse
   d. High income
   e. Stable housing
6. Elderly people have:
   a. More tolerance to the adverse effects of alcohol
   b. Less tolerance to the adverse effects of alcohol
   c. Increase in body water
   d. Increased hepatic blood flow
   e. None of the above
7. Which of the following is a common consequence of substance misuse among elderly individuals who experience homelessness?
   a. Improved mental health
   b. Decreased risk of chronic diseases
   c. Enhanced social support
   d. Further exacerbation of homelessness
   e. Increased access to healthcare services
8. Alcohol-related health problems in elderly people include:
   a. Decreased risk of coronary heart disease
   b. Increased risk of falls
   c. Decreased risk of Alzheimer's disease
   d. Decreased risk of prescribed drug interactions
   e. None of the above
9. Many physical or psychological conditions in the elderly:
   a. May mimic drug and alcohol misuse
   b. May show signs of craving
   c. May be present
   d. Shows denial
   e. None of the above

10. Older people receive:
    a. Less prescribed medications of benzodiazepines
    b. More prescribed medications of benzodiazepines
    c. The same amount of medications as other age groups
    d. More major tranquilliser medications
    e. None of the above
11. In elderly people:
    a. There are no clear recommended sensible drinking limits.
    b. There is greater vulnerability to the harmful effects of alcohol.
    c. Routine screening for alcohol problems is not useful.
    d. Alcohol and drug problems are the same.
    e. None of the above is correct.

ALCOHOL, DRUGS, AND THE ELDERLY

Addiction to illicit drugs and alcohol in elderly individuals is a growing concern. This demographic faces unique challenges and risks associated with alcohol and drug consumption due to factors such as changes in metabolism, medication interactions, and underlying health conditions (NIDA, 2024). It seems that older adults tend to metabolise substances at a slower rate, and their brains may exhibit increased sensitivity to drugs (Colliver et al., 2006). This slower metabolism can result in higher blood concentrations of drugs and alcohol, leading to an increased risk of adverse effects and toxicity. Substance misuse among the elderly can have significant negative impacts on physical health, cognitive function, mental well-being, and overall quality of life.

Three distinct groups of older substance misusers have been identified: "early-onset misusers," "late-onset misusers," and "intermittent misusers," or binge drinkers.

- *Early-onset misusers*, also known as "survivors," have a long history of alcohol and/or drug misuse, often starting at a young age. They typically have a family history of alcohol use disorder and may experience significant health issues, such as psychiatric illness, cirrhosis, and organic brain syndromes (Menninger, 2002). This group faces a reduced lifespan, with estimates suggesting a decrease of 10 to 15 years due to the health risks associated with heavy drinking (Institute of Alcohol Studies, 2007).
- *Late-onset misusers*, or "reactors," begin problematic substance use later in life, often in response to traumatic life events, such as the loss of a loved one, loneliness, or retirement. This group may experience significant life changes, including loss of employment, reduced income, and familial conflict.
- *Intermittent misusers*, or binge drinkers, use alcohol occasionally and may consume to excess, leading to problems. Both late-onset misusers and intermittent misusers have a higher chance of managing their substance misuse if they have access to appropriate treatment, such as counselling and general support (Institute of Alcohol Studies, 2007).

These categorisations highlight the diverse pathways and factors contributing to substance misuse among older adults, emphasising the importance of tailored interventions and support services to address their unique needs.

Elderly individuals often take multiple medications for various health conditions, and the addition of psychoactive substances, such as alcohol or illicit drugs, can exacerbate the risk of adverse drug interactions. These interactions can occur due to pharmacokinetic factors, where the absorption, distribution, metabolism, or excretion of one substance is altered by another. Additionally, pharmacodynamic interactions may occur, where the combined effects of substances lead to amplified or unexpected effects on the body. Over 80% of individuals in a study reported daily use of at least one prescription medication, and close to half reported using more than five medications or supplements. This indicates that approximately 1 in 25 people in this age bracket may be at risk of experiencing a significant drug–drug interaction (Qato et al., 2008).

Older women are particularly vulnerable to the adverse effects of alcohol due to their biological and physiological characteristics. Research suggests that women may be more prone to developing alcohol-related problems later in life compared to men (NIDA, 2015)

This vulnerability is compounded by the fact that older women, more than any other demographic, frequently use psychotropic medications for psychological issues. The findings of the study (Peltier et al., 2020) suggest that as women go through the menopausal transition, there is a notable period of instability in their alcohol use. This period may involve fluctuations in the frequency, quantity, or patterns of alcohol consumption among women. These changes could be influenced by various factors associated with menopause, such as hormonal fluctuations, changes in mood or stress levels, shifts in social dynamics, or alterations in health status.

The elderly population faces unique challenges regarding the diagnosis and treatment of substance misuse, as many physical and psychological conditions common in this demographic can mimic the signs of drug and alcohol misuse. Long-term prescription of medications, particularly hypnotics, anxiolytics, and analgesics, plays a significant role in the development of substance misuse among older individuals (Royal College of Psychiatrists, 2011). Classic features of substance dependence, such as craving, may be absent in older adults, and individuals may deny or downplay their substance use when directly questioned (McGrath et al., 2005). Ageism, denial, stereotyping, and non-specific symptoms further complicate the identification and management of substance misuse in this population, along with stigma, shame, and social isolation (Royal College of Psychiatrists, 2015). The risk factors associated with alcohol and substance disorder in the elderly are presented in Table 18.1.

Effects of alcohol misuse

Alcohol use disorders in elderly individuals can lead to a variety of physical and psychosocial complications. A family history of alcoholism is a risk factor for early-onset drinkers and may have genetic components. Ageing can heighten sensitivity to alcohol's effects, resulting in a higher blood alcohol concentration from the same amount of alcohol compared to younger individuals (Rassool, 2012). Research suggests that even moderate alcohol consumption may impair older adults, although they may not perceive this impairment (Gilbertson et al., 2009). Furthermore, the concurrent use of prescribed and over-the-counter medications with alcohol can pose significant health risks.

Alcohol use disorders in older individuals can lead to a myriad of physical and psychosocial challenges. Physical complications may include liver or brain damage, heart disease, hypertension, cancer, gastrointestinal issues, "holiday heart syndrome" (arrhythmia after alcohol binge), peripheral neuropathy, osteoporosis, and Wernicke's encephalopathy. Social factors such as social exclusion, isolation, bereavement, lack of support, cognitive decline, and declining health contribute to higher rates of alcohol use among older adults (Royal College of

Table 18.1
Risk factors for substance use disorders in elderly people

Psychosocial problems	Physical risk factors	Practical problems
Bereavement	Chronic pain	Impaired self-care
Decreased social activity	Physical disabilities	Reduced coping skills
Loss of friends	Transitions in living or care situations	Altered financial circumstances
Loss of social status	Poor health status	Forced retirement or change in income
Loss of occupational role	Chronic illness	Reduced mobility
Depression	Taking a lot of medicines and supplements	
Loss of loved ones		
Avoidance coping style History of substance use disorders		
Previous or current mental illness		
Feeling socially isolated		

Source: Adapted from NIDA (2020).

Psychiatrists, 2011). Alcohol also impairs reaction time, increasing the risk of accidents, which is a significant cause of falls – a leading cause of mortality and morbidity in older individuals (Wright & Whyley, 1994). Older individuals with alcohol use disorder are more susceptible to various health complications, such as diabetes, hypertension, heart failure, liver and bone disorders, cognitive impairment, and mood disturbances (Grant et al., 2017).

Alcohol misuse in older age is associated with various psychiatric problems, including depression, anxiety, phobias, and an increased risk of suicide. Withdrawal from alcohol may lead to delirium or acute confusional states, along with manifestations of Korsakoff's syndrome. While cognitive impairment is more common among heavy alcohol users, the relationship between alcohol use and dementia is complex. Studies suggest that heavy alcohol use increases the risk of developing vascular dementia and alcohol-related dementia (Farcnik & Persyko, 2005). Additionally, alcohol can act as a trigger for Parkinson's disease in older individuals, and delirium tremens is associated with higher mortality rates in this age group (Feuerlein & Reiser, 1986). Psychiatric disorders such as schizophrenia may co-exist with alcohol problems in older adults, resulting in complex treatment needs (Dar, 2006). Healthcare professionals should remain vigilant for older individuals who may have been exposed to tuberculosis during childhood and may be at risk for bloodborne infections such as HIV. Accidental misuse of prescription drugs and exacerbation of existing mental health issues are additional risks associated with substance misuse in older adults. For instance, a study (Schepis et al., 2019) found that over 25% of individuals over 50 who misuse prescription opioids or benzodiazepines reported suicidal ideation, compared to only 2% of those who do not use them. This highlights the importance of thorough screening before prescribing such medications to older adults. The signs and symptoms of alcohol misuse in the elderly are presented in Table 18.2.

Illicit psychoactive substances

Despite the emergence of a cohort of recreational and dependent addicts in the elderly, there is limited data that exists on the prevalence of illicit substance misuse among older adults. Illicit drug use among older individuals is on the rise in Europe (EMCDDA, 2010) and the United States (NIDA, 2020). In the European Union (EU), heroin is the primary drug of choice for the majority (65%) of older drug users, followed by cocaine, cannabis, and synthetic stimulants (EMCDDA, 2010). On the

Table 18.2
Signs and symptoms of alcohol misuse in elderly people

Physical	Psychological
• Falls	• Drinking to manage negative experiences
• Bruises	• Anxiety
• Incontinence	• Acute confusional state
• Increased tolerance to alcohol	• Withdrawn
• Poor hygiene	• Depression
• Poor nutrition	• Blackouts
• Increased risk of accidents	• Disorientation
• Increased risk of hypothermia	• Memory loss
• Increased risk of stroke and heart disease	• Dementia
• Increased risk of cancer	• Difficulty in decision-making
• Poor liver functioning	• Impact on family member
• Seizures	
• Gastrointestinal complaints	
• Hypertension	
• Mixing alcohol and medications	

contrary, in the United States, cannabis use among older adults is notably more prevalent than the use of cocaine, inhalants, hallucinogens, methamphetamine, or heroin (Kuerbis et al., 2014). As cannabis, cocaine, and synthetic drug use rise among younger generations, it is anticipated that the number of older adults using these substances will significantly increase in the future. Furthermore, the passage of decriminalisation and medical cannabis legislation may contribute to increased cannabis use among older adults as they seek relief from illness-related side effects (Blazer & Wu, 2009). Consequently, there is a growing cohort of recreational and dependent older users expected in the future.

In the European Union (EU), the majority (65%) of older drug users reported heroin as the primary drug of choice, followed by cocaine, cannabis, and synthetic stimulants (EMCDDA, 2010). In contrast, in the United States, the use of cannabis by older adults is considerably more prevalent than cocaine, inhalants, hallucinogens, methamphetamine, and/or heroin use (Kuerbis et al., 2014). Because cannabis, cocaine, and synthetic drug use is rising in the younger generation, it is likely that the number of older people using these psychoactive substances will increase significantly in the future. In addition, it has been suggested that with the passage of decriminalisation and medical cannabis legislations, the rate of use among older adults may increase as they use it to cope with illness-related side effects (Blazer & Wu, 2009). Thus, the future lies with an increasing elderly cohort of recreational and dependent users.

As regular recreational and dependent users of illicit drugs age, they are more likely to experience increased physical and psychosocial complications associated with the ageing process. Drug use can heighten the risk of, or worsen, conditions related to both the body and brain ageing (Beynon et al., 2009). Among older individuals, drug-related ailments may include cardiopulmonary conditions resulting from injecting drug use, changes in blood pressure, susceptibility to deep vein thrombosis, and infections such as HIV and hepatitis C. Additionally, drug use has been identified as a risk factor for earlier onset of conditions like diabetes, neurological disorders, and cancer (EMCDDA, 2010). Concerning psychological well-being, prolonged use of illicit psychoactive substances has been linked to depression and cognitive impairments (Dowling et al., 2008). Older users may experience common symptoms, such as anxiety, loneliness, memory problems, confusion, disorientation, and dementia.

Addiction to psychoactive substances among the elderly can also stem from "iatrogenic dependence," which refers to the inappropriate prescribing of psychoactive medications by medical practitioners. Older individuals often receive more prescribed medications, and the prevalence of drug misuse is notably higher in women compared to men. Women, especially those who are widowed and less educated and have lower income, poor health, and reduced social support, are at increased risk of dependence (King et al., 1994). Psychoactive drugs such as anxiolytics, hypno-sedatives, tranquillisers, and antidepressants are commonly prescribed for older individuals, and many in this demographic also frequently use over-the-counter medications. A study by Whitcup and Miller (1987) revealed that 21% of patients aged 65 or older admitted to a psychiatric unit had a diagnosis of drug dependence, with benzodiazepine dependence being the most common. Moreover, several non-prescription medicinal preparations available in pharmacies are purchased for their non-medical therapeutic effects. For example, antihistamines may be used for their sedative properties or mixed with methadone or heroin, while the amphetamine derivatives in decongestants can serve as stimulants. Additionally, cough linctus and diarrhoea medications containing opiates may be misused for their psychoactive effects.

Nicotine addiction

Tobacco is the most commonly used psychoactive substance among older people. Older individuals face heightened vulnerability to the consequences of smoking due to the cumulative effects of smoke exposure. The over-60s are also more likely than younger people to have smoked at some time in their lives; however, they are more likely than younger people to have given up. While cardiovascular diseases are the most prevalent health issues linked to smoking, the habit also impacts various other systems, including respiratory, nervous, and integumentary systems, among others (Bassil et al., 2022). Many studies have shown that broken bones tend to take longer to heal if those who are injured have smoked (Hoogendoorn et al., 2002). Research on the effects of vaping nicotine (e-cigarettes) among older adults is limited, but certain risks exist across all age groups. While some studies suggest that e-cigarettes may be less harmful than traditional cigarettes when used as a complete replacement by regular smokers, the evidence is mixed (NIDA, 2020). Smoking cessation among older adults (age ≥65 years) is key to cancer prevention (Henley et al., 2019). Quitting smoking can be particularly challenging for the elderly population. Hence, it is essential for healthcare professionals to actively encourage older patients to quit smoking during every patient–healthcare interaction, providing brief interventions, counselling, and considering replacement therapy options.

Co-occurring disorders

There is limited research on the co-existence of alcohol or substance use disorder and psychiatric disorders in late life. Older people were more likely to have the triple diagnosis of alcoholism, depression, and personality disorder, whereas younger people were more likely to have the single diagnosis of schizophrenia (Speer & Bates, 1992). Cannabis use among older adults has been linked to psychiatric comorbidities. The findings of a study by Choi et al. (2016) revealed that older adults who solely used cannabis had a heightened probability of developing major depressive disorder in their lifetime and over the past year compared to non-users. Moreover, the likelihood of experiencing major depressive disorder increased when cannabis was used in conjunction with other illicit drugs. Similarly, Diep et al. (2022) identified that recent cannabis use was correlated with suicidal thoughts in the preceding two weeks and depression in adults. However, establishing causation in these studies presents a challenge. In elderly individuals with alcohol use disorders, co-occurrence of psychiatric disorders such as schizophrenia can complicate treatment strategies (Dar, 2006). Additionally, there is an elevated prevalence of various forms of dementia, excluding Alzheimer's disease, among older adults with alcohol use disorders (Thomas & Rockwood, 2001).

Healthcare interventions

Healthcare professionals play a vital role as the first point of contact for elderly individuals seeking medical attention. However, due to various factors such as stigma, lack of awareness, or age-related assumptions, many professionals may overlook or underestimate the prevalence of alcohol or substance use disorder among older adults. To address this issue, it is imperative to integrate routine screenings for alcohol and drug use into patient assessments, similar to other vital health parameters like blood pressure or cholesterol levels. By routinely asking about substance use, healthcare providers can identify potential problems early on and initiate appropriate interventions. Substance use disorder among this population can exacerbate existing health conditions and complicate social relationships. Therefore, it is essential to provide tailored care, management, and treatment that consider the unique needs and circumstances of elderly individuals. This may involve interdisciplinary approaches that incorporate medical, psychological, and social support services to address the holistic needs of older adults struggling with alcohol or substance use disorders.

HOMELESSNESS AND SUBSTANCE MISUSE

Homelessness is an increasing problem on a global scale, especially with those who have a history of alcohol and substance use disorder (Magwood et al., 2020). The stressors and challenges associated with homelessness, such as trauma, mental health issues, and lack of social support, can contribute to the onset and exacerbation of substance use disorders. Substance misuse is often both a cause and a result of homelessness, often arising after people lose their housing (National Coalition for the Homeless, 2009). The connection between homelessness and substance use disorder is intricate, influenced by various social, political, and economic factors. Research suggests that a significant proportion of homeless individuals attribute drugs and/or alcohol as major contributors to their homelessness (Didenko & Pankratz, 2007). Additionally, substance use may serve as a means of acceptance within the homeless community. Factors contributing to homelessness include unemployment, financial problems, mental health issues, substance misuse, physical disability, lack of affordable housing, social security benefit regulations, and social isolation due to substance use.

Homelessness, especially sleeping rough, has a profound negative impact on both the physical and psychological health of individual. Alcohol and substance use disorder coupled with poor diet, lack of regular healthcare, and inadequate living conditions exacerbates health issues among this population. Homelessness often leads to increased stress, feelings of worthlessness, and reduced self-esteem, prompting some individuals to turn to alcohol or drugs as a coping mechanism. Substance use may also serve as a form of self-medication for mental health issues, like chronic depression or schizophrenia. Risky behaviours, such as polydrug use and unsafe injecting, are common among homeless individuals, exacerbated by the lack of secure housing. The transient lifestyle associated with homelessness further contributes to risky drug use behaviours due to factors like poor hygiene, insecurity, and lack of personal organisation, impacting both the individual and the broader community (Rowe, 2005). Homelessness is strongly linked to deteriorating physical and mental health, with individuals experiencing high rates of health issues, including HIV/AIDS, hepatitis A, addiction, mental illness, tuberculosis, and other serious conditions (Sleet & Francescutti, 2021). Health complications related to alcohol misuse include gastrointestinal problems, hypertension, cardiac issues, memory loss, accidental injuries, and alcohol-related psychosis. Additionally, homelessness contributes to other health problems, such as malnutrition, dental issues, joint diseases, venereal diseases, and infectious hepatitis (Institute of Medicine, 1988). In addition, these health problems stem from psychosocial and economic factors, such as housing instability, discrimination, barriers to healthcare access, inadequate nutrition and protection, limited social services, and deficient public health infrastructure. Recently, there has been a rise in the incidence of tuberculosis (Self et al., 2021), and this is magnified in the homeless due to poor living conditions and diet. The presence of such an infection may go undetected for a considerable period of time, and a homeless person may present at an accident and emergency department with a chronic cough, fever, and haemoptysis (coughing up blood), and perhaps weight loss.

Homeless individuals struggling with alcohol and substance use disorders often avoid traditional primary healthcare services, instead relying on accident and emergency services during crises. Their willingness to engage with health services is influenced by feelings of alienation from society. Many face barriers to accessing rehabilitation facilities and may be denied shelter if intoxicated. Consequently, accessing rehabilitation and treatment facilities is challenging for those experiencing homelessness. Some areas have established nurse-led outreach teams or specialist services to reach this vulnerable group. Health workers must approach these individuals with sensitivity and strive to build trust while offering health improvement suggestions in a non-alienating manner. Despite legal and policy interventions, homelessness persists without a comprehensive public health approach.

KEY POINTS

- Alcohol misuse and drug misuse in elderly people are common but may be largely under-diagnosed and under-treated.
- Alcohol use disorders in elderly people can cause a wide range of physical and psychosocial problems.
- Three groups of older alcohol misusers have been identified: early-onset drinkers, or "survivors"; late-onset drinkers, or "reactors"; and intermittent or binge drinkers.
- Increased vulnerability due to age-related physiological changes and slower metabolism of substances.
- Higher risk of adverse effects from alcohol and drugs due to chronic illnesses and interactions with medications.
- The reported prevalence and patterns of drug misuse in older people are lower than in the younger population.
- Tobacco is the most commonly used psychoactive substance amongst the elderly.
- Limited research on the effects of substance use among older adults, particularly regarding vaping.
- The nature and pattern of alcohol and drug misuse in older people and the associated psychological and physical comorbidity are different in contrast to younger populations.
- There is limited research on the co-existence of alcohol misuse and psychiatric disorders in late life.
- The relationship of homelessness and substance misuse is complex, as trends in homelessness are clearly affected by changing social, political, and economic factors.
- There has been a rise in the incidence of tuberculosis, and this is magnified in the homeless due to poor living conditions and diet.
- Reluctance to engage with traditional healthcare services, leading to increased use of emergency services during crises.

Activity 18.2

Questions

- List the signs and symptoms of alcohol misuse in older people.
- Identify the type of illicit and prescribed psychoactive substances used.
- Describe the nature and pattern of substance misuse among the homeless.
- List the factors which contribute to becoming homeless.
- Discuss the relationship between homelessness and substance misuse.

References: the elderly and alcohol and drug use

Bassil, N. K., Ohanian, M. L. K., & Bou Saba, T. G. (2022). Nicotine use disorder in older adults. *Clinics in Geriatric Medicine*, 38(1), 119–131. https://doi.org/10.1016/j.cger.2021.07.008.

Beynon, C. M., Roe, B., Duffy, P., & Pickering, L. (2009). Self reported health status, and health service contact, of illicit drug users aged 50 and over: A qualitative interview study in Merseyside, United Kingdom. *BMC Geriatrics*, 9, 45. https://doi.org/10.1186/1471-2318-9-45.

Blazer, D. G., & Wu, L. T. (2009). The epidemiology of at-risk and binge drinking among middle-aged and elderly community adults: National survey on drug use and health. *The American Journal of Psychiatry*, 166(10), 1162–1169. https://doi.org/10.1176/appi.ajp.2009.09010016.

Choi, N. G., DiNitto, D. M., Marti, C. N., & Choi, B. Y. (2016). Relationship between marijuana and other illicit drug use and depression/suicidal thoughts among late middle-aged and older adults. *International Psychogeriatrics*, 28(4), 577–589. https://doi.org/10.1017/S1041610215001738.

Colliver, J. D., Compton, W. M., Gfroerer, J. C., & Condon, T. (2006). Projecting drug use among aging baby boomers in 2020. *Annals of Epidemiology*, 16(4), 257–265. https://doi.org/10.1016/j.annepidem.2005.08.003.

Dar, K. (2006). Alcohol use disorders in elderly people: Fact or fiction? *Advances in Psychiatric Treatment*, 12(3), 173–181. https://doi.org/10.1192/apt.12.3.173.

Diep, C., Bhat, V., Wijeysundera, D. N., Clarke, H. A., & Ladha, K. S. (2022). The association between recent cannabis use and suicidal ideation in adults: A population-based analysis of the NHANES from 2005 to 2018. *Canadian Journal of Psychiatry: Revue Canadienne de Psychiatrie*, 67(4), 259–267. https://doi.org/10.1177/07067437211996112.

Dowling, G. J., Weiss, S. R., & Condon, T. P. (2008). Drugs of abuse and the aging brain. *Neuropsychopharmacology: Official Publication of the American College of Neuropsychopharmacology*, 33(2), 209–218. https://doi.org/10.1038/sj.npp.1301412.

EMCDDA. (2010). *Treatment and Care for Older Drug Users*. Lisbon: European Monitoring Centre for Drugs and Drug Addiction.

Farcnik, K., & Persyko, M. (2005). The association between alcohol use and dementia in the elderly. *The Canadian Alzheimer Disease Review*, 8(1), 13–17.

Feuerlein, W., & Reiser, E. (1986). Parameters affecting the course and results of delirium tremens treatment. *Acta Psychiatrica Scandinavica. Supplementum*, 329, 120–123. https://doi.org/10.1111/j.1600-0447.1986.tb10547.x.

Gilbertson, R., Ceballos, N. A., Prather, R., & Nixon, S. J. (2009). Effects of acute alcohol consumption in older and younger adults: Perceived impairment versus psychomotor performance. *Journal of Studies on Alcohol and Drugs*, 70(2), 242–252. https://doi.org/10.15288/jsad.2009.70.242.

Grant, B. F., Chou, S. P., Saha, T. D., Pickering, R. P., Kerridge, B. T., Ruan, W. J., Huang, B., Jung, J., Zhang, H., Fan, A., & Hasin, D. S. (2017). Prevalence of 12-month alcohol use, high-risk drinking, and DSM-IV alcohol use disorder in the United States, 2001–2002 to 2012–2013: Results from the national epidemiologic survey on alcohol and related conditions. *JAMA Psychiatry*, 74(9), 911–923. https://doi.org/10.1001/jamapsychiatry.2017.2161.

Henley, S. J., Asman, K., Momin, B., Gallaway, M. S., Culp, M. B., Ragan, K. R., Richards, T. B., & Babb, S. (2019). Smoking cessation behaviors among older U.S. adults. *Preventive Medicine Reports*, 16, 100978. https://doi.org/10.1016/j.pmedr.2019.100978.

Hoogendoorn, J. M., Simmermacher, R. K., Schellekens, P. P., & van der Werken, C. (2002). Rauchen ist nachteilig für die Heilung von Knochen und Weichteilen [Adverse effects if smoking on healing of bones and soft tissues]. *Der Unfallchirurg*, 105(1), 76–81. https://doi.org/10.1007/s113-002-8170-8.

Institute of Alcohol Studies. (2007). *Alcohol and the Elderly* St Ives, Cambridge: Institute of Alcohol Studies.

King, C. J., Van Hasselt, V. B., Segal, D. L., & Hersen, M. (1994) Diagnosis and assessment of substance abuse in older adults Current strategies and issues. *Addictive Behaviors*, 19(1) 41–55.https://doi.org/10.1016/0306-4603(94)90050-7

Kuerbis, A., Sacco, P., Blazer, D. G., & Moore, A. A. (2014) Substance abuse among older adults. *Clinics In Geriatri*

Medicine, 30(3), 629–654. https://doi.org/10.1016/j.cger.2014.04.008.

McGrath, A., Crome, P., & Crome, I. B. (2005). Substance misuse in the older population. *Postgraduate Medical Journal*, 81(954), 228–231. https://doi.org/10.1136/pgmj.2004.023028.

Menninger, J. A. (2002). Assessment and treatment of alcoholism and substance related disorders in the elderly. *Bulletin of the Menninger Clinic*, 66, 166–184.

NIDA. (2015). *Alcohol: A Women's Health Issue*. Rockville, MD: National Institute on Alcohol Abuse and Alcoholism.

NIDA. (2020). *Substance Use in Older Adults Drug Facts*. https://nida.nih.gov/publications/drugfacts/substance-use-in-older-adults-drugfacts (accessed 26 March 2024).

Peltier, M. R., Verplaetse, T. L., Roberts, W., Moore, K., Burke, C., Marotta, P. L., Phillips, S., Smith, P. H., & McKee, S. A. (2020). Changes in excessive alcohol use among older women across the menopausal transition: A longitudinal analysis of the study of women's health across the nation. *Biology of Sex Differences*, 11(1), 37. https://doi.org/10.1186/s13293-020-00314-7.

Qato, D. M., Alexander, G. C., Conti, R. M., Johnson, M., Schumm, P., & Lindau, S. T. (2008). Use of prescription and over-the-counter medications and dietary supplements among older adults in the United States. *JAMA*, 300(24), 2867–2878. https://doi.org/10.1001/jama.2008.892.

Rassool, G. H. (2012). Types of substance misuse and risk factors. *Nursing Times*, 108(30–31), 12–14.

Royal College of Psychiatrists. (2011). *Our Invisible Addicts*. First Report of the Older Persons' Substance Misuse. Working Group of the Royal College of Psychiatrists (College Report CR165). London: The Royal College of Psychiatrists, June.

Royal College of Psychiatrists. (2015). *Substance Misuse in Older People: An Information Guide* (Cross-Faculty Report OA/AP/0). London: The Royal College of Psychiatrists.

Schepis, T. S., Simoni-Wastila, L., & McCabe, S. E. (2019). Prescription opioid and benzodiazepine misuse is associated with suicidal ideation in older adults. *International Journal of Geriatric Psychiatry*, 34(1), 122–129. https://doi.org/10.1002/gps.4999.

Speer, D. C., & Bates, K. (1992). Comorbid mental and substance disorders among older psychiatric patients. *Journal of the American Geriatric Society*, 40, 886–890.

Thomas, V. S., & Rockwood, K. J. (2001). Alcohol abuse, cognitive impairment, and mortality among older people. *Journal of the American Geriatrics Society*, 49(4), 415–420. https://doi.org/10.1046/j.1532-5415.2001.49085.x.

Whitcup, S. M., & Miller, F. (1987). Unrecognized drug dependence in psychiatrically hospitalized elderly patients. *Journal of the American Geriatrics Society*, 35(4), 297–301. https://doi.org/10.1111/j.1532-5415.1987.tb04634.x.

Wright, F., & Whyley, C. (1994). *Accident Prevention and Risk-Taking by Elderly People: The Need for Advice*. London: Age Concern Institute of Gerontology.

References: homelessness and substance misuse

Didenko, E., & Pankratz, N. (2007). Substance use: Pathways to homelessness or a way of adapting to street life? *Visions: BC's Mental Health and Addictions Journal*, 4(1), 9–10.

Institute of Medicine (US) Committee on Health Care for Homeless People. (1988). *Homelessness, Health, and Human Needs: Health Problems of Homeless People*. Washington, DC: National Academies Press, p. 3.

Magwood, O., Salvalaggio, G., Beder, M., Kendall, C., Kpade, V., Daghmach, W., Habonimana, G., Marshall, Z., Snyder, E., O'Shea, T., Lennox, R., Hsu, H., Tugwell, P., & Pottie, K. (2020). The effectiveness of substance use interventions for homeless and vulnerably housed persons: A systematic review of systematic reviews on supervised consumption facilities, managed alcohol programs, and pharmacological agents for opioid use disorder. *PLOS One*, 15(1), e0227298. https://doi.org/10.1371/journal.pone.0227298.

National Coalition for the Homeless. (2009). *Substance Abuse and Homelessness*. https://nationalhomeless.org/wp-content/uploads/2014/06/addiction-Fact-Sheet.pdf (accessed 27 March 2024).

Rowe, J. (2005). Laying the foundations: Addressing heroin use among the "street homeless". *Drugs: Education, Prevention and Policy*, 12(1), 47–59.

Self, J. L., McDaniel, C. J., Bamrah Morris, S., & Silk, B. J. (2021). Estimating and evaluating tuberculosis incidence rates among people experiencing homelessness, United States, 2007–2016. *Medical Care*, 59(Suppl 2), S175–S181. https://doi.org/10.1097/MLR.0000000000001466.

Sleet, D. A., & Francescutti, L. H. (2021). Homelessness and public health: A focus on strategies and solutions. *International Journal of Environmental Research and Public Health*, 18(21), 11660. https://doi.org/10.3390/ijerph182111660.

Chapter 19

Young people
Alcohol and drug misuse

Learning outcomes

- Discuss the nature of alcohol and drug problems in young people.
- Identify the factors that contribute to the initiation and continuation of adolescent alcohol and drug misuse.
- Discuss the parental influences on the drinking culture of their children.
- Discuss the factors and motivations for not using drugs.
- Examine the issues of co-occurring disorders in young people.
- List the presenting physical, psychological, and social features of young substance misusers.

Activity 19.1

Please choose one correct answer to the following multiple-choice questions.

1. Early initiation of alcohol and drug use among young people is associated with:
   a. Improved academic performance
   b. Decreased risk of addiction
   c. Higher socio-economic status
   d. Increased risk of addiction and academic problems
   e. Enhanced social skills
2. Parental involvement in preventing alcohol and drug misuse among young people:
   a. Has no impact on their behaviour
   b. Significantly increases the risk
   c. Reduces the risk
   d. Only affects academic performance
   e. Depends on the type of substance
3. Binge drinking among college students is characterised by:
   a. Rarely consuming alcohol in large quantities
   b. Consuming alcohol only on special occasions
   c. Regular consumption of small amounts of alcohol
   d. Consuming large amounts of alcohol over a short period
   e. Abstaining from alcohol entirely

DOI: 10.4324/9781003456674-22

4. Substance misuse among adolescents is often influenced by:
   a. Strict parental supervision
   b. Positive peer relationships
   c. Trauma or adverse childhood experiences
   d. High self-esteem
   e. Limited exposure to peer pressure
5. Date rape among young people is commonly associated with the use of:
   a. Marijuana
   b. Cocaine
   c. Rohypnol (roofies)
   d. Prescription painkillers
   e. Antidepressants
6. Protective factors against alcohol and drug misuse among young people include:
   a. Lack of parental involvement
   b. Participation in community service
   c. Early initiation of substance use
   d. Peer pressure
   e. Exposure to high-risk environments
7. The primary reason young people may engage in substance misuse is to:
   a. Improve cognitive function
   b. Enhance decision-making skills
   c. Cope with stress or emotional issues
   d. Boost self-esteem
   e. Achieve academic success
8. Young people recovering from substance misuse may be at risk of relapse due to:
   a. Strong support system
   b. Access to mental health resources
   c. Exposure to triggers or stressors
   d. High self-esteem
   e. Regular exercise routine
9. Substance misuse among homeless youth is often a result of:
   a. Stable living conditions
   b. Access to healthcare services
   c. Lack of peer influence
   d. Trauma or adverse childhood experiences
   e. High socio-economic status
10. Young people who misuse substances may experience feelings of:
    a. Increased self-worth
    b. Reduced stress and anxiety
    c. Worthlessness and rejection
    d. Enhanced social skills
    e. Improved academic performance
11. Cannabis use among young people is associated with:
    a. Reduced risk of mental health disorders
    b. Increased risk of depression and anxiety
    c. Enhanced cognitive function
    d. Improved social relationships
    e. Higher academic achievement

12. Homeless youth often rely on alcohol or drugs to:
    a. Enhance their physical health
    b. Cope with stressors related to homelessness
    c. Improve their socio-economic status
    d. Build positive peer relationships
    e. Access mental health resources
13. The willingness of homeless youth to engage with health services depends on:
    a. Their stable living conditions
    b. Their access to mental health resources
    c. How distant or alienated they feel from society
    d. Their high socio-economic status
    e. Their level of educational attainment
14. Health complications associated with alcohol misuse among young people may include:
    a. Gastric problems and memory loss
    b. Enhanced cardiovascular health
    c. Improved immune function
    d. Reduced risk of accidents
    e. Increased bone density
15. Substance misuse among young people is often influenced by:
    a. Lack of access to peer support
    b. Stable family relationships
    c. Limited exposure to media influence
    d. Trauma or adverse childhood experiences
    e. High socio-economic status
16. The primary reason young people may engage in substance misuse is to:
    a. Improve cognitive function
    b. Enhance decision-making skills
    c. Cope with stress or emotional issues
    d. Boost self-esteem
    e. Achieve academic success
17. Substance misuse among young people can lead to:
    a. Enhanced mental well-being
    b. Decreased risk of accidents
    c. Improved social relationships
    d. Academic problems and addiction
    e. Reduced risk of chronic diseases
18. Legal and policy interventions have often been employed to address homelessness:
    a. With a comprehensive public health approach
    b. Without considering the health implications
    c. Solely focusing on housing solutions
    d. Ignoring socio-economic factors
    e. In collaboration with private organisations
19. Healthcare professionals should approach homeless youth with:
    a. Stigmatising attitudes
    b. Judgement and criticism
    c. Sensitivity and empathy
    d. Indifference
    e. None of the answers

20. This may lead young people from less-harmful drugs to more-harmful drugs:
    a. Gated drugs
    b. Gateway drugs
    c. Pathway drugs
    d. Stepladder drugs
    e. None of the above
21. Examples of risk-taking behaviours include all of the following except:
    a. Experimentation with illegal drugs
    b. Having sex with contraception
    c. Delinquent activity
    d. "Fast & Furious"–type driving
    e. None of the above

INTRODUCTION

Young people often experiment with alcohol and drugs due to various factors, such as peer pressure, curiosity, or to cope with stress and emotional issues. However, substance misuse among youth can lead to serious health, social, and academic consequences. It can impair cognitive function, increase the risk of accidents, and negatively impact mental health, leading to conditions like depression and anxiety. Substance misuse can also hinder academic performance and disrupt social relationships. The Crime and Justice Survey (Home Office, 2007) identified five vulnerable groups of young people: those who have never been in care, homeless youth, homeless truants, excluded from school, and serious or frequent offenders. These groups face unique challenges, such as instability, lack of support networks, and disengagement from education, increasing their susceptibility to substance misuse and involvement in criminal activities. Substance misuse among young people encompasses a wide range of substances, from readily available and legal ones like tobacco and alcohol to illegal drugs such as ecstasy, cannabis, cocaine, and heroin. While most young people experiment with these substances without experiencing long-term harm, a small minority may develop addiction. Tobacco and alcohol, despite being legal, can have severe health consequences for young people. Synthetic drugs, easily accessible online, and stimulants like crack, cocaine, amphetamines, and ecstasy are popular among youth, particularly within the club scene. There is a misconception among many young people that because alcohol or tobacco is legal, they are less risky, contributing to their use as a means of projecting an "adult image" and being perceived as "cool."

Substance use among young people often follows the "gateway" or "escalation" theory, where trying one psychoactive substance increases the likelihood of experimenting with others. For instance, using cigarettes may predict subsequent use of alcohol and cannabis. There is evidence to suggest that "among both early school leavers and students attending school, having tried cigarettes was a strong predictor of drinking alcohol and using cannabis" (Haase & Pratschke, 2011, p. 39). However, the progressing through the "gateway" may also be due to socio-cultural influences (Siddharth et al., 2016). However, the findings of a study by Nkansah-Amankra and Minelli (2016) showed that early initiation of drug use increased the risk of progression to illicit drugs, but this relationship did not persist into adulthood. This suggests that the "gateway hypothesis" may not fully explain drug use over time. Socio-cultural influences also play a role in this progression through the "gateway." Socio-cultural influences such as peers tend to have the strongest effect on adolescent substance use behaviour (Trucco, 2020). Other factors include availability to use substances, perception of substance use approval, schools, and neighbourhoods. However, research has indicated the neurobiological and behavioural changes resulting from adolescent use of nicotine, alcohol, cannabis, opioids, or their combination (Hamidullah et al., 2020). The review highlights that drug exposure during adolescence could elevate the risk of cognitive deficits, psychopathology, or subsequent substance use disorders, potentially linked to structural and functional brain alterations. Understanding the mechanisms driving these changes could offer new paths for developing therapeutics aimed at preventing and mitigating the harm associated with adolescent substance use.

MOTIVES, ADJUSTMENT, AND RISK-TAKING BEHAVIOUR IN YOUNG PEOPLE

Alcohol and substance misuse in young people should be considered in the context of "normal" adolescent risk-taking behaviours and experimentation. During adolescence, individuals often engage in various forms of risk-taking behaviour as they navigate the transition from childhood to adulthood. Experimentation with alcohol and drug is a common aspect of this developmental stage, driven by factors such as curiosity, peer influence, role models in the family, the mass media, and the desire for novelty and sensation-seeking. Young people may perceive substance use as a way to assert independence, fit in with peer groups, or cope with stress and emotions. Several groups of young people vulnerable to problematic drug use have been identified from a review of the literature on risk factors. Young people facing various vulnerabilities, such as truancy, homelessness, involvement in the criminal justice system, or living in unstable family environments, are particularly susceptible to the risks associated with substance misuse (Lloyd, 1998). These individuals often lack stable support systems and may turn to drugs or alcohol as a coping mechanism or as a means of fitting in with peers. Additionally, factors such as family history of substance use, mental health issues, and experiences of trauma further compound their susceptibility to substance misuse.

Early introduction to substances, such as during early teens, is widely recognised as a risk factor for later substance misuse, along with various other factors, including parental and family substance use problems, school difficulties, early smoking initiation, peer and media influences, family dynamics, social isolation, low self-esteem, unemployment, criminal behaviours, and genetic predispositions. Positive or negative parental views on substance use can impact a young person's risk as well. For instance, hereditary factors play a role in the development of problem drinking, with children of alcoholics being significantly more likely to develop alcohol use disorder themselves compared to those without close relatives with alcohol use disorder (Russell, 1990).

Adolescence is characterised by a natural inclination toward experimentation, adventure, and risk-taking, as well as a tendency to challenge authority. This developmental stage is marked by vulnerability to various environmental factors that shape lifestyle and behaviours (Fullerton & Ursano, 1994). It is a period of identity formation, where peer group membership and approval hold significant importance, often leading to a distancing from family and parental ties. Peer influence becomes particularly influential, especially when young people lack support, understanding, or affection from parental figures and family. Substance misuse among youth is not attributable to a single factor, but rather to a combination of multiple risk factors that interact and contribute to their decision to use alcohol or drugs.

Parental influences play a significant role in shaping their children's drinking culture, with parental alcohol use increasing the risk of initiation and intensity of later adolescent alcohol use (Tildesley & Andrews, 2008). Despite intentions to promote safe drinking, parents with liberal attitudes toward alcohol are more likely to have children who drink at risky levels and experience alcohol-related problems (Mares et al., 2011). On the contrary, parental refusal to serve alcohol and negative alcohol-specific attitudes can deter adolescent drinking and excessive alcohol use (Miller & Plant, 2003). Various parental factors contribute to delayed alcohol initiation and lower levels of later drinking, including parental modelling of drinking behaviour, alcohol-specific communication, disapproval of adolescent drinking, general discipline, rules about alcohol, parental monitoring, parent–child relationship quality, family conflict, and parental support (Ryan et al., 2011). Additionally, young people facing family disruptions, such as divorce or breakup, may be particularly vulnerable to substance misuse as a coping mechanism for distress or feelings of rejection.

Young people experience numerous adjustments in their lives, including navigating transient or turbulent sexual relationships, coming to terms with their sexuality and individual sexual orientation, transitioning from school to work or university, and facing the prospect of unemployment. These adjustments, coupled with the risk of sexual exploitation and disinhibited sexual behaviours, create potentially risky contexts for young individuals. Despite exposure to risky contexts during the transition from adolescence to adulthood, most individuals manage this period satisfactorily through resilience. *Resilience* refers to the behaviours and strategies that young people employ to make decisions against drug use, despite being exposed to drugs and other risk factors (Dillon et al., 2006). Table 19.1 presents

Table 19.1
Risk factors for youth high-risk substance use

Risk factors*	Description
Family history of substance use	Genetic predisposition can increase susceptibility to developing substance use disorders, as individuals may inherit traits that make them more prone to addiction.
Role model and favourable parental attitudes towards the behaviour	If parents or caregivers perceive substance use as acceptable or even encourage it, young people may internalise these attitudes or imitate the behaviour and be more likely to experiment with or engage in substance use themselves.
Poor parental monitoring	Inadequate supervision and lack of parental involvement in a child's life.
Parental substance use	Growing up in an environment where one or both parents misuse substances can normalise this behaviour for youth.
Family rejection	Youth experiencing rejection or discrimination from their families may turn to substance use as a coping mechanism.
Association with delinquent or substance-using peers	Peer influence is a powerful factor in shaping adolescent behaviour.
Lack of school connectedness	Feeling disconnected from school, whether due to academic struggles, social isolation, or a lack of supportive relationships with teachers and peers.
Low academic achievement	Academic difficulties can contribute to feelings of frustration, low self-esteem, and disengagement from school, creating a risk factor for substance use.
Childhood sexual abuse	Traumatic experiences such as childhood sexual abuse can have long-lasting effects on mental health and coping mechanisms.
Mental health issues	Co-occurring mental health disorders, such as depression, anxiety, or ADHD, can increase vulnerability to substance use as individuals may self-medicate to alleviate symptoms or escape from distressing thoughts and emotions.

Source: Risk factors CDC (2022).

the risk factors for youth high-risk substance use. Each of the risk factors listed plays a significant role in increasing the likelihood of youth engaging in high-risk substance use.

Factors influencing drug use and motivations for abstaining from drug use are outlined in Table 19.2. Given that only a minority of substance misusers initiate drug use in adulthood, prioritising prevention and management of adolescent substance misuse is crucial. Addressing the needs of these vulnerable youth requires targeted interventions that address the underlying factors contributing to their risk, provide access to support services, and promote positive coping strategies and healthy behaviours. By addressing these challenges comprehensively, we can work towards preventing substance misuse and promoting the well-being of young people in vulnerable situations.

PRESENTING FEATURES OF SUBSTANCE MISUSE IN YOUNG PEOPLE

In youths, the presenting features of substance misuse often manifest through changes in behaviour, such as increased secrecy or withdrawal, declines in academic performance, and prioritisation of peer groups involved in substance use. Risk-taking behaviours, physical changes like changes in appetite or hygiene, and emotional instability, including mood swings and irritability, are also common. These signs underline the importance of early detection and intervention to address substance use issues and mitigate potential long-term consequences on academic, social, and emotional well-being. Table 19.3 lists the presenting features of substance misuse in young people.

CO-OCCURRING DISORDERS IN YOUNG PEOPLE

Limited research exists on the co-occurrence of mental health issues and substance misuse among young individuals, despite both typically emerging during adolescence and early adulthood. Globally, substance use disorders and mental health problems are the primary contributors to disability among individuals aged 10 to 24 (Gore et al., 2011). Young people aged 15 to 24 are notably more susceptible to

Table 19.2
Reasons for using and motivations for not using drugs

Reasons for using drugs	Motivations to not drugs
To escape from problems	Relating to their lifestyle aspirations and relationships: • Other people's disapproval • Legal consequences • Role as parent • Career aspirations
To alleviate boredom	Relating to the practicalities of being a user: • Availability of time • Financial cost
For the "buzz"	Relating to the physical and psychological effects of drugs: • Personal experiences with drugs • Current health conditions/difficulties • Fear of effect on health • Fear of addiction • Fear of losing control
To feel confident	Relating to some of the perceived benefits of using drugs: • Sources of "buzz" • Sources of support/coping mechanisms
To ease physical pain	
To look "hard"	

Source: Home Office (2007).

Table 19.3
Presenting features of substance misuse in young people

Presenting feature	Description
Changes in behaviour	Adolescents may exhibit sudden changes in behaviour, such as increased secrecy, withdrawal from family and social activities, or unexplained mood swings.
Decline in academic performance	Substance use can lead to a decline in academic performance, including lower grades, absenteeism, and disengagement from school activities.
Peer influence	Adolescents may prioritise spending time with peers who also use substances, leading to changes in social circles and interests.
Risk-taking behaviours	Adolescents are more likely to engage in risky behaviours while under the influence of substances, such as driving under the influence, unsafe sexual practices, or involvement in fights.
Physical changes	Physical signs of substance use in adolescents may include changes in appetite, weight loss or gain, fatigue, red or bloodshot eyes, or changes in personal hygiene.
Petty crime	Associated with intoxication, theft to provide funds, "dealing" as part of more serious association with drug culture.
Emotional instability	Adolescents may experience emotional instability, including mood swings, irritability, anxiety, or depression, which may be exacerbated by substance use.
Withdrawal syndrome	Depression on withdrawal of stimulants; irritability, confusion, mood changes as part of withdrawal syndrome.

experiencing mental health issues and/or substance use disorders than any other age group (Pearson et al., 2013). The most prevalent psychiatric comorbidities include conduct disorders with and without hyperkinetic disorders, followed by depressive, anxiety, and impulse control disorders (Thomasius et al., 2022). Young people with a co-occurring disorder face heightened risks compared to those with either condition alone. These risks include multiple hospital visits, higher rates of suicide attempts, challenges in interpersonal relationships, homelessness, poorer treatment outcomes, involvement with the criminal justice system, and increased risk of premature death (Erskine et al., 2015).

Young people who use cannabis face an elevated risk of developing psychotic illnesses like schizophrenia or bipolar disorder (Royal College of Psychiatrists, 2012), although not all cannabis users will experience these conditions. Evidence suggests that genetic vulnerability, family history of psychosis, or certain personality traits may increase the likelihood of developing psychosis with regular use of potent cannabis (Royal College of Psychiatrists, 2012). Some adolescents may exhibit temporary psychotic symptoms, such as hallucinations and delusions, which may not persist long-term. Synthetic cannabinoids, known as "spice" drugs, have been linked to psychotic symptoms and can trigger acute psychosis in vulnerable individuals or worsen existing psychiatric conditions (Papanti et al., 2013). Moreover, cannabis use can impact the health outcomes of first-episode psychosis in young individuals (González-Blanch et al., 2015), emphasising the need for simultaneous treatment of these comorbidities.

PREVENTION AND THERAPEUTIC INTERVENTIONS

National guidelines in many developed countries now include policies and strategies aimed at preventing alcohol and drug use among adolescents. Prevention efforts often focus on education, promoting healthy coping mechanisms, and fostering supportive environments for young people. Research has enhanced our comprehension of factors that mitigate the risk of youth engaging in various risky behaviours, including substance use. These protective factors include parental or family engagement, family support, parental disapproval of substance use, parental monitoring, and school connectedness (CDC, 2022). Early intervention and access to mental health resources are crucial in addressing substance misuse among youth. It is important for various professionals, including healthcare providers, teachers, probation officers, and school healthcare professionals to be equipped to identify and respond to substance misuse issues among young people. This includes involvement in health education and preventative initiatives. Young vulnerable people who use substances, whether drugs and/or alcohol, are heterogeneous, and it would be excluding to ignore their diversity (Epling & McGregor, 2006). Young people vulnerable to substance misuse, such as experimental or recreational users, those with special educational needs, excluded students, and young offenders, require tailored interventions. Preventative and educational programmes, along with identification and assessment strategies, brief intervention techniques, family work, and social skills training, are essential. However, addressing substance misuse should not be undertaken independently but should instead be integrated with broader issues that impact young people, such as sexual health, mental health, education, family dynamics, and spirituality. Young adults undergoing addiction treatment require comprehensive access to evidence-based assessments, psychosocial interventions, pharmacological treatments, harm reduction strategies, and recovery services (Hadland et al., 2021). These approaches must be tailored to address the specific needs of young adults and should be delivered in the least restrictive setting feasible.

CONCLUSION

The significant consumption of alcohol and other psychoactive drugs among young individuals with mental health issues emphasises the importance of addressing both health concerns simultaneously. However, identifying and diagnosing alcohol and drug misuse in young people is becoming increasingly challenging due to the rising trend of using combinations of substances rather than just one. The proliferation of new psychoactive substances poses a significant public health challenge, particularly for young people. Efforts to educate adolescents about the dangers of these substances, enhance regulatory measures, and provide access to evidence-based prevention and treatment services are essential in mitigating the risks associated with synthetic drug use.

Despite substance misuse being a growing problem, many services are not adequately equipped to address the complex needs of adolescent substance users. In some countries, there is a lack of specialised substance misuse services tailored for young people, leading them to seek assistance from either child psychiatry services or adult substance misuse services, which may not be optimally suited to their needs. Nonetheless, there is a shifting landscape with the commissioning of dedicated young people's substance misuse treatment and the establishment of local service delivery.

KEY POINTS

- Substance misuse in young people ranges from readily available and legal substances, such as tobacco, alcohol, and volatile substances, to more uncommon and illegal substances, such as ecstasy, cannabis, cocaine, or heroin.
- Emerging trends: there is a growing concern over the use of new psychoactive substances or synthetic drugs among youth due to their accessibility and potentially harmful effects.
- Adolescents are particularly vulnerable to substance use due to ongoing brain development, peer pressure, curiosity, and societal influences.
- Substance misuse in young people should be considered in the context of "normal" adolescent risk-taking behaviours and experimentation.
- There is a progression from legal substances like alcohol and tobacco to more illicit drugs, known as the gateway theory. Although there is no conclusive evidence of this theory.
- Substance use among youth is often linked with engaging in risky behaviours, such as unsafe sex, driving under the influence, and criminal activities.
- There are relatively well-established associations between several risk and protective factors and problematic drug use among young people.
- Parental attitudes, behaviours, and family dynamics play a significant role in influencing a young person's substance use.
- Several groups of young people vulnerable to problematic drug use have been identified from a review of the literature on risk factors.
- Protective factors: factors such as parental involvement, family support, and school connectedness can mitigate the risk of substance use among youth.
- Substance use often co-exists with mental health disorders among young people, exacerbating the complexity of treatment.
- Young people who use cannabis are also at a higher risk of developing a psychotic illness, such as schizophrenia or bipolar disorder.
- Prevention and intervention: early identification, education, and intervention strategies are crucial in addressing substance use among young people.
- A holistic multi-agency outcomes-focused approach would be undertaken to enhance the prevention of substance misuse by children and young people.

Activity 19.2

Questions

- Discuss the prevalence of substance misuse in young people.
- Examine the factors that contribute to the initiation and continuation of adolescent alcohol and drug misuse.
- Discuss the factors and motivations for not using drugs.
- The presentation of features of substance misuse of young people may be divided into physical, psychological, and social features. List the features.
- Examine the co-occurring disorders issues for young people.

References

CDC. (2022). *High-Risk Substance Use Among Youth*. Centers for Disease Control and Prevention. https://www.cdc.gov/healthyyouth/substance-use/index.htm#:~:text=Risk%20factors%20for%20youth%20high-risk%20substance%20use%20can,school%20connectedness%208%20Low%20academic%20achievement%20More%20items (accessed 28 March 2024).

Dillon, L., Chivite-Matthews, N., Grewal, I., Brown, R., Webster, S., Weddell, E., Brown, G., & Smith, N. (2006). *Risk, Protective Factors and Resilience to Drug Use: Identifying Resilient Young People and Learning from Their Experience*. London: Home Office.

Epling, M., & McGregor, J. (2006). Vulnerable young people and substance misuse. In G. H. Rassool (Ed.), *Dual Diagnosis Nursing*. Oxford: Blackwell Publications.

Erskine, H. E., Moffitt, T. E., Copeland, W. E., Costello, E. J., Ferrari, A. J., Patton, G., Degenhardt, L., Vos, T., Whiteford, H. A., & Scott, J. G. (2015). A heavy burden on young minds: The global burden of mental and substance use disorders in children and youth. *Psychological Medicine*, 45(7), 1551–1563. https://doi.org/10.1017/S0033291714002888.

Fullerton, C. S., & Ursano, R. J. (1994). Preadolescent peer friendships: A critical contribution to adult social relatedness? *Journal of Youth Adolescence*, 23, 43–63. https://doi.org/10.1007/BF01537141.

González-Blanch, C., Gleeson, J. F., Koval, P., Cotton, S. M., McGorry, P. D., & Alvarez-Jimenez, M. (2015). Social functioning trajectories of young first-episode psychosis patients with and without cannabis misuse: A 30-month follow-up study. *PLOS One*, 10(4), e0122404. https://doi.org/10.1371/journal.pone.0122404.

Gore, F. M., Bloem, P. J., Patton, G. C., Ferguson, J., Joseph, V., Coffey, C., Sawyer, S. M., & Mathers, C. D. (2011). Global burden of disease in young people aged 10–24 years: A systematic analysis. *Lancet*, 377(9783), 2093–2102. https://doi.org/10.1016/S0140-6736(11)60512-6.

Haase, T., & Pratschke, J. (2011). Risk and protection factors for substance use among young people. A comparative study of early school-leavers and school-attending students. *Research Digest*, 6(2), 36–44.

Hadland, S. E., Yule, A. M., Levy, S. J., Hallett, E., Silverstein, M., & Bagley, S. M. (2021). Evidence-based treatment of young adults with substance use disorders. *Pediatrics*, 147 (Suppl 2), S204–S214. https://doi.org/10.1542/peds.2020-023523D.

Hamidullah, S., Thorpe, H. H. A., Frie, J. A., Mccurdy, R. D., & Khokhar, J. Y. (2020). Adolescent substance use and the brain: Behavioral, cognitive and neuroimaging correlates. *Frontiers in Human Neuroscience*, 14, 298. https://doi.org/10.3389/fnhum.2020.00298.

Home Office. (2007). *Identifying and Exploring Young People's Experiences of Risk, Protective Factors and Resilience to Drug Use*. Home Office Development and Practice Reports. London: Home Office.

Lloyd, C. (1998). Risk factors for problem drug use: Identifying vulnerable groups. *Drugs: Education, Prevention and Policy*, 5(3), 217–232.

Mares, S. H., van der Vorst, H., Engels, R. C., & Lichtwarck-Aschoff, A. (2011). Parental alcohol use, alcohol-related problems, and alcohol-specific attitudes, alcohol-specific communication, and adolescent excessive alcohol use and alcohol-related problems: An indirect path model. *Addictive Behaviors*, 36(3), 209–216. https://doi.org/10.1016/j.addbeh.2010.10.013.

Miller, P., & Plant, M. (2003). The family, peer influences and substance use: Findings from a study of UK teenagers. *Journal of Substance Use*, 8(1), 9–26. https://doi.org/10.1080/1465989021000067209.

Nkansah-Amankra, S., & Minelli, M. (2016). "Gateway hypothesis" and early drug use: Additional findings from tracking a population-based sample of adolescents to adulthood. *Preventive Medicine Reports*, 4, 134–141. https://doi.org/10.1016/j.pmedr.2016.05.003.

Papanti, D., Schifano, F., Botteon, G., Bertossi, F., Mannix, J., Vidoni, D., Impagnatiello, M., Pascolo-Fabrici, E., & Bonavigo, T. (2013). "Spiceophrenia": A systematic overview of "spice"-related psychopathological issues and a case report. *Human Psychopharmacology*, 28(4), 379–389. https://doi.org/10.1002/hup.2312.

Pearson, C., Janz, T., & Ali, J. (2013). *Health at a Glance: Mental and Substance Use Disorders in Canada* (Statistics Canada Catalogue No. 82-624-X). Electronic document: 82-624-x2013001-2-eng.pdf (PDF, 4.99 MB). https://publications.gc.ca/collections/collection_2013/statcan/82-624-x/82-624-x2013001-2-eng.pdf.

Royal College of Psychiatrists. (2012). *Cannabis and Mental Health*. London: Royal College of Psychiatrists.

Russell, M. (1990). Prevalence of alcoholism among children of alcoholics. In M. Windle & J. S. Searles (Eds.), *Children of Alcoholics: Critical Perspectives*. New York: Guilford, pp. 9–38.

Ryan, S. M., Jorm, A. F., Kelly, C. M., Hart, L. M., Morgan, A. J., & Lubman, D. I. (2011). Parenting strategies for reducing adolescent alcohol use: A Delphi consensus study. *BMC Public Health*, 11, 13. https://doi.org/10.1186/1471-2458-11-13.

Siddharth, S., Naresh, N., Sunil, G., Preeti, P., & Debasish, B. (2016). From one substance dependence to another: Are gateway violations common? *Indian Journal of Social Psychiatry*, 32(2), 171–173.

Thomasius, R., Paschke, K., & Arnaud, N. (2022). Substance-use disorders in children and adolescents. *Deutsches Arzteblatt International*, 119(25), 440–450. https://doi.org/10.3238/arztebl.m2022.0122.

Tildesley, E. A., & Andrews, J. A. (2008). The development of children's intentions to use alcohol: Direct and indirect effects of parent alcohol use and parenting behaviors. *Psychology of Addictive Behaviors*, 22, 326–339. https://doi.org/10.1037/0893–0164X.22.3.326.

Trucco, E. M. (2020). A review of psychosocial factors linked to adolescent substance use. *Pharmacology, Biochemistry, and Behavior*, 196, 172969. https://doi.org/10.1016/j.pbb.2020.172969.

Part 4

Role, prevention, and strategies for change

Chapter 20

Generic role in response to alcohol and drug misuse

Learning outcomes

- Discuss the rationale for working with alcohol and drug misusers.
- Describe some of the roles and interventions of health, social care, and criminal justice system professionals in working with alcohol and drug misusers.

Activity 20.1

Questions

- Have you come into contact with alcohol and drug misusers, or have you included alcohol and drug misusers in your caseload?
- Identify the number of contacts you have made during the past month.
- If contact was made, how many were alcohol or drug misusers or both?
- Reflect on your own roles, whether generic or specialist, in working with substance misusers.
- What are the challenges in working with substance misusers?

Activity 20.2

Please choose one correct answer to the following multiple-choice questions

1. Which of the following is true regarding the role of health and social care professionals in responding to alcohol and drug misuse?
   a. Their role primarily involves direct intervention and treatment of alcohol and substance use disorders.
   b. They have a limited role in addressing substance misuse, mainly focusing on referral to specialist services.
   c. They play a crucial role in early identification, screening, and provision of brief interventions for individuals affected by alcohol and substance use disorders.
   d. Their role is confined to providing education and awareness programmes in the community.
   e. They are responsible for implementing law enforcement measures to curb alcohol and substance use disorders.

DOI: 10.4324/9781003456674-24

2. What is a core aspect of the "core business" for primary and community health services and social care services regarding substance misuse?
   a. Developing new medications for treating alcohol and substance use disorders
   b. Conducting large-scale public health campaigns to prevent substance misuse
   c. Early identification, screening, and provision of brief psychosocial interventions for individuals affected by substance misuse
   d. Providing long-term residential treatment for individuals with alcohol and severe substance use disorders
   e. Conducting research on the socio-economic impacts of substance misuse
3. What is the pressing need for health and social care professionals in responding to alcohol and drug misuse?
   a. To implement strict punitive measures for individuals engaged in substance misuse
   b. To focus solely on providing treatment for individuals with severe substance use disorders
   c. To enhance their knowledge and clinical expertise in alcohol and substance use disorder
   d. To develop community-based recreational programmes to divert individuals from substance misuse
   e. To prioritise administrative tasks over direct patient care in alcohol and substance use disorders cases
4. How do health and social care professionals contribute to the prevention of substance misuse?
   a. By exclusively focusing on treating individuals already affected by alcohol and substance use disorders
   b. By providing early identification and brief interventions for individuals at risk of substance misuse
   c. By avoiding involvement in community outreach programmes related to substance misuse prevention
   d. By implementing punitive measures against individuals engaged in substance misuse
   e. By conducting research on the societal impacts of substance misuse without implementing preventive measures
5. Which of the following accurately describes the role of health and social care professionals in community-based substance misuse services?
   a. They primarily focus on providing inpatient services for alcohol and substance use disorders.
   b. They are responsible for conducting large-scale public health campaigns to prevent alcohol and substance misuse.
   c. They play a key role in providing a range of services, including advice, needle exchange facilities, and counselling for substance misusers.
   d. They have minimal involvement in providing support and interventions for individuals affected by substance misuse.
   e. They focus solely on providing pharmacological interventions for substance misuse without offering psychosocial support.
6. How do health and social care professionals contribute to the treatment of alcohol and substance use disorders?
   a. By prioritising administrative tasks over direct patient care
   b. By offering pharmacological interventions exclusively without psychosocial support
   c. By actively engaging in comprehensive treatment programmes tailored to individual needs
   d. By conducting research on alcohol and substance use disorders without implementing treatment strategies
   e. By avoiding involvement in the treatment of alcohol and substance use disorders altogether

7. What is the primary focus of health and social care professionals when responding to alcohol and substance use disorders in the communities?
   a. Implementing punitive measures against individuals engaged in substance misuse
   b. Providing comprehensive treatment programmes for severe substance use disorders
   c. Early identification, screening, and provision of brief interventions for individuals affected by alcohol and substance use disorders
   d. Conducting research on substance misuse without implementing preventive measures
   e. Advocating for stricter laws and regulations against alcohol and substance misuse
8. What is the role of accident and emergency nurses in addressing alcohol and drug misuse?
   a. They focus solely on providing immediate medical treatment for individuals experiencing substance-related emergencies.
   b. They play a minimal role in identifying and addressing alcohol and substance use disorders among patients.
   c. They actively engage in early identification and brief interventions for individuals presenting with substance-related issues in the emergency department.
   d. Their role is limited to administrative tasks and does not involve direct patient care in alcohol and substance use disorders cases.
   e. They advocate for stricter laws and regulations against substance misuse among the general population.
9. What role do prison healthcare nurses play in addressing alcohol and drug misuse among incarcerated individuals?
   a. They focus solely on providing medical care and do not address substance misuse issues among inmates.
   b. They actively engage in screening, assessment, and provision of treatment for alcohol and substance use disorders among prisoners.
   c. Their role is limited to administrative tasks and does not involve direct patient care in alcohol and substance misuse cases.
   d. They advocate for stricter punitive measures against inmates engaged in alcohol and substance misuse.
   e. They conduct research on substance misuse without implementing preventive measures or treatment strategies within prison settings.
10. How do probation officers contribute to addressing substance misuse in the community?
    a. They have minimal involvement in identifying or addressing substance misuse issues among probationers.
    b. They actively engage in early identification, screening, and provision of brief interventions for individuals on probation affected by alcohol and substance misuse.
    c. Their role is limited to enforcing strict punitive measures against individuals engaged in alcohol and substance misuse.
    d. They provide comprehensive treatment programmes exclusively for individuals with alcohol and substance use disorders.
    e. They conduct research on substance misuse without implementing preventive measures or treatment strategies among probationers.
11. What role do health and social care professionals play in harm reduction strategies for substance misuse?
    a. They primarily focus on punitive measures to deter individuals from substance misuse.
    b. They provide comprehensive treatment programmes without considering harm reduction.
    c. They actively engage in harm reduction approaches, such as providing needle exchange programmes and safe injection sites.
    d. They advocate for stricter laws and regulations against substance misuse.
    e. They conduct awareness campaigns highlighting the dangers of substance misuse without providing tangible support.

INTRODUCTION

Health and social care professionals play a critical role in addressing alcohol and substance use disorders within their respective fields. From primary healthcare settings to residential facilities, these professionals, as frontline responders, have a role in providing support, intervention, and treatment to individuals grappling with alcohol and substance use disorders. Health and social care professionals, including nurses, midwives, social workers, general practitioners, addiction specialists, prison healthcare nurses, probation officers, community-based nurses, and psychologists, are often the first point of contact for individuals struggling with alcohol and substance use disorders. It is essential to recognise that managing early-stage substance use is not solely the responsibility of specialist workers; rather, the active involvement of diverse health and social care professionals is crucial (Rassool & Marshall, 2001). This chapter examine some of the generic roles of health and social care professionals in working with individuals with alcohol and substance use disorders.

RATIONALE FOR WORKING WITH ALCOHOL AND DRUG USERS

Given the increasing prevalence of alcohol and drug misuse and the normalisation of psychoactive substances in society, it is likely that only a minority of individuals struggling with alcohol and substance use will initially seek help from specialist drug and alcohol agencies. Instead, many will first come into contact with primary care services, medical and psychiatric services, social services, voluntary agencies, and the criminal justice system. This highlights the importance of a multi-disciplinary response to alcohol and drug problems, involving both generic workers and specialists. From a public health perspective, several areas pose significant threats to the nation's health due to substance misuse, including smoking, alcohol-related diseases, blood-borne infections, and drug-related deaths from overdose and blood-borne viruses. Many of the medical problems can be directly linked to alcohol and drug use, and they include cancer (tobacco), heart disease (tobacco, cocaine, MDMA [ecstasy], amphetamines, and steroids), HIV and hepatitis C (injection drug use), and alcohol (anaemia, cancer, cardiovascular disease, cirrhosis, dementia, depression, seizures, gout, high blood pressure, infectious disease, nerve damage, and pancreatitis). It is also important to recognise that alcohol and drug misuse often co-occur with mental health issues, such as depression, anxiety, marital difficulties, and personality disorders. Therefore, generic workers in various sectors – such as healthcare, social services, and criminal justice – play a crucial role in identifying and addressing substance misuse issues early on. They can provide initial support, referrals to specialist services when needed, and integrated care that addresses both substance use and co-occurring conditions. This collaborative approach is essential for effectively addressing the complex health and social challenges associated with alcohol and drug misuse in communities.

The significant health and social issues linked to substance misuse underline the urgent requirement for members of the primary healthcare team, including nurses, social workers, and individuals within the criminal justice system, to address the needs of those struggling with substance use. Intervening early in the lifestyles and behaviours of substance misusers can help mitigate the associated health, social, and familial harms. Early intervention strategies implemented by healthcare and social care professionals can have a profound impact on preventing substance misuse from evolving into a chronic problem. These strategies also aim to reduce alcohol-related harm, promote responsible drinking practices, and decrease drug-related deaths from overdose and blood-borne viruses. However, the effectiveness of these interventions heavily depends on policies that acknowledge the necessity of coordinating services among different agencies. Commitment to working within integrated care pathways is crucial for ensuring that the holistic and intricate needs of individuals grappling with alcohol and drug misuse are adequately addressed.

Generic workers play a crucial role in addressing alcohol and substance use issues due to their accessibility and presence in various community settings, including schools, healthcare facilities, and social service agencies. Their holistic approach to care enables them to address not only alcohol and substance use disorders but also underlying mental health concerns, trauma, and social determinants of health, providing comprehensive support to individuals in need. Moreover, their early intervention efforts, stigma reduction strategies, and ability to facilitate referrals and coordinate care contribute to more effective support systems for those struggling with substance use, ensuring timely access to appropriate services tailored to individual needs. Additionally, generic workers' deep engagement within communities enable them to understand and address unique social and cultural factors influencing substance use behaviours. Through community engagement, prevention efforts, and advocacy, they play a vital role in raising awareness, advocating for policy changes, and mobilising resources to prevent substance use disorders and promote healthier behaviours among vulnerable populations. Their non-clinical, empathetic approach fosters a supportive environment that encourages individuals to seek help, ultimately contributing to improved outcomes and well-being for individuals and communities affected by alcohol and substance use issues. Table 20.1 presents the rationale for working with alcohol and drug users.

GENERIC ROLE IN RESPONSE TO ALCOHOL AND DRUG MISUSE

The effective management of alcohol and substance misuse necessitates a multi-professional approach, involving collaboration between various healthcare professionals, social workers, and those in the criminal justice system. Liaison with specialist substance misuse services and other relevant agencies is crucial for comprehensive care delivery. Roles within the substance misuse field range from generic to specialist addiction workers and professionals whose duties may bring them into contact with alcohol substance users. It is essential for health, social care and criminal justice professionals, across hospital and community settings, to prioritise early recognition and the provision of effective care, prevention, and health education. The skills and competencies of professionals in this field can be adapted to meet the needs of both substance users and non-users, highlighting the versatility of roles within generic and addiction services. The workforce can be envisaged as a continuum from specialist to generic roles, spanning various sectors, with each role requiring specific competencies tailored to their level and frequency of contact with alcohol and substance users. Ultimately, addressing drug and alcohol problems is considered core business for many services,

Table 20.1
Rationale for working with alcohol and drug users

Rationale	Explanation
Public health impact	Addressing substance use issues is crucial for improving public health outcomes and reducing the burden on healthcare systems.
Accessibility	First point of contact for individuals struggling with alcohol and substance use disorders. Present in a variety of settings, such as schools, community centres, healthcare facilities, and social service agencies, making them more accessible to individuals in need of support.
Health equity	Providing support and treatment services to alcohol and drug users promotes health equity by ensuring access to care for vulnerable populations.
Early intervention	Well-positioned to identify signs of substance use early on and intervene before the problem escalates. Offering support, guidance, and resources, they can help individuals address their alcohol substance use issues before they become more severe and entrenched.
Referral and coordination	May not provide specialised addiction treatment themselves; they can facilitate referrals to appropriate services and coordinate care across different providers. This ensures that individuals receive comprehensive support tailored to their specific needs, including medical treatment, counselling, peer support, and social services.
Prevention efforts	Reducing alcohol and substance use initiation and promoting healthier behaviours among vulnerable populations, such as youth, families, and marginalised communities. Through education, outreach, and community-based interventions, they can help prevent alcohol and substance use disorders from developing in the first place.
Holistic care	While specialised addiction treatment professionals focus primarily on alcohol and substance use disorders, generic workers are trained to address a wide range of psychosocial issues. Provide holistic care that addresses underlying mental health concerns, trauma, family dynamics, housing instability, unemployment, and other social determinants of health that may contribute to substance use.
Stigma reduction	Often interact with individuals in a non-clinical, non-stigmatising environment. Their approachable behaviour and empathetic attitude can help reduce the stigma.
Community engagement	Deeply embedded within their communities and understand the unique social and cultural factors that influence alcohol and substance use behaviours. Engage with community members, raise awareness about alcohol and substance use issues, advocate for policy changes, and mobilise resources to address underlying systemic issues contributing to addictive behaviours.

emphasising the importance of a collaborative and inclusive approach in tackling alcohol and substance misuse issues. Examples of the types of roles that might fall within each category include specialist addiction nurses and drug and alcohol workers. Generic workers who have a substance misuse function within their portfolio of responsibilities include social workers, youth workers, while generic workers with occasional substance misuse portfolio include prison officers, teachers, probation officer. The roles of nurses and other health and social care professionals are derived from literature sources, such as Public Health England and the Royal College of Nursing (2017).

HOSPITALS INCLUDING EMERGENCY DEPARTMENTS

Nurses play a critical role in hospital-based alcohol and drug liaison services, particularly within emergency departments. Their responsibilities include conducting specialised screening and assessments of patients with alcohol or drug-related health issues in both inpatient and outpatient settings. Nurses also provide interventions for prescribing and withdrawal management during hospitalisation, along with brief interventions to promote health and harm reduction, facilitating referrals to specialist drug and alcohol treatment services when necessary. Additionally, they offer education and training to hospital staff to improve their ability to identify and effectively manage patients with alcohol and drug problems. Nurses also respond to adverse effects resulting from new psychoactive substance (NPS) use and report such cases to the appropriate systems for further action.

Alcohol and drug misusers frequently seek care at accident and emergency (A&E) departments due to various physical and psychological complications resulting from substance use (Gossop et al., 1995). These individuals often rely on A&E as their primary or initial point of contact with health services, particularly following accidental overdoses and crises. Furthermore, chronic effects of sustained heavy drinking lead to admissions with conditions like chronic liver disease, pancreatitis, gastrointestinal bleeding, cardiac arrhythmia, and cancer (Institute of Alcohol Studies, 2015). Individuals who frequently attend A&E for alcohol-related reasons tend to experience alcohol dependence associated with multiple and complex needs, diverse patterns of drinking and other substance use, and varied health and social problems (Wolf et al., 2020). In summary, A&E staff play a crucial role in managing a range of situations related to alcohol and substance misuse, including overdose or coma cases, management of intoxicated clients and disruptive behaviours, withdrawal management (e.g. preventing opiate withdrawal in pregnant women), alcohol or drug-related accidents, respiratory failure (common after opiate overdose), self-harm incidents, and drug-induced psychosis or other mental health problems. With their swift intervention and specialised care, A&E departments contribute significantly to reducing drug-related deaths and providing essential support to individuals in crisis due to alcohol and substance misuse. In general and surgical wards, patients who misuse psychoactive substances may be admitted for health issues that may or may not be directly associated with drug and alcohol use. The are guidelines that are intended for both medical and nursing staff to act as a resource in the management of patients with drug misuse issues (Peagram, 2017).

PRIMARY CARE: COMMUNITY-BASED NURSES

In this section, community-based nurses encompass a diverse range of roles, including community mental health nurses, primary care mental health workers, nurses in sexual health, occupational nurses, health visitors, district nurses, practice nurses, and school nurses. In primary care settings, individuals with problematic alcohol and drug use can receive effective management with specialised support, often provided by experienced nurses. Through shared care schemes, nurses and treatment workers offer various services, including advice on management and pharmacological interventions, key working for those in recovery, alcohol and drug identification with brief advice, and education and training for primary care staff. Additionally, they play a crucial role in bridging primary care and specialist alcohol and drug services, ensuring seamless coordination of care for patients.

COMMUNITY MENTAL HEALTH NURSES

Community mental health nurses play a critical role in addressing the complex needs of clients with psychiatric disorders and substance misuse within various community settings. Their caseload often includes individuals struggling with both illicit psychoactive substances and prescribed medications. These nurses are involved in activities, such as recognising substance misuse, liaising with primary healthcare providers for detoxification and relapse prevention, providing counselling, and offering education on alcohol, drugs, and HIV prevention. However, they face ethical dilemmas in simultaneously encouraging medication compliance while discouraging substance use. This ambivalence may lead to referrals to specialist addiction services rather than direct intervention. Despite possessing the skills to intervene, community mental health nurses may feel de-skilled due to role confusion and legitimacy issues. Additionally, inherent differences in treatment philosophies and goals between substance use disorders and psychiatric disorders may contribute to reluctance in intervention. Overall, challenges such as feelings of frustration, inadequacy, and negative views on treatment outcomes may impact nurses' willingness to address substance misuse effectively (Rassool, 1998; Gafoor & Rassool, 1998). Health-related issues stemming from alcohol and drug misuse encompass a range of concerns, including comorbidities, withdrawal symptoms from alcohol, benzodiazepines, or opiates, blood-borne infections, and psychosis induced by substances like amphetamines or cocaine. Interventions targeting these problems involve multifaceted approaches, such as assessing mental health and substance use issues, providing counselling, implementing harm reduction strategies, facilitating relapse prevention, utilising cognitive therapy, offering health education, exploring alternative therapies for rational substance use, promoting non-drug interventions, supporting home detoxification, and preventing further misuse of drugs and alcohol.

PRACTICE NURSE

Practice nurses are strategically positioned to screen for drug misuse and assess individuals at risk of harmful alcohol consumption, enabling the delivery of health information and brief interventions. Studies suggest that practice nurses are perceived as more understanding and approachable when seeking advice on alcohol use compared to other healthcare professionals (Lock, 2004). The National Institute for Health and Care Excellence (NICE, 2010) recommends alcohol screening as part of routine practice to identify individuals at increased risk of harm and provide brief advice. Early detection and intervention for alcohol and drug problems are emphasised, as evidence indicates their beneficial impact (Kaner et al., 2007). Additionally, some primary healthcare staff, including practice nurses, collaborate with specialist alcohol treatment agencies to provide more complex alcohol interventions, such as assisted alcohol withdrawal and psychological and pharmacological interventions (NICE, 2011). This collaborative approach ensures comprehensive support for individuals with alcohol-related concerns within primary care settings. There is growing evidence to support the effectiveness of nurse-led brief interventions in primary care settings. Interventions led by primary care nurses have shown significant improvements across various outcome categories, including reduced tobacco use (Lukewich et al., 2022). In a study conducted by Owen et al. (2000), it was found that practice nurses were willing to provide advice on sensible drinking and routinely took alcohol intake histories, particularly within well-woman and well-man clinics. However, fewer nurses tended to take alcohol histories in other clinics, such as those for hypertension or diabetes. The authors suggested that this discrepancy might stem from a lack of awareness regarding the role of alcohol in conditions like hypertension. Research by Lock and Kaner (2004) indicates that nurses demonstrate more consistent provision of brief interventions to patients compared to general practitioners (GPs), despite screening fewer patients overall. This highlights the valuable role of practice nurses in preventing alcohol and drug-related problems. By actively engaging in these interventions, practice nurses contribute significantly to promoting healthier behaviours and addressing substance misuse issues among their patients.

MIDWIVES OR OBSTETRIC NURSES

Nurses trained in pregnancy and post-natal care within the context of substance use disorders play a crucial role in addressing specific considerations for pregnant individuals with substance use issues. They provide comprehensive knowledge on the potential anomalies and developmental defects resulting from substance exposure and liaise with various healthcare professionals and partner organisations. Additionally, they advise both service users and prescribers on appropriate clinical management, screen for and manage blood-borne viruses (BBVs), apply safeguarding procedures, and offer guidance on contraception methods. Nurses also support mothers during the post-natal period while assessing risks associated with substance use and ensuring proper care for both the mother and the newborn/infant child.

The prevalence of women misusing alcohol and drugs, particularly those of childbearing age, has risen significantly in recent decades. Accurately identifying pre-natal drug exposure is crucial, not only to comprehend the scope of the issue, but also to facilitate appropriate medical and psychosocial interventions (Lester et al., 2004). This identification enables healthcare professionals to provide timely support and interventions to both the mother and the unborn child, reducing the risk of adverse outcomes and promoting optimal health for both. Midwives play a crucial role in supporting pregnant women who misuse substances, encouraging them to make positive changes in their behaviour. Interventions include promoting harm reduction strategies, advocating for cervical cytology screening during antenatal care, and closely monitoring newborns for withdrawal symptoms in cases of opiate dependence. Additionally, midwives provide health education on maternal health; antenatal screenings for hepatitis C, hepatitis B, and HIV; antenatal counselling; smoking cessation support; HIV prevention; management of withdrawal symptoms; antenatal care; post-natal care; and support for both mother and child. They also facilitate liaison with specialist services. Midwives are particularly well-positioned to deliver evidence-based behavioural support programmes, such as very brief advice (VBA), addressing alcohol and drug use among pregnant women. By offering comprehensive care and guidance, midwives contribute to the well-being of both mother and child during pregnancy and beyond.

However, pregnant women who misuse drugs or alcohol may delay seeking antenatal care, increasing health risks for both themselves and their babies. This delay is often attributed to factors such as lack of awareness of pregnancy due to menstrual disturbances or amenorrhea resulting from drug use, or simply a lack of motivation. To mitigate these risks, it is recommended that pregnant women with substance misuse issues receive close supervision and care from maternity services, following evidence-based guidelines. Some areas have established specialist drug and alcohol midwifery teams, which facilitate shared care between maternity services and substance misuse treatment services. These multidisciplinary approaches aim to provide comprehensive support to pregnant women wit
substance misuse issues, addressing both their me
ical needs and broader psychosocial concerns, ult
mately promoting the health and well-being of bo
mother and baby.

HEALTH VISITORS

Health visitors often encounter diverse client grou
including families and significant others, who mi
use substances such as alcohol, tobacco, and bo
prescribed and illicit drugs. This presents a mul
faceted challenge for health visitors as they work
support the health and well-being of individuals ar
families within their communities. While health vi
itors primarily focus on child health up to the age
5, their role extends beyond just providing care
children, encompassing preventative health educ
tion for the entire family. Interventions undertak
by health visitors include offering advice, counse
ling, health education and promotion, and har
reduction strategies. Some primary healthcare trus
have designated specialist health visitors for dru
and alcohol, who supplement existing services b
working with families and providing drug counse
ling services across all age groups. The roles of the
specialists vary but may involve identifying risks f
individuals living with substance misusers, conduc
ing needs assessments, and developing care plans f
families. They also collaborate with homeless ar
socially excluded drug misusers while liaising wi
various agencies, such as the Area Child Protectic
Committee, social services, midwifery services, ge
eral healthcare services, school nurses (if applic
ble), and specialist alcohol and drug teams. Throu
these multidisciplinary collaborations, speciali
health visitors contribute to addressing the compl
needs of families affected by substance misuse.

Alcohol and substance misuse can significant
impact parenting by diverting time and energy aw
from children and prioritising the addiction ov
the needs of the child. This can lead to neglect, la
of supervision, and inconsistent caregiving. Ch
dren of parents who misuse substances may exp
rience negative health outcomes, including foet
alcohol spectrum disorders, neonatal abstinen
syndrome, visual impairments, behavioural issu
and an increased risk of sudden infant death or acc
dental injury. Building resilience is crucial in mi
gating these adverse effects, and health visitors pl
a vital role in identifying and supporting families

strengthen resilient factors (Jenkins, 2015). By providing education, resources, and assistance, health visitors help families navigate challenges associated with substance misuse and promote the well-being of children in these environments. Health visitors play a vital role in providing support, guidance, and interventions to mitigate the impact of substance misuse on individuals, families, and communities, ultimately aiming to improve health outcomes and promote healthier lifestyles.

NURSE-LED CLINICS IN GENITOURINARY MEDICINE

Nurse-led clinics in genitourinary medicine (GUM) have been established to provide comprehensive care for patients with sexual health concerns. Individuals who misuse drugs and alcohol often access GUM services due to concerns related to blood-borne infections, HIV status, or sexually transmitted infections. Injecting drug users, in particular, exhibit high-risk behaviours, including unsafe sexual practices while under the influence. Those with HIV-positive status require specialised care for both substance use and HIV-related disease. Nurses in sexual health settings must collaborate closely with substance misuse and general healthcare services. Interventions include conducting drug and alcohol histories, sexual assessments, pre- and post-test counselling, general counselling, health education, and implementing harm reduction strategies.

OCCUPATIONAL HEALTH NURSE

The misuse of psychoactive substances in the workplace poses significant concerns for management, professional organisations, and occupational health staff, leading to absenteeism, accidents, and decreased workforce efficiency. The opioid epidemic has significant implications for the workplace, requiring occupational health nurses to be vigilant about the serious risks linked to opioid prescribing (Higgins & Simons, 2019). Occupational health services provided at workplaces are essential for addressing the healthcare needs of employees and play a crucial role in public health strategies, including reducing health inequalities and social exclusion. Occupational health nurses (OHNs) play a crucial role in promoting employee well-being and productivity through preventative health measures. This may involve addressing substance use issues and providing counselling and crisis intervention services for a wide range of issues including immunisations, stress management, smoking cessation support (Amaral, 2024). The health and safety executive recommends that organisations implement drug and alcohol policies to ensure a healthy and safe working environment. Research indicates that implementing policies addressing tobacco smoking or alcohol use in the workplace can result in various benefits. These include reduced absenteeism rates, enhanced safety performance, decreased maintenance and air-conditioning costs, improved productivity, increased morale among non-smoking employees, fewer accidents, and a reduced risk of losing skilled workers prematurely due to retirement or death (McEwen, 1991). Such policies contribute to fostering a healthier and more supportive work environment while promoting the well-being and retention of employees.

DISTRICT NURSE

District nurses, who provide comprehensive nursing care to patients in various non-hospital settings, including homes, GP surgeries, and residential care homes, also have a significant role in prevention and harm reduction related to drug and alcohol misuse. Their interventions encompass early identification and recognition of substance misuse, health education, and generic assessment of substance use–related health problems. However, a study by Peckover and Chidlaw (2007) revealed that district nurses face challenges and limitations in providing care to drug and alcohol misusers, primarily due to limited knowledge and experience with this client group. The authors identified issues such as prejudice and perceived risk which influence service provision and may result in suboptimal care for individuals struggling with substance misuse. Addressing these challenges is crucial to ensure that district nurses can effectively support and provide appropriate care to patients with drug and alcohol-related issues in community settings.

SCHOOL NURSE

The use of tobacco, alcohol, and illicit drugs among young people and schoolchildren is a significant public health concern, prompting the development of various support and prevention initiatives. In the

UK, Alcohol Concern has created a toolkit aimed at assisting young people who are experiencing or at risk of alcohol-related harm. Meanwhile, in the United States, the National Association of School Nurses (NASN) has taken a proactive role in promoting health and preventing prescription drug misuse among youth. To address the risk of overdose-related deaths, NASN advocates for the inclusion of opioid overdose management, including the use of naloxone, in school emergency preparedness plans. The school nurse is identified as a key leader in emergency preparedness and response, responsible for facilitating access to naloxone and managing drug-related incidents at school. Additionally, school nurses often provide health education and promotion, including drug and sex education, as part of the personal, social, and health education curriculum. Their interventions may involve offering advice, information, and health counselling to parents and children; promoting health; and referring individuals to specialist or non-specialist agencies as needed. Ultimately, school nurses play a crucial role in contributing to school policies on alcohol and drugs, ensuring a comprehensive approach to promoting student well-being and safety.

GENERAL PRACTITIONERS AND ADDICTION SPECIALISTS

In recent years, there has been a significant rise in the involvement of doctors from diverse professional backgrounds in working with individuals who misuse drugs and alcohol. General practitioners (GPs) serve as the initial point of contact for many patients grappling with substance use issues, positioning them ideally to identify and address such problems through appropriate interventions. Recognising the importance of primary care–based interventions, the Royal College of General Practitioners underlines GPs' responsibility in providing medical care to patients with drug or alcohol problems, highlighting the potential for these interventions to mitigate physical, psychological, and social harm for both individuals and communities. Additionally, the Royal College of Psychiatrists and Royal College of General Practitioners (2005) outlines key competencies for doctors in this domain, spanning advice, identification, assessment, patient management, training, supervision, teaching, research, audit, and management and service development. However, the findings of a study (Coste et al., 2020) indicated that patients looked to their general practitioners (GPs) to take a leading role in addressing alcohol use disorder through attentive listening, providing information, and offering support. A non-judgemental attitude from GPs was crucial, as it enabled participants to open up about their struggles, marking a significant step towards seeking treatment.

In the United States, addiction specialists play a pivotal role in addressing substance use and addiction. These specialists, certified by organisations such as the American Board of Addiction Medicine (ABAM) or the American Board of Psychiatry and Neurology (ABPN), possess the necessary expertise to provide prevention, screening, intervention, and treatment services (ASAM, 2017). Meanwhile, in the UK, doctors serve as addiction psychiatrists or consultant addiction psychiatrists, offering strategic leadership and expert clinical advice to multidisciplinary substance misuse practitioners. The role of addiction specialist doctors in recovery-oriented treatment systems is delineated in resources provided by organisations such as the Royal College of Psychiatrists, the Royal College of General Practitioners, & Public Health England (2014), outlining essential functions that contribute to effective care delivery and support for individuals on the path to recovery.

CLINICAL PSYCHOLOGISTS

Clinical psychologists are integral members of specialist drug and alcohol services, contributing significantly to the treatment of alcohol and drug misuse. Their expertise lies in conducting assessments and administering various psychological treatments tailored to the individual's needs. These treatments may include counselling, relapse prevention strategies, motivational interventions, and solution-based therapy. Clinical psychologists also actively participate in multidisciplinary and multi-agency care planning, collaborating with other healthcare professionals to ensure comprehensive and holistic care for individuals struggling with substance misuse. Their role is essential in addressing the psychological aspects of addiction and supporting individuals on their journey to recovery.

SOCIAL WORKERS

Social workers in local authority social service departments are instrumental in addressing alcohol and drug misuse within various community and residential settings. Given the complex interplay between substance misuse and various social issues such as child abuse, domestic violence, homelessness, and poverty, social workers play a vital role in addressing these multifaceted challenges. Social workers trained in addictions often work in specialised treatment settings, offering interventions such as community care assessment, case management, therapy (both group and individual), family counselling, advocacy for housing and employment needs, and community resource development. Additionally, they collaborate closely with other health and social care professionals to provide comprehensive support to individuals and families affected by alcohol and drug misuse.

CRIMINAL JUSTICE SETTINGS

Nurses play important roles within various criminal justice settings, including police custody healthcare services, liaison and diversion services, and drug and alcohol arrest referral schemes. They are positioned to offer a range of services, such as screening, assessment, and provision of brief interventions to promote health and harm reduction. Additionally, nurses provide medical and psychosocial support for substance misuse, mental and physical health issues, including interventions addressing risks associated with new psychoactive substances (NPS), and advice on opioid substitution therapy (OST). They also contribute to release plans, focusing on relapse prevention, overdose risk management, and addressing co-existing mental and physical health concerns, along with other vulnerabilities, such as housing, domestic violence, and self-harm risk, ensuring a holistic approach to care for individuals transitioning from custody to the community.

HOSPITAL AND COMMUNITY PHARMACISTS

Hospital pharmacists play an important role in advising clinicians on medication management for alcohol and drug misusers, including those on substitute medications, and providing guidance on psychoactive substance interactions. They liaise with various healthcare professionals across hospital, community, and primary care settings. Community pharmacists also serve as vital points of contact within primary healthcare, offering services such as dispensing controlled drugs prescriptions, monitoring for interactions and adverse reactions, supplying clean injecting equipment, and referring clients to treatment agencies. They play a key role in identifying inappropriate prescribing and monitoring misuse potential of over-the-counter medications. There is evidence to suggest that experienced pharmacists demonstrate better overall management of drug misuse, possess greater knowledge about pain management and pharmacotherapy, and encounter fewer obstacles when screening for opioid misuse and providing interventions (Hoppe et al., 2019).

ALCOHOL CARE TEAM

Over the past three decades, there has been a notable rise in dedicated alcohol liaison nurse services, alcohol care teams, and alcohol nurse specialists both within hospitals and in the community. Their primary objective is to enhance the care and discharge processes for patients grappling with alcohol-related issues. The teams have demonstrated significant benefits in reducing acute hospital admissions, readmissions, and mortality rates while enhancing the quality and efficiency of alcohol care services (Moriarty, 2020). Alcohol care teams operating across acute departments, such as accident and emergency (A&E), are pivotal in ensuring prompt access to brief interventions and appropriate services within 24 hours of identifying alcohol-related problems. These interventions typically involve structured advice sessions lasting 20 to 40 minutes, tailored feedback on health risks associated with alcohol consumption, practical guidance on reducing alcohol intake, and the provision of written materials to support the advice, as recommended by NICE guidelines (2016). The key components of alcohol care team, based on the UK model (Moriarty et al., 2010; NICE, 2016; Williams et al., 2014), include:

- A clinician-led, multidisciplinary alcohol care team, with integrated alcohol treatment pathways across primary, secondary, and community care
- Coordinated alcohol policies for emergency departments and acute medical units
- A seven-day alcohol specialist nurse service
- Addiction and liaison psychiatry services
- An alcohol assertive outreach team for frequent hospital attenders

- Specialist consultant hepatologists and gastroenterologists with expertise in liver disease
- Collaborative, multidisciplinary, person-centred care
- Quality metrics, national indicators, and audit
- Workforce planning, training, and accreditation
- Research, education, and health promotion for the public and healthcare professionals
- Formal links with local authority, public health, clinical commissioning groups, patient groups, and other key stakeholders

The comprehensive approach to alcohol care encompasses a clinician-led, multidisciplinary team operating across primary, secondary, and community care settings. Coordinated policies are implemented in emergency departments and acute medical units, supported by a specialised alcohol nurse service available seven days a week. Additional services include addiction and liaison psychiatry, assertive outreach for frequent hospital attendees, and expertise from hepatologists and gastroenterologists. Collaborative, person-centred care is emphasised, alongside quality metrics, workforce planning, research, education, and formal links with stakeholders to promote public health and improve outcomes. Alcohol specialist nurses may represent a highly cost-effective mechanism. There is evidence to suggest that the alcohol liaison services or alcohol care teams have a significant role in reducing the length of time alcohol-dependent patients spend in hospital, which saves money, and addressing their alcohol misuse improves their health by reducing the likelihood of readmission (Public Health England, 2014).

SPECIALIST ADDICTION NURSES

Historically, various occupational titles, such as alcohol nurse, drug dependency nurse, chemical substance nurse, and others, were assigned to professionals working with individuals experiencing drug and alcohol misuse. However, the formalisation of addiction nursing as a distinct clinical specialty within mental health nursing began in the mid-1980s. The concept of addiction nursing was introduced by Rassool (1996, 1997) in the UK, defining it as a specialised branch of mental health nursing focused on providing care and treatment interventions for individuals whose health issues stem directly from the use and misuse of psychoactive substances, as well as other addictive behaviours, such as eating disorders and gambling.

The scope of professional practice in addiction nursing encompasses clinical practice, which involves nursing care and a variety of psychosocial intervention strategies, including complementary therapies. Additionally, addiction nurses are involved in education, policymaking, and research, contributing to the care and interests of their clients. A notable aspect of their expanded role is the prescribing of drugs (Rassool, 2004). Addiction nurses work in both residential and community settings, where they have been instrumental in developing innovative healthcare initiatives and community-oriented programmes for individuals struggling with drug and alcohol misuse. Many recent developments in addiction care have been nurse-led, such as smoking cessation clinics, mobile methadone clinics, outreach programmes for drug-using commercial sex workers, and satellite clinics for homeless drinkers. Moreover, addiction nurses have played a significant role in the development of multiprofessional post-graduate educational programmes in addictive behaviours (Rassool & Gafoor, 1997; Rassool, 2000).

The significant role of specialist addiction nurses in alcohol and drug treatment services has been extensively documented (Rassool & Gafoor, 1997). The roles of the nurse in relation to drug and alcohol have been articulated in a document from the World Health Organization/International Council of Nurses (WHO/ICN, 1991). These roles are provider of care, educator/resource, counsellor/therapist, advocate, promoter of health, researcher, supervisor/leader, and consultant. The role of the nurse includes the delivery of direct support and treatment to individuals grappling with alcohol and substance use disorders, offering guidance and fostering supportive environments for patients, their families, and colleagues. Their role as counsellors and therapists focuses on addressing emotiona and psychological needs, while as educators, they empower diverse groups with valuable health information to prevent alcohol and substance use anc promote healthier lifestyles. They act as advocate lobbying for policy changes and improved care aiming to reduce the demand for abused drugs anc enhance support systems. They initiate health promotion campaign for broader policy and legislatio changes to mitigate the societal impacts of alcoho and substance use. Their role as researchers advanc knowledge on interventions and prevention strategies, guiding evidence-based approaches to addressing alcohol and substance misuse. Being supervisor leaders, and consultants offers guidance, mentorshi and specialised expertise to ensure high-quality car delivery, fostering supportive working environments for professionals and non-professionals alike.

Recent literature on the role of addiction nurses (Public Health England and Royal College of Nursing, 2017) indicates that addiction nurses utilise their expertise to provide comprehensive care and support to patients with alcohol problems. They employ specialised skills and knowledge to assess patients' physical and mental health, develop personalised care plans, and deliver various interventions tailored to individual needs. These interventions may include behavioural counselling, education about alcohol misuse, and medication management. Addiction nurses are also authorised to prescribe medications, monitor patients' adherence, and address any side effects. Additionally, they play a crucial role in facilitating referrals to other services for further treatment as needed. A recent study examined the Primary Care Alcohol Nurse Outreach Service (PCANOS in Glasgow (Mohan et al., 2022), which employ addiction nurses to collaborate closely with Deep End GP practices, serving Scotland's most deprived populations. Patients with alcohol-related health issues who have had limited engagement with other alcohol services are referred by their GPs to PCANOS. Addiction nurses conduct home visits over a 12-week period, providing specialised care aimed at reducing patients' alcohol consumption levels and facilitating their connection with other community-based alcohol services for long-term support. Overall, addiction nurses contribute significantly to the diagnosis, treatment, and support of individuals struggling with alcohol and substance-related issues, enhancing their overall well-being and recovery journey. A brief description of the roles is shown in Table 20.2.

Table 20.2
Roles of addiction nurses

Provider of care	Create caring and supportive environments
	Offer direct support and treatment
	Support of families and colleagues
	Interventions to address their substance use disorders
	Prescribe medications
Counsellor/ therapist	Focus on addressing the emotional and psychological needs of individuals
	Through therapy sessions, provide guidance, support, and coping strategies to help individuals navigate the challenges associated with substance use and work towards recovery
Educator/ resource	Disseminate valuable health information to diverse groups, including community organisations, schools, and professionals
	Empower individuals with knowledge about the risks associated with substance use
	Provide information on prevention strategies, healthier lifestyles, and available support services
Advocate	Lobby for policy changes and improved care to reduce the demand for misused drugs
	Enhance support systems for individuals affected by substance misuse
	Raise awareness about the societal impacts of substance misuse, and advocate for policies that prioritise prevention, treatment, and harm reduction
Health promoter	Health education and promotion
	Campaign for broader policy and legislation changes
	Work to foster environments conducive to healthier behaviours
	Promote community engagement, and advocate for resources to support prevention and treatment initiatives
Researcher	Advancing knowledge about effective interventions and prevention strategies
	Contribute to the development of evidence-based approaches to addressing substance use disorders, guiding clinical practices and policy decisions
Supervisor/ leader	Provide guidance, mentorship, and oversight to professionals and non-professionals involved in addressing substance misuse
	Ensure high-quality care delivery; foster supportive working
Consultant	Specialised expertise and support to professionals within the field of alcohol and drug
	Provide guidance on clinical practices, programme development, and policy implementation
	Enhance the capacity of care providers to deliver effective interventions and support services

KEY POINTS

- Health and social care professionals, whether in primary healthcare or residential settings, typically serve as the initial point of contact for individuals exhibiting potential or early signs of alcohol and drug issues.
- Recognising the importance of a multidisciplinary team comprising various health and social care professionals to address the complex needs of individuals struggling with alcohol and substance use disorders.
- The significant health and social challenges associated with substance misuse underline the urgent requirement for members of the primary healthcare team, including nurses, social workers, and professionals, within the criminal justice system, to address the needs of individuals affected by drug and alcohol misuse.
- Within the drug and alcohol field, a diverse range of roles exists, encompassing not only specialist workers but also professionals whose duties bring them into contact with individuals experiencing drug and alcohol misuse.
- These roles within the field of drug and alcohol services are distinguished by the level and frequency of interaction with individuals affected by substance misuse.
- Emphasising the role of health and social care professionals in prevention efforts through education, awareness campaigns, and community outreach programmes aimed at reducing the incidence of alcohol and substance use disorders
- The role of the generic worker is to conduct systematic screening and initial assessments to identify individuals at risk of or currently experiencing alcohol and drug misuse, enabling early brief interventions and referrals.
- Multidisciplinary alcohol care team with integrated treatment pathways across care settings. Coordinated policies for emergency and acute care units. Specialised nurse service, addiction and liaison psychiatry, and assertive outreach teams. Collaborative, person-centred care with quality metrics, workforce training, research, and community links.
- Addiction nurses contribute significantly to the diagnosis, treatment, and support of individuals struggling with alcohol and substance-related issues, enhancing their overall well-being and recovery journey.

References

Amaral, F. V. (2024). *What Is an Occupational Health Nurse? (Duties and Salary)*. https://www.indeed.com/career-advice/finding-a-job/occupational-health-nurse (accessed 30 March 2024).

ASAM. (2017). *What Is an Addiction Specialist?* Rockville, MD: American Society of Addiction Medicine.

Coste, S., Gimenez, L., Comes, A., Abdelnour, X., Dupouy, J., & Escourrou, E. (2020). Discussing alcohol use with the GP: A qualitative study. *BJGP Open*, 4(2). https://doi.org/10.3399/bjgpopen20X101029.

Gafoor, M., & Rassool, G. H. (1998). The co-existence of psychiatric disorders and substance misuse: Working with dual diagnosis patients. *Journal of Advanced Nursing*, 27(3), 497–502. https://doi.org/10.1046/j.1365-2648.1998.00545.x.

Gossop, M., Marsden, J., Edwards, C., Wilson, A., Segar, G., Stewart, D., & Lehmann, P. (1995). *The October Report. The National Treatment Outcome Research Study: A Report Prepared for the Task Force*. London: Department of Health.

Higgins, S. A., & Simons, J. (2019). The opioid epidemic and the role of the occupational health nurse. *Workplace Health & Safety*, 67(1), 36–45. https://doi.org/10.1177/2165079918796242.

Hoppe, D., Ristevski, E., & Khalil, H. (2019). The attitudes and practice strategies of community pharmacists towards drug misuse management: A scoping review. *Journal of Clinica Pharmacy and Therapeutics*, 45(3), 430–452.

Institute of Alcohol Studies. (2015). *Alcohol's Impact on Emergency Services*. London: Institute of Alcohol Studies, p. 27.

Jenkins, M. (2015). Substance use: The role of the health visitor in supporting families. *Journal of Health Visiting*, 3(7), 374–380.

Kaner, E. F. S., Beyer, F., Dickinson, H. O., Pienaar, E., Campbell, F., Schlesinger, C., Heather, N., Saunders, J., & Burnand, B (2007). Effectiveness of brief alcohol interventions in primar care populations. *Cochrane Database of Systematic Reviews* 2007(2), CD004148. https://doi.org/10.1002/14651858 CD004148.pub3.

Lester, B. M., Andreozzi, L., & Appiah, L. (2004). Sub stance use during pregnancy: Time for policy to catch u with research. *Harm Reduction Journal*, 1, 5. https://do org/10.1186/1477-7517-1-5.

Lock, C. A. (2004). Alcohol and brief intervention in primar health care: What do patients think? *Primary Health Car Research and Development*, 5, 162–178.

Lock, C. A., & Kaner, E. F. S. (2004). Implementation of brief alcohol interventions by nurses in primary care: Do non-clinical factors influence practice? *Family Practice,* 2(3), 270–275.

Lukewich, J., Martin-Misener, R., Norful, A. A., Poitras, M. E., Bryant-Lukosius, D., Asghari, S., Marshall, E. G., Mathews, M., Swab, M., Ryan, D., & Tranmer, J. (2022). Effectiveness of registered nurses on patient outcomes in primary care: A systematic review. *BMC Health Services Research,* 22(1), 740. https://doi.org/10.1186/s12913-022-07866-x.

McEwen, J. (1991). Interventions in the workplace. In I. Glass (Ed.), *The International Handbook of Addiction Behaviour.* London: Routledge.

Mohan, A., Sharp, C., Mitchell, D., Eadie, D., & Fitzgerald, N. (2022). *Exploring the Management of Alcohol Problems in Deep End Practices in Scotland.* Scottish Health Action on Alcohol Problems (SHAAP). https://www.shaap.org.uk/downloads/405-alcohol-management-deep-end-2022/view-document/405.html (accessed 1 April 2024).

Moriarty, K. J. (2020). Alcohol care teams: Where are we now? *Frontline Gastroenterology,* 11(4), 293–302. https://doi.org/10.1136/flgastro-2019-101241.

Moriarty, K. J., Cassidy, P., Dalton, D., Farrell, M., Gilmore, I., Hawkey, C., Keaney, F., Moore, K., Owens, L., Rhodes, J., Shenker, D., & Sheron, N. (2010). Alcohol Related Disease: Meeting the Challenge of Improved Quality of care and Better Use of Resources. A Joint Position Paper on behalf of the British Society of Gastroenterology/Alcohol Health Alliance UK and British Association for Study of the Liver, p. 9. www.alcohollearningcentre.org.uk/_assets/bsg_alc_disease_10.pdf (accessed 24 June 2024).

NICE. (2010). *Alcohol-Use Disorders: Preventing Harmful Drinking* (PH24). London: National Institute for Health and Care Excellence.

NICE. (2011). *Alcohol Use Disorder: The NICE Guideline on Diagnosis, Assessment and Management of Harmful Drinking and Alcohol. National Clinical Practice.* London: National Institute for Health and Care Excellence.

NICE. (2016). *Alcohol Care Teams: Reducing Acute Hospital Admissions and Improving Quality of Care.* Published on behalf of the British Society of Gastroenterology and Bolton NHS Foundation Trust. http://www.nice.org.uk/localPractice/collection (accessed 31 March 2024).

Owen, L., Gilmore, I. T., & Pirmohamed, M. (2000). General practice nurses' knowledge of alcohol use and misuse: A questionnaire survey. *Alcohol and Alcoholism,* 35(3), 259–262.

Peagram, S. (2017). *Drug Misuse Management in the Acute Hospital Setting – Guidelines* (PAT/T 21 v.3). Doncaster and Bassetlaw Teaching Hospitals. https://www.dbth.nhs.uk/wp-content/uploads/2017/07/PAT-T-21-v-3-Drug-Misuse-Management-in-the-Acute-Hospital-Setting-Guidelines-final.pdf (accessed 30 March 2024).

Peckover, S., & Chidlaw, R. G. (2007). Too frightened to care? Accounts by district nurses working with clients who misuse substances. *Health & Social Care in the Community,* 15(3), 238–245. https://doi.org/10.1111/j.1365-2524.2006.00683.x.

Public Health England. (2014). *Alcohol Care in England's Hospitals: An Opportunity Not to Be Wasted.* London: Public Health England, p. 6.

Public Health England and Royal College of Nursing. (2017). *The Role of Nurses in Alcohol and Drug Treatment Services: A Resource for Commissioners, Providers and Clinicians* (PHE Publications Gateway No. 2017349). London: Public Health England.

Rassool, G. H. (1996). Addiction nursing and drug and alcohol: A slow response to partial accommodation. *Journal of Advanced Nursing,* 24(2), 425–427.

Rassool, G. H. (1997). Addiction nursing-towards a new paradigm: The UK experience. In G. H. Rassool & M. Gafoor (Eds.), *Addiction Nursing-Perspectives on Professional and Clinical Practice.* Cheltenham: Nelson Thornes.

Rassool, G. H. (1998). Health care professionals and drug and alcohol. In G. H. Rassool (Ed.), *Substance Use and Misuse: Nature, Context and Clinical Interventions.* Oxford: Blackwell Publications.

Rassool, G. H. (2000). Addiction: Global problem and global response complacency or commitment? *Journal of Advanced Nursing,* 32(3), 505–508.

Rassool, G. H. (2004). Prescription for change: Perspectives on prescribing authority for addiction nurses in the United Kingdom. *Journal of Addictions Nursing,* 15(4), 193–197.

Rassool, G. H., & Gafoor, M. (Eds.). (1997). *Addiction Nursing-Perspectives on Professional and Clinical Practice.* Cheltenham: Nelson Thornes.

Rassool, G. H., & Marshall, F. (2001). Substance use and misuse: A public health perspective. *Nursing Research,* 6(6), 906–918.

Royal College of Psychiatrists and Royal College of General Practitioners. (2005). *Roles and Responsibilities of Doctors in the Provision of Treatment for Drug and Alcohol Misusers* (Council Report CR131). London: Royal College of Psychiatrists and Royal College of General Practitioners.

Royal College of Psychiatrists, Royal College of General Practitioners Substance Misuse and Associated Health, & Public Health England. (2014). *The Role of Addiction Specialist Doctors in Recovery Orientated Treatment Systems. A Resource for Commissioners, Providers and Clinicians* (PHE Gateway No. 2014112). London: Public Health England.

WHO/ICN. (1991). *Role of the Nurse in relation to Substance Misuse.* Geneva: Internation Council of Nurses.

Williams, R., Aspinall, R., Bellis, M., Camps-Walsh, G., Cramp, M., Dhawan, A., Ferguson, J., Forton, D., Foster, G., Gilmore, I., Hickman, M., Hudson, M., Kelly, D., Langford, A., Lombard, M., Longworth, L., Martin, N., Moriarty, K., Newsome, P., O'Grady, J., Pryke, R., Rutter, H., Ryder, S., Sheron, N., & Smith, T. (2014). Addressing liver disease in the UK: A blueprint for attaining excellence in health care and reducing premature mortality from lifestyle issues of excess consumption of alcohol, obesity, and viral hepatitis. *Lancet,* 384(9958), 1953–1997. https://doi.org/10.1016/S0140-6736(14)61838-9.

Wolf, C., Curry, A., Nacht, J., & Simpson, S. A. (2020). Management of alcohol withdrawal in the emergency department: Current perspectives. *Open Access Emergency Medicine: OAEM,* 12, 53–65. https://doi.org/10.2147/OAEM.S235288.

Chapter 21

Public health approaches to substance misuse

Learning outcomes

- Have an awareness of the relevant literature on the key concepts, theories, and current debates that inform prevention, health education, and promotion practices.
- Describe the types of prevention strategies.
- Examine the strengths and limitations of the four pillars model approaches.
- Discuss the various health education approaches to alcohol and drug misuse.
- Critically reflect on your own role and experiences as a health educator.
- Discuss your role in the rational use of psychoactive substances.
- Have an understanding of health-promoting institutions in relation to substance misuse.

Activity 21.1

There is only one answer to the following multiple-choice questions.

1. Which of the following statements best describes the primary aim of public health approaches to substance misuse?
   a. To promote constructive lifestyles among individuals
   b. To delay or avoid the onset of substance misuse
   c. To provide treatment exclusively for those already affected by substance misuse
   d. To advocate for policy changes related to substance use
   e. All of the above
2. Select the statement that accurately represents the role of public health policies in addressing substance misuse.
   a. Public health policies focus solely on individual-level interventions.
   b. Public health policies aim to reduce the societal impacts of substance misuse.
   c. Public health policies are primarily concerned with punishing substance users.
   d. Public health policies have no impact on preventing substance misuse.
   e. None of the above.
3. Which of the following is not a key component of the government alcohol strategy?
   a. Promoting sensible drinking
   b. Reducing the harm caused by alcohol
   c. Assisting families affected by alcohol-related issues
   d. Focusing solely on the minority of harmful drinkers
   e. All of the above

DOI: 10.4324/9781003456674-25

4. High-risk groups susceptible to substance misuse include:
   a. Individuals with strong social support networks
   b. Non-smokers
   c. Pregnant women
   d. Athletes
   e. None of the above
5. Which statement accurately describes primary prevention efforts in substance misuse?
   a. Encouraging drinking behaviour
   b. Reducing the demand for substance misuse
   c. Targeting individuals who have tried psychoactive substances
   d. Providing health information to individuals currently using substances
   e. All of the above
6. Secondary prevention aims to:
   a. Promote healthy lifestyles among individuals
   b. Reduce and limit health and social harms associated with substance misuse
   c. Encourage substance use among vulnerable populations
   d. Prevent the onset of substance misuse
   e. None of the above
7. Tertiary prevention seeks to:
   a. Prevent substance misuse among at-risk populations
   b. Limit and reduce further complications arising from substance misuse
   c. Promote treatment exclusively for substance users
   d. Encourage substance use as a coping mechanism
   e. All of the above
8. Which statement accurately describes selective prevention programmes?
   a. They target individuals who have not yet tried psychoactive substances.
   b. They aim to reduce the influence of risk factors associated with substance misuse.
   c. They focus on individuals currently receiving treatment for substance misuse.
   d. They advocate for policy changes related to substance use.
   e. None of the above.
9. Rational use of psychoactive substances involves:
   a. Extravagant prescribing practices
   b. Over-prescribing medications to individuals
   c. Ensuring the right drug is administered to the right patient, at the right dose, and for the right duration
   d. Incorrect prescribing practices
   e. None of the above
10. Indicated prevention programmes target:
    a. General population groups
    b. Individuals currently receiving treatment for substance misuse
    c. Individuals who have not yet tried psychoactive substances
    d. Individuals with strong social support networks
    e. None of the above
11. Public health education programmes aim to:
    a. Impart knowledge about substance misuse
    b. Provide treatment exclusively for substance users
    c. Identify alcohol and drug users
    d. Meet alcohol and drug education requirements
    e. All of the above

12. Which of the following is not a universal prevention activity?
    a. Schools-based prevention programmes
    b. Mass media campaigns
    c. Selective prevention programmes
    d. Community outreach initiatives
    e. All of the above
13. Irrational prescribing practices may include:
    a. Extravagant prescribing
    b. Over-prescribing medications
    c. Providing appropriate doses of medication
    d. Correct prescribing practices
    e. None of the above
14. An alternative to medication for addressing substance misuse is:
    a. Pharmacological therapies
    b. Increasing the dosage of medications
    c. Counselling and relaxation therapies
    d. Continuing the same medication regimen
    e. None of the above
15. The goal of public health approaches to substance misuse is to:
    a. Promote substance use among vulnerable populations
    b. Limit access to treatment services
    c. Reduce the societal impacts of substance misuse
    d. Increase the stigma associated with substance use
    e. None of the above

INTRODUCTION

In today's society, health and social care professionals play a crucial role in promoting health, education, prevention, and harm reduction related to alcohol and drug misuse. The new public health represents a modern approach to improving the health of individuals and communities through evidence-based scientific, technological, and management strategies (Tulchinsky & Varavikova, 2010). It encompasses a wide range of interventions and initiatives aimed at addressing various health issues and promoting well-being on both individual and population levels. A public health approach to addressing these issues involves collaboration across various sectors, including health, social services, education, and criminal justice. Health and social care professionals have opportunities in every patient encounter to provide information and support for healthcare and harm reduction practices, including those related to tobacco smoking, alcohol, psychoactive drugs, and sexual health. Prevention efforts aim to promote constructive lifestyles and delay or prevent the onset of alcohol and drug misuse through diver strategies. Health promotion is now recognised an essential component of public health policy ar is integrated into health and education service Additionally, harm reduction strategies focus c minimising the negative consequences of substanc misuse, particularly in areas such as injection pra tices and sexual health.

The WHO/UNODC (2007) global initiative c the primary prevention of substance abuse proje aimed to reduce the use of psychoactive substanc and related problems among young people aged to 24 years. The initiative, implemented in multip countries, showed positive outcomes overall, wi some areas experiencing a decrease in psychoacti substance use among youth or a delay in the age onset. The four pillars model, encompassing preve tion, treatment, enforcement, and harm reductic (Drug Alliance Policy, p. 1), has been proposed a comprehensive strategy to address substance mi use. The COVID-19 pandemic has worsened ri factors associated with substance use disorders ar has presented significant challenges to healthca systems and public health policies worldwide, necessitating innovative treatment and prevention approaches to mitigate its impact (Ornell et al., 2020). Individuals with substance use disorders (SUD) represent a vulnerable population at heightened risk of contracting the virus due to a combination of clinical, psychological, and psychosocial factors. This chapter explores the relationships between public health, health education, and prevention concepts within the context of substance misuse, with a focus on health-promoting hospitals, schools, and workplaces.

PUBLIC HEALTH, HEALTH EDUCATION, AND PREVENTION

Since the late 1980s, prevention and treatment have gained significant attention on political and service agendas. Public health campaigns have been launched to raise awareness about the risks associated with tobacco smoking, drunk driving, and the misuse of various substances, including over-the-counter drugs, alcohol, prescribed medications, and illicit drugs. This has led to increased emphasis on the public health triangular model, which highlights the interaction between the host (the individual), the agent (the substance), and the environment (Rassool & Marshall, 2001). Prevention efforts now target the person, the substance, and the environment, employing strategies such as influence and persuasion, competency development, and environmental improvements to encourage healthy choices and promote health-oriented policies (Macpherson, 2001).

Health education and health promotion are integral components of professional practice, encompassing a range of activities from providing advice to implementing structured interventions. Health promotion aims to empower individuals to take control of their health and improve their overall well-being by making informed decisions and accessing appropriate health services. According to the World Health Organization (WHO, 1986), health promotion involves enabling people to increase control over their health and achieve physical, mental, and social well-being. While this definition provides a broad framework, it may lack specificity in the context of preventing alcohol and drug misuse.

In the context of substance misuse prevention, health education plays a crucial role in promoting healthier lifestyles and enabling individuals to make informed choices regarding tobacco smoking, alcohol consumption, and drug use. Health education within the realm of health promotion seeks to equip individuals with the knowledge and skills necessary to identify and address their health needs, as well as to navigate the environmental and socio-political factors influencing their health behaviours (WHO, 1986). By incorporating health education into broader health promotion efforts, professionals can effectively address substance misuse and promote overall well-being within communities.

In public health, health education activities are often categorised into three levels: primary, secondary, and tertiary prevention. However, this three-stage model may be too restrictive to fully address the complexities of prevention and public health policies. Another dimension to consider is the harm reduction approach, which aims to minimise both the risk of individuals engaging in substance misuse and the harm associated with substance misuse. Core elements of effective, research-based prevention programmes include structure, content, and delivery. *Structure* refers to how the programme is organised and constructed, while *content* pertains to the information, skills, and strategies presented in the programme. *Delivery* encompasses how the programme is selected or adapted and implemented, as well as how it is evaluated within a specific community (NIDA, 2003).

PRIMARY PREVENTION

Primary prevention aims to reduce the demand for and prevent the initiation of illegal drug use, alcohol consumption, and tobacco smoking. This includes efforts to discourage alcohol consumption among young people and high-risk groups, thereby delaying the onset of substance use. Primary prevention approaches encompass both individual and environmental strategies. In individual approaches, young people are provided with knowledge, skills, attitudes, and resources regarding the harms of substance misuse. Peer education is highlighted as particularly effective, involving young people in both receiving and providing information (WHO, 2000). Primary prevention encompasses environmental approaches aimed at creating supportive environments for young people, involving family, peers, and community resources to foster positive attachments and resilience. Strengthening parent–child communication and providing access to social, educational, and health services are essential components. Promoting positive social norms is emphasised as part of creating safe and supportive environments (WHO, 2000). Primary prevention efforts involve health education, media campaigns, and community mobilisation, targeting not only non-users but also experimental, recreational, and dependent users. Vulnerable groups such as binge drinkers, pregnant women, youth offenders, injecting drug users, prisoners, sex workers, and the homeless require particular attention due to their heightened risk behaviours.

In a study of the factors that influence the effectiveness of primary prevention of substance use (Mardaneh Jobehdar et al., 2021), universal prevention programmes generally showed greater effectiveness compared to selective and indicated programmes. Among different settings, school-based interventions were reported as particularly effective. In family settings, selective programmes demonstrated higher efficacy. Additionally, interventions delivered by specialists were more effective than those by laypeople or peers. Multidisciplinary interventions involving contributions from multiple professionals were associated with increased effectiveness. Afuseh et al. (2020) suggested that identifying age-related risk factors for the development of substance use disorders is important for recognising individuals who may be at risk. The authors recommended that the development of a comprehensive list of risk factors within each age group is essential for creating age-specific, evidence-based screening tools and tailoring appropriate individual interventions.

SECONDARY PREVENTION

Secondary prevention of alcohol and substance use disorders involves interventions aimed at individuals who are at risk of developing such disorders or who have already initiated substance use but have not yet developed severe problems. Secondary prevention of substance misuse involves identifying individuals at risk of adverse outcomes due to substance misuse and intervening early to mitigate harm. It focuses on reducing the negative consequences associated with substance use, such as health problems and social dysfunction, through strategies such as early recognition, targeted interventions, and rehabilitation. Key components include promoting rational use of medications, providing health education on safer substance use practices, and advocating for safer sexual behaviours. Overall, secondary prevention aims to prevent the escalation of substance-related problems and promote healthier outcomes for individuals and communities.

TERTIARY PREVENTION

The tertiary level of prevention aims to minimise complications and dysfunctions by providing effective care, treatment, and rehabilitation services. Its goal is to restore individuals to an optimal level of

Table 21.1
Key aspects of secondary prevention I of substance misuse

Key aspects	Description
Early recognition	Prompt identification of individuals who are experiencing harmful effects or are at risk of adverse outcomes due to substance misuse.
Intervention	Implementation of targeted interventions aimed at addressing substance-related issues and preventing the progression to more severe problems.
Rehabilitation	Provision of support and resources for individuals to address substance-related disabilities or dysfunctions and facilitate their recovery process.
Rational use of prescribed medication	Ensuring appropriate and responsible use of prescription medications to minimise the risk of substance misuse or dependence.
Health information	Providing education and guidance on safer alcohol and drug use practices to reduce the likelihood of adverse health effects.
Safer sexual practices	Promoting awareness of the link between substance misuse and risky sexual behaviours, and advocating for safer sexual practices to prevent the transmission of blood-borne viruses, such as HIV and hepatitis infections.

functioning and prevent relapse. Tertiary prevention involves engaging residential and community facilities to address alcohol- or drug-related problems, focusing on treatment rather than prevention. This level of prevention is primarily conducted by specialist addiction services, distinguishing it from primary and secondary prevention efforts. Preventive interventions for health and social care professionals primarily involve primary and secondary approaches, encompassing assessment, intervention, and evaluation. It is important to recognise the impracticality of completely eradicating substance use across the entire population. Instead, professionals should focus on health education to mitigate the harm associated with ongoing substance use and misuse. This approach acknowledges the limitations while aiming to reduce the negative consequences of substance use.

FRAMEWORK FOR CLASSIFYING PREVENTION

Prevention initiatives are often categorised into universal, selective, and indicated prevention programmes, with the aim of addressing substance misuse. Universal programmes focus on promoting health and preventing the onset of substance use among individuals, communities, or schools. These initiatives may include schools-based programmes, mass media campaigns, or community-wide interventions targeting children and young people (Cance et al., 2023; Mrazek & Haggerty, 1994). Selective prevention programmes target specific groups at increased risk of substance use problems, aiming to reduce risk factors, enhance protective factors, and prevent substance use initiation (Edmonds et al., 2005). Indicated prevention programmes, also known as harm reduction, target individuals already exhibiting problematic substance use, offering specialised interventions tailored to their needs.

Prevention programmes targeting substance use and its adverse effects are typically tailored to specific settings, age groups, and populations, with the aim of being evidence-based (NIDA, 2014).

- Reduce risk factors and enhance protective factors
- Help people avoid or delay the onset of drug use
- Stop substance use from progressing into higher-risk substance use or a substance use disorder
- Reduce harms related to substance use and misuse, such as injuries or infections

Prevention programmes are also structured to address the needs of individuals at different life stages, including pre-natal, early childhood, adolescence, and adulthood (LeNoue & Riggs, 2016). These programmes are often implemented in various settings, such as family homes, healthcare facilities, and community settings.

HEALTH EDUCATION INTERVENTIONS

Health education plays a crucial role in empowering individuals to make informed choices and adopt healthier lifestyles, particularly in relation to substance misuse. Beyond simply providing information, health education aims to facilitate behavioural change by promoting alternatives to substance use and fostering awareness of the associated risks. This shift towards comprehensive education and prevention strategies involves the provision of advice and brief interventions by healthcare professionals, emphasising early recognition and minimal interventions. Early recognition and minimal interventions are also part of the process of preventive health education (Babor & Grant, 1992; WHO, 1986) to mitigate health-related harms. By equipping individuals with the knowledge and skills to navigate substance-related issues, health education contributes to reducing the prevalence of substance misuse and its associated negative consequences.

Patients in hospital and primary healthcare settings often express dissatisfaction with the information and advice they receive regarding healthier lifestyle choices, such as sensible drinking practices and smoking cessation. Research suggests that individuals welcome clearer guidance in these areas to support their efforts towards a healthier life (Hartz et al., 1991). Early recognition and minimal interventions can be effectively integrated into brief assessments, which encompass taking a comprehensive drug, alcohol, and tobacco history, conducting risk assessments, and providing counselling. These practices, outlined in Chapters 24 and 26, enable healthcare professionals to identify substance use patterns early and deliver targeted interventions to promote healthier behaviours. The National Institute of Clinical Excellence (NICE, 2007) outlines

Table 21.2
Prevention programmes in specific settings

Programme	Descriptions
Family-based programmes	Aim to support parents and caregivers in accessing resources and developing skills linked to positive substance use outcomes in children. Examples include the nurse–family partnership, an intensive parenting intervention offering home nurse visits to new and expecting parents. Provision of parenting classes focused on early child development and fostering nurturing relationships with children.
School-based programmes	Designed to equip students with social, emotional, cognitive, and substance-refusal skills. Provision of social and emotional skills training to children, connecting at-risk youth with positive mentors. Organising after-school activities to engage students in constructive pursuits.
Community-based programmes	Collaboration with community organisations and leaders to identify and address local-level risk factors for substance use. Develop strategies to mitigate their impact. Prioritise evidence-based interventions tailored to a community's specific needs and resources. Fostering a proactive approach to substance misuse prevention at the grassroots level.
Population-specific programmes	Target groups with shared circumstances or characteristics, such as housing status, ethnicity, gender, or geographic location, to address unique challenges and leverage strengths that may influence substance use outcomes. These programmes tailor interventions to meet the specific needs of each group, such as providing housing, education, and healthcare for young people experiencing homelessness to mitigate risk factors associated with substance use.
Prevention strategies	Implemented in healthcare settings, enable clinicians to identify patients who may be at risk for substance use disorders and to facilitate their access to appropriate care and support services. Involve routine screening for substance use during primary care visits, particularly in paediatric settings, to detect potential issues early on and intervene effectively.
Workplaces and criminal justice settings	Programmes can also be tailored for workplaces and criminal justice settings.

Source: Contents based on NIDA (2014).

appropriate means for implementing both generic and specific interventions to support attitude and behaviour changes at population and community levels. At the community level, primary healthcare teams play a crucial role in promoting preventive health behaviours. This involves not only targeting individuals but also assisting the community as a whole in making lifestyle and behaviour changes. Mobilising the community is a key element of this approach, as highlighted in suggestions for nurses as primary healthcare workers documented by the World Health Organization (WHO, 1986). However, it is important to recognise that the strategy of preventive health education cannot be solely implemented by nurses in isolation.

A successful strategy for encouraging the community to adopt healthier lifestyles and behaviours necessitates establishing positive partnerships with influential stakeholders within the community. These partnerships should involve collaboration with community leaders, members of the public, social services, education services, non-statutory and voluntary agencies, police services, and the media. Research suggests that the effectiveness of drug campaigns and safer sex strategies depends on grass-roots prevention campaigns facilitated by credible, trained peers (Kelly & Murphy, 1991). Within this framework, emphasis is also placed on promoting overall health and increasing individual awareness to maintain a healthier lifestyle. This can involve the development of alternative activities, such as physical and recreational activities, stress reduction techniques, and other coping skills. Helping individuals make informed choices about the responsible use of legal psychoactive substances is also part of this process. A variety of approaches has been used in an attempt to prevent and reduce substance misuse demand. Table 21.3 summarises the models, goals, and interventions of health education in relation to alcohol and drugs.

THE PREVENTION, TREATMENT, ENFORCEMENT, AND HARM REDUCTION APPROACH

The prevention, treatment, enforcement, and harm reduction (four pillars model) approaches have been implemented in many countries. The prevention plan aims to mitigate harm associated with substance use at individual, family, neighbourhood, and community levels. It seeks to delay the onset of first substance use, reduce the incidence and prevalence of problematic substance use and dependence, and enhance public health, safety, and order. The treatment pillar of the plan encompasses a spectrum of interventions and support programmes designed to empower individuals with addiction to make healthier decisions. By reducing preventable deaths, illnesses, and injuries, and by fostering social integration, treatment not only improves individual health but also contributes to community well-being. Embracing the principles of harm reduction, the plan prioritises minimising harm associated

Table 21.3
Health education/public health approaches to substance misuse

Approach	Goals	Health education Intervention	Examples
Public health/medical problems	Reduction of morbidity and mortality.	Prevention of ill health. Clinical interventions.	Public health/medical problems.
Behaviour change	Change of life-style and behaviour.	Media campaign. Health information: controlled drinking, safer drug use, and safer sex. Alcohol and driving.	Prevent non-smokers to start smoking. Persuade smokers to stop. Counselling. Harm reduction: reducing or minimising ill effect or harm from alcohol and drug.
Educational	Changing attitude. Increase knowledge and awareness. Develop skills in decision-making and resilience.	Health information on smoking, drinking, and drug-taking. Learning coping skills and stress management.	Information about effects of substance misuse and health-related problems. Provision of resources. Referral to specialist services.
Consumer empowerment	Enabling individuals to identify their health concerns.	Advocacy. Meeting specific health and socio-economic needs.	Clients identify health needs, types, and access to services. Community anti-drug campaign.
Social change	Enabling changes to health and social policies. Bringing changes to the social environment. Improvement in health and social equality in access to services and treatment interventions.	Lobbying. Political and social actions.	Alcohol and drug policy in the workplace. Limit of marketing and advertising of alcohol and tobacco. Decriminalisation of drugs. Labelling on alcohol beverages.

Source: Adapted from Rassool and Gafoor (1997).

with substance misuse and acknowledges that abstinence may not be immediately achievable for all individuals. Instead, it advocates for a pragmatic approach focused on incremental progress towards healthier outcomes, recognising that small steps can lead to significant improvements in both individual and community health. The enforcement pillar of the drug policy prevention plan is geared towards upholding public safety and order through the implementation of legal measures and regulatory enforcement. This pillar aims to deter illegal drug activities, including production, trafficking, and distribution, thereby reducing the availability of illicit substances within communities.

The four pillars model has been found to be effective in reducing the number of drug users consuming street drugs, a significant drop in overdose deaths, a reduction in crime, and a reduction in the infection rates for HIV and hepatitis (Kerr et al., 2005; MacPherson, 2001). Evidence-based interventions have been crafted to address immediate factors contributing to the risk of substance use disorder (SUD), such as behavioural issues, trauma, and inadequate parental involvement (Fishbein & Sloboda, 2023). Additionally, at the population level, a range of broader approaches exists. These encompass enforcing policies related to the accessibility and availability of substances like tobacco, alcohol, and cannabis, along with policies addressing systemic issues like child poverty, family economic instability, and systemic racism, which are underlying factors exacerbating the SUD crisis (Fishbein & Sloboda, 2023). Apart from interventions directed at individuals and families, community-based strategies have demonstrated efficacy in decreasing substance use disorder and enhancing overall health outcomes.

A review of evidence commissioned by the European Monitoring Centre for Drugs and Drug Addiction (EMCDDA) (Sumnall et al., 2017) presents an overview of their findings in relation to prevention strategies. Various interventions have been evaluated for their effectiveness in preventing drug use among young people. School-based prevention programmes, particularly those with manualised approaches, have demonstrated effectiveness, while brief interventions delivered in schools or healthcare settings have shown limited impact. Universal family interventions involving both parents and children may prevent cannabis use, though evidence on other drug use is inconclusive. Mass media campaigns alone have generally been ineffective, but structured interventions delivered online show promise, especially when targeted at schools or family groups. Selective mentoring interventions may not directly prevent drug use among high-risk youth, but certain approaches within mentoring programmes could indirectly improve engagement in skill-building activities. In addition to these interventions, motivational interviewing, cognitive behavioural therapy, and multicomponent approaches, including parental and behavioural skills training, have shown potential in reducing cannabis and other drug use, particularly among specific groups with mental health disorders like attention-deficit hyperactivity disorder or disruptive behavioural disorders. Overall, a combination of approaches, including targeted school-based programmes, family interventions, and tailored therapeutic interventions, may offer the most effective strategy in preventing drug use among young people.

RATIONAL USE OF PSYCHOACTIVE SUBSTANCE

The term "rational use" refers to the appropriate utilisation of medications, ensuring that the correct drug is administered to the right patient, in the correct dosage, and for the appropriate duration of therapy, while also ensuring that the associated risks are acceptable (WHO, 1989). Licit (prescribed and over-the-counter) as well as illicit psychoactive substances pose significant public health concerns, with nearly half of all medicines globally being used irrationally, leading to adverse drug reactions, drug resistance, prolonged illness, mortality, and financial burden, particularly in developing countries, where patients often bear the cost of medications out of pocket (WHO, 2004a). While opioids have established roles in managing acute and cancer-related pain, their use in chronic pain management remains contentious. Opioid analgesics like fentanyl, morphine, and pethidine are commonly utilised worldwide. Despite the presence of clear guidelines recommending restrictions on their use, many patients with chronic pain continue to receive prescriptions for potent opioids (Castellanos et al., 2020). This practice has been identified as a contributing factor to the ongoing opioid epidemic.

In recent years, concerns have escalated regarding the appropriate utilisation and distribution of psychoactive drugs due to escalating consumption rates reported in various countries, primarily attributed to over-prescription, irrational use, and increased adverse effects, leading to both psychological and physical dependence. Commonly prescribed psychoactive drugs like hypnotics, sedatives, and tranquilisers are frequently misused, resulting in health-related problems and dependence. The rise of self-care approaches, consumerism, and popular demands for increased self-control have contributed to the misuse of over-the-counter drugs, many of which contain alcohol, hallucinogenic compounds, and narcotics like codeine, known to be addictive. Moreover, the availability and accessibility of medications through the internet underscore the necessity for heightened public health education regarding the appropriate use of psychoactive substances and other drugs (Rassool, 2005).

The proliferation of compounds sold over the internet poses a significant risk, as some of these substances have addictive potential and can even be life-threatening. Additionally, there appears to be a concerning parallel between the therapeutic use of psychoactive substances and their non-medical or recreational use. *Irrational use* of psychoactive substances refers to their usage that deviates from established good clinical practice. This irrational prescribing, also known as "pathological" prescribing, occurs when the criteria in the prescribing process are not met. Examples of such irrational prescribing include extravagant prescribing, over-prescribing, incorrect prescribing, multiple prescribing, indiscriminate use of injections, and under-prescribing of sedative-hypnotic drugs and antibiotics (Rassool, 2000; WHO, 2004b).

Prescribing and medication management have expanded the role and authority of healthcare professionals within the multidisciplinary teams. The nursing, midwifery, medical, and pharmaceutical professions are all participants in medication management and other intervention strategies, and this would enhance the provision of a more comprehensive and streamlined service and improve the quality of care. The process of rational prescribing and the rational use of drugs includes assessing healthcare needs of the patient (making a diagnosis), planning and setting goals for care, administering and monitoring the effects of medications, providing patient education and discharge planning, interdisciplinary collaboration, evaluating desired and adverse effects of medications, and documenting the process (Manias & Street, 2000; Rassool, 2005).

Healthcare professionals bear a professional obligation to ensure the rational use of psychoactive drugs, emphasising the importance of promoting such usage and educating healthcare providers in this domain (Ghodse & Khan, 1988; Rassool & Winnington, 1993). Their proficiency and clinical acumen regarding various medications sand the repercussions of their misuse serve as a foundation for effective nursing interventions (Rassool & Winnington, 1993). Non-pharmacological therapies like counselling and relaxation techniques may serve as viable alternatives to medication containing psychoactive substances. While addressing the issue of psychoactive drug misuse, it is essential to also consider the appropriate utilisation of therapeutic medications (Rassool & Winnington, 1993).

HEALTH-PROMOTING HOSPITALS

Over the past two decades, the concept of "health-promoting hospitals" has gradually emerged in Europe, with a focus on enhancing health and preventing disease. The Budapest Declaration on Health Promoting Hospital (WHO, 1991) emphasises that health-promoting hospitals not only provide high-quality medical services but also promote health perspectives and activities among staff, patients, relatives, and the wider community. This movement seeks to utilise hospitals as platforms for promoting positive health within their own environments and in the broader community. By shifting the focus from illness to health-oriented approaches, hospitals can implement health education and promotion activities for both staff and patients. Several initiatives aimed at creating health-promoting hospitals are underway, with key principles derived from the Ottawa Charter for Health Promoting Hospitals (WHO, 1992) serving as a strategic basis. Hospitals that become part of the International Network of Health Promoting Hospitals strive to deliver top-notch, comprehensive medical and nursing services. They achieve this by incorporating health promotion activities into their corporate identity and daily practice for patients, staff, and the community (WHO, 1998). In line with this, the WHO (2003) has established five standards to delineate the principles and actions that should characterise care in every hospital. The five standards address management policy; patient assessment, information, and intervention; promoting a healthy workplace; and continuity and cooperation. The standards include:

- The health improvement/promotion policies or initiatives which are an integral part of an organisation's quality management system (for example, alcohol and drug policy)
- Initiatives to support patient treatment, improve prognosis, and promote patients' health and well-being
- Initiatives that ensure patients are informed about planned activities that enable them to participate actively in such activities, and that facilitate integration of health improvement/promotion initiatives in all patient care
- Policies or initiatives that support a healthy and safe environment for staff or promote staff health and well-being
- Initiatives involving other health, social care, education, and criminal justice sectors

Alcohol and drug policies are now part of many health and social care institutions. Health-promoting hospitals have been shown to have a positive impact on patient loyalty Wartiningsih et al., 2020). By implementing these standards and guidelines, public sector hospitals can improve patient satisfaction, strengthen patient–provider relationships, and ultimately foster greater loyalty among patients. This commitment to health promotion and patient-centred care not only benefits individual patients but also contributes to the overall improvement of healthcare delivery within the community.

HEALTH PROMOTION: SUBSTANCE MISUSE AND THE WORKPLACE

The workplace serves as an ideal setting for engaging a significant number of adults in prevention and health promotion efforts aimed at addressing tobacco smoking, alcohol use, and drug misuse. Workplace health programmes encompass a coordinated and comprehensive array of strategies aimed at meeting the health and safety needs of all employees. These programmes typically include various initiatives, policies, benefits, environmental supports, and connections to the surrounding community. The overarching goal of workplace health programmes is to promote the well-being of employees by addressing a wide range of health-related concerns, including physical health, mental health, safety, and overall quality of life. These programmes may include activities such as health screenings, wellness initiatives, ergonomic assessments, safety trainings, access to healthcare resources, and support for health behaviours both at work and in employees' person lives.

Examples of workplace health programme com ponents and strategies include (CDC, 2016):

- Educational sessions on health
- Availability of nearby fitness centres f employees
- Implementation of corporate policies encoura ing healthy habits, such as a campus-wide ban c tobacco use
- Provision of health insurance coverage for pr ventive screenings
- Promotion of a healthy workplace environmen including offering healthy food options in ven ing machines or cafeterias
- Ensuring a safe work environment free fro known health and safety hazards, with mech nisms in place to address emerging issues as the occur

However, the implementation of health-promotir programmes in the workplace has benefitted th organisations from the reduction of stress, absente ism, and sickness among staff, reduced staff turnove and an increase in organisational efficiency. Accor ing to an OECD analysis (2020), 68% of partic pating companies stated that they provided stre and mental health programmes. Additionally, 80 of companies reported implementing measures expand the health-related choices available to ind viduals. These measures include offering healthi food options in cafeterias and providing addictic management programmes. Workplace health pr motion initiatives have demonstrated numero benefits for both employees and companies. The include enhancing productivity, reducing sickne absences, fostering positive working relationship boosting employee morale, and cultivating a favou able public image for organisations that impleme such programmes (Kuhn & Chu, 2022). Gossc and Grant (1990) outlined three primary focuses employee drug education activities:

- "Impersonal" information
- Employee participation
- Health promotion activities

It is expected that organisations will promote th involvement of all staff members, managemer trade unions, and professional organisations decision-making processes related to healthcare policy. Healthcare professionals play an important role in shaping the development of occupational health services and policies concerning health in the workplace, including educational programmes addressing substance misuse.

HEALTH-PROMOTING SCHOOLS

Young people are among the high-risk groups prone to experimenting with legal and illicit psychoactive substances. To address this, primary prevention initiatives are vital in motivating young individuals to refrain from drug experimentation. Health-promoting schools are integral to the WHO Global Schools Health Initiative, initiated in 1995. A *health-promoting school* is defined as one where all members of the school community collaborate to provide pupils with comprehensive and positive experiences and structures aimed at promoting and safeguarding their health (WHO, 1995). This involves integrating health into both formal and informal curricula, establishing a safe and healthy school environment, offering appropriate health services, and engaging families and the wider community in health promotion efforts. The WHO model emphasises the continuous strengthening of the school's capacity as a healthy setting for living, learning, and working. Health-promoting schools focus on:

- Caring for oneself and others, creating conditions conducive to health
- Making healthy decisions and taking control of life circumstances
- Preventing leading causes of death, disease, and disability
- Influencing health-related behaviours through knowledge, skills, and attitudes
- Building the capacity for peace, education, social justice, sustainable development, and more

The primary objective of school health education is to foster behaviours and environments conducive to health. Skills-based drug education, a key element of comprehensive drug prevention programmes in schools, focuses on equipping young individuals with the knowledge, attitudes, and skills necessary to resist drug use and maintain their decisions to abstain from drugs. The plan of action for addressing substance misuse among young people involves training teachers, supporting innovative drug education projects, developing school policies on managing drug-related incidents, and implementing interdepartmental publicity campaigns and treatment services. Schools should adopt policies that encompass a range of responses to address substance misuse, with prevention being the primary focus, while offering treatment and rehabilitation to those who have already been involved with psychoactive substances, rather than punitive measures (Parsons et al., 2002).

CONCLUSIONS

The role of nurses and other healthcare professionals in addressing substance misuse encompasses supporting, educating, preventing, and providing care, all falling under the umbrella term of "health intervention." These professionals are involved in both primary and secondary prevention initiatives, making substance use prevention, health education, and promotion integral components of health and educational policies. Effective alcohol and drug education is not substance-focused but rather focuses on personal and social development within the context of general health promotion strategies aimed at eliminating the societal factors contributing to substance abuse. Successful health promotion activities rely on a coordinated approach that utilises existing prevention strategies, involving healthcare professionals, schools, families, and other stakeholders in efforts to prevent and reduce the impact of substance misuse. Additionally, ensuring the ongoing education of compassionate practitioners is paramount in addressing substance misuse effectively.

KEY POINTS

- Health education, prevention, and harm reduction are increasingly forming part of the role of health and social care professionals.
- Every encounter with a patient affords an opportunity to transmit knowledge about healthcare and harm reduction in relation to tobacco smoking, alcohol, psychoactive drugs, and sexual health.
- Health promotion has emerged as an integral part of public health policy and now forms an important part of the health and education services.
- Health promotion includes the provision of information on healthier lifestyles for patients

and how to make the best use of health services, with the intention of enabling people to make rational health choices and of ensuring awareness of the factors determining the health of the community.

- Health education activities have been viewed as existing on three levels: primary, secondary, and tertiary prevention.
- Alcohol and drug policy is now part of many hospital health and social care policies.
- Health-promoting schools are part of the WHO Global Schools Health strategy.
- The primary goal of school health education is to help individuals adopt behaviours and create conditions that are conducive to health.
- The importance of promoting the rational use of psychoactive drugs and the need to educate healthcare professionals in this area has been recognised.
- A comprehensive workplace health promotion scheme empowers social partners from both inside and outside workplace enterprises for the health maintenance of workers and their families and creates healthy working environments for the same.

Activity 21.2

Questions

- What is meant by the terms *health education*, *health promotion*, and *prevention*?
- What is meant by the terms *rational use* and *irrational use*?
- Describe two systems for classifying prevention programmes.
- Reflect on the terms *rational prescribing* and *rational use of drugs*. What do they mean to you now?
- List some examples of effective prevention programmes that have been adopted at your place of work (if appropriate) or at the community level.
- Describe the features of workplace prevention programmes.
- Examine the strengths and limitations of the four pillars model approaches.
- Examine your local/institutional alcohol and drug policy.

References

Afuseh, E., Pike, C. A., & Oruche, U. M. (2020). Individualized approach to primary prevention of substance use disorder: Age-related risks. *Substance Abuse Treatment, Prevention, and Policy,* 15(1), 58. https://doi.org/10.1186/s13011-020-00300-7.

Babor, T. F., & Grant, M. (Eds.). (1992). *Project Identification and Management of Alcohol-related Problems. Report on Phase II: A Randomized Clinical Trial of Brief Interventions in Primary Health Care.* Geneva: World Health Organization.

Cance, J. D., Adams, E. T., D'Amico, E. J., Palimaru, A., Fernandes, C. S. F., Fiellin, L. E., Bonar, E. E., Walton, M. A., Komro, K. A., Knight, D., Knight, K., Rao, V., Youn, S., Saavedra, L., Ridenour, T. A., & Deeds, B. (2023). Leveraging the full continuum of care to prevent opioid use disorder. *Prevention Science: The Official Journal of the Society for Prevention Research,* 24(Suppl 1), 30–39. https://doi.org/10.1007/s11121-023-01545-x.

Castellanos, J. P., Woolley, C., Bruno, K. A., Zeidan, F., Halberstadt, A., & Furnish, T. (2020). Chronic pain and psychedelics: A review and proposed mechanism of action. *Regional Anesthesia and Pain Medicine,* 45(7), 486–494. https://doi.org/10.1136/rapm-2020-101273.

CDC. (2016). *Workplace Health Model.* Centers for Disease Control and Prevention. https://www.cdc.gov/workplacehealthpromotion/model/index.html#:~:text=Examples%20of%20workplace%20health%20program%20components%20and%20strategies,accessible%20through%20vending%20machines%20or%20cafeterias%20More%20items (accessed 2 April 2024).

Edmonds, K., Sumnall, H. R., McVeigh, J., Bellis, M. A., McGrath, Y., & Wilkinson, L. (2005). *Drug Prevention Among Vulnerable Young People.* https://www.researchgate.net/publication/259502706_Drug_Prevention_among_Vulnerable_Young_People (accessed 1 April 2024).

Fishbein, D. H., & Sloboda, Z. (2023). A national strategy for preventing substance and opioid use disorders through evidence-based prevention programming that Fosters healthy outcomes in our youth. *Clinical Child and Family Psychology Review,* 26(1), 1–16. https://doi.org/10.1007/s10567-022-00420-5.

Ghodse, A. H., & Khan, I. (1988). *Psychoactive Drugs: Improving Prescribing Practices.* Geneva: World Health Organization, pp. 22–35.

Hartz, C., Plant, M., & Watts, M. (1991). *Alcohol and Health.* London: Medical Council on Alcoholism.

Kelly, J. A., & Murphy, D. A. (1991). Some lessons learned about risk reduction after ten years of the HIV/AIDS epidemic. *AIDS Care,* 3(3), 251–257. https://doi.org/10.1080/09540129108253070.

Kerr, T., Tyndall, M., Li, K. Montaner, J., & Wood, E. (2005). Safer injection facility use and syringe sharing in injection drug users. *The Lancet,* 366(9482), 316–318.

Kuhn, K., & Chu, C. (2022). Health-promoting workplaces. In S. Kokko & M. Baybutt (Eds.), *Handbook of Settings-Based Health Promotion.* Cham: Springer, pp. 167–176. https://doi.org/10.1007/978-3-030-95856-5_9.

LeNoue, S. R., & Riggs, P. D. (2016). Substance abuse prevention. *Child and Adolescent Psychiatric Clinics of North America,* 25(2), 297–305. https://doi.org/10.1016/j.chc.2015.11.007.

Macpherson, D. (2001). *A Four-Pillar Approach to Drug Problems in Vancouver.* https://www.researchgate.net/publication/242480594_A_Four-Pillar_Approach_to_Drug_Problems_in_Vancouver (accessed 1 April 2024).

Manias, E., & Street, A. (2000). Legitimation of nurses' knowledge through policies and protocols in clinical practice. *Journal of Advanced Nursing,* 32(6), 1467–1475. https://doi.org/10.1046/j.1365-2648.2000.01615.x.

Mardaneh Jobehdar, M., Razaghi, E. M., Haghdoost, A. A., Baleshzar, A., Khoshnood, K., Ghasemzadeh, M. R., & Motevalian, S. A. (2021). Factors that influence the effectiveness of primary prevention of substance use: A review of reviews. *Iranian Journal of Psychiatry and Behavioral Sciences,* 15(4), e116288. https://doi.org/10.5812/ijpbs.116288.

Mrazek, P. J., & Haggerty, R. J. (Eds.). (1994). *Reducing Risks for Mental Disorders: Frontiers for Preventive Intervention Research.* Washington, DC: National Academy Press.

NICE (National Institute of Clinical Excellence). (2007). *Behaviour Change.* London: NICE. www.nice.org.uk/PH006.

NIDA. (2003). *Preventing Drug Use Among Children and Adolescents.* National Institute on Drug Abuse. www.drugabuse.gov/publications/preventing-drug-use-among-children-adolescents-in-brief (accessed 1 April 2024).

NIDA. (2014). *Prevention.* https://nida.nih.gov/research-topics/prevention (accessed 1 April 2024).

Ornell, F., Moura, H. F., Scherer, J. N., Pechansky, F., Kessler, F. H. P., & von Diemen, L. (2020). The COVID-19 pandemic and its impact on substance use: Implications for prevention and treatment. *Psychiatry Research,* 289, 113096. https://doi.org/10.1016/j.psychres.2020.113096.

Parsons, C., Stears, D., & Thomas, C. (2002). *Models of Health Promoting Schools in Europe. United Kingdom-The Eco-Holistic Model of The Health Promoting School.* Copenhagen: WHO Regional Office for Europe.

Rassool, G. H. (2000). Addiction: Global problem and global response complacency or commitment? *Journal of Advanced Nursing,* 32(3), 505–508.

Rassool, G. H. (2005). Nursing prescription: The rational use of psychoactive substances. *Nursing Standard,* 19(2), 45–51.

Rassool, G. H., & Marshall, F. (2001). Substance use and misuse: A public health perspective. *Nursing Research,* 6(6), 906–918.

Rassool, G. H., & Gafoor, M. (1997). *Addiction Nursing: Perspectives on Professional and Clinical Practice.* Cheltenham: Nelson-Thornes.

Rassool, G. H., & Winnington, J. (1993). Using psychoactive substances. *Nursing Times,* 89(47), 38–40.

Sumnall, H. R., Bates, G., & Jones, L. (2017). *Evidence Review Summary: Drug Demand Reduction, Treatment and Harm Reduction.* European Monitoring Centre for Drugs and Drug Addiction (EMCDDA). Liverpool: Public Health Institute, Liverpool John Moores University.

Tulchinsky, T. H., & Varavikova, E. A. (2010). What is the "new public health"? *Public Health Review,* 32, 25–53. https://doi.org/10.1007/BF03391592.

Wartiningsih, M., Supriyanto, S., Widati, S., Ernawaty, E., & Lestari, R. (2020). Health promoting hospital: A practical strategy to improve patient loyalty in public sector. *Journal of Public Health Research,* 9(2), 1832. https://doi.org/10.4081/jphr.2020.1832.

WHO. (1986). Ottawa charter for health promotion. *Journal of Health Promotion,* 1, 1–4.

WHO. (1989). *Report of the World Health Organization Meeting on Nursing/Midwifery Education in the Rational Use of Psychoactive Drugs* (DMP/PND/89.5). Geneva: WHO.

WHO. (1991). *Europe. Budapest Declaration on Health Promoting Hospitals. HPH Networking Documents.* Geneva: WHO Regional Office for Europe.

WHO. (1992). *Europe: Health Promoting Hospitals. Networking Documents.* Geneva: WHO Regional Office for Europe.

WHO. (1995). *WHO's Expert Committee Recommendation on Comprehensive School Health Education and Promotion.* Geneva: WHO.

WHO. (1998). *Health Promotion Glossary.* Geneva: World Health Organization.

WHO. (2000). *Primary Prevention of Substance Abuse. A Workbook for Project Operators* (WHO/MSD/MDP/00.17). Department of Mental Health and Substance Dependence. Noncommunicable Diseases and Mental Health. Geneva: WHO.

WHO. (2003). *Developing Standards for Health Promotion in Hospitals.* Copenhagen: World Health Organization, WHO Regional Office for Europe. www.euro.who.int/Document/IHB/hphstandardsfinrpt.pdf.

WHO. (2004a). *Promoting Rational Use of Medicines Saves Lives and Money.* The International Conference on Improving Use of Medicines, Thailand. Geneva: World Health Organization, 30 March–2 April.

WHO. (2004b). *Healthy Workplaces.* Copenhagen: World Health Organization Regional Office for Europe.

WHO/UNDOC. (2007). *Outcome Evaluation Summary Report: WHO/UNODC Global Initiative on Primary Prevention of Substance Abuse.* Geneva: World Health Organization.

Chapter 22

Strategies in helping people to change

Learning outcomes

- Discuss the nature of motivation and readiness to change.
- Examine the reasons tat people change.
- Describe one model of helping people to change.
- Discuss the strengths and limitations of the trans-theoretical stages of change model.

INTRODUCTION

Healthcare professionals must embrace the challenge of becoming agents of change, guiding, motivating, educating, coaching, and supporting individuals in overcoming alcohol or drug addiction throughout their journey of change. This requires healthcare providers to grasp the nature of change, assess individuals' readiness for change, and communicate effectively to facilitate behavioural change. The concept of a change agent has been embraced by health and social care professionals, whose role involves helping individuals understand why change is necessary and how it benefits them. Change agents play a key role in guiding and facilitating transformative changes within organisations or frameworks. They must actively listen to the concerns, perspectives, and needs of all stakeholders involved in the change process. By doing so, they gain valuable insights into the challenges and opportunities associated with the proposed changes.

Increasing patient motivation to change is grounded in various theories and models that provide frameworks for understanding behaviour change. These include the health action model, health belief model, theory of reasoned action, trans-theoretical stages of change model, social learning theory, social cognitive theory, theory of planned behaviour, community development, and models of organizational change. Each of these theories offers unique insights into the factors influencing behaviour change and provides strategies for promoting motivation and facilitating the process of change. By drawing from these theories and models, healthcare professionals can tailor interventions to address the specific needs and circumstances of individual patients, ultimately enhancing their motivation to adopt healthier behaviours. When planning work on behaviour change with individuals, NICE (2007) suggested that a number of concepts drawn from the psychological literature are helpful. These concepts include:

- Outcome expectancies (helping people develop accurate knowledge about the health consequences of their behaviours)
- Personal relevance (emphasising the personal salience of health behaviours)
- Positive attitude (promoting positive feelings towards the outcomes of behaviour change)
- Self-efficacy (enhancing people's belief in their ability to change)
- Descriptive norms (promoting the visibility of positive health behaviours in people's reference groups – that is, the groups they compare themselves to, or aspire to)
- Subjective norms (enhancing social approval for positive health behaviours in significant others and reference groups)
- Personal and moral norms (promoting personal and moral commitments to behaviour change)

DOI: 10.4324/9781003456674-26

- Intention formation and concrete plans (helping people form plans and goals for changing behaviours over time and in specific contexts)
- Behavioural contracts (asking people to share their plans and goals with others)
- Relapse prevention (helping people develop skills to cope with difficult situations and conflicting goals)

This chapter will focus on two models: the health action model and the transtheoretical stages of change model. Both models are relevant in the prevention of alcohol and drug misuse and helping people change their health behaviour.

MOTIVATION AND READINESS TO CHANGE

Change is often perceived as a process rather than an isolated event, and individuals may exhibit resistance to change even when it involves straightforward behavioural adjustments, such as adhering to medication regimens. For instance, a study revealed that over a third of patients fail to adhere to prescribed medications for conditions like high blood pressure and cholesterol within six months (Chapman et al., 2005). Similarly, some individuals grappling with alcohol and drug issues not only resist change but also lack motivation to contemplate altering their consumption habits. This resistance to change can stem from various factors, including personality traits, psychosocial circumstances, and environmental and cultural influences.

Among the major theories and models of behaviour change, the transtheoretical model (TTM), also known as the stages of change model, stands out as one of the most extensively applied and researched. Introduced by Prochaska and DiClemente (1983, 1986), the TTM categorises individuals into different stages based on their readiness to change their behaviour. Within the TTM framework, various types of pre-contemplators have been identified, characterised by the "4Rs": reluctance, rebellion, resignation, and rationalisation. Reluctant pre-contemplators are individuals who, due to a lack of awareness or inertia, are not inclined to consider change, as they have not fully grasped the impact of the problem. Rebellious pre-contemplators, on the other hand, are heavily invested in their substance use and decision-making autonomy, thus resisting external influence and advice. Resigned pre-contemplators have lost hope in the possibility of change, feeling overwhelmed by the complexities of addiction and having made unsuccessful attempts to quit or control their substance use in the past. Rationalising pre-contemplators, meanwhile, are adept at justifying their behaviour, often believing they have all the answers and providing reasons that their substance use is not problematic or why change is unnecessary. In some cases, individuals may not pursue change because they perceive it as unattainable.

In a study by Matzger et al. (2005) investigating reasons for behaviour change among problem drinkers, findings suggested that "hitting rock bottom," experiencing traumatic events, and having spiritual or religious experiences were cited as motivations for reducing alcohol consumption. Surprisingly, interventions by family members (such as receiving warnings from a spouse) or medical doctors were found to have negative associations with positive outcomes. Instead, evidence indicates that a community reinforcement and family training (CRAFT) approach, which focuses on teaching behavioural change skills for use at home, was the most effective method for engaging unmotivated drinkers in treatment (Miller et al., 1999). From a psychoanalytic perspective, resistance to change may stem from individuals' fear of perceived threats associated with change. These threats include the relinquishment of infantile wishes and fantasies, anxiety, guilt, fears of disrupting vital relationships, defence mechanisms, unconscious beliefs contributing to pathology, as well as feelings of devotion and loyalty to early figures and stable internal self-concepts (Eagle, 1999).

There is a prevailing consensus that incremental changes are typically recommended for individuals seeking to alter their alcohol and drug use behaviours. However, evidence suggests that radical, sweeping, and comprehensive changes may sometimes be easier for people to adopt than small, incremental adjustments (Ornish, 2002). In the context of alcohol and drug misuse, some individuals may benefit from incremental changes, while others may require more radical transformations. However, whether the paradox exists that large changes are easier than small ones in the addiction field remains inconclusive. Table 22.1 presents some of the reasons that individuals may initiate change.

The motivation and readiness to change one's lifestyle and behaviours are influenced by both internal and external factors (Mason, 2018; Rollnick et al., 1999). Alcohol and drug misusers must have

Table 22.1
Why do people change?

Key factors	Description
Experience	Experience of pain or frustration prompts realisation that current behaviour is ineffective.
Hitting "rock bottom"	Recognition of hitting "rock bottom" varies for individuals in the case of alcohol and substance use disorder.
Recognition of ineffective behaviour	When individuals realise that their current actions or behaviours are not yielding desired outcomes or causing distress, they may be motivated to change.
Humility	Humility leads to acknowledgement of need for change.
Desire for improvement	People may seek change to enhance their quality of life, achieve personal growth, or pursue greater fulfilment.
Intrinsic motivation	Intrinsic motivation, driven by internal desires, is crucial for long-term change.
External pressures	External pressures offer short-term assistance, but intrinsic motivation is essential for lasting change.
Reward	Accumulation of small victories fosters belief in ability to change, which is rewarding or reinforcing.
Meaningful connections	Meaningful connections with others provide support and encouragement.
Social support	Social support through groups, family, or counselling aids in the change process.
Competence	Developing a sense of competence instils hope for change.

the desire and readiness to adopt new behaviours, which requires conviction and confidence (Rollnick et al., 1999). "Confidence" refers to the belief in one's ability to adopt new behaviours, while "conviction" pertains to the belief that change is important and worthwhile. Without these core beliefs, individuals lack the motivation to take action and make necessary changes. Motivated individuals seeking behaviour change require a different approach from those who are unmotivated (NICE, 2007). The latter may need additional information about the benefits of change and a realistic plan of action. It is crucial to acknowledge that interventions aimed at changing one behaviour may inadvertently lead to another undesirable behaviour. For instance, giving up heroin use may result in increased alcohol consumption. Tailoring intervention strategies to individual needs and addressing potential unintended consequences are essential.

THE HEALTH ACTION MODEL

The health action model (Tones, 1987; Tones et al., 1990) integrates various health-related theories, such as the health belief model and the theory of reasoned action, emphasising the importance of an ecological and multifactorial approach in preventing alcohol and drug misuse. This model elucidates how factors like knowledge, beliefs, values, attitudes, drives, and normative pressures interact to shape individual intentions to act, while also considering environmental circumstances, information, and pe sonal skills that facilitate the translation of intentio into health actions. Tones et al. (1990) undersco the model's recognition of three key influence on decision-making: environmental, interpersona and intrapersonal factors, along with the availabili of post-decisional support. It delineates the stag individuals undergo during behavioural change an serves as a framework for various interventions b health educators, comprising behavioural intentio and socio-cultural and environmental factors.

In the health action model, behavioural inte tion, or an individual's readiness to act, is infl enced by a complex interplay of cognitive facto such as knowledge and beliefs, motivating facto like values and attitudes, and normative pressur from social norms and significant others. The mod also considers the broader physical, cultural, an socio-economic environment, as well as the acqu sition of relevant knowledge and skills, which ca either facilitate or hinder the translation of inte tion into action. Feedback loops play a crucial ro in this process, as experiences during health actio can either reinforce or deter further action (Ton et al., 1990). Therefore, providing environment and social support is vital once an individual con mits to behaviour change. Nonetheless, the mod acknowledges potential barriers, such as enviro mental factors, knowledge deficits, and skill def ciencies, highlighting the importance of addressi these challenges. To effectively prevent alcoh and drug misuse, a comprehensive strategy mu consider individual, educational, environmental, political, and socio-cultural factors, employing an integrated community-based approach.

TRANSTHEORETICAL STAGES OF CHANGE MODEL

The transtheoretical model (Prochaska et al., 1992; Prochaska & Velicer, 1997) offers an integrative framework for understanding behavioural change. Its central construct, the stages of change, delineates the temporal dimension of health behaviour change, encompassing emotions, cognitions, and actions. Initially devised in the context of smoking cessation research, this model has since been applied to various behaviours, including alcohol and drug interventions, exercise, weight control, and HIV prevention measures. In this model, change is conceptualised as a process wherein individuals progress through different stages of readiness for change. These stages include pre-contemplation, contemplation, action, maintenance, termination, or relapse. Effective intervention strategies are tailored to individuals' specific stage of change, ensuring alignment with their readiness and motivation levels. Figure 22.1 depicts a model of the process of change.

Pre-contemplation

During the *pre-contemplation* stage, individuals lack awareness or insight into their problematic behaviour. They may be unaware of the need for change despite engaging in high-risk behaviours. Often perceived as resistant or unmotivated, pre-contemplators tend to avoid discussions or thoughts regarding the targeted health behaviour (Prochaska et al., 1992). Some individuals in this stage may deny the need for change altogether or feel resigned, lacking hope for any potential improvement.

Contemplation

During the *contemplation* stage, individuals seriously consider changing their behaviour. They are aware of both the advantages and disadvantages of such a change but may hesitate or doubt their ability to follow through. Ambivalence arises as individuals weigh the costs and benefits of changing. Some may remain in this stage for extended periods, a phenomenon known as chronic contemplation or behavioural procrastination. Individuals in this stage often exhibit high levels of ambivalence, showing interest in learning about change but struggling to commit to a decision.

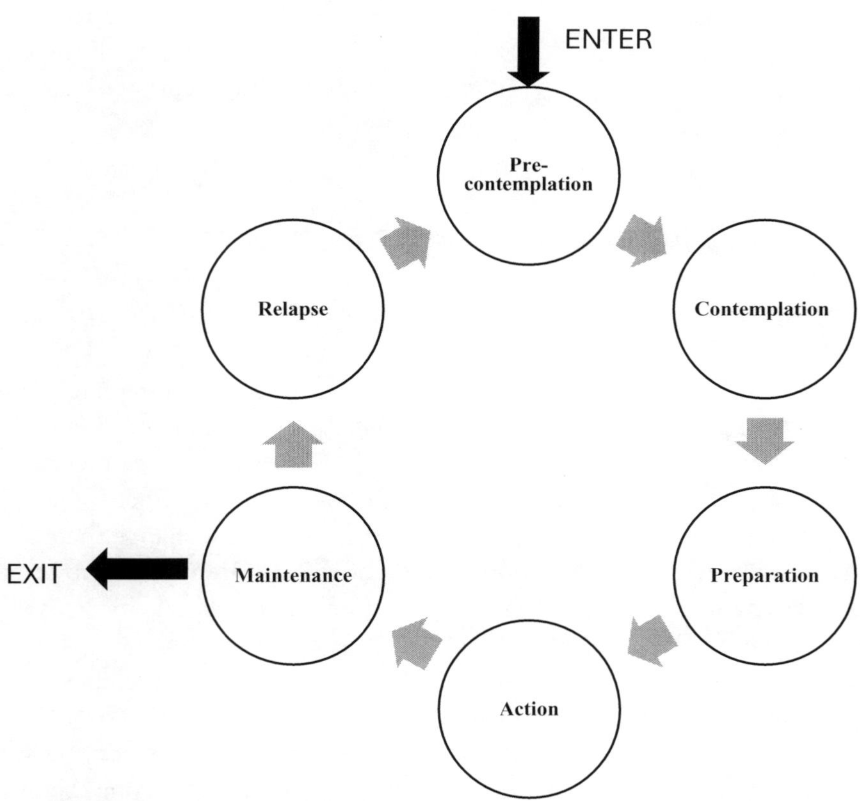

FIGURE 22.1 A model of the process of change.

Preparation

During the *preparation* stage, individuals are actively planning and making final adjustments in preparation for changing their behaviour. They are committed to taking action in the immediate future, typically within the next month. Sometimes, external incidents serve as catalysts for change, such as pressure from a partner, recent illness, or involvement with the criminal justice system. Although some residual ambivalence may remain, individuals in this stage often have a sense of self-efficacy, believing they can overcome ambivalent behaviours. The preparation stage is considered a transitional phase rather than a stable one, as individuals intend to progress to action within the next 30 days.

Action

Action is the stage where individuals have actively implemented specific, tangible changes in their lifestyles and behaviours. It marks the phase where individuals have successfully taken steps to reduce their high-risk behaviours. However, it is also a critical stage where the risk of relapse is significant, requiring ongoing effort and vigilance to maintain the changes made.

Maintenance

At this stage, individuals are actively engaged in maintaining the positive changes they have made during the action phase. They are focused on preventing relapse and consolidating the gains achieved through their efforts. Maintainers exhibit high levels of self-efficacy and are less prone to temptation or relapse compared to those in the action stage.

Termination or relapse

In the termination phase, individuals have gained adequate self-efficacy to eliminate the risk of lapse or relapse. Their former lifestyles and behaviours are no longer perceived as desirable. Most substance misusers experience relapse on the journey to permanent cessation or stable reduction of high-risk behaviours. In relapse, the individual reverts back to old behaviours which can occur during either action or maintenance, and the individual will experience an immediate sense of failure that can seriously undermine their self-confidence.

This model of change operates in a circular rather than a linear fashion, as depicted in Figure 22.1. Individuals may cycle through multiple iterations of contemplation, action, and relapse before reaching the stages of maintenance and/or termination or exiting the system without achieving freedom from substance misuse. The "revolving-door schema" illustrates how individuals enter and exit the stages at various points, often experiencing multiple cycles. Relapse is considered a normal part of the process, and individuals who experience relapse may need to develop better strategies for anticipating high-risk situations, managing environmental triggers, and coping with unexpected stressors in order to progress to the termination stage. A crucial aspect of this model is the recognition that counselling outcomes can be enhanced when there is alignment between the client's stage of change and the type of counselling interventions offered.

MATCHING INTERVENTIONS

The stages of change model is highly practical for selecting suitable interventions, as outlined in Chapter 26 regarding various intervention strategies. By pinpointing an individual's stage in the change process, intervention strategies can be customised to align with their readiness to change. A condensed overview of the stages of change model and corresponding intervention strategies is provided in Table 22.2.

KEY POINTS

- Healthcare professionals need to accept the challenge to become agents of change, nudging, motivating, educating, and supporting individuals throughout the process of change.
- There are a number of theories or models that are in the prevention of alcohol and drug misuse and helping people change their health behaviours.
- Individuals are resistant to change, albeit when a simple behavioural change is vital, such as taking medications.
- Individuals may not change because they believe they cannot change.
- The health action model shows the stages a person goes through during the process of behaviour

Table 22.2
Summary of stages of change model and intervention strategies

Stages of change	Individual stage	Intervention models
Pre-contemplation	Denial	Support
	Rationalisation	Locus of control
	Feeling of no control	Health belief model
	Not thinking about change	Motivational interviewing
	Lack of awareness of severity of consequences	
	Resistance to change	
Contemplation	Weighing benefits and costs of proposed change	Counselling
		Motivational interviewing
Preparation	Deciding on action	Counselling
	Making the steps necessary to prepare for action	Cognitive behavioural therapy
		Motivational interviewing
Action	Taking a definitive action to change	Cognitive behavioural therapy
		12-step programme
Maintenance	Maintaining new behaviour over time	Counselling
		Support
		Cognitive behavioural therapy (relapse prevention)
		12-step programme
Termination/relapse	Self-efficacy	Support
	Re-cycling – learning from relapse	Self-help groups
		Motivational interviewing

change and can act as a framework for a range of possible interventions by health educators.
- The health action model is divided into two main sections: behavioural intention and socio-cultural and environmental factors.
- Motivation and readiness to change require both conviction and confidence.
- The transtheoretical model is an integrative model of behaviour change.
- Its most popular construct has been the stages of change, which reflects the temporal dimension of health behaviour change and involves emotions, cognitions, and behaviour.
- The transtheoretical model construes change as a process involving progress through a series of six stages: pre-contemplation, contemplation, action, maintenance, termination or relapse.
- Individuals will be at different stages in this process of change, and intervention strategies should match their particular stage

Activity 22.1 Helping people change.

State whether the following statements are true or false by ticking the appropriate boxes.

Statements	True	False
In the transtheoretical model of change, *pre-contemplators* are individuals who have been thinking about change.		
Reluctant pre-contemplators are those who, through lack of knowledge or inertia, do not want to consider change.		

Statements	True	False
Rebellious pre-contemplators do not have a heavy investment in drug-taking or drinking.		
Resigned pre-contemplators have given up hope about the possibility of change.		
Rationalising pre-contemplators have plenty of reasons that drinking or drug-taking is a problem.		
Many individuals have made many attempts to quit or control their drinking or drug-taking.		
Having traumatic events and having spiritual/religious experiences were given as reasons for cutting down on alcohol.		
There is no evidence to suggest that radical, sweeping, comprehensive changes are often easier for people than small, incremental ones.		
Confidence relates to the person's belief that they have the ability to adopt a new behaviour.		
Conviction is a belief that a new behaviour is important and worth the effort to achieve it or why change is needed.		
In the health belief model, there is omission of environmental circumstances, information, and personal skills that may facilitate the translation of intentions into health actions.		
In the stage of change model, behavioural change is viewed as a process with individuals at various levels of motivation or stages of "readiness" to change.		
The stage model of change is a linear model.		
Most substance misusers experience relapse on the journey to permanent cessation or stable reduction.		

Activity 22.2

There is only one correct answer to the following multiple-choice questions.

1. According to the transtheoretical model, which stage involves individuals who are unaware of the need for behavioural change?
   a. Pre-contemplation
   b. Contemplation
   c. Preparation
   d. Action
   e. Maintenance
2. In which stage of change are individuals seriously contemplating a change in behaviour but may still be undecided?
   a. Pre-contemplation
   b. Contemplation
   c. Preparation
   d. Action
   e. Maintenance

3. Which stage involves individuals making specific, overt changes in their behaviour?
   a. Pre-contemplation
   b. Contemplation
   c. Preparation
   d. Action
   e. Maintenance
4. During which stage do individuals plan and make final adjustments before taking action in the immediate future?
   a. Pre-contemplation
   b. Contemplation
   c. Preparation
   d. Action
   e. Maintenance
5. Which stage is characterised by individuals continuing with desirable actions and working to prevent relapse?
   a. Pre-contemplation
   b. Contemplation
   c. Preparation
   d. Action
   e. Maintenance
6. In the transtheoretical model, what distinguishes individuals in the maintenance stage from those in the action stage?
   a. Higher levels of self-efficacy
   b. Less frequent temptation to relapse
   c. Greater motivation for change
   d. Increased awareness of the need for change
   e. Stronger social support
7. Which stage of change involves individuals entering and exiting the change process multiple times?
   a. Pre-contemplation
   b. Contemplation
   c. Preparation
   d. Action
   e. Maintenance
8. According to the transtheoretical model, relapse is considered:
   a. A failure in the change process
   b. An inevitable part of the change process
   c. A sign of lack of motivation
   d. A result of external influences
   e. A temporary setback
9. The stages of change model emphasises:
   a. Linear progression through the stages
   b. Immediate and permanent behaviour change
   c. The importance of external motivation
   d. Matching interventions to individual readiness
   e. The inevitability of relapse
10. Which stage of change involves individuals actively seeking information and considering making a change?
   a. Pre-contemplation

b. Contemplation
c. Preparation
d. Action
e. Maintenance

11. What is the primary focus of intervention strategies based on the transtheoretical model?
a. Changing external circumstances
b. Addressing past failures
c. Increasing external motivation
d. Matching interventions to readiness to change
e. Promoting immediate action

12. According to the transtheoretical model, what role does relapse play in the change process?
a. It indicates a lack of commitment to change
b. It is a natural and anticipated part of change
c. It suggests the need for more intensive interventions
d. It signifies a return to the pre-contemplation stage
e. It leads to termination of the change process

Activity 22.3

Questions

- Discuss the nature of motivation and readiness to change.
- List the reasons that people change.
- Can you apply the models of helping people to change in your work or speciality?
- Reflect on how you would apply this model of change to your patient or client.

References

Chapman, R. H., Benner, J. S., Petrilla, A. A., Tierce, J. C., Collins, S. R., Battleman, D. S., & Schwartz, J. S. (2005). Predictors of adherence with antihypertensive and lipid-lowering therapy. *Archives of Internal Medicine,* 165(10), 1147–1152. https://doi.org/10.1001/archinte.165.10.1147.

Eagle, M. (1999). Why don't people change? A psychoanalytic perspective. *Journal of Psychotherapy Integration,* 9, 3–32. https://doi.org/10.1023/A:1023254726930.

Mason, P. (2018). *Health Behavior Change: A Guide for Practitioners* (3rd ed.). Edinburgh: Churchill Livingstone.

Matzger, H., Kaskutas, L. A., & Weisner, C. (2005). Reasons for drinking less and their relationship to sustained remission from problem drinking. *Addiction,* 100(11), 1637–1646. https://doi.org/10.1111/j.1360-0443.2005.01203.x.

Miller, W. R., Meyers, R. J., & Tonigan, J. S. (1999). Engaging the unmotivated in treatment for alcohol problems: A comparison of three strategies for intervention through family members. *Journal of Consulting and Clinical Psychology,* 67(5), 688–697. https://doi.org/10.1037//0022-006x.67.5.688.

NICE. (2007). *Behaviour Change.* London: NICE (National Institute of Clinical Excellence). www.nice.org.uk/PH006.

Ornish, D. (2002). *Intensive Lifestyle Changes in Management of Coronary Heart Disease: Harrison's Advances in Cardiology.* New York: McGraw-Hill.

Prochaska, J. O., & DiClemente, C. C. (1983). Stages and processes of self-change of smoking: Toward an integrative model of change. *Journal of Consulting and Clinical Psychology,* 51(3), 390–395. https://doi.org/10.1037/0022-006X.51.3.390.

Prochaska, J. O., & DiClemente, C. C. (1984). Self-change processes, self-efficacy and decisional balance across five stages of smoking cessation. *Progress in Clinical and Biological Research,* 156, 131–140.

Prochaska, J. O., & DiClemente, C. C. (1986). Towards a comprehensive model of change. In W. R. Miller & N. Heather (Eds.), *Treating Addictive Behaviors: Processes of Change*. New York: Plenum.

Prochaska, J. O., DiClemente, C. C., & Norcross, J. C. (1992). In search of how people change. Applications to addictive behaviors. *The American Psychologist, 47*(9), 1102–1114. https://doi.org/10.1037//0003-066x.47.9.1102.

Prochaska, J. O., & Velicer, W. F. (1997). The transtheoretical model of health behavior change. *American Journal of Health Promotion: AJHP,* 12(1), 38–48. https:/doi.org/10.4278/0890-1171-12.1.38.

Rollnick, S., Mason, P., & Butler, C. (1999). *Health Behavior Change A Guide for Practitioners*. Edinburgh: Churchill Livingstone.

Tones, K. (1987). Devising strategies for preventing drug misuse: The role of the health action model. *Health Education Research*, 2(4), 305–317.

Tones, K., Tilford, S., & Keeley-Robinson, Y. (1990). *Health Education: Effectiveness, Efficiency and Equity*. London: Chapman and Hall.

Chapter 23

Working with diversity

Cultural competence

Learning outcomes

- Define *culture* and *cultural competence*.
- Identify the goals of culturally competent services.
- Discuss how an understanding of culture allows us to provide culturally competent care.
- Describe culturally competent attitudes, knowledge, and skills.
- Describe the challenges and problems in the provision and delivery of culturally competent care.

Activity 23.1

Please state whether the following statements are true or false by ticking the appropriate box.

Statements	True	False
Culture is an important component and determinant of health.		
The provision of culturally competent care is not a legal and a moral requirement for nurses.		
Understanding culture allows us to be more aware of cultural differences and stereotypes.		
The "world view" of health and illness and their causes are not determined by cultural factors.		
There are no differences among Black and minority ethnic communities and differences between members of the same ethnic group.		
Cultural and religious beliefs should be applied equally to members of a particular Black and minority ethnic group.		
The goals of culturally competent care are cultural awareness, cultural knowledge, cultural skill, and cultural encounters.		
Awareness of one's own beliefs, practices, and perceptions is important in delivering culturally competent care.		

DOI: 10.4324/9781003456674-27

Statements	True	False
Ethnocentrism among professionals shapes the experience of substance misuse services by Black and minority ethnic users.		
Unaddressed ethnocentrism can lead to misdiagnosis, mistreatment, and insufficient treatment.		
Transcultural counselling is being an expert on any given culture.		

Activity 23.2

There is only one correct answer to the following multiple-choice questions.

1. What is *culture*?
   a. A set of rules and norms shared by a particular group of people
   b. A genetic predisposition to certain behaviours
   c. An individual's personal preferences
   d. A biological trait passed down through generations
   e. A universal concept with no variation across societies
2. What does *cultural competence* refer to?
   a. Understanding and respecting people from different cultural backgrounds
   b. Enforcing one's own cultural norms on others
   c. Avoiding interactions with people from diverse backgrounds
   d. Treating everyone the same regardless of cultural differences
   e. Ignoring cultural differences altogether
3. Why is cultural competence important in healthcare?
   a. It allows healthcare providers to impose their cultural beliefs on patients
   b. It ensures that all patients receive identical treatment
   c. It enhances communication and trust between healthcare providers and patients from diverse backgrounds
   d. It creates barriers to effective care delivery
   e. It promotes discrimination based on cultural differences
4. Black and ethnic minority communities are
   a. A heterogeneous group with varying values, attitudes, and religious beliefs
   b. A homogeneous group with varying values, attitudes, and religious beliefs
   c. A special group with varying values, attitudes, and religious beliefs
   d. A group with a high prevalence of substance misuse
   e. None of the above
5. What does cultural competence aim to achieve?
   a. Assimilation of diverse cultures into a dominant culture.
   b. Preservation of cultural homogeneity.
   c. Recognition and respect for cultural differences.
   d. Ignorance of cultural backgrounds.
   e. Exclusion of minority cultures from mainstream services.

6. How does understanding culture enhance care provision?
   a. By promoting a one-size-fits-all approach
   b. By ignoring cultural differences
   c. By improving communication and trust
   d. By enforcing stereotypes
   e. By prioritising one culture over others
7. Culturally competent attitudes include:
   a. Ethnocentrism
   b. Stereotyping
   c. Respect for diversity
   d. Cultural imposition
   e. Discrimination
8. What is one key aspect of cultural competence?
   a. Ignoring cultural differences to maintain neutrality
   b. Being dismissive of patients' cultural beliefs and practices
   c. Recognising and valuing diversity
   d. Assuming that one's own cultural norms are superior
   e. Refusing to adapt to patients' cultural preferences
9. Which of the following is NOT a potential barrier to cultural competence?
   a. Language barriers
   b. Lack of awareness of one's own cultural biases
   c. Stereotyping and cultural assumptions
   d. Embracing cultural humility
   e. Insensitivity to cultural differences
10. Which of the following statements about culturally competent care is false?
    a. It recognises and respects diversity.
    b. It promotes ethnocentrism.
    c. It adapts services to meet cultural needs.
    d. It improves health outcomes.
    e. It addresses language barriers.
11. What are common challenges in delivering culturally competent care?
    a. Lack of diversity in patient populations
    b. Cultural competence training for staff
    c. Language barriers
    d. Ignorance of cultural differences
    e. None of the above
12. What is a potential consequence of neglecting cultural competence in care delivery?
    a. Increased patient satisfaction
    b. Better health outcomes
    c. Reduced trust between patients and providers
    d. Improved communication
    e. Enhanced understanding of diverse perspectives
13. How does cultural competence contribute to holistic care?
    a. By prioritising one culture over others
    b. By ignoring cultural differences
    c. By considering the influence of culture on health beliefs and practices
    d. By enforcing stereotypes
    e. By adhering strictly to clinical guidelines

14. How can healthcare providers enhance their cultural competence?
    a. By assuming that all patients have similar cultural backgrounds
    b. By avoiding interactions with patients from diverse cultures
    c. By engaging in ongoing education and training on cultural diversity
    d. By imposing their cultural beliefs on patients
    e. By ignoring patients' cultural preferences during treatment
15. What is the first step towards cultural competence?
    a. Embracing one's own cultural biases
    b. Dismissing the importance of cultural diversity
    c. Acknowledging and respecting cultural differences
    d. Assuming that all patients share the same cultural norms
    e. Avoiding discussions about cultural differences with patients
16. How can healthcare providers demonstrate cultural competence in practice?
    a. By imposing their cultural beliefs on patients
    b. By ignoring patients' cultural preferences
    c. By adapting their approach to meet patients' cultural needs
    d. By assuming that all patients share the same cultural norms
    e. By avoiding interactions with patients from diverse cultures
17. How can healthcare providers avoid cultural stereotyping and assumptions?
    a. By assuming that all patients share the same cultural norms
    b. By engaging in ongoing self-reflection and awareness of cultural biases
    c. By imposing their own cultural beliefs on patients
    d. By avoiding discussions about cultural differences with patients
    e. By disregarding patients' cultural preferences during treatment
18. Ethnocentric health interventions are
    a. A belief that one's way of life is superior to others
    b. A belief that one's view of the world is more desirable
    c. A belief that shapes the experiences of professionals
    d. All of the above
19. Intercultural therapy and counselling recognise
    a. The importance of internal realities of culture
    b. The importance of internal realities of beliefs
    c. The importance of external realities of beliefs of the patient's life
    d. All of the above
    e. B and C only

INTRODUCTION

Health is recognised as a cultural concept, as culture plays a pivotal role in shaping individuals' perspectives on health, illness, and healthcare. This acknowledgement underlines the significance of understanding cultural factors in healthcare provision. Culture shapes the way individuals and groups' world view interact with each other and navigate their environments. Culture significantly impacts health outcomes through its influence on individuals' beliefs, behaviours, access to healthcare, and responses to illness. Cultural factors shape health beliefs and practices, affecting how individuals perceive and seek healthcare. They also influence health behaviours, perceptions of illness and wellness, and attitudes towards mental health and addictive behaviours. Additionally, cultural norms regarding family, social support, and access to resources play crucial roles in determining health outcomes.

The demand for culturally competent approaches in drug and alcohol services is increasingly recognised, necessitating the development of appropriate services and the demonstration of cultural competence among staff. Nurses, in particular, are mandated by legal and moral standards outlined in *The Code: Professional standards of practice and behaviour for nurses and midwives* (NMC, 2018) to provide culturally competent care. Furthermore, services for individuals struggling with alcohol and drug misuse are required to adopt race equality schemes (NTA, 2002) to ensure the elimination of discrimination and the promotion of equal opportunities across various demographic factors. As populations become more diverse globally, health, social care, and criminal justice agencies face the challenge of evolving culturally competent systems to effectively meet the needs of these communities within integrated service provisions. Understanding and addressing cultural differences are crucial in healthcare and social care settings. Therefore, this chapter aims to explore the impact of cultural diversity on health and social care while proposing a framework for the establishment of culturally competent care system.

CULTURE

In order to grasp cultural competence, it is important to define culture. *Culture* encompasses various aspects, with multiple definitions reflecting its complexity. Leininger (1991) describes *culture* as the shared beliefs, values, and practices transmitted throughout a society, influencing how individuals live, make decisions, and interact. Cross et al. (1989) expand on this, defining *culture* as the integrated pattern of human behaviour encompassing thoughts, communications, actions, customs, beliefs, values, and institutions within racial, ethnic, religious, or social groups. UNESCO (2001) adds the spiritual component, framing culture as a set of distinctive feature – spiritual, material, intellectual, and emotional – encompassing art, literature, lifestyles, values, traditions, and beliefs. Understanding culture is pivotal in recognising how individuals interpret their world views and respond to them. It fosters awareness of cultural pluralism, differences, and stereotypes. Moreover, culture profoundly impacts health, healthcare provision, and delivery. Cultural factors shape perceptions of health, illness, and their causes, influencing how individuals seek and respond to healthcare. Therefore, cultural competence is essential in providing effective and responsive care.

Cultural factors, including beliefs and spiritual aspects, significantly influence attitudes and behaviours related to substance use and misuse. Culture shapes individuals' perceptions and expectations regarding substance misuse issues they may encounter (Heath, 2001). Additionally, cultural norms and religious beliefs can act as protective factors against substance use initiation, while societal changes and acculturation may contribute to alcohol and drug misuse. Understanding cultural health behaviours is crucial for breaking down barriers and promoting equity in healthcare delivery. Substance misuse services must develop practices and procedures to provide culturally competent care, recognising and respecting diverse cultural backgrounds and beliefs. This approach is essential for effectively addressing substance misuse issues and improving health outcomes across diverse communities.

CULTURAL COMPETENCE

The concept of cultural competence lacks a universally agreed-upon definition and is often intertwined with related terms, such as *cultural awareness, sensitivity, appropriateness,* and *specificity* (Rassool, 2006a). Wilson et al. (2013) define *cultural competence* as the acquisition and maintenance of culture-specific skills. This definition emphasises the practical nature of cultural competence, focusing on its importance for individuals to effectively function and interact within diverse cultural contexts. Cultural competence involves acquiring the necessary skills to navigate different cultural backgrounds and interact effectively with people from various cultural backgrounds. Cultural competence can be seen as an overarching term that encapsulates the ability to effectively meet the needs of diverse communities. Cultural appropriateness serves as the means through which cultural competence is achieved, with cultural sensitivity and specificity serving as foundational components for culturally appropriate practices (Sangster et al., 2002). Cultural competence, as described by Papadopoulos et al. (1998), involves the capacity to deliver effective healthcare while considering individuals' cultural beliefs, behaviours, and needs. In the context of substance misuse, Rassool (2006) defines *cultural competence* as the willingness and ability of the workforce, services, and the system to value cultural diversity and be culturally responsive in providing services to diverse communities. Additionally, in a study by Sangster et al. (2002) on delivering drug services to Black and minority ethnic communities, cultural competence is described as the ability to meet the diverse needs of a community.

The distinction made between cultural competence as an overarching term and cultural appropriateness as the mechanism through which it is achieved is insightful. It highlights the importance of not only understanding diverse cultural backgrounds but also adapting practices and approaches to suit specific cultural contexts. Additionally, the recognition of cultural sensitivity and specificity as foundational components emphasises the need for healthcare providers to possess not only an awareness of cultural differences but also the ability to tailor their interactions and interventions accordingly.

ALCOHOL AND DRUG MISUSE: CULTURAL AND RELIGIOUS DIVERSITY

Due to cultural and religious diversity, variations exist in the nature and extent of substance misuse among culturally and linguistically different communities. These differences stem from a range of cultural factors, including beliefs, attitudes, values, customs, and practices related to alcohol and substance use. Cultural and religious beliefs shape attitudes towards alcohol and drugs. For example, in some cultures, alcohol consumption may be prohibited or discouraged due to religious teachings, while in others, moderate alcohol use may be accepted or even celebrated as part of cultural rituals or drinking to get drunk (Mackinnon et al., 2017). Social norms play a pivotal role, as cultures vary in their acceptance and normalisation of substance use, leading to differing rates of misuse. Moreover, cultural perceptions contribute to stigma and shame surrounding alcohol and substance misuse, deterring individuals from seeking help within their communities. Access to treatment is hindered by cultural and linguistic barriers, leading to underutilisation of services among minority groups. Additionally, coping mechanisms and experiences of trauma intersect with cultural backgrounds, influencing vulnerability to alcohol and substance misuse. For instance, cultures emphasising communal support may have lower rates of substance use as coping mechanisms, while refugees or immigrants facing acculturation challenges may be at heightened risk.

In the United States, drug use rates vary among different ethnic groups, with the highest rates observed among American Indian. Alaska Native individuals had the highest prevalence of illicit drug use in the past year, followed closely by multiracial individuals. The use of marijuana is highest among American Indian or Alaska Native or multiracial people. American Indian or Alaska Native individuals had the highest likelihood of experiencing a substance use disorder (Center for Behavioral Health Statistics and Quality, 2022). White people were more likely than people in all other racial or ethnic groups to be alcohol users. The prevalence of tobacco product use or nicotine vaping was higher among American Indian or Alaska Native people.

In the UK, the data reveals significant differences in illicit drug use across demographic groups (NHS Digital, 2021). White British and Black adults exhibit higher rates of illicit drug use compared to Asian adults. Within the White British population, men are more likely than women to have used illicit drugs. Black women, White British women, and women from the White other group are more inclined to have used illicit drugs compared to Asian women. Asian men were more likely to have used illicit drugs compared with Asian women. Individuals from ethnic minority groups tend to drink less and are more prone to abstain from alcohol compared to their White British counterparts (Institute of Alcohol Studies, 2020). However, certain groups exhibit relatively high rates of higher-risk drinking behaviours, such as older Irish men and men belonging to the Sikh religion. Additionally, some ethnic minority communities experience greater alcohol-related harm. For instance, White Irish men face elevated rates of alcoholic liver disease and other alcohol-related illnesses, while Sikh men experience higher rates of liver cirrhosis (Institute of Alcohol Studies, 2020). In Australia, Aboriginal and Torres Strait Islander people, although less likely to drink than the general population, are more likely to consume alcohol at risky levels for long-term harm (The Department of Health and Aged Care, 2020). These disparities emphasise the importance of recognising and addressing unique risk factors and health outcomes within different ethnic communities to develop targeted interventions and support services.

CHALLENGES FOR PROVIDERS OF CULTURALLY COMPETENT CARE

Health and social care providers encounter significant challenges in delivering services to alcohol and drug users from culturally and linguistically diverse communities. These challenges are particularly pronounced in recognising and assessing substance misuse due to cultural variations in symptom presentation and cases involving a "dual diagnosis" of substance misuse and psychiatric disorders (Rassool, 2006b). Culturally and linguistically diverse communities comprise a heterogeneous group with varying values, attitudes, religious beliefs, and customs that influence patterns of substance misuse. It is valuable to avoid applying cultural and religious beliefs stereotypically to members of specific minority ethnic groups, as there are often differences within and between these communities. This cultural diversity, characterised by variations in lifestyles, health behaviours, religion, and language, profoundly impacts alcohol and drug use patterns. Recognising and navigating these complexities are essential for providing effective and culturally sensitive support and intervention for individuals from diverse backgrounds.

Generally, individuals from culturally and linguistically different communities are underrepresented in seeking treatment and advice for drug and alcohol problems. These barriers are varied and can be specific to certain higher-risk groups, such as Irish Travellers (Institute of Alcohol Studies, 2020). Individuals from ethnic minority backgrounds face various barriers when seeking help for alcohol-related issues. Some of the barriers experienced by ethnic minorities include awareness of health implications of excessive drinking, not being aware what support is available, difficulties navigating services and problems not being recognised by professionals, stigma and exclusion, lack of trust in the confidentiality of services, and community shame and stigma, especially among communities where there is a religious restriction on alcohol (e.g. Islam) (Gleeson et al., 2019). For instance, in the UK, problem drinking may go unnoticed among women and young individuals from South Asian ethnic groups due to religious prohibitions against alcohol consumption (Joseph Rowntree Foundation, 2010). However, the utilisation of services varies across different ethnic groups. Fernandez's study (2004) in the UK revealed that many clients from the Bengali community preferred community/outpatient detoxification over inpatient detoxification, considering it a quicker and simpler method to become "clean." This preference was appealing to users, while clinicians deemed Asian clients suitable for outpatient detoxification due to their uncomplicated drug profiles and minimal drug histories (Fernandez, 2004).

The idea of cultural competence extends beyond individual-focused anti-racism training and is integrated into all aspects of service provision, delivery, and the overall care system. This signifies a significant progression, emphasising the importance of understanding and respecting the cultural backgrounds, beliefs, and values of those receiving care. Cultural competence involves adapting services to cater to the diverse needs of various cultural groups, ensuring equal access to high-quality care for everyone. By embracing cultural competence within the healthcare system, providers can effectively address the distinct challenges encountered by ethnically and culturally diverse populations, ultimately enhancing health outcomes and minimising disparities. Cross et al. (1989) list five essential elements that contribute to an institution's or agency's ability to become more culturally competent. These include:

- Valuing diversity
- Having the capacity for cultural self-assessment
- Being conscious of the dynamics inherent when cultures interact
- Having institutionalised cultural knowledge
- Having developed adaptations of service delivery reflecting an understanding of cultural diversity

The five elements essential for culturally competent drug services, as outlined by Sangster et al. (2002), should permeate every level of an organisation, encompassing policymaking, administration, and practice. Moreover, these elements should be evident in the attitudes, structures, policies, and services of the organisation. A summary of these core elements is presented in Table 23.1.

GOALS OF CULTURALLY COMPETENT CARE

The goals of culturally competent care, as identified by Campinha-Bacote et al. (1996), Kavanagh and Kennedy (1992), and Tervalon and Murray-Garcia (1998), encompass four key elements: cultural awareness, cultural knowledge, cultural skill, and cultural encounters.

- *Cultural awareness* involves recognising and accepting cultural differences, fostering an appreciation for diversity.
- Cultural knowledge entails actively seeking out diverse world views and explanatory models of

Table 23.1
Cultural competence and service delivery in substance misuse services

- Cultural ownership and leadership (the extent to which race and ethnicity are considered important by a service).
- Symbols of accessibility (something that shows Black and minority ethnic people that they are welcomed by a service, for example, posters, leaflets, culturally specific newspapers, and magazines.
- Familiarity with, and ability to meet, the distinct needs of communities.
- Holistic, therapeutic, and social help.
- A range of services.
- Black and minority ethnic workers.
- Community attachment and ownership and capacity building (the process through which the skills and structures needed to provide drug services are developed).

Source: Adapted from Sangster et al. (2002).

disease, which can facilitate mutual understanding between cultures.

- Cultural skill involves learning how to culturally assess patients beyond mere factual information, such as understanding issues from their perspective, reducing resistance and defensiveness, and acknowledging and learning from mistakes in communication.
- Cultural encounters involve actively engaging and working with individuals from different cultural backgrounds, which can challenge and dispel stereotypes, providing valuable real-world experiences that may contradict academic knowledge. It is essential to remain open-minded and humble, letting go of stereotypes and embracing the individuality of each patient in the pursuit of culturally competent care.

MODEL OF CULTURAL COMPETENCE

A model that provides a valuable framework for understanding and assessing intercultural competence, particularly in nursing education and practice, is the Purnell model for cultural competence (Purnell & Paulanka, 2003). The Purnell model is a comprehensive framework utilised in nursing and various other fields to assess cultural competence. It encompasses aspects of cultures, individuals, healthcare, and healthcare professionals, providing a holistic approach to understanding and addressing cultural diversity. Another model to promote the inclusion of cultural competence in nursing and healthcare sciences education has been developed by Papadopoulos et al. (1998). A model of cultural competence is shown in Figure 23.1.

The model comprises four progressive stages, beginning with cultural awareness, which involves critically examining personal values and beliefs to understand their influence on health beliefs and practices. Cultural knowledge follows, where exposure to diverse cultural communities enhances understanding of their health behaviours and challenges. Cultural sensitivity, the third stage, emphasises viewing clients as equal partners, fostering trust, acceptance, and respect. Finally, cultural competence integrates awareness, knowledge, and sensitivity to effectively address diverse needs, including assessment, diagnosis, and clinical skills. This stage also entails recognising and challenging racism and discrimination. The model combines multicultural and anti-racist perspectives, fostering a broader understanding of inequalities and promoting skill development for change at the patient/client level (Papadopoulos et al., 1998).

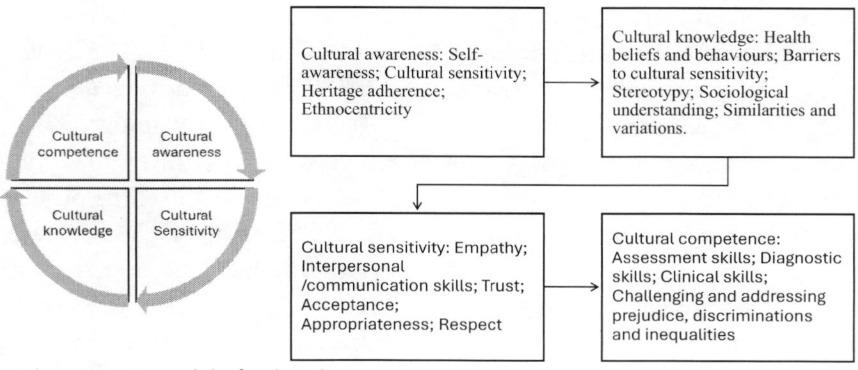

FIGURE 23.1 A model of cultural competence.

Health and social care professionals may not feasibly acquire knowledge of all culturally and linguistically diverse communities, but they can develop an appreciation for diversity and deliver culturally sensitive care to heterogeneous populations. However, it is essential for professionals to possess cultural knowledge and an understanding of the traditions specific to the populations they serve. The ultimate objective of interventions is to provide culturally competent care that reduces barriers and enhances health outcomes.

HEALTHCARE APPROACHES: CLINICAL AND EDUCATIONAL

The Nursing and Midwifery Council in England sets professional standards for registered nurses and midwives, emphasising the importance of treating individuals with kindness, respect, and compassion, delivering fundamental care effectively, avoiding assumptions, recognising diversity and individual choice, and upholding human rights (NMC, 2018). Similarly, the General Social Care Council is dedicated to promoting equality and diversity in service provision and employment policies. The General Medical Council outlines principles for good medical practice, and other healthcare professionals, such as psychologists, pharmacists, and occupational therapists, also have guidance on promoting equality and diversity in their respective fields.

Health and social care professionals must recognise the influence of their own beliefs, practices, and perceptions on the care they provide to clients from diverse cultural backgrounds. Being aware of one's own values and those of the healthcare system is crucial for culturally competent nursing (Leonard & Plotnikoff, 2000). Burr (2002) identified some stereotypical views held by qualified and experienced healthcare professionals of South Asian patients, warning against the dangers of imposing one's own values on others. Such imposition implies a belief in the superiority of one's own values and expectations for conformity to the majority culture. Additionally, some ethnic and racial groups may feel disempowered in the face of institutionalised racism and privilege experienced by dominant groups (Singer & Clair, 2003).

Respecting the belief systems of individuals and acknowledging their influence on health behaviour are fundamental aspects of culturally competent care. Misunderstandings and intolerance often arise from a lack of understanding and sensitivity in asking questions. Health and social care professionals must recognise their own cultural expectations and refrain from imposing them on individuals from different cultures. It is imperative for professionals to confront and challenge their own prejudices and negative perceptions of culturally and linguistically diverse communities. Furthermore, they should consider the diverse ethnic and cultural backgrounds of their patients to ensure the delivery of safe and effective care. Culturally competent approaches are vital for ensuring equitable access to substance misuse services and improving healthcare outcomes. Healthcare professionals who possess cultural knowledge and competence can deliver care that meets the unique needs of diverse communities. Gerrish (2000) advocates for individualised care, which emphasises equity, holism, respect for individuality, partnership-building between patients and professionals, and promotion of independence. This approach involves a comprehensive assessment of physical, psychological, social, and spiritual needs, which can be applied across various cultural contexts.

Some ethnocentric health interventions are clearly biased towards the dominant culture, and mainstream counselling may be inappropriate for some culturally and linguistically different communities. Ethnocentrism is a belief that one's way of life and view of the world are inherently superior to others' and more desirable (Leininger & McFarland, 2002). Studies have shown the predominance of Eurocentric counselling and support by treatment staff and staff ignorance of cultural factors that impact on drug use and drug treatment (Abdulrahim et al., 1994; NTA, 2003). The literature also has shown how ethnocentrism among professionals shapes the experience of mental health services by Black and minority ethnic users (Littlewood & Lipsedge, 1989). Unaddressed ethnocentrism can compromise nurse–patient relationships and lead to misdiagnosis, mistreatment, and insufficient treatment (Greipp, 1995). This is also applicable to professionals in the substance misuse services.

Members of culturally and linguistically different communities often have limited knowledge or experience of counselling processes (Rassool, 2006, 2016, 2024). While a client-centred approach is commonly advocated in the literature, it may not always align with the preferences of these clients. A transcultural approach, on the other hand, may be more suitable as part of therapeutic interventions for managing alcohol and drug problems within these communities. Transcultural therapy or counselling is recommended for addressing mental health and substance use issues, recognising the internal cultural realities (beliefs, values, attitudes, religion, and language) of both the therapist and the patient while being sensitive to the external realities of the patient's life (e.g. poverty, refugee status, racism, sexism). Emphasising the importance of understanding and addressing both unconscious cultural aspects and overt differences, transcultural therapy aims for successful therapeutic outcomes (Kareem & Littlewood, 2000). D'Ardenne and Mahtani (1999) highlight that *transcultural counselling* involves valuing and acknowledging culture without necessarily requiring expertise in every cultural context. However, despite the recognition of culturally competent nursing as a theoretical strategy, there is considerable evidence indicating that nurses often fail to deliver sensitive and appropriate care to minority ethnic patients. The practical application and understanding of the elements involved in cultural competence are sometimes unclear or underutilised (Kirkham, 1998). To effectively meet the objectives of cultural competence policies, it is crucial to critically examine existing policies and procedures related to cultural sensitivity and competence. By doing so, improvements can be made to enhance the experiences of Black and ethnic minority service users (Loudon et al., 1999).

Professional development is crucial for cultivating a workforce capable of delivering culturally competent care. Research by Bhui et al. (2007) highlights a scarcity of evidence regarding the effectiveness of cultural competency training and service delivery, particularly in mental healthcare. To address this gap, the educational curriculum for nurses, allied health professionals, and social care workers should encompass cultural awareness, knowledge, and sensitivity. Additionally, it should confront prevalent societal issues, such as stereotyping, discrimination, and racism, while examining institutional factors affecting minority cultures (Bhui et al., 2007). Classroom discussions that challenge biases and language use, such as dichotomous terms like "us" and "them," contribute to enhancing student cultural understanding (Browne et al., 2002). Ultimately, cultivating inherent care, appreciation, and respect for others allows professionals to exhibit warmth, empathy, and authenticity, thereby promoting culturally congruent behaviours and attitudes. However, attaining comprehensive cultural competence may demand more than just education and training, prompting the need for continual evaluation and improvement of professional approaches.

CONCLUSION

Conducting a population-based assessment of local needs can facilitate the delivery of accessible and effective services rooted in cultural competence. Understanding cultural variations allows for the development of interpersonal skills that avoid prejudice, stereotypes, biases, and clinical uncertainty. In mental health, progress and change rely on an inclusive process involving various stakeholders, such as politicians, policymakers, service providers, service users, carers, and importantly, Black and minority ethnic communities themselves (Sashidaran, 2002). Substance misuse among culturally and linguistically diverse communities must be examined within socio-political contexts, including the pervasive influence of racism. Addressing issues related to alcohol and drug problems in these communities involves navigating complexities such as language barriers, cultural norms, gender dynamics, religious beliefs, familial values, health perceptions, stigma, confidentiality concerns, oppression, and racism (Rassool, 1997).

Effectively working with these client groups does not necessitate expertise in every ethno-cultural group but rather demands cultural flexibility, acceptance, and understanding, viewing each patient or client as an individual (Rassool, 1995). Essential to this approach is cultivating openness to cultural diversity and recognising the relativity of one's own beliefs, values, and culture. There is an urgent imperative to equip nurses and other healthcare professionals in the substance misuse field with cultural competence and race-related knowledge to enable them to deliver care in a culturally sensitive manner. Furthermore, professional and regulatory bodies, along with educational institutions, should establish standards of care and core competencies that promote culturally competent practices and integrate diversity and cultural issues into curricula.

KEY POINTS

- The provision of culturally competent care has been advocated for by professionals.
- Culture is related to health, healthcare provision, and delivery.

- Understanding cultural health behaviour can reduce barriers and promote equity in the delivery of health and social care.
- Cultural competence describes an ability to meet the needs of diverse communities.
- Cultural appropriateness provides the mechanism through which cultural competence is achieved.
- Cultural sensitivity and cultural specificity form the building blocks for culturally appropriate ways of working.
- There are major challenges facing health and social care providers in the provision and delivery of services for alcohol and drug users from culturally and linguistically different communities.
- Health and social care professionals must be aware of their own beliefs, practices, and perceptions, as these may have an impact on the care they provide to clients from diverse cultural backgrounds.
- If cultural competence policy objectives are to be met, it is essential to examine policies and procedures regarding cultural sensitivity and competence to improve the experiences of culturally and linguistically different communities.
- The educational curriculum of nurses and allied health and social care professionals should include cultural awareness, cultural knowledge, and cultural sensitivity.

Activity 23.3

Questions

- Define *culture*.
- Define *cultural competence*.
- Discuss the four-stage model of cultural competence.
- List the barriers in the provision of culturally competent care.
- Identify the core elements needed in the development and provision of culturally competent drug services for culturally and linguistically different communities.

References

Abdulrahim, D., White, D., Phillips, K., Boyd, G., Nicholson, J., & Elliot, J. (1994). *Ethnicity and Drug Use: Towards the Design of Community Interventions* (Vol. 1). AIDS Research Unit. London: University of East London.

Bhui, K., Warfa, N., Edonya, P., McKenzie, K., & Bhugra, D. (2007). Cultural competence in mental health care: A review of model evaluations. *BMC Health Services Research, 7*, 15. https://doi.org/10.1186/1472-6963-7-15.

Browne, A. J., Johnson, J. L., Bottorff, J. L., Grewal, S., & Hilton, B. A. (2002). Cultural diversity: Recognizing discrimination in nursing practice. *The Canadian Nurse,* 98(5), 24–27.

Burr, J. (2002). Cultural stereotypes of women from South Asian communities: Mental health care professionals' explanations for patterns of suicide and depression. *Social Science & Medicine (1982)*, 55(5), 835–845. https://doi.org/10.1016/s0277-9536(01)00220-9.

Campinha-Bacote, J., Yahle, T., & Langenkamp, M. (1996). The challenge of cultural diversity for nurse educators. *Journal of Continuing Nursing Education*, 27(2), 59–64.

Center for Behavioral Health Statistics and Quality. (2022). *2021 National Survey on Drug Use and Health: Methodological Summary and Definitions.* https://www.samhsa.gov/data/report/2021-methodological-summary-and-definitions (accessed 3 April 2024).

Cross, T. L., Bazron, B. J., Dennis, K. W., & Isaacs, M. R. (1989). *Towards a Culturally Competent System of Care.* CASSP Technical Assistance Center. Washington, DC: Georgetown University Child Development Center.

D'Ardenne, P., & Mahtani, A. (1999). *Transcultural Counselling in Action.* London: Sage.

Department of Health and Aged Care. (2020). *Alcohol and Aboriginal and Torres Strait Islander Peoples.* https://www.health.gov.au/topics/alcohol/alcohol-throughout-life/alcohol-and-aboriginal-and-torres-strait-islander-peoples (accessed 3 April 2024).

Fernandez, J. (2004). Cultural considerations: Improving community involvement. *Substance Misuse Management in General Practice, Net Work*, 8, 9 September.

Gerrish, K. (2000). Individualized care: Its conceptualization and practice within a multiethnic society. *Journal of Advanced Nursing*, 32(1), 91–99. https://doi.org/10.1046/j.1365-2648.2000.01455.x.

Gleeson, H., Thom, B., Bayley, M., & McQuarrie, T. (2019). *Rapid Evidence Review: Drinking Problems and Interventions in Black and Minority Ethnic Communities* [Internet]. Alcohol Change UK. https://alcoholchange.org.uk/publication/rapid-evidence-review-drinking-problems-and-interventions-in-black-and-minority-ethnic-communities (accessed 3 April 2024).

Greipp, M. E. (1995). Culture and ethics: A tool for analysing the effects of biases on the nurse-patient relationship. *Nursing Ethics,* 2(3), 211–221. https://doi.org/10.1177/096973309500200304.

Heath, D. B. (2001). Culture and substance abuse. *The Psychiatric Clinics of North America,* 24(3), 479–viii. https://doi.org/10.1016/s0193-953x(05)70242-2.

Institute of Alcohol Studies. (2020). *Ethnic Minorities and Alcohol.* https://www.ias.org.uk/wp-content/uploads/2020/12/Ethnic-minorities-and-alcohol.pdf (accessed 3 April 2024).

Joseph Rowntree Foundation. (2010). *Ethnicity and Alcohol: A Review of the UK Literature.* York: Joseph Rowntree Foundation.

Kareem, J., & Littlewood, R. (2000). *Intercultural Therapy.* Oxford: Blackwell.

Kavanagh, K. H., & Kennedy, P. H. (1992). *Promoting Cultural Diversity: Strategies for Health Care Professionals.* Newbury Park, CA: SAGE Publications, Inc.

Kirkham, S. R. (1998). Nurses' descriptions of caring for culturally diverse clients. *Clinical Nursing Research,* 7(2), 125–146. https://doi.org/10.1177/105477389800700204.

Leininger, M., & McFarland, M. (2002). *Transcultural Nursing: Concepts, Theories, Research, and Practice* (3rd ed.). New York: McGraw-Hill.

Leininger, M. M. (Ed.). (1991). *Culture Care Diversity and Universality: A Theory of Nursing.* New York: National League of Nursing.

Leonard, B. J., & Plotnikoff, G. A. (2000). Awareness: The heart of cultural competence. *Advanced Practice in Acute and Critical Care,* 11(1), 51–59.

Littlewood, R., & Lipsedge, M. (1989). *Aliens and Alienists: Ethnic Minorities and Psychiatry.* London: Unwin Hyman.

Loudon, R., Anderson, M., Gill, P., & Greenfield, S. (1999). Educating medical students for work in culturally diverse societies. *JAMA,* 282(9), 875–880.

Mackinnon, S. P., Couture, M. E., Cooper, M. L., Kuntsche, E., O'Connor, R. M., Stewart, S. H., & DRINC Team (2017). Cross-cultural comparisons of drinking motives in 10 countries: Data from the DRINC project. *Drug and Alcohol Review,* 36(6), 721–730. https://doi.org/10.1111/dar.12464.

NHS Digital. (2021). *Illicit Drug Use.* https://www.ethnicity-facts-figures.service.gov.uk/health/alcohol-smoking-and-drug-use/illicit-drug-use-among-adults/latest/#:~:-text=Black%20women%20%289.7%25%29%2C%20White%20British%20women%20%286.2%25%29%20and,illicit%20drugs%20compared%20with%20White%20British%20women%20%286.2%25%29 (accessed 3 April 2024).

NTA. (2002). *Race Equality Scheme and Workplan.* London: National Treatment Agency.

NTA. (2003). *Black and Minority Ethnic Communities: A Review of the Literature on Drug Use and Related Service Provision.* London: National Treatment Agency.

Nursing and Midwifery Council (NMC). (2018). *The Code: Professional Standards of Practice and Behaviour for Nurses and Midwives.* https://www.nmc.org.uk/globalassets/sitedocuments/nmc-publications/nmc-code.pdf (accessed 3 April 2024).

Papadopoulos, I., Tilki, M., & Taylor, G. (1998). *Transcultural Care: A Guide for Health Care Professionals.* Wiltshire: Quay Books.

Purnell, L. D., & Paulanka, B. J. (2003). *Transcultural Health Care: A Culturally Competent Approach* (2nd ed.). Philadelphia: F.A. Davis.

Rassool, G. H. (1995). The health status and health care of ethno-cultural minorities in the United Kingdom: An agenda for action. *Journal of Advanced Nursing,* 21(2), 199–201.

Rassool, G. H. (1997). Ethnic minorities and substance misuse. In G. H. Rassool & M. Gafoor (Eds.), *Addiction Nursing: Perspectives on Professional and Clinical Practice.* Cheltenham: Stanley Nelson.

Rassool, G. H. (2006a). Black and ethnic minority communities: Substance misuse and mental health: Whose problems anyway. In G. H. Rassool (Ed.), *Dual Diagnosis Nursing.* Oxford: Blackwell Publications.

Rassool, G. H. (2006b). *Dual Diagnosis Nursing.* Oxford: Blackwell Publications.

Rassool, G. H. (2016). *Islāmic Counselling: An Introduction to Theory and Practice.* East Sussex: Routledge.

Rassool, G. H. (2024). *Islāmic Counselling and Psychotherapy: From Theory to Practice* (2nd ed.). Oxford: Routledge.

Sangster, D., Shiner, M., Sheikh, N., & Patel, K. (2002). *Delivering Drug Services to Black and Minority Ethnic Communities* (DPAS/P16). London: Home Office Drug Prevention and Advisory Service (DPAS).

Sashidaran, S. P. (2002). *Inside Outside: Improving Mental Health Services for Black and Minority Ethnic Communities in England.* London: Department of Health.

Singer, M., & Clair, S. (2003). Syndemics and public health: Reconceptualizing disease in bio-social context. *Medical Anthropology Quarterly,* 17(4), 423–441. https://doi.org/10.1525/maq.2003.17.4.423.

Tervalon, M., & Murray-Garcia, J. (1998). Cultural humility versus cultural competence: A critical distinction in defining physician training outcomes in multicultural education. *Journal of Health Care Poor Underserved,* 9(2), 117–125.

UNESCO. (2001). UNESCO Universal Declaration on Cultural Diversity. https://en.unesco.org/about-us/legal-affairs/unesco-universal-declaration-cultural-diversity (accessed 3 April 2024).

Wilson, J., Ward, C., & Fischer, R. (2013). Beyond culture learning theory: What can personality tell us about cultural competence? *Journal of Cross-Cultural Psychology,* 44(6), 900–927.

Part 5

Care planning and intervention strategies

Chapter 24

Framework for assessment, risk assessment, and screening

Learning outcomes

- Describe briefly the client's journey.
- Identify the types of assessment.
- Describe the aims and purpose of screening or initial assessment.
- Describe the aims and purpose of triage screening.
- Describe the aims and purpose of comprehensive assessment.
- Have an awareness of the barriers in assessing those with comorbidity.
- Identify and assess possible risk behaviours.
- Carry out assessment to identify and prioritise needs.
- Carry out a comprehensive substance misuse assessment.
- Discuss issues related to confidentiality and records keeping.

Activity 24.1

There is only one correct answer to the following multiple-choice questions.

1. What does the client's journey typically involve in the context of assessment?
   a. A single assessment session
   b. A continuous process from initial contact to intervention
   c. A written report summarising the client's background
   d. A final assessment conducted by a senior clinician
   e. A questionnaire filled out by the client
2. Which of the following is NOT a type of assessment commonly used in client evaluation?
   a. Screening
   b. Triage
   c. Comprehensive
   d. Preliminary
   e. Continuous
3. What is the primary aim of screening or initial assessment?
   a. To provide a diagnosis
   b. To identify potential risk behaviours
   c. To establish a therapeutic relationship
   d. To determine treatment duration
   e. To secure insurance coverage

DOI: 10.4324/9781003456674-29

4. Triage screening primarily serves to:
   a. Determine the severity of the client's condition
   b. Initiate immediate treatment
   c. Identify the client's preferred treatment approach
   d. Establish a timeline for intervention
   e. Conduct a preliminary diagnosis
5. What is the primary goal of comprehensive assessment?
   a. To gather detailed information about the client's life circumstances
   b. To assess the client's psychological stability
   c. To diagnose specific mental health disorders
   d. To evaluate the effectiveness of previous treatments
   e. To recommend medication
6. Which of the following is a potential barrier when assessing individuals with comorbidity?
   a. Lack of confidentiality
   b. Limited access to assessment tools
   c. Difficulty in prioritising needs
   d. Misinterpretation of risk behaviours
   e. Overreliance on self-reporting
7. What is a key aspect of identifying and assessing possible risk behaviours?
   a. Conducting a physical examination
   b. Relying solely on the client's self-report
   c. Exploring family history
   d. Collaboration with law enforcement agencies
   e. Reviewing medical records
8. What is the purpose of prioritising needs during assessment?
   a. To determine the client's eligibility for treatment
   b. To allocate resources effectively
   c. To establish a diagnosis
   d. To ensure confidentiality
   e. To expedite the assessment process
9. Which of the following is a component of a comprehensive substance misuse assessment?
   a. Assessing family dynamics
   b. Evaluating academic achievement
   c. Identifying substance abuse patterns
   d. Reviewing financial records
   e. Monitoring medication adherence
10. What are some issues related to confidentiality and record-keeping in assessment?
    a. Ensuring client anonymity
    b. Maintaining accurate records
    c. Sharing information with third parties without consent
    d. Storing records in a secure location
    e. All of the above
11. Which stage of the assessment process involves gathering detailed information about the client's background and current situation?
    a. Screening
    b. Triage screening
    c. Comprehensive assessment
    d. Initial assessment
    e. Follow-up assessment

12. What is the primary goal of triage screening?
    a. To diagnose mental health disorders
    b. To determine the severity of the client's condition
    c. To identify potential risk behaviours
    d. To establish a therapeutic relationship
    e. To monitor treatment progress
13. When assessing individuals with comorbidity, which of the following is a common challenge?
    a. Limited access to assessment tools
    b. Lack of awareness of risk behaviours
    c. Difficulty in prioritising needs
    d. Inadequate training of assessors
    e. Overreliance on self-reporting
14. Which aspect of assessment involves discussing issues related to confidentiality and record-keeping?
    a. Initial assessment
    b. Comprehensive assessment
    c. Follow-up assessment
    d. Triage screening
    e. Continuous assessment
15. How does comprehensive assessment differ from screening?
    a. Comprehensive assessment is shorter in duration.
    b. Screening focuses on specific issues, while comprehensive assessment gathers detailed information.
    c. Comprehensive assessment requires specialised training.
    d. Screening involves only self-reporting by the client.
    e. Comprehensive assessment does not involve risk assessment.

INTRODUCTION: TREATMENT JOURNEY

The process of assessment and care planning is integral to effective clinical practice, providing a structured foundation for delivering care and interventions. It is considered a fundamental component within the systematic approach to healthcare provision. Evaluation of care is essential within this framework to ensure the quality and effectiveness of interventions. Negotiating a written care plan with the patient is a good practice as it promotes transparency and collaboration in decision-making. The client journey through the drug treatment system encompasses all stages of their engagement with services, from referral to discharge and ongoing care. This journey is described by the National Treatment Agency (NTA, 2005) as comprising four overlapping components:

- Engagement
- Treatment delivery (including maintenance)
- Community integration (which underpins both delivery and treatment maintenance or completion)
- Treatment completion (for all those who choose to be drug-free and who can benefit)

This framework guides assessment and care planning, which should be specifically targeted and focused on setting goals and objectives, and monitoring outcomes in relation to these four stages in the client journey (NTA, 2006). The phases of the treatment journey are presented in Figure 24.1.

In clinical practice, the treatment journey for clients experiencing alcohol- or drug-related issues is recognised as a cyclical process, encompassing engagement, retention, follow-up, re-engagement of dropout clients, and completion of treatment. However, clients may not follow a linear progression through these phases, as they might enter or exit treatment at various stages during their substance use careers. The delivery of care and treatment should be responsive to individual needs across different care settings. This involves the capacity to

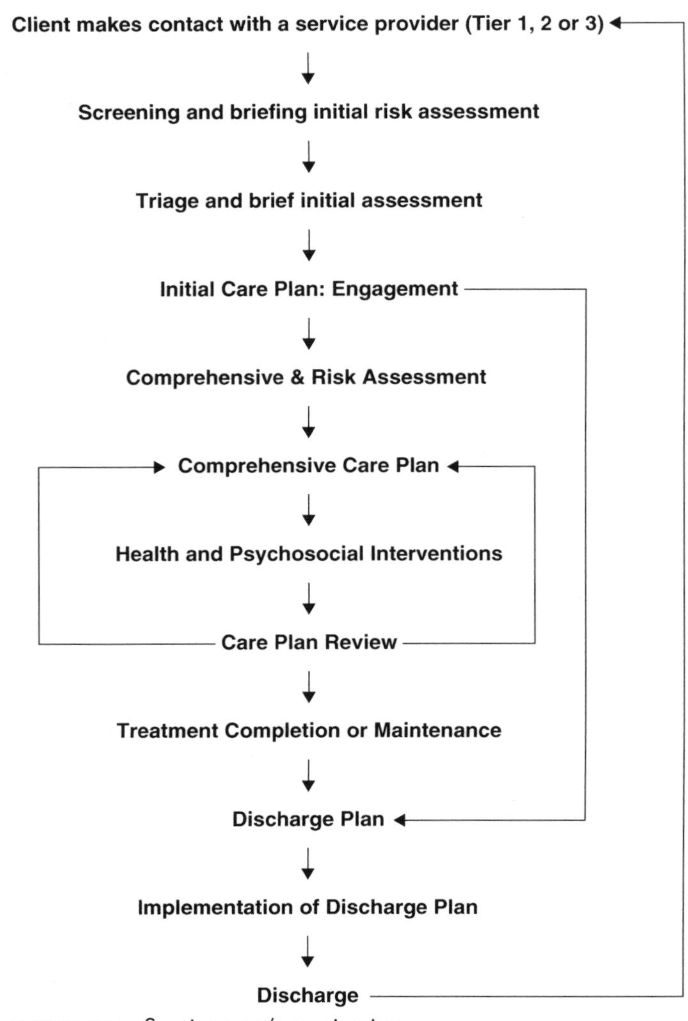

FIGURE 24.1 Service user's service journey.

assess needs, diagnose conditions, formulate personalised care plans, implement interventions, and continually evaluate the effectiveness of care provided. Collaboration among healthcare team members is emphasised to ensure comprehensive and coordinated care delivery. An essential aspect of effective practice is empowering individuals and their caregivers to actively participate in all aspects of care planning, delivery, and evaluation. This collaborative approach promotes patient autonomy and ensures that care is tailored to meet the specific needs and preferences of each individual.

ASSESSMENT

Assessment is a pivotal stage within the systematic approach to care and interventions, serving as a dynamic and interpersonal process where patients gain insight into their addiction and associated health needs. It involves a comprehensive analysis of an individual's physical/medical, psychosocial, and spiritual requirements through the collection of data, typically conducted via interviewing and recording medical/nursing and psychosocial history.

The primary purposes of assessment include gathering information for care and health or social interventions, addressing urgent medical and psychological issues, providing feedback on substance misuse levels, and establishing rapport with the client. The maintenance of rapport, empathy, genuineness, and non-judgemental attitudes is crucial during assessment, as they facilitate effective communication and relationship building. Research indicates that the initial clinical encounter significantly impacts attitude change, commitment enhancement, and goal clarification for individuals struggling with alcohol use (Edwards et al., 2003). Consequently, the assessment process should yield a written document that serves as a basis for discussing care planning, setting goals and objectives, implementing the care plan, and evaluating its efficacy. This documentation ensures continuity of care and facilitates ongoing monitoring and adjustment as needed.

LEVELS OF ASSESSMENT

In practice, three levels of assessment have been identified in practice: screening or initial assessment, triage, and comprehensive assessment.

SCREENING OR INITIAL ASSESSMENT

Screening or initial assessment is a concise process designed to ascertain whether an individual has issues related to drug and alcohol use, as well as health-related problems and risk behaviours. Typically conducted in generic settings such as hospitals or primary healthcare facilities, this type of assessment is crucial for identifying substance misuse issues among patients presenting with conditions like overdose, self-harm, lost prescriptions, withdrawal seizures, delirium tremens, and withdrawal syndrome in A&E departments. The outcome of screening determines the level of interventions needed and the urgency of referral to alcohol or drug treatment services. Screening assessments can also serve as a catalyst for motivating substance misusers to transition from pre-contemplation to the contemplation stage of change through brief opportunistic interventions. Moreover, the assessment process provides an opportunity for health education and the promotion of harm reduction strategies. One commonly used tool for screening is the CAGE questionnaire, consisting of four straightforward questions that can be easily incorporated into routine assessments. A positive response to two or more questions on the CAGE questionnaire is indicative of problem drinking. This simple yet effective tool aids in quickly identifying individuals who may require further evaluation and intervention for alcohol-related issues. This short questionnaire concentrates on the consequences rather than on the quantity or frequency of alcohol use. It includes the following questions.

1. Have you ever felt that you should cut down your drinking?
2. Have people annoyed you by criticising your drinking?
3. Have you ever felt bad or guilty about your drinking?
4. Have you ever had a drink first thing in the morning to steady your nerves or get rid of a hangover (eye-opener)?

A number of screening instruments have been introduced to assess alcohol and drug problems and comorbidity. Table 24.1 presents a summary of screening instruments for alcohol and drug problems. Table 24.2 presents the fast alcohol screening test (FAST).

INITIAL AND COMPREHENSIVE ASSESSMENT

Initial assessment typically occurs when an individual with alcohol or substance use problems initially interacts with generic services. This initial encounter provides an opportunity to gather essential information about the individual's substance use, as well as their overall health and social circumstances. During this assessment, the focus is on establishing a baseline understanding of the individual's needs and determining the appropriate level of care or intervention required. This initial assessment sets the stage for further engagement with specialised substance misuse services and guides the development of a comprehensive care plan tailored to the individual's specific needs. Alcohol and drug misusers with complex needs require assessment that is comprehensive and multi-professional to plan effective care and treatment. Comprehensive assessment is carried out when a client may (NTA, 2006):

- Require structured and/or intensive intervention.
- Have significant psychiatric and/or physical comorbidity.
- Have a significant level of risk of harm to self or others.
- Be in contact with multiple service providers.
- Have a history of disengagement from drug treatment services.
- Be pregnant or have children "at risk."

The process of taking a drug and alcohol history involves conducting a detailed assessment of an individual's current substance use patterns. Initially, the assessment aims to understand the individual's perceptions of their drug and/or

Table 24.1
Screening tools for alcohol and drug problems

CAGE	This easy-to-use patient questionnaire is a screening test for problem drinking and potential alcohol problems.	Ewing, 1984
AUDIT: The Alcohol Use Disorders Identification Test	Brief self-report questionnaire (WHO) to identify people whose alcohol consumption has become hazardous or harmful to their health.	Babor & Higgins-Biddle, 2001
CUAD: The Chemical Use, Abuse, and Dependence Scale	Brief (20 minutes to administer), reliable, and validated tool for the identification of substance use disorders in severely mentally ill inpatients.	McGovern & Morrison, 1992
FAST: Fast Alcohol Screening Test	Brief four-item questionnaire. FAST is potentially the shortest screening tool.	Hodgson et al., 2002
DAST – 10: The Drug Abuse Screening Test	Self-report questionnaire for measuring the severity of drug (not alcohol) dependence.	Skinner, 1982
DALI: The Dartmouth Assessment of Lifestyle Instrument	An 18-item interviewer-administered tool (on average, 6 minutes to complete). It was developed primarily to detect alcohol, cannabis, and cocaine use disorders.	Rosenberg et al., 1998
MMSE: Mini-Mental State Examination	Brief quantitative measure to screen for cognitive impairment, to estimate its severity, to follow cognitive changes over time, and to document response to treatment.	Folstein et al., 1975
PRISM: The Psychiatric Research Interview for Substance and Mental Disorders	Diagnostic interview based on *DSM-IV*. More reliable for assessing psychiatric disorders in those who have comorbid substance use disorders.	Hasin et al., 1998
SATS: The Substance Abuse Treatment Scale	To evaluate treatment progress or as an outcome measure. The scale is intended for assessing a person's stage of substance misuse treatment.	McHugo et al., 1995

Source: Adapted from Crawford and Crome (2001).

Table 24.2
The Fast Alcohol Screening Test (FAST)

1. How often do you have eight or more drinks on one occasion?
   __ Never __ Less Than Monthly __ Monthly __ Weekly __ Daily or Almost Daily
2. How often during the last year have you been unable to remember what happened the night before because you had been drinking?
   __ Never __ Less Than Monthly __ Monthly __ Weekly __ Daily or Almost Daily
3. How often during the last year have you failed to do what was normally expected of you because of your drinking?
   __ Never __ Less Than Monthly __ Monthly __ Weekly __ Daily or Almost Daily
4. Has a relative or friend, a doctor, or other health worker been concerned about your drinking or suggested you cut down?
   __ No __ Yes, but not in the last year. __ Yes, in the last year.

Scoring FAST:
Score questions 1, 2, and 3 as follows:

- Never – 0 points
- Less than monthly – 1 point
- Monthly – 2 points
- Weekly – 3 points
- Daily or almost daily – 4 points

Score question 4 as follows:

- No – 0 points
- Yes, but not in the last year – 2 points
- Yes, in the last year – 4 points

The maximum score is 16. A total score of 3 indicates hazardous drinking.
If a person answered "never" on the first question, he or she is not a hazardous drinker, and the remaining questions are not necessary.
If a person answers "weekly" or "daily or almost daily" on the first question, he or she is considered a hazardous drinker, and the rest of the questions are skipped.
If a person answers "monthly" or "less than monthly" to the first question, the other three questions are needed to complete the screening for hazardous drinking.

Source: Hodgson et al. (2002).

alcohol consumption. Subsequently, the focus shifts towards gathering information about the following aspects:

- *Current pattern of alcohol and substance use.* This includes the frequency, duration, and intensity of substance use.
- *Types of drugs used.* Identification of specific substances consumed by the individual.
- *Quantities of substances used.* Determining the amount of drugs or alcohol consumed by the individual.
- *Level of dependence.* Assessing the extent of reliance on substances and the presence of withdrawal symptoms or medical complications.
- *Risk behaviours.* Identifying any behaviours associated with substance use that may pose a risk to the individual's health or safety.
- *Associated problems.* Exploring any physical, psychological, or social issues arising from alcohol and substance use disorder.
- *Source of help.* Understanding the individual's access to support services or resources for addressing substance use concerns.
- *Source of access to psychoactive substances.* Investigating how the individual obtains drugs or alcohol.
- *Withdrawal symptoms.* By asking about withdrawal symptoms, healthcare professionals can gauge the level of dependence on substances and assess the potential risks associated with withdrawal.
- *Periods of abstinence and relapse.* Documenting any periods of sobriety or recurrence of substance use.

By addressing these components comprehensively, healthcare professionals can gain valuable insights into the individual's substance use history, which informs the development of tailored interventions and treatment plans. This structured approach ensures that the assessment is thorough and encompasses all relevant aspects of the individual's substance use behaviour. An outline of the assessment of substance use is shown in Table 24.3.

Assessment of substance misuse often focuses solely on an individual's negative aspects, such as weaknesses, risks, and problems. However, including an assessment of positive aspects can enhance self-efficacy and self-esteem. Acknowledging strengths may reduce resistance to engagement with services and positively influence coping strategies and treatment outcomes. A strengths-based approach highlights successful strategies used in managing substance misuse and psychiatric symptoms, such as previous coping mechanisms for remaining drug- or alcohol-free. Comprehensive assessment is an ongoing process, spanning several weeks and involving information gathering from various sources, including partners, significant others, key workers, doctors, and nurses. While self-report or checklist assessments of substance misuse levels have limitations, additional collateral data and laboratory investigations can provide confirmation of substance use or abstinence. Accountability for completing comprehensive assessments

Table 24.3
Assessment of substance use

• Statement of the need/problem	Consider the individual's concerns, issues, needs, or problems.
• Current drug and alcohol use	Type, quantity, frequency, and route of administration (drug).
• Pattern of drug or alcohol use	Details of drug/alcohol-taking for past week/month.
• Current use of other substances	Prescribed, illicit, or over-the counter drugs.
• Level of dependence	Any withdrawal symptoms. Evidence of increasing tolerance.
• Associated problems	Any medical, psychiatric, social, or legal problems.
• Risk behaviours	Source of injecting equipment. Sharing of equipment. Knowledge about sterilisation and needle exchange services. Sexual behaviour when intoxicated.
• Periods of abstinence/relapse	Duration, periods of abstinence – voluntary or enforced. Reasons for lapse or relapse.
• Sources of help	Social support systems. Statutory agencies. Local authorities. Voluntary agencies. Self-help groups.
• Coping strategies and strengths	Previous strategies in coping with use of alcohol and drug use. Achievements, strengths, and positive aspects of the individual.

Source: Rassool and Winnington (2006)

should be clear, with named key workers typically leading each case. This approach ensures thorough evaluation and facilitates tailored interventions for individuals struggling with substance misuse.

ASSESSMENT OF SUBSTANCE MISUSE AND PSYCHIATRIC DISORDERS

Individuals with co-occurring disorders, experiencing both substance misuse and psychiatric disorders, present complex and multiple needs that pose challenges for comprehensive assessment. Before conducting a full assessment, certain observations may indicate the presence of substance misuse and/or mental health problems, warranting further investigation. These indicators serve as cues for healthcare professionals to delve deeper into the assessment and diagnosis process. Table 24.4 provides a summary of these indicators for further assessment, guiding clinicians in recognising potential signs of substance misuse and mental health issues. These observations help ensure a more thorough evaluation of individuals with comorbidity, facilitating appropriate interventions and treatment planning tailored to their specific needs. Table 24.4 presents the indicators for further assessment.

Table 24.4
Indicators for further assessment

- Use of psychoactive substances to control thoughts and feelings
- Self-medication of psychoactive substances for alleviating mental health problems
- Use of psychoactive substances to balance or reduce side-effects of prescribed medications
- Misuse of prescription and over-the-counter drugs
- Unable to reduce alcohol and/or drug use
- Previous detoxification and/or rehabilitation
- Symptoms of withdrawal
- High tolerance of psychoactive substances
- Drug-seeking behaviour
- Self-harm
- Frequency of mood swings and sadness
- Anger and impulsiveness
- Over suspiciousness

Source: Adapted from Rassool and Winnington (2006).

Assessing individuals with both substance misuse and psychiatric disorders presents significant challenges, as substance use can obscure psychiatric symptoms or alter diagnosis. Distinguishing between the effects of psychoactive substances and symptoms of mental health issues adds complexity to the assessment process. Many psychiatric symptoms may be temporary and related to substance misuse withdrawal or intoxication rather than indicating a true "dual diagnosis." Given these complexities, it may be more practical for workers to address immediate symptoms until the individual has recovered from drug intoxication or withdrawal. Consequently, it is unlikely that a comprehensive assessment can be completed during the initial contact with individuals experiencing dual diagnosis. Instead, ongoing assessment and management are necessary to accurately evaluate and address the individual's needs over time.

The assessment process for individuals with comorbid substance misuse and mental health disorders is influenced by factors such as the lack of knowledge, skills, and attitudes among healthcare professionals (Rassool & Winnington, 2006). This lack of expertise may lead to under-recognition of comorbid conditions, as individuals may go unnoticed in both drug and alcohol services and mental health services. The segregation of mental health and substance misuse services further perpetuates this issue, with staff often focusing on their respective areas of expertise. Mental health workers may identify mental health problems but overlook substance misuse issues, while workers in drug and alcohol services may focus solely on substance misuse and fail to recognise underlying mental health concerns. Consequently, the assessment process may become centred on establishing primacy between mental health and substance misuse, rather than addressing the individual's comprehensive needs. Individuals with comorbid conditions may struggle to fit within the expectations of both drug and alcohol services and mental healthcare systems, leading to a lack of adequate support and treatment. This phenomenon of individuals falling through the gaps of the healthcare system is referred to as "system misfits" (Bachrach, 1986).

A key aspect of working with patients experiencing comorbidity is the ability to conduct a comprehensive assessment encompassing various domains. This includes evaluating mental health history and current symptoms, as well as assessing both current and historical substance use and misuse. Additionally, assessing physical health, social needs, and recognising diversity among individuals with dual diagnosis are crucial components of the assessment process. One notable feature of a co-occurring disorder's assessment is the use of "timelines." Timelines involve recording the sequence of events for both substance misuse and mental health problems over a specified period. This approach provides invaluable information, especially in determining which event occurred first – substance misuse or mental health issues (Moore & Rassool, 2001). Understanding the chronological order of events can help identify potential causal relationships and guide treatment prioritisation. The art of completing a substance misuse assessment relies on incorporating essentially the following elements (Rassool & Winnington, 2006):

- Assessment of history and current nature of the type and frequency of psychoactive substances used
- Assessment of mental health history and current symptoms
- Assessment of current physical health
- Assessment of level and nature of risks in evidence
- Assessment of social needs (housing, employment, social networks)
- Assessment with self-awareness of diversity issues and cultural competence

A number of screening instruments have been introduced to assess comorbidity Crawford & Crome, 2001).

RISK ASSESSMENT

Risk assessment and management are integral components of good practice in substance misuse services. The emphasis on risk assessment and management has emerged in response to various factors, including perceived shortcomings in community care policies, critiques of existing practices following inquiries into tragedies involving individuals with serious mental illness, government initiatives aimed at reducing self-harm and enhancing community management of individuals with mental illness, and the imperative for mental health providers to mitigate the rising costs associated with litigation and complaints (Doyle, 2004).

Conducting risk assessment should be considered good practice as part of the overall assessment process.

Risk assessment aims to identify factors that indicate the likelihood of harm to oneself or others, particularly in the context of alcohol and substance misuse. This information is crucial for developing comprehensive care plans and implementing appropriate management strategies. The severity of substance misuse, including the use of multiple psychoactive substances, increases the risk of overdose and suicide. Involving the individual being assessed, relevant professionals, and informal caregivers or significant others is essential for a thorough risk assessment process. Individuals may not always disclose risky behaviours or self-harm tendencies, emphasising the importance of gathering information from multiple sources. Risk assessment is an ongoing process, with critical points for further assessment occurring before individuals are discharged from the hospital, referred to other agencies or services, or returned to the care of informal caregivers. These assessments ensure that interventions are tailored to address emerging risks and promote the safety and well-being of individuals receiving care. The principal elements of risk assessment and management are:

- Risk of suicide or self-harm – ideas, plans, and intentions
- Risk of overdose, polydrug use, and unsafe injecting practices
- Risk of harm or violence to others
- Risk of harm or abuse/exploitation by others
- Risk of severe self-neglect
- Risk related to physical condition

While there is no specific method for predicting risky behaviour, several factors have been identified in the literature as associated with an increased likelihood of engaging in such behaviours. These factors encompass patterns of past and current psychosocial and physical problems that may serve as indicators of risk behaviours. A summary of these predisposing and precipitating risk factors is presented in Table 24.5.

Assessment of an individual's risk of violence towards others is a critical aspect that must be communicated to informal carers, relevant agencies, and key individuals involved in their care and support. When such risk is identified, it is essential to ensure that the individual receives adequate personal care, supervision, and treatment to mitigate potential harm. In assessing the risk of harm or violence towards others, it is important to consider the potential victims of the perpetrator. Exploring

Table 24.5
Predictors of risk

Precipitating factors	Predisposing risk factors
• Specific plan	• Previous history of harm to self or others
• Neurological (organic disorders)	• Family history of harm or mental illness
• Continuing high suicidal and behavioural intent	• Borderline or impulsive personality
• Hopelessness	• Social exclusion
• Hallucinations and persecutory delusions	• Lack of support network
• Social isolation	• Past sexual or physical abuse
• Recent loss or separation	• Depression
• Recent psychiatric hospitalisation	• Schizophrenia
• Relationship breakdown	• Substance misuse
• Unemployment	
• Imprisonment or threat of imprisonment	
• Homelessness	
• Cultural and diversity issues (e.g. shame)	
• Intoxication with alcohol or drugs	
• Poor compliance with medication or treatment programmes	
• Poor communications between professionals	

Source: Adapted from Evans and Sullivan (2001)

issues related to the likely victims and their awareness of the risks posed to them and others is crucial for developing effective risk management strategies. Additionally, practitioners must pay attention to the individual's vulnerability to various forms of danger or exploitation, including sexual, financial, occupational, and familial risks, especially when their judgement or cognitive functioning is significantly impaired.

Assessing the risk of self-harm and attempted suicide among individuals with co-occurring disorders is important, as they are more likely to pose a risk to themselves than to others. This assessment involves examining factors such as previous self-harm incidents, their frequency, seriousness, intentionality, and the individual's current intentions, plans, access, and means to carry out self-harm (Rassool & Winnington, 2006). Conducting this assessment requires a sensitive and non-judgemental approach, despite the challenges practitioners may face in discussing such sensitive topics. It is important to debunk the myth that addressing "risky behaviours" or self-harm may encourage individuals to engage in them. Instead, acknowledging these thoughts and feelings allows practitioners to work with individuals through techniques such as anger management, individual therapy, and group work (Rethink & Turning Point, 2004). An examination of the "risky behaviours" should include the following questions:

- Does the individual have a suicide plan or serious intentions?
- How specific is the plan?
- What method will be used?
- Does the individual have the means to carry out the plan?
- When will the "risky behaviour" happen?

Effective risk management should aim to minimise risk without disempowering individuals. This can be achieved through open discussion, standardised assessment, and the development of up-to-date, jointly owned care plans. Collaboration and communication are key to ensuring the success of these strategies (O'Rourke & Bird, 2001). Risk assessment should be evidence-based, and risk management should be systematically planned by multidisciplinary teams to enable more effective interventions. Consultation and communication between team members and relevant personnel from other agencies or services regarding risk assessment and management are essential aspects of good clinical practice. Furthermore, proper documentation and information sharing are fundamental when assessing an individual's future potential risk. Keeping accurate records and sharing relevant information among healthcare professionals ensures that all team members are informed and can work together to address and mitigate risks effectively.

TESTING FOR CURRENT DRUG AND ALCOHOL USE

Self-reported assessment indicating current drug and/or alcohol use may prompt the need for laboratory investigations to aid in early identification and diagnosis. These investigations contribute objective information to the overall assessment. Various bodily fluids can be tested for drugs and alcohol, including serum, urine, exhaled air, and hair. Urine analysis is commonly used to assess drug use and can be conducted using two main methods: immunoassay tests and gas chromatography. While immunoassay tests are based on detecting antibodies to ingested drugs, gas chromatography is more accurate. Hair testing is another method that can detect drugs deposited within the growing hair follicle and covers longer periods than a single urine test, though it is more expensive (McPhillips et al., 1997). Saliva drug testing is capable of detecting up to ten drugs, including amphetamine, cocaine, opiates, marijuana, and benzodiazepines. However, these tests only indicate whether drugs are present or absent and do not measure the amount of drugs in the body. The detection periods for urine drug screening are outlined in Table 24.6.

Several blood tests can be conducted to assess the presence of drugs or alcohol in an individual's system. Essential investigations include liver function tests (LFT), gamma-glutamyl transferase (GGT), aspartate transaminase (AST), and mean corpuscular volume (MCV). These tests provide valuable information about an individual's alcohol consumption and potential liver damage. A summary of special blood tests for drugs and alcohol is provided in Table 24.7. Additionally, individuals who engage in injecting drug use and share needles or other paraphernalia are at risk of cross-infections. Therefore, blood tests may also be performed to determine the presence of HIV and hepatitis B and C infections. It is imperative that these tests are accompanied by

Table 24.6
Detection periods for urine drug screening

Substances	Detection times
Cannabinoids (marijuana)	
• Single use	2 days
• Moderate use (3 times per week)	2 weeks
• Daily use	2–4 weeks
• Heavy use (daily)	Up to 12 weeks
Alcohol	7–12 hours
Amphetamines	2–3 days
Short-acting benzodiazepines	3–5 days
Long-acting benzodiazepines	Up to 30 days
Buprenorphine	Up to 11 days
Cocaine metabolites	2–4 days
Codeine/morphine/propoxyphene (Heroin is detected in urine as the 48-hour metabolite morphine.)	1–2 days
Fentanyl	2–3 days
Heroin or morphine	1–3 days
Methadone	3–4 days
Oxycodone	1–3 days
Methaqualone	7 days+
Methadone (maintenance dosing)	7–9 days (approximate)
Norpropoxyphene	6–48 hours
Phencyclidine (PCP)	8 days (approximate)

Source: Adapted from Sissons (2023).

Table 24.7
Special laboratory alcohol and drug tests

Tests	Detected substance(s)	Observations
Gamma glutamyl transferase (GGT)	Alcohol	Elevated before liver damage. More likely to have liver damage at higher readings.
Liver functions tests (LFT)	Alcohol and drug	Liver damage due to alcohol.
Full blood count	Alcohol	Mean red blood cells raised in heavy chronic drinkers.
Aspartate transaminase (AST)	Alcohol	Suggests alcohol-related liver damage.
Uric acid	Alcohol	Increase of urates and possibly gout.
Haemoglobin	Drug and alcohol	Anaemia due to poor nutrition or vitamin deficiencies.
Tests for HIV, hepatitis B and C	Drug	History of injecting.

Source: Rassool and Winnington (2006)

pre-test and post-test counselling to ensure individuals are informed about the implications of the results and provided with appropriate support.

CONFIDENTIALITY

Confidentiality is a fundamental duty in healthcare practice, governed by legal and ethical obligations. However, exchanging and sharing information is essential for effective health and social care processes. This must be done while adhering to confidentiality codes and supported by clear policies and procedures. Maintaining patient privacy and building trusting relationships enhance their willingness to seek care. Information provided in confidence should not be disclosed without the patient's consent, especially in sensitive areas like sexual, reproductive, and public health and psychiatric disorders, which may lead to stigmatisation. Patients should be assured that information will not be disclosed to family or employers without their consent. As part of the assessment process, clients should be informed about how their information may be shared, and the consequences. Information in the care plan can be shared with named participants, including the user. However, in exceptional circumstances where disclosure may compromise safety, certain information may be withheld from the user, ensuring protection for all involved parties.

Informed consent is an ongoing agreement by an individual to receive treatment, undergo procedures, or participate in research. This agreement implies that the risks, benefits, and alternatives have been adequately explained to them (Royal College of Nursing, 2011). It is essential that informed consent is documented, accessible in the client's notes, and subject to regular review. Moreover, a user's decision to provide informed consent for the disclosure of information should also be subject to regular review. Any disclosure should occur within the professional codes of conduct of the service providers.

RECORD-KEEPING (CASE NOTES)

Record-keeping is a fundamental practice in health and social care services, applicable across all settings. These records may encompass every episode of care for an individual or focus solely on the current episode. They should include diagnostic documentation, such as blood tests, X-rays, and ECG results. It is imperative that record-keeping be simple, accurate, legible, and regularly updated. Clinical records must be kept confidential and securely stored, whether in paper or electronic format. Electronic medical records, while offering convenience, require robust policies to safeguard patient confidentiality, including strict access controls and security measures. Electronic patient records are accessible to authorised staff across hospital and community-based services, with access strictly controlled via password protection. In some jurisdictions, legislation grants patients or their legal guardians the right to request access to their health records. It is important to recognise that record-keeping involves considerations by third parties, including courts of law and other healthcare or social care professionals, highlighting the critical role these records play in ensuring continuity of care and accountability within the healthcare system.

Nurses' regulatory standards for practice underscore the significance of maintaining clear and accurate patient records. Patient records serve as crucial evidence of the assessments and interventions

Table 24.8
Key principles for maintaining patient records

Key principles	Descriptions
Timeliness	Records should be completed promptly after the event or as soon as possible.
Authentication	All records, whether handwritten or digital, must be signed, timed, and dated, with digital entries traceable to the person providing care.
Competence with electronic systems	Healthcare professionals should stay updated on electronic systems used in their workplace, including security, confidentiality, and proper usage.
Accuracy and honesty	Records must be accurate, be free from falsification, and provide comprehensive information about care given and future arrangements.
Clarity and avoidance of jargon	Jargon and speculation should be avoided to ensure records are understandable to all parties.
Patient involvement	Whenever possible, patients should be involved in record-keeping and should understand the content of their records.
Readability	Records should be clear and legible, even when photocopied or scanned.
Record alterations	If changes are necessary, the original entry should remain visible, and the new entry should be signed, timed, and dated.
Secure storage	Records must be stored securely and should only be destroyed according to local policy.

Source: Contents adapted from Royal College of Nursing (2023).

conducted, facilitating continuity of care by allowing other healthcare professionals to readily access patients' current care plans and treatments (Brooks, 2021). It is essential for nurses to adhere to the policies and procedures governing patient record maintenance, which can vary across healthcare organisations. Thus, nurses must diligently review and comply with these guidelines to ensure proper record-keeping practices are followed. According to the Health and Care Professions Council (HCPC, 2021), healthcare professionals have a duty to maintain full, clear, and accurate records for individuals they care for, treat, or provide services to. These records are crucial for safeguarding continuity of care, ensuring appropriate treatment, meeting legal requirements, and providing evidence for decision-making processes. The specific records, formats, and retention periods vary depending on the healthcare setting and subject matter. Adherence to organisational and regulatory guidelines is essential for proper record-keeping practices. Table 24.8 presents the key principles for maintaining patient records (Royal College of Nursing, 2023).

KEY POINTS

- The progression through the drug treatment system has been described as the client journey and covers all stages of a person's involvement with services, from referral to discharge and continuing care.
- Assessment and care planning are a continuing process and a foundation for good clinical practice.
- There are three levels of assessment: screening, initial, and comprehensive assessment.
- Screening or initial assessment is a brief process that aims to determine whether an individual has a drug and alcohol problem, health-related problems, and risk behaviours.
- Initial assessment usually takes place during substance misusers' first contacts with substance misuse services.
- Initial assessment involves a complete assessment including a client's readiness to engage in treatment, risk behaviours, and the urgency to access treatment.
- Alcohol and drug misusers with complex needs require assessment that is comprehensive and multi-professional to plan effective care and treatment.
- Taking a drug and alcohol history is a detailed assessment of the current presentation of an individual's drug and alcohol pattern of use.
- Assessment all too often focuses only on the individual's negative aspects of substance misuse, such as an individual's weaknesses, risks, and problems.
- Clinical assessment for those with substance misuse and psychiatric disorders is difficult because substance misuse can mask psychiatric symptoms or distort diagnosis.

- Many individuals with dual diagnosis remain unnoticed in both drug and alcohol services and mental health services.
- Risk assessment is an ongoing process, and there are several critical points when practitioners need to conduct further assessment of "risky behaviours."
- The exchange and sharing of information have to be done in observing the code of practice regarding confidentiality and underpinned by clear policies and procedures.
- Record-keeping is a basic health and social care practice and is applicable to all services.

References

Babor, T. F., & Higgins-Biddle, J. C. (2001). *Brief Intervention for Hazardous and Harmful Drinking: A Manual for Use in Primary Care* (Document No. WHO/MSD/MSB/01.6b). Geneva: World Health Organization.

Bachrach, L. (1986). The context of care for the chronic mental patient with substance abuse. *Psychiatric Quarterly,* 87(58), 3–14.

Brooks, N. (2021). How to undertake effective record-keeping and documentation. *Nursing Standard,* 36. https://doi.org/10.7748/ns.2021.e11700.

Crawford, V., & Crome, I. (2001). *Co-existing Problems of Mental Health and Substance Misuse (Dual Diagnosis): A Review of Relevant Literature.* London: Royal College of Psychiatrists.

Doyle, M. (2004). Organisational responses to crisis and risk: Issues and implications for mental health nurses. In T. Ryan (Ed.), *Managing Crisis and Risk in Mental Health Nursing* (2nd ed.). Cheltenham: Nelson Thornes, pp. 40–56.

Edwards, G., Marshall, E. J., & Christopher, C. H. (2003). *The Treatment of Drinking Problems: A Guide for the Helping Professions.* Cambridge: Cambridge University Press.

Evans, K., & Sullivan, J. M. (2001). *Dual Diagnosis: Counseling the Mentally Ill Substance Abuser* (2nd Ed.), New York: Guilford Press.

Ewing, J. A. (1984). Detecting alcoholism: The CAGE questionnaire. *JAMA,* 252(14), 1905–1907. https://doi.org/10.1001/jama.252.14.1905.

Folstein, M. F., Folstein, S. E., & McHugh, P. R. (1975). "Mini-mental state": A practical method for grading the cognitive state of patients for the clinician. *Journal of Psychiatric Research,* 12(3), 189–198. https://doi.org/10.1016/0022-3956(75)90026-6.

Hasin, D., Trautman, K., & Endicott, J. (1998). Psychiatric research interview for substance and mental disorders: Phenomenologically based diagnosis in patients who abuse alcohol or drugs. *Psychopharmacology Bulletin,* 34(1), 3–8.

Health & Care Professions Council (HCPC). (2021). *Record Keeping.* London: HCPC. https://www.hcpc-uk.org/standards/meeting-our-standards/record-keeping/ (accessed 5 April 2024).

Hodgson, R., Alwyn, T., John, B., Thom, B., & Smith, A. (2002). The fast alcohol screening test. *Alcohol and Alcoholism,* 37(1), 61–66.

McGovern, M. P., & Morrison, D. H. (1992). The chemical use, abuse, and dependence scale (CUAD): Rationale, reliability, and validity. *Journal of Substance Abuse Treatment,* 9(1), 27–38. https://doi.org/10.1016/0740-5472(92)90007-b.

McHugo, G. J., Drake, R. E., Burton, H. L., & Ackerson, T. H. (1995). A scale for assessing the stage of substance abuse treatment in persons with severe mental illness. *The Journal of Nervous and Mental Disease,* 183(12), 762–767. https://doi.org/10.1097/00005053-199512000-00006.

McPhillips, M. A., Kelly, F. J., Barnes, T. R. E., Duke, P. J., Gene-Cos, N., & Clark, K. (1997). Detecting comorbid substance misuse among people with schizophrenia in the community: A study comparing the results of questionnaires with analysis of hair and urine. *Schizophrenia Research,* 25, 141–148.

Moore, K., & Rassool, G. H. (2001). Synthesis of addiction and mental health nursing: An approach to community interventions. In G. H. Rassool (Ed.), *Dual Diagnosis: Substance Misuse and Psychiatric Disorders.* Oxford: Blackwell Publishing.

NTA. (2005). *Treatment Effectiveness Strategy.* London: National Treatment Agency.

NTA. (2006). *Care Planning Practice Guide.* London: National Treatment Agency.

O'Rourke, M., & Bird, L. (2001). *Risk Management in Mental Health: A Practical Guide to Individual Care and Community Safety.* London: Mental Health Foundation Publications.

Rassool, G. H., & Winnington, J. (2006). Framework for multidimensional assessment. In G. H. Rassool (Ed.), *Dual Diagnosis Nursing.* Oxford: Blackwell Publications.

Rethink and Turning Point. (2004). *Dual Diagnosis Toolkit: Mental Health and Substance Misuse. A Practical Guide for Professionals and Practitioners.* London: Rethink and Turning Point.

Rosenberg, S. D., Drake, R. E., Wolford, G. L., Mueser, K. T., Oxman, T. E., Vidaver, R. M., Carrieri, K. L., & Luckoor, R. (1998). Dartmouth assessment of lifestyle instrument (DALI): A substance use disorder screen for people with severe mental illness. *The American Journal of Psychiatry,* 155(2), 232–238. https://doi.org/10.1176/ajp.155.2.232.

Royal College of Nursing. (2011). *Informed Consent in Health and Social Care Research: RCN Guidance for Nurses.* London: Royal College of Nursing.

Royal College of Nursing. (2023). *Record Keeping: The Facts.* https://www.rcn.org.uk/Professional-Development/publications/rcn-record-keeping-uk-pub-011-016 (accessed 5 April 2024).

Sissons, B. (2023). What to know about urine drug tests. *Medical News Today.* https://www.medicalnewstoday.com/articles/323378 (accessed 5 April 2024).

Skinner, H. A. (1982). The drug abuse screening test. *Addictive Behaviors,* 7(4), 363–371. https://doi.org/10.1016/0306-4603(82)90005-3.

Chapter 25

Care planning

Principles and practice

Learning outcomes

- Define what is a *care plan*.
- Identify the key principles in care planning.
- Differentiate between initial and comprehensive care plans.
- Describe the stages of a patient's treatment journey.
- Understand and discuss the need for patient involvement in the care planning process.
- Identify skills in developing a therapeutic relationship to help engage patients in the assessment and care planning processes.
- Discuss the importance of multi-agency working, information sharing, and communication throughout the assessment and care planning processes.

Activity 25.1

There is only one correct answer to the following multiple-choice questions.

1. What is a *care plan*?
   a. A summary of medical history
   b. A document outlining patient's preferences for care
   c. A comprehensive strategy for providing individualised care
   d. A list of medications prescribed to the patient
   e. A report on patient's treatment progress
2. What are the key principles in care planning?
   a. Ambiguity and confusion
   b. Secrecy and isolation
   c. Collaboration and transparency
   d. Incompetence and negligence
   e. Miscommunication and misinformation
3. The planning phase of the client's treatment journey involves:
   a. The development of a care plan
   b. The implementation of intervention
   c. The evaluation of intervention
   d. The part of an integrated system
   e. None of the above

DOI: 10.4324/9781003456674-30

4. How do initial and comprehensive care plans differ?
   a. Initial plans are more detailed.
   b. Comprehensive plans are developed later in the treatment process.
   c. Comprehensive plans cover a shorter time frame.
   d. There is no difference between initial and comprehensive care plans.
   e. Initial plans involve fewer stakeholders.
5. What are the stages of a patient's treatment journey?
   a. Assessment, diagnosis, treatment, discharge
   b. Referral, consultation, intervention, follow-up
   c. Engagement, retention, follow-up, completion
   d. Initial assessment, ongoing assessment, discharge planning
   e. Screening, assessment, treatment, evaluation
6. Why is patient involvement important in the care planning process?
   a. It increases paperwork for healthcare providers.
   b. It allows patients to dictate their own treatment without professional input.
   c. It enhances treatment adherence and outcomes.
   d. It delays the care planning process.
   e. It reduces the responsibility of healthcare providers.
7. Considerations of the client's cultural and ethnic background enables:
   a. The provision of a comprehensive care plan
   b. The provision of culturally competent care
   c. The provision of measurable goals
   d. The provision of achievable goals
   e. None of the above
8. A care plan should include:
   a. SMART goals or objectives
   b. Treatment interventions
   c. Risk behaviour and management
   d. B and C only
   e. All of the above
9. Which of the following statements regarding patient involvement in care planning is true?
   a. Patient involvement is optional and not essential for effective care planning.
   b. Patient involvement ensures that care plans align with patients' preferences and needs.
   c. Patient involvement increases healthcare costs and delays treatment.
   d. Patient involvement leads to decreased patient satisfaction and adherence.
   e. Patient involvement only applies to certain patient populations and not others.
10. What are the skills needed to develop a therapeutic relationship to engage patients in the assessment and care planning processes?
   a. Isolation and detachment
   b. Active listening and empathy
   c. Authoritative demeanour and control
   d. Limited communication and indifference
   e. Judgemental attitude and criticism
11. What is the role of information sharing in the assessment and care planning processes?
   a. To hoard information and limit access
   b. To facilitate collaboration and coordination among healthcare professionals
   c. To create barriers and hinder communication
   d. To manipulate information for personal gain
   e. To ensure patients are kept in the dark about their care

12. The effectiveness of the care plan is based on the
    a. Engagement of the client in the assessment process
    b. Client's active involvement in the formulation of the care plan
    c. Client's sense of ownership of the care plan
    d. A and B only
    e. All of the above
13. Reviewing a care plan provides a framework within which:
    a. The key worker can decide whether a goal has been achieved
    b. The client can decide whether a goal has been achieved
    c. Information on unmet needs are provided
    d. A and C only
    e. All of the above
14. If the client has been found to have urgent health needs during initial assessment:
    a. Engagement of the client is necessary.
    b. Engagement of the client in treatment is necessary.
    c. A comprehensive care plan should be formulated.
    d. An initial care plan should be formulated.
    e. Refer the client to specialist service.
15. A comprehensive care plan underlies:
    a. Planning of structured pharmacological or psychosocial interventions
    b. Delivery of structured pharmacological or psychosocial interventions
    c. Its development by a key worker or the multidisciplinary team
    d. A and B only
    e. All of the above
16. Node-link mapping is a technique for:
    a. Visually displaying thoughts
    b. Visually displaying feelings
    c. Visually displaying actions
    d. A and C only
    e. All of the above
17. Why is multi-agency working important in the assessment and care planning processes?
    a. It increases bureaucracy and delays decision-making.
    b. It allows each agency to work independently without coordination.
    c. It enhances collaboration, pooling of resources, and holistic care.
    d. It creates confusion and conflicts among agencies.
    e. It decreases accountability and responsibility.
18. Engagement is concerned with:
    a. The development of a therapeutic alliance between staff and client
    b. Intervening with the client's immediate needs
    c. Understanding the client and their view
    d. All of the above
    e. None of the above
19. The long-term or continuing care stage is reached when there are:
    a. Changes in drug and alcohol misuse
    b. Changes in physical and psychological health
    c. Changes in offending behaviour and social functioning
    d. Changes in one or more of the aforementioned domains of functioning
    e. There is a relapse period

CARE PLANNING AND TREATMENT JOURNEY

The planning phase of a patient's treatment journey involves creating a personalised care plan based on their needs, serving as a road map for their treatment. Care planning is crucial for structured alcohol and drug interventions and includes identifying patient needs, implementing care, coordinating integrated care, and evaluating its effectiveness. Having a personal care plan outlining treatment interventions is considered good practice. The patient journey often begins with primary healthcare or generic services like A&E departments or emergency departments, where screening and risk assessment for drug and alcohol problems are conducted. Interventions may include providing health information, harm reduction strategies, and referrals to specialist services based on patient needs. The progression of the patient journey is outlined, emphasising the importance of tailored care planning in guiding patients through their treatment

WHAT IS A CARE PLAN?

A *care plan* is a structured document developed collaboratively between the patient and healthcare or social care professionals focusing on identified needs, goals, strengths, and risks. It serves as a task-oriented plan of action aimed at guiding interventions to address the patient's needs. The care plan monitors changes in the patient's progress and provides valuable information to other professionals involved in the patient's care. The effectiveness of the care plan relies on active engagement from the patient throughout the assessment and planning process. It should be perceived as a contractual agreement between the patient and care providers, promoting accountability. Regular review and evaluation of the care plan are essential, either at predetermined intervals or upon request from the patient, their carer, or a member of the care team.

KEY PRINCIPLES IN CARE PLANNING

The initial step in care planning involves conducting an accurate and comprehensive assessment, which serves as the foundation for determining appr priate healthcare interventions and support. Ca planning principles are rooted in addressing t holistic needs of the individual, establishing tre ment goals and targets, defining interventions treatment modalities, and ensuring accountabili and responsibility in delivering care. A comprehe sive care plan, developed collaboratively with t patient, should encompass patient needs identifi across four key domains (NTA, 2006b):

- Drug and alcohol misuse
- Physical and psychological health
- Offending behaviour
- Social functioning

Table 25.1 shows the four key domains and asso ated health and social care outcomes.

Every service user should have a personalis care plan that considers their unique needs, dev oped collaboratively with the patient and signi cant others. The plan should reflect evidence-bas practices and interventions, ensuring continuity aftercare. It must be patient-centred, with conte agreed upon by both the patient and the servi provider. Additionally, cultural and ethnic bac grounds should be considered to provide cultural competent care.

A care plan should include SMART goals (sp cific, measurable, achievable, realistic, and time-lir ited) with stated target dates for evaluation. Ea goal should be patient-centred and accompanied evidence-based treatment interventions. Referenc to risk behaviours, risk management, and em gency planning should be explicit. Interventi strategies must be specific, not generic, and appr priate to the individual's needs. The responsibili for carrying out interventions lies with the agen and service provider, with input from the patie and other involved parties. Effective planning care for individuals requires effective communic tion and coordination among agencies and servi providers. This facilitates the sharing of informati and ensures a smooth transition between servic It is essential to establish clear guidelines regardi the dissemination of information to third parti A care plan should include a contingency plan case the desired outcomes are not achieved. Regul monitoring, review, and evaluation of the care pl are crucial, with input from the patient, their sign icant others, or the care team. Reviewing the ca plan helps assess goal achievement, identify unmet needs, and evaluate the effectiveness of interventions. Adjustments to intervention strategies may be necessary to improve goal attainment. The principles of care planning aim to optimise patient outcomes and are summarised in Table 25.2.

Table 25.1
Four key domains

Domains	
Alcohol and drug	Drug use, including types of drugs, quantity and frequency of use, pattern of use, route of administration, source of drugs (including preparation), and prescribed medication. Alcohol use, including quantity and frequency of use, pattern of use, whether in excess of "safe" levels, and alcohol dependence symptoms.
Physical and psychological health	Physical problems, including complications of drugs and alcohol use, blood-borne infections, risk behaviours, liver disease, abscesses, overdose, and enduring severe physical disabilities. Pregnancy may also be an issue. Psychological problems include personality problems or disorders, self-harm, history of abuse or trauma, depression and anxiety, and severe psychiatric comorbidity. Contact with mental health services will need to be recorded.
Criminal involvement and offending	Legal issues, including arrests, fines, outstanding charges and warrants, probation, imprisonment, violent offences, and criminal activity. Involvement with workers in the criminal justice system, for example, probation workers.
Social functioning	Social issues, including childcare issues, partners, domestic violence, family, housing, education, employment, benefits, and financial problems.

Source: NTA (2006a).

Table 25.2
Key principles in care planning

Key principles	
Client-centred approach	• Client-directed. • Holistic needs of client. • Involved in decision-making on the components of the care plan and how it will be delivered.
Diversity	• Reflect the cultural and ethnic background, gender, and sexuality.
Goals	• Need to reflect the outcome of the assessment. • Based on philosophy of care. • SMART – specific, measurable, achievable, realistic, and time-bound. • Taking account of individual's current state and motivation. • Short-term and long-term goals.
Intervention strategies	• Type of interventions. • Pharmacological and psychosocial interventions. • Harm reduction.
Risk management	• Identification of risk factors as per assessment. • Risk management and contingency plan.
Communication and liaison	• Sharing of information in line with service policies on confidentiality and the sharing of information.
Key worker	• Developing, implementing, and evaluating a care plan • Deliver heath and psychosocial interventions.
Promoting and enhancing engagement	• Where an individual has been difficult to engage in treatment and rehabilitation, the plan should identify a plan for promoting and enhancing their engagement.
Monitor	• Monitor plan and changes in client's needs.
Review	• Identity their review date.

KEY ISSUES IN PLANNING AND DELIVERING CARE

The care programme approach (CPA) is a framework used in mental health services for assessing, planning, implementing, and evaluating care. While NHS England's "Care Programme Approach – Improvement position statement" replaces CPA with the community mental health framework, it acknowledges CPA's principles, intending to integrate them into the new approach (National Collaborating Centre for Mental Health, 2019). This new strategy emphasises delivering mental health support within the community and integrating it with place-based care. Key aspects include ensuring quality assessments, accessible interventions, flexible care transitions, and integration with community assets to enhance individuals' mental well-being. The framework suggests replacing the CPA in community mental health services while preserving its fundamental theoretical principles rooted in effective care coordination and high-quality care planning.

The CPA is designed to facilitate effective collaboration among various agencies, ensuring a seamless service for individuals with severe mental health issues. By addressing both health and social care needs through an integrated approach, CPA aims to provide comprehensive support. It involves systematic assessments of health and social care needs, development of agreed care plans, allocation of a dedicated care coordinator, and regular reviews of progress. This holistic approach encompasses management, treatment, care, and support, fostering connections across social work or care services, health, education, employment, housing, criminal justice, and voluntary agencies. This enables individuals to access a range of services tailored to their needs. When effectively implemented, the CPA facilitates multi-disciplinary staff to develop a consensus plan of care, reducing inter-professional conflicts, and enhancing opportunities for collaborative efforts (Simpson, 2006). For patients with concurrent substance misuse and psychiatric disorders, an "enhanced" version of CPA is applied, which incorporates a contingency plan to ensure ongoing care and support. This plan encompasses instructions for crisis management and contact details for assistance during non-working hours.

For patients with co-occurring disorders, particularly dual diagnosis, it is a requirement to have a designated care plan coordinator. This individual assumes a leadership role in formulating the care plan, representing the entire team and other involved service providers. In the case of young substance misusers, the responsibility for care planning and delivering treatment interventions may fall under child and adolescent mental health services, social services, or a young offenders team.

INITIAL CARE PLAN

During initial or triage assessment, if a patient is found to have urgent health needs, an initial care plan may be devised before a comprehensive assessment. This plan should encompass identifying health or social care needs, setting goals, and planning interventions. This initial care planning stage provides an opportunity to engage patients in treatment through the delivery of harm reduction strategies and ensuring expedited treatment delivery. Immediate needs, such as rapid prescribing referrals and urgent housing concerns, should be addressed in the initial care plan (NTA, 2006b). A designated key worker is responsible for developing the patient's initial care plan and ensuring either a comprehensive assessment is conducted or an appropriate referral to another service provider is made. Table 25.3 provides examples of care plan contents.

COMPREHENSIVE CARE PLAN

Comprehensive assessment forms the foundation for planning and implementing structured pharmacological or psychosocial interventions. Node-link mapping, also known as mapping, is a technique that may aid in the development of a care plan. It visually represents thoughts, feelings, and actions as nodes, with named links depicting the relationships between them (Dees et al., 1994). Node-link mapping offers a framework for key workers and patients to explore problems, identify goals, develop plans, and take specific actions to address those goals (NTA, 2006b). The comprehensive care plan may be developed by a key worker alone or in collaboration with other members of the multidisciplinary team. It includes goal-setting based on the four key domains identified through initial and ongoing comprehensive assessment, along with intervention strategies. The planning of interventions is guided by the needs or goals identified in the comprehensive assessment process.

Table 25.3
Examples of care plan contents

Background	Goal	Interventions
A client presents to a drug service with a history of amphetamine use. In an initial assessment, she is found to be street homeless.	Client to make contact with housing services and obtain temporary housing.	Referral to specialist vulnerable housing worker. Completion of assessment of substance misuse.
A client who is new to treatment presents with a history of self-harm and is under the care of a community psychiatric nurse (CPN).	To coordinate mental health interventions with substance misuse interventions.	To reduce the frequency of self-harming behaviour. To stabilise client mood and reduce drug and/or alcohol use.
A client who is new to treatment identifies a history of sharing injecting paraphernalia. The client is very anxious about hepatitis C and worried about having a test.	To increase the client's knowledge of blood-borne viruses in preparation for taking an HCV antibody test within three months and to stop needle sharing within three months.	To attend the HCV education group the service provides and to discuss the issue in key working sessions.
A client is using crack cocaine weekly, although stable on a daily methadone prescription.	To reduce crack cocaine, use by 50% over the next three months, as evidenced by production of 50% cocaine-free oral fluid tests.	Relapse prevention techniques. Drug diaries. Psycho-education. Skills development to manage cravings and high-risk situations. Weekly oral fluid tests.
A client is now stable on buprenorphine daily and has been for three months. The client has abstinence as an eventual goal.	To reduce the dose over the next three months.	Relapse prevention techniques. Monitoring.

Source: Adapted from NTA (2006b).

PLANNING INTERVENTIONS

The planning of interventions is guided by the needs or goals identified in the care planning process, which encompasses the engagement stage, intervention delivery stage, and long-term treatment and continuing care stage. Each stage involves various intervention strategies tailored to the individual's needs. These strategies include pharmacological treatment, harm reduction approaches, motivational interviewing, individual cognitive behavioural counselling, lifestyle modifications, relapse planning and prevention techniques, and family education. By addressing these diverse strategies, the care plan aims to provide comprehensive support and promote the individual's well-being over the long term.

STAGE OF ENGAGEMENT

Engagement in mental health services revolves around fostering and maintaining a therapeutic alliance between staff and patients. Approaching patients with confrontation or judgement may hinder their willingness to engage with treatment services. Instead, the focus should be on understanding the patient's perspective, responding to their behaviour and language, and recognising their unspoken needs to build trust and authenticity (Price, 2002). This can be achieved through non-confrontational, empathetic, and respectful interactions that acknowledge the patient's subjective experiences of substance misuse. The strength of the therapeutic alliance is influenced by the patient's perception of the service's value, the staff's social marketing of the services, and addressing the patient's immediate needs (Rassool, 2006). Issues related to alcohol and drug misuse are typically addressed after a working alliance has been established, as immediate needs such as emergency care, accommodation, finances, and legal matters often take precedence for the patient at the initial stage of engagement. Guidelines that will help promote engagement with the service provider are presented in Table 25.4.

During the engagement stage, motivational interviewing (see Chapter 26) principles are applied to facilitate change, relying on consistent communication and a collaborative relationship between staff and patient. The goal is to empower the patient, fostering self-awareness and enhancing motivation and commitment to change, all while avoiding

Table 25.4
Promoting engagement

Key areas	Descriptions
Empathy and understanding	Foster a supportive and non-judgemental environment where individuals feel understood, valued, and respected. Empathy plays a crucial role in building trust and rapport, a non-confrontational approach.
Accessible services	Ensure services are easily accessible, both physically and in terms of communication channels, to encourage individuals to seek help without barriers.
Tailored approach	Adopt a personalised approach to care, acknowledging the unique needs and preferences of each individual. Tailoring interventions to match their specific circumstances enhances engagement.
Clear communication	Use clear, jargon-free language when discussing treatment options, goals, and care plans. Effective communication helps individuals understand their condition and the proposed interventions.
Collaborative decision-making	Involve individuals in decision-making processes regarding their care and treatment. Collaborative decision-making empowers individuals and increases their investment in the treatment process.
Meeting initial needs	Provide assistance in fulfilling immediate necessities, like access to food, shelter, housing, and clothing. Offer support in navigating social security's benefit entitlements, if appropriate.
Meeting legal needs	Offer aid and support in addressing legal concerns.
Holistic support	Offer comprehensive support that addresses not only clinical needs but also social, emotional, practical concerns, and spiritual dimension. A holistic approach acknowledges the interconnectedness of various aspects of an individual's life.
Continuity of care	Maintain continuity of care by establishing consistent points of contact and ensuring smooth transitions between different levels of care or service providers. Involve family or carers wherever possible.
Cultural competence	Recognise and respect cultural differences, beliefs, and values when delivering care. Cultural sensitivity promotes inclusivity and ensures services are relevant and acceptable to diverse populations.

confrontational or resistant interactions. Various straightforward techniques outlined by the Department of Health (2002) can be employed for this purpose:

- Education about substances and the problems that may be associated with misuse, including the effects on mental health.
- Presentation of objective assessment data (for example, liver function tests, urinalysis).
- Balance sheets, on which the patient lists the pros and cons of continued use/abstinence.
- Exploration of barriers to the attainment of future goals.
- Reframing problems or past events emphasising the influence of substance misuse.
- Reviewing medication and the use of an optimal medication regime.

Engagement frequently persists throughout the patient's treatment journey, involving interventions such as harm reduction strategies, providing pertinent health and social care information related to their substance misuse and treatment, and involving significant others to bolster patient support during treatment.

INTERVENTIONS DELIVERY STAGE

During this stage, the focus is on maintaining the apeutic relationships and convincing the patie of the value and benefits of treatment. It may ta several months before a patient is ready to recei active treatment interventions for their substan misuse. It is crucial to agree on the anticipat treatment goal at the outset of care planning a to target intermediate goals that aim to reduce t harm caused by drug and alcohol misuse, witho prematurely emphasising complete cessation. So patients may opt to reduce their substance misu necessitating pharmacological intervention for sa detoxification. Patients require significant suppo during this phase, and detoxification should not pursued without concurrent interventions. Inte ventions at this stage encompass various treatme modalities, including pharmacological manag ment, health education, motivational interviewi psychosocial interventions, harm reduction stra egies, relapse prevention techniques, occupation therapy, welfare advice, community prescribi initiatives, and employment services. In drug trea ment delivery, there is a heightened emphasis enhancing service users' physical and mental healt particularly those with hepatitis C infections and individuals misusing alcohol (NTA, 2006a). Initial review timetables should be agreed upon between the patient and key worker, with subsequent reviews scheduled based on local policies and patient needs (NTA, 2006b). Changes in healthcare needs, situations, or crises often prompt reviews of the care plan. However, the care plan, including its goals and associated interventions, should be monitored and reviewed as necessary.

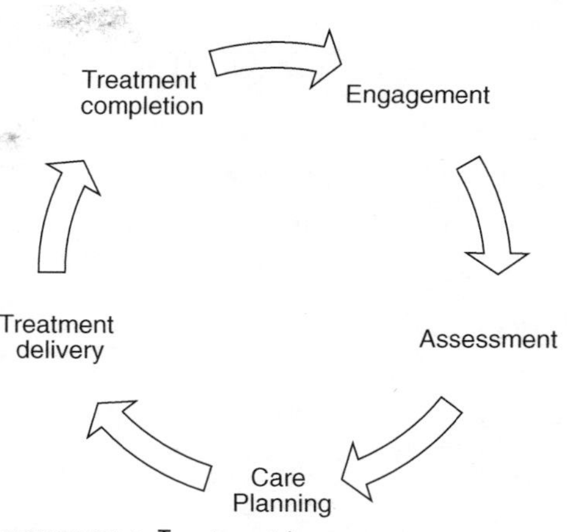

FIGURE 25.1 Treatment journey.

LONG-TERM OR CONTINUING CARE STAGE

This phase marks the completion stage, occurring when patients have achieved changes in one or more of the following domains: drug and alcohol misuse, physical and psychological health, offending behaviour, and social functioning. During this stage, interventions are focused on assisting patients in maintaining the achieved changes throughout their treatment journey. Substance misuse, whether of alcohol or drugs, is characterised by chronic relapse. Therefore, it is crucial to offer interventions aimed at preventing and managing future relapses once a patient has reduced their misuse or achieved abstinence. It is important for both patients and staff to accept relapse without perceiving it as weakness or failure. If sustained substance use occurs, reverting to the motivation for change stage is necessary, and attention must be given to developing new action plans. The principles and strategies of "relapse prevention" for substance misuse aim to identify high-risk situations and proactively rehearse coping strategies (see Chapter 26 for more details).

During this completion stage, patients should continue receiving community integration interventions initiated during the intervention delivery phase to address specific social needs, facilitating successful reintegration into the wider community (NTA, 2006b). Encouraging patients to establish or maintain contact with self-help groups such as Narcotics Anonymous (NA), Alcoholics Anonymous (AA), or non-12-step equivalents is essential at this stage. Additionally, efforts should focus on addressing social needs, such as housing, relationships, and childcare, while supporting training, education, employment, and life opportunities. Although this stage may mark the end of the treatment journey road map for some patients, in clinical practice, due to the relapse rate among substance misusers, patients may often find themselves returning to an earlier stage of the treatment journey.

KEY POINTS

- The planning phase of the patient's treatment journey involves the development of a care plan for the patient based on their needs.
- Care planning provides a "road map" of the patient's treatment journey and is a key component of structured alcohol and drug treatment interventions.
- Care planning and care coordination are key components of an integrated system of treatment for drug and alcohol misusers.
- The patient journey may start with primary healthcare services or generic services.
- The care planning process, an essential component of the patient treatment journey, is a method for setting goals based on the needs identified by assessment and planning interventions to meet those goals with the patient.
- A care plan is a structured and task-oriented plan of action between the patient and the health or social care professional.
- The effectiveness of the care plan is based on the engagement of the service user throughout the assessment and care planning process, and the patient must be actively involved in the formulation of the care plan.
- The first step in care planning is accurate and comprehensive assessment.
- Every service user should have a documented care plan which is individualised to the patient's needs, is developed with the patient and significant others, reflects evidence-based practice

and interventions, and provides for continuity of aftercare.

- Identifying health or social care needs, setting goals, and planning interventions should be part of the initial care plan.
- The comprehensive care plan is based on the key principles of care planning.
- The planning of interventions is based upon th needs or goals identified in the care planni process.
- The process includes the engagement stage, inte ventions delivery stage, and long-term treatme and continuing care stage.

Activity 25.2

Write an outline of a care plan for the following scenarios.

- A 25-year-old unmarried man, currently unemployed, has been injecting heroin for the past two years. Despite undergoing methadone treatment, he persists in using illicit heroin. Previous attempts at outpatient detoxification have proven ineffective. Despite his substance use, he maintains a stable relationship and has previously held down several jobs. He has been offered full-time employment contingent on achieving sobriety. While he expresses motivation for detoxification, he is reluctant to consider any plans beyond this stage.
- Miriam is a 28-year-old individual, was prescribed temazepam and dihydrocodeine following a car accident. She has frequented the accident and emergency (A&E) department on multiple occasions, appearing intoxicated. There is a rising pattern of reported lost or misplaced prescriptions, along with a surge in crises situations where SE seeks additional prescriptions.
- John is a 42-year-old man who works as a construction worker. He has a history of heavy alcohol use, which has escalated over the past few years due to stress at work and relationship issues. His drinking has led to frequent absences from work and conflicts with his partner. John's family and friends have expressed concerns about his health and well-being.
- Sarah is a 25-year-old university student studying engineering. She has been struggling with stress and anxiety due to academic pressure and relationship issues. Seeking relief, Sarah turned to synthetic drugs, particularly synthetic cannabinoids, which she began using sporadically to cope with stress and unwind after exams. Over time, Sarah's occasional use escalated into regular consumption, leading to detrimental effects on her physical health, academic performance, and relationships.

References

Dees, S. M., Dansereau, D. F., & Simpson, D. D. (1994). A visual representation system for drug abuse counselors. *Journal of Substance Abuse Treatment,* 11(6), 517–523. https://doi.org/10.1016/0740-5472(94)90003-5.

Department of Health. (2002). *Mental Health Policy Implementation Guide Dual Diagnosis Good Practice Guide.* London: Department of Health.

National Collaborating Central for Mental Health. (2019). *The Community Mental Health Framework for Adults and Older Adults.* NHS England and NHS Improvement and the National Collaborating Central for Mental Health. https://www.england.nhs.uk/wp-content/uploads/2019/09/community-mental-health-framework-for-adults-and-older-adults.pdf (accessed 6 April 2024).

NTA. (2006a). *Models of Care for Treatment of Adult Dr Misusers: Update 2006.* London: National Treatme Agency.

NTA. (2006b). *Care Planning Practice Guide.* London: Natio Treatment Agency.

Price, P. (2002). Nursing interventions in the care of dually dic nosed patients. In G. H. Rassool (Ed.), *Substance Misuse a Psychiatric Disorders.* Oxford: Blackwell Publishing.

Rassool, G. H. (2006). Understanding dual diagnosis: overview. In G. H. Rassool (Ed.), *Dual Diagnosis Nursi* Oxford: Blackwell Publishing.

Simpson, A. (2006). Shared care and inter-professional pr tice. In G. H. Rassool (Ed.), *Dual Diagnosis Nursing.* Oxfo Blackwell Publishing.

Chapter 26

Psychosocial and pharmacological interventions

Learning outcomes

- Discuss the principle of psychosocial interventions.
- Describe the range of psychosocial interventions in the treatment of substance misusers.
- Describe the range of pharmacological interventions in the treatment of substance misusers.
- Have an understanding of the use of complementary therapies.
- Discuss the effectiveness of treatment interventions for alcohol and drug misuse.

Activity 26.1 Psychosocial and pharmacological interventions.

Please state whether the following statements are true or false. Reflect on the statements and give reason(s) for choosing a particular option.

Statements	True	False
Psychosocial and pharmacological interventions for the treatment of alcohol and drug misuse can be delivered across all four tiers of the models of care.		
Pharmacological interventions are categorised as detoxification, medications for relapse prevention, and nutritional supplements.		
There is no evidence to suggest that drug misuse treatment is effective in terms of reduced substance misuse.		
There is evidence of the effectiveness of psychosocial and pharmacotherapies in achieving reductions in drinking and alcohol problems.		
The nature and severity of the complex needs of substance misusers are likely to influence the type and range of interventions.		
The goals of psychosocial interventions are to improve the psychosocial well-being of alcohol and drug users.		
The effectiveness of a therapeutic alliance is crucial to the delivery of any treatment intervention and patient outcomes.		
Brief interventions comprise of a single brief advice session or several short (15–30 minutes) counselling sessions.		

DOI: 10.4324/9781003456674-31

Statements	True	False
There is no evidence for the effectiveness of brief interventions in a variety of settings for alcohol and tobacco.		
The effectiveness of counselling does not lie with the technique or approach used but with the actual counsellor.		
Matching counselling techniques to a client's goals is crucial in determining successful outcomes.		
Motivational interviewing has been found to increase the effectiveness of more extensive psychosocial treatments for substance misusers.		
There is no evidence that contingency management is a useful treatment for "non-responsive" clients.		
In relapse prevention, clients may need support to identify risks associated with their substance misuse.		

Activity 26.2

There is only one correct answer to the following multiple-choice questions.

1. What is the primary focus of psychosocial interventions in the treatment of substance misuse?
   a. Biological changes
   b. Pharmacological interventions
   c. Psychological and social factors
   d. Genetic predispositions
   e. Environmental influences
2. Which of the following best describes psychosocial interventions in the treatment of substance misuse?
   a. Sole reliance on medication
   b. Involves addressing only physical health
   c. Focuses on psychological and social factors
   d. Involves isolation from social support
   e. Emphasises genetic determinants
3. The term "psychosocial" is the:
   a. Connection of social and family networks
   b. Connections with social and cultural factors
   c. Connections between psychological and medical experience
   d. Connections between psychological and social experience
   e. None of the above
4. One of the principles of good practice in psychosocial interventions is based on:
   a. The assessment of needs or goals
   b. The assessment of health and social care needs
   c. The enabling of decision-making
   d. The contact between a service provider and the client
   e. None of the above

5. Key working is a basic:
   a. Intervention to reduce alcohol or drug-related harm
   b. Delivery mechanism for a range of psychosocial components
   c. Provision of alcohol and drug misuse–related advice and information
   d. All of the above
   e. None of the above
6. The aim of brief interventions is:
   a. To motivate those at risk to change their substance use behaviour
   b. To help the client understand their substance misuse problems
   c. To encourage clients to reduce or give up their substance use
   d. All of the above
   e. None of the above
7. Brief interventions are intended to:
   a. Treat clients with alcohol and drug dependence
   b. Treat clients at risk of alcohol problems
   c. Treat clients with chronic drug problems
   d. Treat clients in primary care only
   e. None of the above
8. Motivational enhancing technique originates from:
   a. Cognitive behavioural theory
   b. Psychodynamic theory
   c. Theory of change
   d. School of family therapy
   e. None of the above
9. Motivational interviewing is employed:
   a. When clients present showing no or little commitment to change
   b. When clients present showing readiness to change
   c. As non-directive counselling
   d. When pharmacological interventions have failed
   e. None of the above
10. Motivational interviewing is a technique that:
    a. Does not require an in-depth counselling knowledge
    b. Involves a judgemental approach
    c. Uses closed questioning with the client
    d. Expresses sympathy with the client
    e. None of the above
11. The principles of motivational interviewing:
    a. Express empathy and develop discrepancy
    b. Roll with resistance
    c. Support self-efficacy
    d. All of the above
    e. None of the above
12. Contingency management is the process of:
    a. Using medical reinforcers to increase desired behaviours
    b. Using negative reinforcers to increase desired behaviours
    c. Using positive reinforcers to increase desired behaviours
    d. Engagement with the service to increase desired behaviours
    e. None of the above

13. Pharmacological interventions in the treatment of substance misuse primarily target:
    a. Psychological factors
    b. Genetic predispositions
    c. Environmental influences
    d. Biological changes
    e. Social support networks
14. Complementary therapies used in substance misuse treatment typically:
    a. Are the sole form of treatment
    b. Focus solely on medication
    c. Include psychological interventions only
    d. Are used in conjunction with conventional treatments
    e. Ignore psychological and social factors
15. The effectiveness of treatment interventions for alcohol and drug misuse is influenced by:
    a. Genetic factors only
    b. Environmental factors only
    c. Pharmacological interventions only
    d. Psychological and social factors
    e. Complementary therapies only
16. Which aspect is essential to consider when discussing the principle of psychosocial interventions?
    a. Biological factors
    b. Medication dosage
    c. Psychological and social factors
    d. Genetic make-up
    e. Environmental toxins
17. Which range of interventions is commonly included in psychosocial treatments for substance misuse?
    a. Only pharmacological interventions
    b. Sole reliance on genetic testing
    c. Incorporation of complementary therapies
    d. Addressing psychological and social factors
    e. Ignoring environmental influences
18. The range of pharmacological interventions in the treatment of substance misuse primarily targets:
    a. Environmental factors
    b. Social support networks
    c. Biological changes
    d. Genetic predispositions
    e. Psychological factors
19. Complementary therapies in substance misuse treatment are typically used:
    a. Exclusively
    b. In isolation from other treatments
    c. In conjunction with conventional treatments
    d. After psychological interventions fail
    e. Without considering social support networks

20. Which factor significantly contributes to the effectiveness of treatment interventions for alcohol and drug misuse?
    a. Pharmacological interventions alone
    b. Ignoring psychological and social factors
    c. Considering genetic predispositions only
    d. Addressing psychological and social factors
    e. Excluding complementary therapies
21. When discussing the principle of psychosocial interventions, what should be emphasised?
    a. Biological factors only
    b. Ignoring psychological and social factors
    c. Considering pharmacological interventions only
    d. Addressing psychological and social factors
    e. Neglecting environmental influences
22. Psychosocial interventions in substance misuse treatment typically involve:
    a. Sole reliance on medication
    b. Addressing only biological changes
    c. Involvement of psychological and social factors
    d. Ignoring genetic predispositions
    e. Excluding environmental influences

INTRODUCTION

Psychosocial interventions for alcohol and drug misuse comprise various approaches, including brief interventions, counselling, cognitive behavioural therapy (CBT), family therapy, social skills training, supportive work, and complementary therapies. These strategies aim to address the psychological, social, and behavioural aspects of substance misuse to promote recovery and reduce harm. On the other hand, pharmacological interventions involve treatments such as detoxification, medications for relapse prevention, and nutritional supplements. These interventions target the physiological aspects of substance use disorders and can help manage withdrawal symptoms, prevent relapse, and support overall health during recovery. Treatment for drug misuse, specially methadone, has shown effectiveness in reducing substance consumption and criminal behaviour among a significant portion of individuals, with clients often displaying improved behaviour during treatment compared to before admission (Gerstein & Harwood, 1990).

Research indicates that medication combined with behavioural therapy or counselling is the preferred initial approach for treating opioid addiction, including addiction to prescription pain relievers, heroin, or fentanyl (NIDA, 2023). Medications are also effective in treating alcohol and nicotine addiction. For individuals addicted to stimulants or cannabis, behavioural therapies are the primary treatment approach, as no medications are currently available (NIDA, 2023). Treatment should be individualised to address each patient's specific drug use patterns and associated medical, mental, and social issues. There is evidence to suggest that drug misuse treatment is effective in terms of reduced substance misuse, improvements in personal and social functioning, reduced public health and safety risks and reduced criminal behaviour (McLellan et al., 1996; Prendergast et al., 2002; NTA, 2006a). Research indicates the effectiveness of both psychosocial interventions and pharmacotherapies in reducing drinking and alcohol-related problems among individuals with alcohol use disorder (NTA, 2006b).

Alcohol and drug misuse often entail multifaceted challenges spanning medical, psychosocial, social, and legal domains, necessitating intervention strategies tailored to individual service users' needs. The nature and severity of these needs play an important role in determining the appropriate types and range of interventions. The willingness of the client to acknowledge the need for change and engage voluntarily is also pivotal. Service providers must establish clear policies, procedures, goals, and objectives that are transparent to both staff and clients, while remaining adaptable to facilitate personalised treatment planning and implementation.

Establishing an explicit treatment alliance, potentially through a contract and regular reviews, is essential for measuring expected outcomes and overall progress. The format of these reviews may vary based on local policies, ranging from informal discussions to more formal assessments.

PSYCHOSOCIAL INTERVENTIONS

Psychosocial interventions aim to enhance the psychosocial well-being of individuals struggling with alcohol and drug use. The term "psychosocial" underscores the interconnectedness between psychological aspects (thoughts, emotions, behaviour) and broader social experiences (relationships, culture). These interventions encompass a diverse range of approaches, including brief interventions, counselling, motivational interviewing, solution-focused therapy, and more. The National Institute for Care and Health Excellence (NICE, 2007a) provides guidelines covering psychosocial interventions for adults and young people dealing with opioid, cannabis, or stimulant misuse, applicable across various treatment settings, including inpatient, residential, community-based, and within prison services.

PRINCIPLES OF PSYCHOSOCIAL INTERVENTIONS

One fundamental principle of effective practice in psychosocial interventions is the comprehensive assessment of health and psychosocial care needs, guiding decision-making regarding appropriate interventions. Key working, a core component of good practice, entails regular contact between service providers and patients and serves as a fundamental delivery mechanism for various psychosocial components. These interventions encompass regular reviews of care plans and treatment goals, provision of advice and information on alcohol and drug misuse, efforts to reduce harm associated with substance use, motivation enhancement, relapse prevention strategies, and assistance with addressing social issues, such as family conflicts, housing, and employment challenges.

The effectiveness of treatment interventions heavily relies on establishing a strong therapeutic alliance with the patient, which significantly impacts patient outcomes. This alliance hinges on various factors, including the ability to engage the patient effectively, demonstrating warmth and tru and adapting the intervention style to align wi the patient's preferences. It is essential to addre difficult emotions and understand the patien emotional context, including their motivation le els (Roth & Pilling, 2007). Furthermore, treatme goals should be collaboratively established betwe the key worker and the patient, rather than impose ensuring they are patient-directed and based mutual agreement. The psychosocial interventio are presented in Table 26.1.

BRIEF INTERVENTIONS

Brief interventions are aimed at motivating indivi uals at risk to change their substance use behavio typically through a single advice session or a series short counselling sessions. They seek to raise awar ness of the risks associated with alcohol or drug u and encourage individuals to reduce or cease th substance use. While not intended to treat alcoh and drug dependence, brief interventions targ individuals with problematic or risky substan use (WHO, 2005). These interventions may al facilitate acceptance of more intensive treatme or referral to specialised services for those wi severe dependence. Screening tools are common employed to identify suitable candidates for inte vention based on hazardous levels of substance u (Heather & Kaner, 2001). Table 26.2 presents t elements of brief intervention.

The acronym "FRAMES" encapsulates the el ments of effective brief interventions: feedbac responsibility, advice, menu, empathy, and self-e ficacy (Bien et al., 1993). These interventions c be administered in a supportive, non-judgemen manner by health or social services worke Research indicates that positive approaches in bri interventions yield better outcomes compared confrontational styles. Strong evidence supports t effectiveness of brief interventions in reducing alc hol consumption among hazardous and harmf drinkers, as well as tobacco use. Additionally, the is growing evidence supporting their effectivene for addressing other substance use disorders. T National Institute for Health and Care Excellen (NICE, 2007b) guideline on psychosocial inte ventions recommends offering opportunistic bri interventions focused on motivation to individu in limited contact with drug services, such as tho attending needle and syringe exchanges or prima

Table 26.1
The principles of psychosocial interventions

Key principles	Descriptions
Person-centred approach	Tailoring interventions to meet the unique needs, preferences, and circumstances of each individual
Holistic perspective	Recognising the interconnectedness of psychological, social, and environmental factors influencing substance use behaviours
Collaborative relationship	Establishing a therapeutic alliance between the individual and the treatment provider, based on trust, respect, and mutual understanding
Strengths-based focus	Identifying and building upon an individual's existing strengths, resources, and resilience to support recovery
Flexibility and adaptability	Tailoring interventions to respond to the evolving needs and circumstances of the individual throughout the treatment process
Evidence-based practice	Utilising interventions grounded in empirical research and proven effectiveness for addressing substance misuse
Harm reduction	Prioritising strategies aimed at minimising the negative consequences of substance use, even if complete abstinence is not immediately achievable
Culturally competent care	Acknowledging and respecting cultural diversity, and adapting interventions to be culturally sensitive and relevant
Continuum of care	Providing comprehensive and coordinated care across various treatment settings, including prevention, early intervention, treatment, and aftercare support

Table 26.2
Elements of effective brief interventions

	Acronym	Elements	Counselling responses
F	Feedback	Feedback of personal risk or impairment	Your difficulty in getting to work on time may be related to your alcohol or drug use. Sharing results of assessments (such as cognitive testing, liver function tests).
R	Responsibility	Emphasis on personal responsibility for change	It is your responsibility to make a decision about stopping substance misuse for the next two weeks.
A	Advice	Clear advice to change	It is recommended that you stop drinking or using drugs for the next two weeks to see if that makes a difference.
M	Menu	Menu of alternative change options	If you cannot reduce or stop your substance misuse, there are other options, such as AA or NA, or referral to the specialist service.
E	Empathy	Therapeutic empathy as a counselling style	I understand that this will be difficult for you because you feel alcohol helps you to unwind after a stressful working day.
S	Self-efficacy	Enhancement of patient self-efficacy or optimism	Considering how difficult you find this, I am confident that you have the abilities or strengths to consider changing your behaviour.

care settings, when concerns about drug misuse are identified. These interventions should:

- Normally consist of two sessions each lasting 10 to 45 minutes
- Explore ambivalence about drug use and possible treatment, with the aim of increasing motivation to change behaviour
- Provide non-judgemental feedback

NICE (2007b) also advised service providers to regularly furnish individuals with drug misuse information regarding self-help groups rooted in 12-step principles, such as Alcoholics Anonymous, Narcotics Anonymous, and Cocaine Anonymous. The WHO Brief Intervention Study Group (1996) investigated 1,260 men and 299 women who drank at levels posing a risk of alcohol-related problems without prior alcohol dependence history. Their findings suggested the resilience of brief interventions across diverse healthcare settings and socio-cultural groups. Notably, employing a self-help manual proved superior to minimal advice alone, and the provision of a brief intervention was deemed preferable to no therapeutic intervention (Heather et al., 1986; Heather, 1998).

COUNSELLING

Counselling encompasses a range of psychological support, from general assistance to specific behavioural and cognitive behavioural techniques. It provides a private and confidential space for clients to address underlying issues related to alcohol or drug problems, such as past trauma, relationship difficulties, and mental health concerns. The goal of counselling is to explore and address these underlying problems that contribute to or result from substance misuse. Client-centred techniques, including clarification, exploration, reflection, and summarisation, are employed to facilitate the expression of feelings and thoughts. Counselling focuses on the client's needs and experiences, rather than providing direct advice or direction. Successful therapy often depends on the rapport and connection between the counsellor and the client, emphasising acceptance, respect, and trust-building. Velleman (2001) outlines a six-stage approach to counselling substance misusers, emphasising trust-building, problem exploration, goal-setting, empowerment, maintenance of changes, and closure. The effectiveness of counselling lies not only in the techniques used but also in the therapeutic relationship between the counsellor and the client. The counselling skills are presented in Table 26.3.

MOTIVATIONAL INTERVIEWING

Matching counselling techniques to a client's goals is essential for successful outcomes, as no single approach suits all clients. Motivational interviewing is particularly useful when clients display little or no commitment to change. Rollnick and Miller (1995) characterise motivational interviewing directive client-centred counselling for eliciting behaviour change by helping clients explore and resolve ambivalence. Unlike non-directive counselling, motivational interviewing is more focused and goal-directed, with the counsellor taking a directive approach to address and resolve ambivalence, which is its central purpose. MI has proven effective in enhancing motivation for behavioural change among patients with various behaviourally influenced health problems (Bischof et al., 2021). Additionally, MI has been successful in promoting treatment adherence and optimising medical interventions.

MI has been extensively and successfully utilised among individuals with alcohol and other drug problems to enhance engagement and reduce substance use (Miller & Rollnick, 2013). This technique does not demand an in-depth counselling background but rather employs a non-judgemental approach, open-ended questioning, and reflective listening. MI aims to bolster the patient's self-esteem, self-efficacy, and awareness of their issues. It elicits self-motivational statements from the patient, emphasising their motivated behaviour while recognising that the responsibility for change lies with the patient. The four principles of MI are to express empathy, develop discrepancy, roll with resistance, and support self-efficacy. Various tools and strategies, including pencil-and-paper exercises, structured questions, and focused reflections, have been developed to apply these principles effectively (Mason, 2006). MI has been shown to enhance the effectiveness of more extensive psychosocial treatments for alcohol problems and to improve outcomes for drug-related issues (NTA, 2006a, 2006b).

CONTINGENCY MANAGEMENT

Contingency management (CM) involves employing positive reinforcers to encourage desired behaviours. By offering incentives such as vouchers, privileges, prizes, or modest financial rewards, contingent upon desired behaviours, such as abstinence or engagement with treatment, this approach motivates individuals to make positive changes in their substance use patterns. Research indicates that CM is particularly effective when targeted towards changing the use of a single illicit drug and has been successful in engaging "non-responsive" patients who may not have responded to traditional interventions. The principles of CM (NICE, 2007b) are presented in Table 26.4.

CM, integrated into structured care plans alongside other interventions, has garnered robust support as an effective approach, particularly noted

Table 26.3
Counselling skills

Techniques	Explanations	Examples
Empathy	Incorporating acceptance and understanding. Seeing the world view of the other person.	I understand how you are feeling about reducing your alcohol consumption. That must be difficult for you.
Active listening	Involves paying attention to a client's verbal and non-verbal messages. Listening in a way that conveys respect, interest, and empathy.	
Open-ended questions	The "how," "what," or "why" questions. Open-ended questions encourage clients to express their feelings and share information about their situation.	Can you tell me more about that? How do you feel about that? Why do you feel you are at risk for HIV?
Reflective	Encouraging a client to express and explore. Repetition of the last few words or a significant word or phrase can be reflected.	I feel that a part of me is . . . missing.
Focusing	Attempting to redirect the patient in an understanding manner.	
Affirming	Reinforcing or complimenting the client on the positive actions they have taken.	You have managed to reduce your alcohol consumption. This is a positive step in managing to do safer injecting practices.
Correcting misperceptions	Providing correct information to the patient in a sensitive way that does not put the patient on the defensive. Acknowledging misinformation and correcting it.	
Summarising	Presenting the main points to the client.	

Table 26.4
The principles of contingency management

- Providing incentives, typically in the form of vouchers exchangeable for goods or services chosen by the service user, or privileges like take-home methadone doses, contingent upon drug-negative test results (e.g. free from cocaine or non-prescribed opioids), is recommended.
- The screening frequency should begin with three tests per week for the initial three weeks, followed by two tests per week for the subsequent three weeks, and then one test per week until stability is attained.
- Vouchers should initially have a nominal value and increase with each consecutive period of abstinence.
- While urinalysis is the preferred testing method, oral fluid tests may be considered as an alternative.
- For individuals at risk of physical health complications, including transmittable diseases due to drug misuse, material incentives like shopping vouchers should be considered to promote harm reduction.
- These incentives can be provided on a one-off basis or over a limited duration, contingent upon adherence to or completion of each intervention.

Source: Contents adapted from NICE (2007b).

in the NICE guideline for its strong evidence base and positive outcomes. Contingency management has shown remarkable effectiveness in promoting behaviour change among individuals struggling with substance use disorder (Proctor, 2022). Several studies have provided evidence supporting the effectiveness of contingency management when targeted towards changing the use of a single illicit drug. One study by Petry et al. (2000) examined the efficacy of CM in promoting abstinence from cocaine use among cocaine-dependent individuals. The researchers found that participants who received CM interventions, such as vouchers contingent on cocaine-negative urine samples, showed significantly higher rates of cocaine abstinence compared to those who did not receive CM. Similarly, Silverman et al. (1996) conducted a study on the effectiveness of CM in reducing drug use among opioid-dependent individuals. They observed that participants who received CM interventions, such as vouchers contingent on opioid-negative urine samples, demonstrated higher rates of opioid abstinence compared to those who did not receive CM. Furthermore, high-certainty evidence shows that financial incentives, whether monetary or vouchers, effectively improve smoking cessation rates at long-term follow-up in diverse populations. These incentives help precipitate, reinforce, and sustain behavior change, demonstrating their efficacy in promoting smoking cessation. Notley et al. (2019)

These studies offer robust evidence supporting the efficacy of CM, especially when aimed at altering the consumption of particular illicit substances. They highlight its effectiveness in reaching individuals who may have been unresponsive to conventional interventions.

CUE EXPOSURE

Cue exposure targets conditioned responses like craving by exposing individuals to stimuli associated with substance use. Childress et al. (1988) highlighted the phenomenon of "cue reactivity," showing physiological and subjective responses in opiate and cocaine users exposed to drug-related cues. These responses include changes in skin temperature and withdrawal-like symptoms, indicating the presence of conditioned craving.

The typical method involves exposing drug or alcohol users to cues associated with substance use, such as showing a cocaine user white powder or drug paraphernalia or presenting an alcohol user with a beer bottle. Simultaneously, efforts are made to diminish the urge to use. Cue exposure serves to decrease the desire triggered by the cue, allowing individuals to practice coping strategies like relaxation. This process can boost self-efficacy, enhancing the likelihood of employing these coping mechanisms during future encounters with real-life cues (Monti et al., 1989). While cue exposure demonstrates potential as a method for treating alcohol addiction, especially when integrated with coping and communication skills training within a comprehensive cognitive behavioural therapy programme, its efficacy in addressing drug addiction is less substantiated (Conklin & Tiffany, 2002).

The virtual reality cue exposure therapy (VR-CET) programme has shown promise in reducing alcohol craving by immersing individuals in environments that resemble conditioned contexts and contain relevant cues (Karimpour Vazifehkhorani et al., 2022). By paying attention to various cues and contexts within the virtual environment, individuals can confront and gradually extinguish conditioned responses associated with alcohol use. Moreover, the treatment's effectiveness may be enhanced when the virtual environment closely resembles real-life situations where alcohol consumption typically occurs. This approach allows for targeted exposure to cues that trigger craving, facilitating the development of coping mechanis and reducing the likelihood of relapse.

RELAPSE PREVENTION

Relapse prevention, a cognitive behavioural tec nique, focuses on teaching individuals copi skills to manage triggers and prevent relapse. Th approach involves identifying specific situatio where coping inadequacies occur and emplo ing techniques such as instruction, modelli role-playing, and behavioural rehearsal to tea coping strategies. Gradual exposure to stress situations allows individuals to develop adapti mastery over time. A relapse prevention plan tailored to the individual's identified risk facto which may include support to recognise risks ass ciated with substance misuse. Key components o relapse prevention plan often include assertiven training and fostering social inclusion. Figure 26 provides the key elements of relapse preventi skills training.

Relapse prevention skills training typically cove the following areas:

- *Self-monitoring for high-risk situations*. Identifyi triggers and high-risk situations whereby indivi uals learn to recognise situations, emotions, a thoughts that may lead to relapse.
- *Coping strategies*. Techniques are taught to effe tively manage triggers and cravings, such as rela ation techniques, distraction methods, and ur surfing.
- *Assertiveness training*. Individuals learn to asse ively communicate their needs and boundar in social situations to reduce peer pressure a stress.
- *Problem-solving skills*. Strategies are taught address problems and challenges that may ar during recovery, enabling individuals to find co structive solutions.
- *Lifestyle balance*. Emphasis is placed on ma taining a healthy lifestyle through activities su as exercise, nutrition, sleep hygiene, and leisu pursuits.
- *Social support*. Building a support network friends, family, peers, or support groups is enco aged to provide encouragement, accountabili and assistance during difficult times.
- *Developing a relapse prevention plan*. Individ als create a personalised plan outlining speci

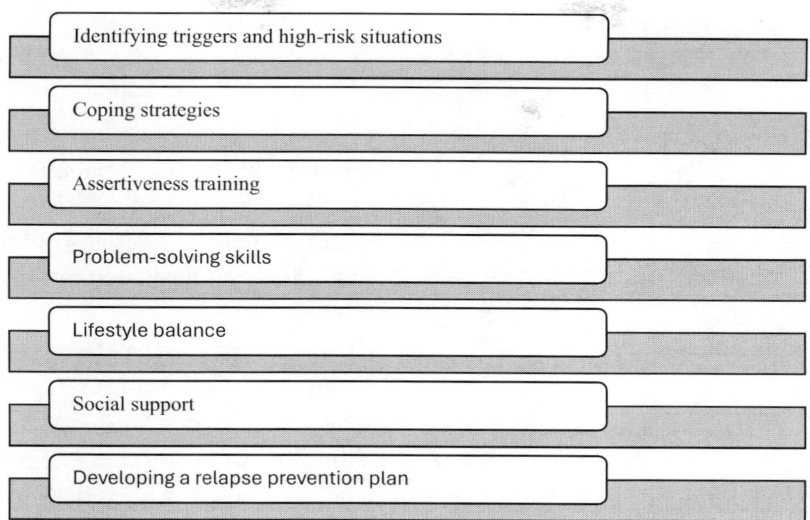

FIGURE 26.1 Relapse prevention skills training.

strategies and resources to utilise when faced with high-risk situations or cravings.

These areas are integral to equipping individuals with the skills and resources necessary to maintain abstinence and prevent relapse in the long term.

Numerous research studies have provided evidence supporting the effectiveness of relapse prevention (RP) programmes in the treatment of substance use disorders. A meta-analysis conducted by Irvin et al. (1999) examined 26 controlled trials of RP interventions for alcohol and drug dependence. The analysis found that RP programmes were associated with significant reductions in relapse rates and increased periods of abstinence compared to control conditions. Cognitive Behaviour Therapy (CBT) for alcohol and other drugs is well-established and effective compared to minimal/usual care. Combining CBT with motivational interviewing, contingency management, or pharmacotherapy also shows efficacy. However, no form of CBT consistently outperforms other empirically-supported treatments. Magill et al. (2023). In a study by McCrady (2000) evaluating the effectiveness of psychological interventions for alcohol use disorder, such as brief interventions and relapse prevention, was classified as efficacious. A Cochrane review (Hajek et al., 2013) also discussed regarding relapse prevention in smokers. The authors concluded that there is insufficient evidence to support the use of any specific behavioural intervention to help smokers who have successfully quit for a short time to avoid relapse. The verdict is strongest for interventions focused on identifying and resolving tempting situations, as most studies were concerned with these.

MARITAL AND FAMILY THERAPIES

Marital and family therapies involve examining the role of significant others in the addictive process and addressing drug misuse within the family context. These interventions aim to identify sources of stress related to drug misuse and support families in developing more effective coping behaviours. The effectiveness of marital therapy in addressing substance use disorders is supported by various studies and clinical trials. Research has shown that involving spouses or partners in treatment can lead to better outcomes, including reduced substance use and improved relationship functioning. For example, a meta-analysis conducted by Powers et al. (2008) found that marital therapy significantly reduced substance use and improved relationship satisfaction among couples affected by substance use disorders.

Another study by Fals-Stewart et al. (2004) demonstrated that couples-based interventions were more effective than individual therapy in reducing substance use and promoting abstinence. Additionally, research has shown (Hogue et al., 2022) that systemic family therapy is well-established as a standalone treatment for addressing substance use disorders. Additionally, behavioural family therapy and behavioural couple therapy are considered probably efficacious as standalone treatments and well-established when integrated into multicomponent treatment approaches. These results highlight the effectiveness of family-based interventions in addressing substance misuse within a broader treatment context.

SOLUTION-FOCUSED BRIEF THERAPY

Solution-focused brief therapy (SFBT) (De Shazer et al., 1986; De Shazer & Dolan, 2012), based on Ericksonian principles, prioritises positive aspects of a person's life rather than focusing solely on pathology. Solution-focused brief therapy emphasises the identification and utilisation of the client's strengths and resources rather than dwelling on weaknesses or problems. The therapy is future-focused, aiming to help clients envision and work towards their desired future outcomes rather than analysing past issues extensively. Rather than analysing problems in depth, the therapist and client collaborate to co-construct solutions. This involves exploring exceptions to the problem, times when the issue was less severe or absent, and identifying small steps towards positive change. SFBT is typically brief, aiming for practical, tangible results in a relatively short period. Sessions often focus on setting specific, achievable goals and monitoring progress towards them. The therapist takes a collaborative stance, working alongside the client rather than adopting a directive approach. The client is seen as the expert in their own life, with the therapist facilitating the exploration of possibilities and solutions. SFBT pays attention to language patterns and communication styles, often utilising techniques such as reframing, scaling questions, and miracle questions to evoke change and promote a positive outlook. The therapy acknowledges that even small changes can lead to significant improvements. Therefore, the focus is on identifying and amplifying these small changes to facilitate larger shifts in behaviour and outlook.

TRADITIONAL, MINNESOTA MODEL, 12-STEP-ORIENTED MODEL

The approach of treating substance misuse as a spiritual and medical disease has its roots in self-help groups like Alcoholics Anonymous (AA), which originated in the United States in 1933. These groups emphasise reaching out to other individuals struggling with alcohol use disorder to support each other in maintaining sobriety. Over time, this philosophy led to the establishment of similar groups, such as Narcotics Anonymous (NA) for drug users and Al-Anon and Families Anonymous (FA) for the families of those affected by substance abuse. AA groups are widespread, with meetings available throughout the week in most cities. They convene in various community and institutional settings, including church halls, hospitals, prisons, and clinics. Importantly, the use of such premises does not compromise the core values of these abstinence-based groups, which include group identity, open confession, and confidential sharing of personal information among members.

While AA is often described as spiritual rather than religious, it emphasises belief in a higher power rather than a specific deity, making it inclusive to individuals of various beliefs, including atheists. This openness contributes to the welcoming atmosphere of AA groups, where individuals can find support and guidance in their journey towards recovery. The 12-step model is presented in Table 26.5.

A meta-analysis of the role of AA in treatment outcomes found that the more involved one is with the process, the better the drinking outcome (Tonigan et al., 1996). However, research findings indicate a positive relationship between participation in Alcoholics Anonymous (AA) and existential well-being,

Table 26.5
The 12-step model

- Admitted we were powerless over alcohol, that our lives had become unmanageable.
- Came to believe that a Power greater than ourselves could restore us to sanity.
- Made a decision to turn our will and our lives over to the care of God as we understood Him.
- Made a searching and fearless moral inventory of ourselves.
- Admitted to God, to ourselves, and to another human being the exact nature of our wrongs.
- Were entirely ready to have God remove all these defects of character.
- Humbly asked Him to remove our shortcomings.
- Made a list of all persons we had harmed, and became willing to make amends to them all.
- Made direct amends to such people wherever possible, except where to do so would injure them or others.
- Continued to take a personal inventory and, when we were wrong, promptly admitted it.
- Sought through prayer and meditation to improve our conscious contact with God as we understood Him, praying only for knowledge of His will for us and the power to carry that out.
- Having had a spiritual experience (awakening) as the result of these steps, we tried to carry this message to alcoholics, and to practice these principles in all our affairs.

which, in turn, predicts subjective well-being, including life satisfaction, positive affect, and negative affect (Wnuk, 2022). The 12-step model has been adapted to align with Islāmic principles and values, creating a framework tailored for Muslim individuals seeking recovery from addiction (Rassool, 2024)

SOCIAL INTERVENTIONS

The social model of intervention highlights the dynamic interplay between an individual's internal experiences and their surrounding networks and communities. Notably, there is growing acknowledgement of the pivotal role families can play in substance misuse treatment. This involvement is instrumental in enhancing substance-related outcomes for the individual and mitigating the adverse effects of substance misuse on other family members (Copello et al., 2006). This intervention model revolves around empowering and supporting both the individual and their family social networks in devising strategies to address specific social challenges and difficulties. Advocacy also emerges as a significant component, particularly in assisting individuals with housing, childcare, and welfare benefits issues. Such support directly impacts an individual's capacity to tackle their alcohol or drug problems effectively. The mounting evidence base supports the effectiveness of both family-focused and social network–focused interventions. Importantly, these approaches either equal or surpass outcomes achieved through individual interventions (Copello et al., 2006).

COMPLEMENTARY THERAPIES

Complementary therapies are gaining traction within allopathic healthcare systems worldwide, particularly in the addiction field. Among these, acupuncture has garnered significant interest. Acupuncture's primary aim is to clear blockages in the body's meridians, facilitating the flow of Chi, considered the vital energy of all beings. Both physical and psychological issues can impede this energy flow. Auricular acupuncture, pioneered at Lincoln Hospital in New York in the early 1970s, is the most recognised form of acupuncture used in addiction treatment. It involves stimulating specific points on the ear to address various substance misuse and addictive behaviours. Auricular acupuncture has shown promise in treating addiction to substances such as cigarettes, alcohol, opiates (including methadone detoxification), cocaine, crack cocaine, and tobacco. Additionally, it has been utilised effectively in preventing relapse among individuals struggling with addiction. While some clinical studies have reported positive findings regarding the use of acupuncture to treat drug dependence, it is important to approach these results with caution. The available data do not conclusively establish acupuncture as an effective treatment for drug addiction (Xiang et al., 2015). The evidence supporting acupuncture's effectiveness in detoxification treatment is largely anecdotal, and despite its use in some clinics and drug court programmes, acupuncture is still considered an alternative medicine (Spray & Jones, 1995). Auricular acupuncture is not a magic solution to substance misuse treatment but can be a complementary tool in the detoxification process.

Aromatherapy involves harnessing the natural essences of aromatic plants to promote healing of the body, mind, and spirit. These essential oils are extracted from plants through methods such as distillation and solvent extraction. Each oil possesses unique properties, and they are often combined to provide comprehensive treatment. However, due to potential contraindications of certain oils with specific conditions, aromatherapy should only be administered by qualified practitioners. Massage is frequently paired with aromatherapy to enhance relaxation and promote a sense of calmness in clients. This combination can be particularly beneficial in the context of substance misuse, offering individuals a reprieve from stress and providing a therapeutic outlet (Mc Donald & Rassool, 1997). Many clients attending substance misuse services find aromatherapy to be a welcoming and effective form of therapy. Miller and Walker (1997) advocate for making therapies that offer hope freely available, suggesting that treatments should be practiced and reimbursed until proven ineffective or harmful. Despite the potential benefits, there is currently a lack of literature specifically addressing the use of aromatherapy in the addiction field. This underscores the need for further research to explore the efficacy and potential applications of aromatherapy in treating substance misuse.

Reflexology is among the most popular complementary therapies utilised by nurses, as reported by Trevelyan (1996). This practice involves massaging the hands, feet, or head to address physical, psychological, and emotional ailments. In the context of substance misuse treatment, reflexology is offered alongside other complementary treatments. During a reflexology session, the practitioner assesses for imbalances and energy blockages in the feet or hands. Using compression massage techniques, they apply pressure with their thumbs and fingers to specific reflex points. The practitioner maintains focus throughout the session, facilitating the flow of Chi, or vital energy. Many clients find relaxation in the massage alone, enjoying the opportunity to unwind in a peaceful environment. However, reflexology has been shown to have a moderating effect on anxiety and fatigue (Cai et al., 2022). There is no specific evidence regarding reflexology's effectiveness in treating substance misuse, as there is limited research directly addressing this topic.

Complementary therapies offer valuable options for substance misuse services, providing additional avenues of care for individuals in this client group. However, it is essential to conduct more research to assess the safety and effectiveness of these therapies fully. Some types of complementary therapies are contraindicated for some culturally and linguistically different communities due to their belief systems.

PHARMACOLOGICAL INTERVENTIONS

Effective pharmacological treatment involves prescribing a spectrum of medications. The need for pharmacological treatment and the type of treatment depend on the consequences of substance misuse. The aims of pharmacological interventions are:

- To reduce harms associated with illicit psychoactive substances, by prescribing a substitute opiate-based medication (for example, methadone)
- To reduce withdrawal syndromes
- To enable the maintenance of abstinence
- To enable the prevention of relapse
- To prevent complications of substance misuse (for example, use of vitamins) and in the treatment of co-existing substance misuse and psychiatric disorders

The management of withdrawal syndromes associated with alcohol, opiates, and hypno-sedatives often requires pharmacological interventions to alleviate symptoms and reduce associated risks. Alcohol and hypno-sedatives withdrawal can be particularly dangerous, with significant mortality and morbidity rates if left untreated. In these cases, pharmacological treatments are crucial for mana ing withdrawal symptoms effectively and prever ing severe complications. Methadone maintenan therapy is commonly used as a substitute for op ates, providing stabilisation for individuals by alle ating withdrawal symptoms, reducing cravings, a minimising adverse effects. This allows clients function without experiencing the negative effe of opiate withdrawal. Naltrexone, a long-acti opiate antagonist, is utilised in relapse preventi by blocking the effects of opiate use. It can he individuals maintain abstinence by reducing t rewarding effects of opiates if relapse occurs. Bo methadone and buprenorphine have demonstrat efficacy in achieving positive outcomes and are re ommended by guidelines, such as those from t National Institute for Health and Care Excellen (NICE, 2007c), for the treatment and prevention withdrawals from heroin and for maintenance pr grammes. These medications can help individu stabilise their condition, reduce withdrawal sym toms, and support long-term recovery from opia addiction.

METHADONE

Methadone is a synthetic opioid medication p marily used in the treatment of opioid dependen particularly heroin addiction. Methadone is long-acting opioid agonist, meaning, it activates t same opioid receptors in the brain as heroin or oth opioids. However, methadone's effects last mu longer, typically between 24 and 36 hours, whi helps stabilise individuals and reduce cravings wit out causing the euphoria or "high" associated wi shorter-acting opioids. However, methadone is n an effective treatment for other psychoactive su stances. For clients with a history of relapse a treatment dropout, methadone is the treatment choice. Methadone maintenance treatment (MM involves the daily administration of methado under medical supervision to individuals with op oid dependence. MMT aims to stabilise patien reduce opioid use, prevent withdrawal symptor and minimise the risk of overdose.

Methadone is utilised in detoxifying opia addicts due to its effectiveness in eliminating wit drawal symptoms. Many individuals on methado maintenance treatment require continuous thera for years without adverse effects. While remai ing physically dependent on methadone, patier experience freedom from the chaotic lifestyles associated with heroin use. Methadone has many advantages, such as:

- Stabilisation of opioid effects
- Reduction in illicit drug use
- Improved social functioning
- Lower mortality rates
- High retention in treatment
- Cost-effectiveness and accessibility

The baseline dose of methadone is administered to alleviate withdrawal symptoms, ensure comfort, and minimise the risk of overdose. Dose reduction strategies depend on individual assessments and treatment plans. Rapid reduction can occur over 7 to 21 days, while slower reductions may extend over several months, particularly for individuals with complex social or other needs. Generally, higher doses allow for greater reductions, while lower doses necessitate more gradual reductions to minimise withdrawal symptoms. Reduction intervals can vary, such as daily, alternate days, or weekly, and adjustments may be made to maintain stability and control anxiety. Psychological support should accompany any delays in reduction, and progress should be regularly monitored and discussed with the multidisciplinary team.

Methadone has been extensively studied for its effectiveness in treating opioid dependence. Numerous studies have shown that methadone maintenance treatment (MMT) is associated with a significant reduction in illicit opioid use. For example, a meta-analysis published in the Cochrane Database of Systematic Reviews concluded that MMT is effective in retaining individuals in treatment and reducing heroin use compared to no treatment or placebo (Mattick et al., 2009). The findings of a study (Teoh Bing Fei et al., 2016) showed that methadone maintenance therapy effectively reduced heroin use, injection practices, and criminal activity while improving social functioning and physical symptoms. However, it did not reduce sex-related HIV risk behaviours. Methadone maintenance has been associated with a reduction in mortality rates among individuals with opioid dependence. The findings of a study (Degenhardt et al., 2009) showed that MMT was associated with a significant decrease in all-cause mortality compared to no treatment or detoxification. Methadone treatment has been shown to improve retention rates in substance use treatment programmes. Higher retention rates are associated with better treatment outcomes, including reduced drug use and improved social functioning (Connock et al., 2007). Overall, the evidence supports the effectiveness of methadone maintenance treatment in reducing opioid use, improving social functioning, reducing mortality rates, and increasing retention in treatment programmes for individuals with opioid dependence.

NALTREXONE

Naltrexone hydrochloride, known simply as naltrexone, is a long-acting opioid antagonist primarily employed in the treatment of alcohol and opiate addiction. This medication works by blocking the effects of opioids in the brain, thereby reducing cravings and preventing relapse in individuals recovering from addiction. It is often used as part of a comprehensive treatment plan that includes counselling, support groups, and other therapeutic interventions. By helping curb the desire for opioids or alcohol, naltrexone can aid individuals in maintaining abstinence and achieving long-term recovery. It can be administered orally or as an implant and has minimal adverse effects. Naltrexone should not be confused with naloxone, which is used in emergency cases of overdose rather than for longer-term dependence control.

There is ample evidence to suggest the effectiveness of naltrexone pharmacotherapy in preventing relapse in individuals with alcohol and opioid addiction. The COMBINE study (Anton et al., 2006) demonstrated that naltrexone, either alone or in combination with behavioural therapy, significantly reduced heavy drinking days and increased abstinence rates compared to placebo in individuals with alcohol use disorder. Meta-analyses of naltrexone and acamprosate consistently show their efficacy for treating alcohol use disorders (Maisel et al., 2013). The findings of a Cochrane review (Minozzi et al., 2016) showed that naltrexone is effective in preventing relapse to opioid use after detoxification, particularly when adherence to treatment is ensured. Recommendations for managing individuals undergoing naltrexone treatment for opioid addiction include immediate intervention for unblocked opioid use (such as detoxification or switching to buprenorphine) and increased clinical attention for blocked use (including direct observation of naltrexone ingestion, dose adjustment, or intensified treatment contact) (Sullivan et al., 2007). These strategies aim to address relapse and support recovery effectively. In a multicentre, randomised, placebo-controlled clinical trial evaluating the efficacy of naltrexone depot for treating alcohol dependence, participants receiving naltrexone showed substantial improvements compared to those on placebo. Specifically, the naltrexone group experienced significantly fewer heavy drinking days and higher rates of abstinence (Kranzler et al., 2013). This suggests that naltrexone depot is effective in reducing alcohol consumption and promoting abstinence in individuals with alcohol dependence.

BUPRENORPHINE AND NON-OPIATES

Buprenorphine is licensed in numerous countries for treating drug dependence. Administered as a sublingual tablet once daily, it has an effective duration exceeding 24 hours. Compared to methadone, it induces lower euphoria at higher doses, entails lesser risk of physical dependence, and boasts a milder withdrawal profile. Buprenorphine also exhibits reduced potential for misuse and less respiratory depression, rendering it safer in overdose situations. Evidence suggests that buprenorphine is linked with a decreased risk of fatal overdose, particularly during the initial weeks of treatment initiation (NICE, 2007c). Buprenorphine's dual mechanism of action can paradoxically worsen withdrawal symptoms if used concurrently with methadone or other opiates. It should be administered at least 24 hours after the last methadone dose and at least four hours following heroin use to prevent exacerbating withdrawal symptoms. Additionally, buprenorphine is reported to have a lower overdose potential compared to methadone, rendering it a safer option in this regard.

Non-opiate treatments, such as lofexidine and clonidine, offer satisfactory options for managing opiate withdrawal symptoms. Lofexidine effectively reduces withdrawal effects, like chills, sweating, stomach cramps, muscle pain, sleep difficulties, and runny nose. Unlike opiates, it is less prone to misuse or diversion on the black market. Lofexidine can be safely administered under supervision in various settings, including inpatient, residential, and community settings. Evidence suggests that treatment regimes utilising alpha2 adrenergic agonists like clonidine and lofexidine, as well as methadone dose reduction over approximately 10 days, demonstrate similar efficacy in managing withdrawal from heroin or methadone (Gowing et al., 2001). Clonidine, although not licensed for opiate withdrawal treatment, serves as a non-opiate option for managing withdrawal symptoms. However, its substantial hypotensive effect necessitates blood pressure monitoring and potential treatment modification or withdrawal in case of symptomatic hypotension (Gowing et al., 2016).

KEY POINTS

- There are a wide range of psychosocial and pharmacological interventions for the treatment of alcohol and drug misuse.
- There is evidence to suggest that substance misuse treatment is effective in terms of reduced substance misuse, improvements in personal and social functioning, reduced public health and safety risks, reduced criminal behaviour.
- The delivery of interventions includes regular reviews of care plans and treatment goals, harm reduction approach, promoting readiness to change, preventing relapse, and addressing social problems.
- The effectiveness of a therapeutic alliance is crucial to the delivery of any treatment intervention and patient outcomes.
- Brief interventions comprise of a single brief advice session or several short (15 to 30 minutes) counselling sessions.
- Motivational interviewing is "directive, client-centred counselling for eliciting behaviour change by helping clients to explore and resolve ambivalence."
- Motivational interviewing has been found to increase the effectiveness of more extensive psychosocial treatments for alcohol problems and improved outcomes for drug-related problems.
- NICE has recommended that drug services should introduce contingency management programmes to reduce illicit drug use and/or promote engagement with services for people receiving methadone maintenance treatment.
- Clients may need support to identify risks associated with their substance misuse, and a relapse prevention plan is based on the identified risk factors.
- Marital behavioural therapy in particular and various other combinations of family approaches

have demonstrated effectiveness in reducing dropout and relapse rates.

- The key role that families can play in substance misuse treatment, in terms of preventing and/or influencing the course of the substance misuse problem, is in improving substance-related outcomes for the user and also helping to reduce the negative effects of substance misuse problems on other family members.
- Auricular acupuncture has been used during detoxification.
- Aromatherapy is welcomed by most clients attending services.
- Reflexology is one of the many complementary treatments on offer to clients who present with substance misuse problems.
- Complementary therapies can be of great value in substance misuse services.
- Effective pharmacological treatment involves prescribing a spectrum of medications.
- Methadone treatments are the most widely used type of treatment for opiate addiction throughout the world.

Activity 26.3

Questions

- What does the acronym "FRAMES" stand for?
- List the six stages in the counselling process.
- What are the advantages in using methadone?
- How would you develop a plan of relapse prevention?

References

Anton, R. F., O'Malley, S. S., Ciraulo, D. A., Cisler, R. A., Couper, D., Donovan, D. M., Gastfriend, D. R., Hosking, J. D., Johnson, B. A., LoCastro, J. S., Longabaugh, R., Mason, B. J., Mattson, M. E., Miller, W. R., Pettinati, H. M., Randall, C. L., Swift, R., Weiss, R. D., Williams, L. D., Zweben, A., & COMBINE Study Research Group. (2006). Combined pharmacotherapies and behavioral interventions for alcohol dependence: The COMBINE study: A randomized controlled trial. *JAMA,* 295(17), 2003–2017. https://doi.org/10.1001/jama.295.17.2003.

Bien, T. H., Miller, W. R., & Tonigan, J. S. (1993). Brief interventions for alcohol problems: A review. *Addiction,* 88(3), 315–336.

Bischof, G., Bischof, A., & Rumpf, H. J. (2021). Motivational interviewing: An evidence-based approach for use in medical practice. *Deutsches Arzteblatt International,* 118(7), 109–115. https://doi.org/10.3238/arztebl.m2021.0014.

Cai, D. C., Chen, C. Y., & Lo, T. Y. (2022). Foot reflexology: Recent research trends and prospects. *Healthcare,* 11(1), 9. https://doi.org/10.3390/healthcare11010009.

Childres, A. R., Mc Lellan, A. T., Ehrman, R., & O'Brien, C. P. (1988). Classically conditioned responses in opioid and cocaine dependence: A role in relapse? In B. A. Ray (Ed.), *Learning Factors in Substance Abuse* (DHHS Publication No. 88–1576). Washington, DC: U.S. Government Printing Office, pp. 25–43.

Conklin, C. A., & Tiffany, S. T. (2002). Applying extinction research and theory to cue-exposure addiction treatments. *Addiction,* 97(2), 155–167. https://doi.org/10.1046/j.1360-0443.2002.00014.x.

Connock, M., Juarez-Garcia, A., Jowett, S., Frew, E., Liu, Z., Taylor, R. J., Fry-Smith, A., Day, E., Lintzeris, N., Roberts, T., Burls, A., & Taylor, R. S. (2007). Methadone and buprenorphine for the management of opioid dependence: A systematic review and economic evaluation. *Health Technology Assessment,* 11(9), I–IV. https://doi.org/10.3310/hta11090.

Copello, A. G., Templeton, L., & Velleman, R. (2006). Family interventions for drug and alcohol misuse: Is there a best practice? *Current Opinion in Psychiatry,* 19(3), 271–276. https://doi.org/10.1097/01.yco.0000218597.31184.41.

Degenhardt, L., Randall, D., Hall, W., Law, M., Butler, T., & Burns, L. (2009). Mortality among clients of a state-wide opioid pharmacotherapy program over 20 years: Risk factors and lives saved. *Drug and Alcohol Dependence,* 105(1–2), 9–15. https://doi.org/10.1016/j.drugalcdep.2009.05.021.

De Shazer, S., Berg, I. K., Lipchik, E. V. E., Nunnally, E., Molnar, A., Gingerich, W., & Weiner-Davis, M. (1986). Brief therapy: Focused solution development. *Family Process,* 25(2), 207–221.

De Shazer, S., & Dolan, Y. (2012). *More Than Miracles: The State of the Art of Solution-Focused Brief Therapy.* New York: Haworth Press.

Fals-Stewart, W., O'Farrell, T. J., & Birchler, G. R. (2004). Behavioral couples therapy for substance abuse: Rationale, methods, and findings. *Science & Practice Perspectives,* 2(2), 30–41. https://doi.org/10.1151/spp042230.

Gerstein, D. R., & Harwood, H. J. (Eds.). (1990). *Treating Drug Problems: Volume 1: A Study of the Evolution, Effectiveness, and Financing of Public and Private Drug Treatment Systems.*

Institute of Medicine (US) Committee for the Substance Abuse Coverage Study. Washington, DC: National Academies Press (US). https://www.ncbi.nlm.nih.gov/books/NBK235506/.

Gowing, L., Farrell, M., Ali, R., & White, J. M. (2001). Alpha2 adrenergic agonists for the management of opioid withdrawal. *The Cochrane Database of Systematic Reviews*, 1, CD002024. https://doi.org/10.1002/14651858.CD002024.

Gowing, L., Farrell, M., Ali, R., & White, J. M. (2016). Alpha$_2$-adrenergic agonists for the management of opioid withdrawal. *The Cochrane Database of Systematic Reviews*, 2016(5), CD002024. https://doi.org/10.1002/14651858.CD002024.pub5.

Hajek, P., Stead, L. F., West, R., Jarvis, M., Hartmann-Boyce, J., & Lancaster, T. (2013). Relapse prevention interventions for smoking cessation. *The Cochrane Database of Systematic Reviews*, 8, CD003999. https://doi.org/10.1002/14651858.CD003999.pub4.

Heather, N. (1998). Using brief opportunities for change in medical settings. In W. Miller & N. Heather (Eds.), *Treating Addictive Behaviors*. New York: Plenum.

Heather, N., & Kaner, E. (2001). *Brief Interventions: An Opportunity for Reducing Excessive Drinking*. Paper presented to Working Group: Health Systems and Alcohol at Ministerial Conference on Young People and Alcohol, Stockholm, Sweden, 19–21 February.

Heather, N., Whitton, B., & Robertson, I. (1986). Evaluation of a self-help manual for media-recruited problem drinkers: Six-month follow-up results. *The British Journal of Clinical Psychology*, 25(Pt 1), 19–34. https://doi.org/10.1111/j.2044-8260.1986.tb00667.x.

Hogue, A., Schumm, J. A., MacLean, A., & Bobek, M. (2022). Couple and family therapy for substance use disorders: Evidence-based update 2010–2019. *Journal of Marital and Family Therapy*, 48, 178–203. https://doi.org/10.1111/jmft.12546.

Irvin, J. E., Bowers, C. A., Dunn, M. E., & Wang, M. C. (1999). Efficacy of relapse prevention: A meta-analytic review. *Journal of Consulting and Clinical Psychology*, *67*(4), 563–570. https://doi.org/10.1037//0022-006x.67.4.563.

Karimpour Vazifehkhorani, A., Attaran, A., Karimi Sarasandrud, A., Faghih, H., & Yeganeh, N. (2022). Effectiveness of cue-exposure therapy on alcohol craving in virtual environment: Based on habit loop. *Addiction & Health*, 14(2), 78–86. https://doi.org/10.22122/AHJ.2022.196454.1288.

Kranzler, H. R., Knapp, C., & Ciraulo, D. A. (2013). Pharmacotherapy of alcoholism. In H. R. Kranzler, D. Ciraulo, & L. Zindel (Eds.), *Clinical Manual of Addiction Psychopharmacology* (2nd ed.). Washington, DC: American Psychiatric Press.

Magill, M., Kiluk, B. D., & Ray, L. A. (2023). Efficacy of cognitive behavioral therapy for alcohol and other drug use disorders: Is a one-size-fits-all approach appropriate? *Substance Abuse and Rehabilitation*, 14, 1–11. https://doi.org/10.2147/SAR.S362864.

Maisel, N. C., Blodgett, J. C., Wilbourne, P. L., Humphreys, K., & Finney, J. W. (2013). Meta-analysis of naltrexone and acamprosate for treating alcohol use disorders: When are these medications most helpful? *Addiction*, 108(2), 275–293. https://doi.org/10.1111/j.1360-0443.2012.04054.x.

Mason, P. (2006). Motivational interviewing. In G. H. Rassool (Ed.), *Dual Diagnosis Nursing*. Oxford: Blackwell Publications.

Mattick, R. P., Breen, C., Kimber, J., & Davoli, M. (2009). Methadone maintenance therapy versus no opioid replacement therapy for opioid dependence. *The Cochrane Database of Systematic Reviews*, (3). https://doi.org/10.1002/14651858.CD002209.

McCrady, B. S. (2000). Alcohol use disorders and the division 12 task force of the American Psychological Association. *Psychology of Addictive Behaviors: Journal of the Society of Psychologists in Addictive Behaviors*, 14(3), 267–276.

McDonald, L., & Rassool, G. H. (1997). Complementary therapies in addiction nursing practice. In G. H. Rassool & M. Gafoor (Eds.), *Addiction Nursing: Perspectives on Professional and Clinical Practice*. Cheltenham: Nelson Thornes.

McLellan, A. T., Woody, G. E., Metzger, D., McKay, J., Durrell, J., Alterman, A. I., & O'Brien, C. P. (1996). Evaluating the effectiveness of addiction treatments: Reasonable expectations, appropriate comparisons. *The Milbank Quarterly*, *74*(1), 51–85.

Miller, W. R., & Walker, D. D. (1997). Should there be aromatherapy for addiction? *Addiction*, 92(4), 486–487. https://doi.org/10.1111/j.1360-0443.1997.tb03384.x.

Miller, W. R., & Rollnick, S. (2013). *Motivational Interviewing: Helping People Change* (3rd ed.). New York: Guilford Press.

Minozzi, S., Amato, L., Jahanfar, S., Bellisario, C., Ferri, M., & Davoli, M. (2020). Maintenance agonist treatments for opiate-dependent pregnant women. *The Cochrane Database of Systematic Reviews*, 11(11), CD006318. https://doi.org/10.1002/14651858.CD006318.pub4.

Monti, P. M., Abrams, D. S., Kadden, R. M. and Cooney, N. L. (1989). *Treating Alcohol Dependence*. New York: Guilford. Press.

NICE. (2007a). *Drug Misuse in Over 16s: Psychosocial Interventions. Clinical Guideline 25*. London: National Institute for Health and Clinical Excellence.

NICE. (2007b). *Drug Misuse: Psychosocial Interventions* (NICE Clinical Guideline 51). London: National Institute for Health and Clinical Excellence.

NICE. (2007c). *Methadone and Buprenorphine for the Management of Opioid Dependence*. (Technology Appraisal Guidance (TA114)). London: National Institute for Health and Clinical Excellence.

NIDA. (2023). *Treatment and Recovery*. https://nida.nih.gov/publications/drugs-brains-behavior-science-addiction/treatment-recovery (accessed 6 April 2024).

Notley, C., Gentry, S., Livingstone-Banks, J., Bauld, L., Perera, R., & Hartmann-Boyce, J. (2019). Incentives for smoking cessation. *The Cochrane Database of Systematic Reviews*, 7(7), CD004307. https://doi.org/10.1002/14651858.CD004307.pub6.

NTA. (2006a). *Treating Drug Misuse Problems: Evidence of Effectiveness*. London: National Treatment Agency.

NTA. (2006b). *Review of the Effectiveness of Treatment for Alcohol Problems*. London: National Treatment Agency.

Petry, N. M., Martin, B., Cooney, J. L., & Kranzler, H. R. (2000). Give them prizes, and they will come contingency management for treatment of alcohol dependence. *Journal of Consulting and Clinical Psychology*, 68(2), 250–257. https://doi.org/10.1037//0022-006x.68.2.250.

Powers, M. B., Vedel, E., & Emmelkamp, P. M. (2008). Behavioral couples therapy (BCT) for alcohol and drug use disorders: A meta-analysis. *Clinical Psychology Review,* 28(6), 952–962. https://doi.org/10.1016/j.cpr.2008.02.002.

Prendergast, M. L., Podus, D., Chang, E., & Urada, D. (2002). The effectiveness of drug abuse treatment: A meta-analysis of comparison group studies. *Drug and Alcohol Dependence,* 67(1), 53–72. https://doi.org/10.1016/s0376-8716(02)00014-5.

Proctor, S. L. (2022). Rewarding recovery: The time is now for contingency management for opioid use disorder. *Annals of Medicine,* 54(1), 1178–1187. https://doi.org/10.1080/07853890.2022.2068805.

Rassool, G. H. (2024). *Islāmic Counselling and Psychotherapy: An Introduction from Theory to Practice* (2nd ed.). Oxford: Routledge.

Rollnick, S., & Miller, W. R. (1995). What is motivational interviewing? *Behavioural and Cognitive Psychotherapy,* 23, 325–334.

Roth, A. D., & Pilling, S. (2007). *The Competences Required to Deliver Effective Cognitive and Behavioural Therapy for People with Depression and with Anxiety Disorders.* London: Department of Health.

Silverman, K., Higgins, S. T., Brooner, R. K., Montoya, I. D., Cone, E. J., Schuster, C. R., & Preston, K. L. (1996). Sustained cocaine abstinence in methadone maintenance patients through voucher-based reinforcement therapy. *Archives of General Psychiatry,* 53(5), 409–415. https://doi.org/10.1001/archpsyc.1996.01830050045007.

Spray, J. R., & Jones, S. M. (1995). The use of acupuncture in drug addiction treatment. *News Briefs.* https://ndsn.org/sept95/guest.html (accessed 7 April 2024).

Sullivan, M. A., Garawi, F., Bisaga, A., Comer, S. D., Carpenter, K. M., Raby, W. N., Anen, S. J., Brooks, A. C., Jiang, H., Akerele, E. O., & Nunes, E. V. (2007). Management of relapse in naltrexone maintenance for heroin dependence. *Drug and Alcohol Dependence,* 91(2–3), 289–292.

Teoh Bing Fei, J., Yee, A., Habil, M. H., & Danaee, M. (2016). Effectiveness of methadone maintenance therapy and improvement in quality of life following a decade of implementation. *Journal of Substance Abuse Treatment,* 69, 50–56. https://doi.org/10.1016/j.jsat.2016.07.006.

Tonigan, S., Connors, G, & Miller, W. R. (1996). The alcoholic anonymous involvement scale (AAI): Reliability and norms. *Psychology of Addictive Behavior,* 10, 75–80.

Trevelyan, T. (1996). A true complement. *Nursing Times,* 95, 5.

Velleman, R. (2001). *Counselling for Alcohol Problems* (2nd ed.). London: Sage Publications.

WHO. (1996). Brief intervention study group. A cross-national trial of brief interventions with heavy drinkers. *American Journal of Public Health,* 86(7), 948–955. https://doi.org/10.2105/ajph.86.7.948.

WHO. (2005). *Brief Intervention for Substance Use: A Manual for Use in Primary Care Department of Mental Health & Substance Dependence.* Geneva: World Health Organization.

Wnuk, M. (2022). The beneficial role of involvement in alcoholics anonymous for existential and subjective well-being of alcohol-dependent individuals? The model verification. *International Journal of Environmental Research and Public Health,* 19(9), 5173. https://doi.org/10.3390/ijerph19095173.

Xiang, A., Zhang, B., & Liu, S. (2015). Role of acupuncture in the treatment of drug addiction. In M. Saad (Ed.), *Complementary Therapies for the Body, Mind and Soul.* InTech. https://doi.org/10.5772/59418.

Chapter 27

Harm reduction approach

Learning outcomes

- Explain what is meant by *harm reduction approach*.
- Discuss the rationale for harm reduction approach.
- Discuss the harm reduction approach to drug, alcohol, tobacco, and blood-borne and HIV infections.
- Explain what is meant by safer drug use and safer sex practice.
- Discuss the advantages and limitations of needle syringe schemes.

Activity 27.1

Please state whether the following statements are true or false. Reflect on the statements and give reason(s) for choosing a particular option.

Statements	True	False
Harm reduction is an integral and important part of the overall HIV prevention strategy.		
Harm reduction cannot work alongside approaches that aim for reductions in drug, alcohol, and tobacco consumption.		
Harm reduction focuses on "safer" drug use and has also been developed as a way of educating young people about drug use.		
Harm reduction approaches nudge more substance misusers to engage in prevention and treatment programmes.		
Engagement in treatment can provide a window of opportunity to minimise harm caused by alcohol and drug misuse.		
Harm reduction does not provide better outcomes for substance misusers.		
A comprehensive alcohol policy needs population-level interventions focusing on the availability and accessibility of alcohol and alcohol harm reduction interventions.		
Currently, the tobacco harm reduction strategy is based on supply-and-demand reduction strategies.		

DOI: 10.4324/9781003456674-32

Statements	True	False
Abstinence-oriented treatment, such as nicotine replacement therapy, may be a viable option for most smokers.		
In the context of HIV and other blood-borne diseases, harm reduction strategies aim to reduce the health and social harms of drug injecting.		
There is no evidence to suggest that harm reduction is effective in HIV prevention programmes.		
There is evidence that needle exchange programmes increased either the number of people using drugs or the frequency of injecting drug use.		
It is important to tailor harm reduction programmes to meet the specific needs of cocaine users.		
Many injecting drug users need access to services in the evening, at night, or on weekends.		

Activity 27.2

There is only one correct answer to the following questions.

1. The harm reduction approach primarily aims to:
   a. Encourage recreational drug use
   b. Eliminate substance use entirely
   c. Reduce the negative consequences of substance use
   d. Enforce strict drug laws
   e. Increase awareness about safe substance use practices
2. The rationale for the harm reduction approach emphasises:
   a. Punishing individuals with substance use disorders
   b. Prioritising complete abstinence as the only solution
   c. Reducing the harms associated with substance use while respecting individual autonomy
   d. Increasing access to illicit drugs for recreational purposes
   e. Promoting healthy lifestyle choices
3. Harm reduction strategies for alcohol may include:
   a. Encouraging excessive drinking to build tolerance
   b. Implementing stricter alcohol advertising regulations
   c. Promoting designated driver programmes
   d. Enforcing mandatory alcohol consumption in public spaces
   e. Advocating for alcohol-free events
4. Safer drug use practices aim to:
   a. Increase the negative consequences of drug use
   b. Promote sharing of needles and syringes
   c. Minimise the negative consequences of drug use through strategies such as using sterile equipment
   d. Encourage recreational drug use without any precautions
   e. Encourage overdose as a means of controlling drug use

5. An advantage of needle syringe schemes is:
   a. Increased risk of blood-borne infections
   b. Stigmatisation of drug users
   c. Access to sterile injection equipment and healthcare services
   d. Limited coverage and opposition from the community
   e. Increased drug-related crimes
6. The harm reduction approach addresses:
   a. Only the legal aspects of substance use
   b. Only the health consequences of substance use
   c. Both the health and social consequences of substance use
   d. Only the economic consequences of substance use
   e. Only the psychological consequences of substance use
7. The harm reduction approach recognises that:
   a. Complete abstinence is the only acceptable outcome
   b. Criminalising substance use is the most effective solution
   c. Reducing substance use is not a realistic goal for everyone
   d. Mandatory treatment is the best approach for all individuals
   e. Only medical interventions are effective in addressing substance use
8. Safer sex practices aim to:
   a. Increase the risk of sexually transmitted infections
   b. Promote unsafe sexual behaviour
   c. Minimise the risk of sexually transmitted infections and unintended pregnancies
   d. Encourage sharing of needles during sexual encounters
   e. Advocate for abstinence-only education
9. Needle syringe schemes are designed to:
   a. Encourage the sharing of needles among drug users
   b. Stigmatise drug users
   c. Provide access to clean injection equipment and healthcare services
   d. Limit access to healthcare for drug users
   e. Promote unsafe injection practices
10. The harm reduction approach acknowledges that:
   a. Substance use disorders are solely the result of individual choice
   b. Substance use disorders are primarily a criminal issue
   c. Substance use disorders have complex causes and require multifaceted interventions
   d. Substance use disorders can only be addressed through punitive measures
   e. Substance use disorders can be eradicated through abstinence-only education
11. Harm reduction strategies for tobacco include:
   a. Encouraging smoking in public places
   b. Limiting access to smoking cessation programmes
   c. Providing education on smoking cessation and access to nicotine replacement therapies
   d. Allowing tobacco companies to freely advertise their products
   e. Implementing higher taxes on tobacco products
12. Safer drug use practices involve:
   a. Encouraging sharing of needles and syringes
   b. Minimising the negative consequences of drug use through strategies such as using sterile equipment
   c. Promoting overdose as a way to control drug use
   d. Encouraging recreational drug use without any precautions
   e. Encouraging the use of contaminated needles and syringes

13. An advantage of needle syringe schemes is:
    a. Increased risk of blood-borne infections
    b. Stigmatisation of drug users
    c. Access to sterile injection equipment and healthcare services
    d. Limited coverage and opposition from the community
    e. Decreased access to healthcare services
14. The harm reduction approach prioritises:
    a. Criminalising substance use
    b. Enforcing strict drug laws
    c. Reducing the harms associated with substance use while respecting individual autonomy
    d. Promoting recreational drug use
    e. Ignoring the negative consequences of substance use
15. Safer sex practices aim to:
    a. Increase the risk of sexually transmitted infections
    b. Promote unsafe sexual behaviour
    c. Minimise the risk of sexually transmitted infections and unintended pregnancies
    d. Encourage sharing of needles during sexual encounters
    e. Advocate for abstinence-only education
16. The first principle of reducing harm involves drawing attention to:
    a. The dangers of drugs and to technique-specific hazards
    b. The dangers of psychoactive drugs
    c. The dangers of needle exchange schemes
    d. The dangers of not using sterile equipment
    e. To reduce the incidence of problem drinking
17. *Alcohol harm reduction* can be broadly defined as measures that aim:
    a. To reduce the incidence of problem drinking
    b. To reduce controlled drinking
    c. To reduce alcohol consumption
    d. To promote zero-tolerance
    e. To reduce the harms
18. Syringe exchange schemes provide:
    a. Paraphernalia
    b. Educational resources
    c. Health interventions
    d. All of the above
    e. A and C only

INTRODUCTION

The broad consensus acknowledges that psychoactive substance misuse is a societal reality, necessitating interventions beyond mere abstinence. Harm reduction, as a strategy, aims to mitigate the negative consequences of substance use, contrasting with primary prevention efforts. It prioritises promoting safer drug use and sex practices to prevent overdose and blood-borne infections transmission. This approach signifies a shift towards addressing substance misuse pragmatically, recognising the potential for incremental improvements leading to significant lifestyle changes, potentially culminating in abstinence. This paradigm shift in policy and strategy reflects a more inclusive and pragmatic approach to tackling substance misuse, emphasising harm reduction as a stepping stone towards improved well-being.

Since the mid-1980s, many Western countries have viewed harm reduction as an integral and important part of the overall HIV prevention strategy and have supported a comprehensive and complementary package of interventions for HIV prevention, treatment, and care among drug users. Three phases of the development of harm reduction have been observed (Erickson, 1999). The first phase stemmed from a growing concern in the 1960s about the health risks associated with tobacco and alcohol use in the population. The second phase began in 1990 with a sharp focus on AIDS prevention among injection drug users. There is a third phase, in which an integrated public health perspective is being developed for all licit and illicit psychoactive substances. The benefits and limitations of the harm reduction approach are presented in Table 27.1.

Harm reduction can work alongside approaches that aim for reductions in drug, alcohol, and tobacco consumption. The principles of harm reduction (Harm Reduction Coalition) are outlined in Table 27.2.

The emphasis on public health in harm reduction has facilitated collaboration between various sectors, including health, social services, criminal justice, and law enforcement. This collaboration has led to increased cooperation and coordination among these systems, resulting in more comprehensive and effective approaches to addressing substance misuse.

Harm reduction strategies encourage individuals who misuse substances to engage with prevention and treatment programmes, thereby promoting healthier behaviours and reducing the risk of harm. By providing support and resources to individuals who may not otherwise seek help, harm reduction interventions create opportunities to minimise the

Table 27.1
Benefits and limitations of the harm reduction approach

Advantages	Limitations
• A society free of substance misuse is unrealistic.	• Provides a disguise for pro-legalisation efforts.
• Is a pragmatic public health approach.	• Encourages illegal use of psychoactive substances.
• Complements approaches that aim for reductions in drug, alcohol and tobacco consumption.	• Encourages drinking behaviour.
• Engages people and motivates them to make contact with substance misuse services.	• Encourages substance misusers from attaining abstinence.
• Reduces harm caused by substance misuse.	• Undercuts abstinence-oriented treatment programmes.
• Promotes controlled use of psychoactive substances.	• Resource constraints.
• Avoids moralistic, stigmatising, and judgemental statements about substance misusers.	
• Reduces accidental death and overdose and saves lives.	
• Reduces the transmission of blood-borne infections.	

Table 27.2
Principles of harm reduction

- Accepts that psychoactive substances are a part of our society, and chooses to minimise their harmful effects rather than to ignore or condemn them.
- Understands that substance misuse is a complex and multifaceted phenomenon that encompasses a continuum of behaviours, ranging from dependence to total abstinence, and acknowledges that some ways of using drugs or alcohol are clearly safer than others.
- Calls for the non-judgemental, non-coercive provision of services and resources to individuals who use drugs and the communities in which they live in order to assist them in reducing attendant harm.
- Ensures that substance misusers and those with a history of substance misuse routinely have a real voice in the creation of programmes and policies designed to serve them.
- Affirms substance misusers themselves as the primary agents of reducing the harms of their substance use, and seeks to empower users to share information and support each other in strategies which meet their actual conditions of use.
- Recognises that the realities of poverty, class, racism, social isolation, past trauma, sex-based discrimination, and other social inequalities affect both people's vulnerability to and capacity for effectively dealing with substance-related harm.
- Does not attempt to minimise or ignore the real and tragic harm and danger associated with licit and illicit drug use.

Source: Harm Reduction Coalition.

negative consequences associated with substance misuse. Engagement in treatment programmes offers an opportunity to address alcohol and substance misuse and its associated harms. Even small reductions in alcohol or drug misuse can lead to significant improvements in health outcomes and overall well-being. Therefore, harm reduction prioritises harm minimisation rather than absolute cessation of substance use, recognising that any reduction in harmful behaviours is beneficial. It is essential to conduct harm reduction within a public health framework that prioritises the health, human rights, and social needs of individuals who use drugs, as well as their families and communities. By addressing the underlying factors contributing to alcohol and substance use disorder and adopting a holistic approach, harm reduction interventions can effectively mitigate harm and promote the well-being of all stakeholders involved.

HARM REDUCTION: DRUG

Harm reduction programmes include supervised consumption of methadone or other opiate substitutes, needle exchange schemes (pharmacy-based needle exchange or other forms of needle exchange), programmes to reduce the risk associated with HIV and hepatitis, health information about safer drug use, and safer sex. Information about safer drug use is providing health information for people who choose to use drugs to do so in the safest possible way. The harm reduction advice about safer drug use is presented in Table 27.3.

Table 27.3
Safer drug use

Choosing safer environments	• Opting for safer places to use drugs can significantly mitigate risks. • Using drugs with friends rather than alone can provide a support network in case of emergencies and reduce the likelihood of adverse reactions going unnoticed. • Avoiding isolated places like abandoned buildings or outdoor areas can enhance safety by reducing the risk of accidents or encounters with law enforcement.
Safer methods of drug administration	• Swallowing pills, smoking, or inhaling substances is generally less risky compared to injection. • Swallowing drugs eliminates the risk of infections associated with injecting. • Smoking or inhaling substances can provide a slower onset of effects, allowing users more time to recognise and respond to potential adverse reactions.
Understanding risks of injection	• Risks, including overdose, infections, abscesses, blood clots, and even death. • It is more dangerous to inject in big veins like the groin or neck. • Understanding these risks is crucial for individuals who choose to inject drugs, as it empowers them to make informed decisions about their health and safety. • Seeking assistance from local needle and syringe exchange programmes can provide access to clean equipment, guidance on safer injection practices, and resources for reducing harm.
Avoiding needle sharing	• Sharing needles, syringes, filters, spoons, and water should always be avoided to prevent the transmission of blood-borne infections, such as HIV and hepatitis B and C. • Even small amounts of blood left on injection equipment can pose significant risks. • Ensuring access to clean, sterile equipment and avoiding sharing with others are critical components of safer drug use. • Ask about hepatitis B vaccination.
Maintaining hygiene	• Keeping hands and injection sites clean, using sterile equipment, and avoiding contamination can reduce the risk of infections and other complications. • Using alcohol swabs to clean the injection site before injection and properly disposing off used equipment afterward are essential hygiene practices.
Avoiding mixing drugs	• Mixing different substances, also known as polydrug use, or drug cocktails, can increase the unpredictability of effects and the risk of adverse reactions. • It is advisable to avoid combining drugs, as doing so can amplify their individual effects and lead to dangerous outcomes.
Minimising alcohol consumption	• Combining alcohol with drug use can potentiate the effects of both substances and increase the risk of respiratory depression, overdose, and other adverse events. • Individuals should be cautious when using alcohol alongside drugs and consider abstaining from alcohol altogether to reduce potential harm.

The primary principle of harm reduction involves highlighting the specific hazards associated with the misuse of various psychoactive substances, particularly for injecting drug users. This approach aims to raise awareness of the risks inherent in injecting practices, including technique-specific hazards and the sharing of equipment. One significant initiative in harm reduction has been the establishment of needle syringe schemes, which offer sterile equipment, guidance on safer injecting techniques, and additional services to individuals who typically use illegal drugs. These schemes provide vital resources and support to minimise the harms associated with injecting drug use. They emphasise safer injecting practices and educate users on techniques to reduce risks. Additionally, they offer information on cleaning and sterilising injecting equipment to prevent the transmission of infections. The procedure of safer injecting and methods of cleaning injecting equipment are typically presented in educational materials provided by needle syringe schemes. These resources outline steps such as using clean needles and syringes for each injection, avoiding needle sharing, proper disposal of used equipment, and disinfection techniques. By promoting safer injecting practices and offering access to sterile equipment, needle syringe schemes play a crucial role in harm reduction efforts, ultimately aiming to protect the health and well-being of injecting drug users and their communities. Table 27.4 outlines the harm reduction of injecting drug users.

Harm reduction measures for drug misusers involve persuading individuals to stop sharing injecting equipment, transitioning from injection to oral drug use, decreasing overall drug use, and ultimately working towards achieving abstinence from drug use altogether. These goals are implemented progressively, with the aim of reducing the negative consequences associated with drug misuse and promoting healthier behaviours and outcome.

Decades of research have underscored the effectiveness of harm reduction strategies (Puzhko et al., 2022; Ruiz et al., 2019) in preventing deaths from overdoses, reducing the transmission of infectious diseases, lowering healthcare costs, and facilitating access to treatment and healthcare services for individuals who use drugs (Coye et al., 2021; Kim et al., 2014; Nassau et al., 2022; Surratt et al., 2020). These initiatives not only improve the health and well-being of affected individuals but also benefit the broader community by promoting safer practices and reducing the societal burden of drug-related harms.

HARM REDUCTION: ALCOHOL

Harm reduction strategies for alcohol focus on minimising the negative consequences associated with alcohol consumption, recognising that complete

Table 27.4
Harm reduction and injecting drug users

Safer injecting use

- Always inject with the blood flow.
- Rotate injection sites.
- Use sterile, new injecting equipment, with the smallest-bore needle possible.
- Avoid neck, groin, breast, feet, and hand veins. Mix powders with sterile water, and filter solution before injecting.
- Always dispose of equipment safely (either in a bin provided or by placing the needle inside the syringe and placing both inside a drinks can).
- Avoid injecting into infected areas.
- Do not inject into swollen limbs, even if the veins appear to be distended.
- Poor veins indicate a poor technique. Try to see what is going wrong.
- Do not inject on your own.
- Learn basic principles of first aid and cardiopulmonary resuscitation in order that you may help friends at times of crisis.

Method cleaning injecting equipment

1. Pour bleach into one cup (or bottle) and water into another.
2. Draw bleach up with the dirty needle and syringe.
3. Expel bleach into sink.
4. Repeat steps 2 and 3.
5. Draw water up through needle and syringe.
6. Expel water into sink.
7. Repeat steps 5 and 6 at least two or three times.

Source: Department of Health (1999).

abstinence may not be feasible or desirable for everyone. These approaches aim to promote safer drinking behaviours and reduce the risks of alcohol-related harm. The health education message advocating for moderate or controlled drinking serves as an alcohol harm reduction strategy, aiming to decrease problem drinking and its negative consequences. Alcohol harm reduction focuses on promoting moderate drinking, preventing problem drinking, and mitigating the adverse outcomes of alcohol misuse through practical approaches. Harm reduction offers a pragmatic approach to alcohol consumption and alcohol-related problems based on three core objectives:

- To reduce harmful consequences associated with alcohol use
- To provide an alternative to zero-tolerance approaches by incorporating drinking goals (abstinence or moderation) that are compatible with the needs of the individual
- To promote access to services by offering low-threshold alternatives to traditional alcohol prevention and treatment

(Marlatt & Witkiewitz, 2002).

Educational interventions, such as those targeting college students, have been successful in reducing alcohol consumption and related issues (Bewick et al., 2008). Screening and brief interventions in primary care settings have also shown promise in decreasing harmful alcohol use (Kaner et al., 2017). Moreover, policy interventions, including increasing alcohol taxes, have been associated with reductions in alcohol-related harm, including mortality and traffic fatalities (Wagenaar et al., 2010). Community-based programmes, such as designated driver initiatives, have effectively lowered alcohol-related motor vehicle crashes and injuries (Shults et al., 2001). Additionally, providing access to treatment and support services for alcohol use disorders has led to improved outcomes, including decreased alcohol consumption and healthcare utilisation (Williams et al., 2017). Table 27.5 details the examples and benefits of an alcohol harm reduction approach.

HARM REDUCTION: TOBACCO

Tobacco harm reduction (THR) is a range of practical policies, regulations, actions, and strategies that

Table 27.5
Examples and benefits of alcohol harm reduction approach

Examples of alcohol harm reduction approach	Benefits of alcohol harm reduction approach
• Promoting safer design of drinking environment • Campaigns against drinking and driving • Serving alcohol in shatter-proof glass to prevent injuries • Training bar staff to serve alcohol responsibly • Minimising violence and antisocial behaviour by managing drinking context • Screening patients for risky drinking behaviours during routine medical appointments • Brief interventions • May involve personalised feedback, goal-setting, and referrals to specialised treatment if necessary • Health education on controlled drinking in educational institutions • Providing shelters for homeless drinkers and intoxicated individuals • Implementing policies such as increased taxation on alcohol, restrictions on alcohol advertising, and marketing • Enforcing laws against underage drinking and drunk driving • Establishing community partnerships to organise alcohol-free events • Promoting designated driver programmes • Providing support services for individuals struggling with alcohol use disorder	• Practical approaches • Realistic approaches • Not based on national policies, legislation, or funding • Delivered by local communities based on local needs • Short-term aim: minimising the impacts of alcohol consumption • Long-term aim: changing drinking cultures, promoting the benefits of responsible drinking, and discouraging harmful drinking • Screening and brief interventions shown to reduce alcohol consumption, decrease the likelihood of developing alcohol-related problems, and improve overall health outcomes for individuals at risk • Community-based programmes creating supportive environments that encourage responsible drinking behaviours, foster social connections, and reduce the stigma associated with seeking help for alcohol-related problems

reduce health risks by providing safer forms of products/substances or encouraging less-risky behaviours (CASAA, 2024). It is around the idea of reducing the health risks associated with tobacco use, primarily by encouraging smokers to switch to less-harmful forms of nicotine consumption. This can include products such as electronic cigarettes (e-cigarettes), nicotine replacement therapies (like patches or gum), and smokeless tobacco products. The rationale behind THR is that while complete abstinence from nicotine is ideal, for many smokers, quitting altogether may be difficult or not immediately achievable. In such cases, transitioning to less-harmful alternatives can still provide significant health benefits by reducing exposure to the harmful chemicals found in tobacco smoke (Harm Reduction, 2022).

Advocates of THR promote switching to less-harmful nicotine delivery methods to reduce smoking-related diseases and deaths. However, ongoing debate and research surround THR, with critics raising concerns about the long-term health effects and potential risks of alternative nicotine products. Research on newer heated tobacco products (HTPs) is limited, with some evidence showing reduced exposure to harmful chemicals but lacking independent evidence proving they are less-harmful than cigarettes or aid in quitting smoking. A UK Cochrane review (Tattan-Birch et al., 2022) highlighted that all safety trials were funded by tobacco companies, with most trials showing unclear or high risk of bias. Independent research on HTPs' effectiveness and safety is deemed necessary. The term "endgame" in the context of tobacco control refers to the ultimate goal of achieving a tobacco-free society. In certain countries like New Zealand and Canada, discussions about "endgame" approaches to achieve a tobacco- and nicotine-free future are gaining momentum. These approaches include strategies like de-nicotinising tobacco products, aiming to gradually phase out nicotine from tobacco products as part of broader efforts to eliminate tobacco and nicotine use (Laugesen et al., 2010; van der Deen et al., 2018).

HARM REDUCTION: HIV AND BLOOD-BORNE INFECTIONS

Harm reduction strategies for preventing HIV transmission among injecting drug users include syringe exchange programmes, methadone maintenance therapy, hepatitis vaccination, promoting safer sexual practices, providing sexual health services, ensuring access to drug and HIV treatment, and offering clinical and home-based care. These interventions aim to reduce health and social risks associated with drug injection while addressing broader health needs. Table 27.6 shows the core package of interventions for HIV among injecting drug users (IDUs).

Table 27.6
Prevention strategies of HIV among IDUs: core package of interventions

Provisions	Descriptions
Syringe exchange programmes	Providing clean needles and syringes to IDUs to reduce the risk of HIV transmission through shared injection equipment
Opioid substitution therapy (e.g. methadone maintenance therapy)	Offering medication-assisted treatment to reduce drug dependency and associated risky injection practices
Hepatitis vaccination	Administering vaccines against hepatitis B and, where applicable, hepatitis C to prevent transmission among IDUs
Promotion of safer sexual practices	Encouraging the consistent use of condoms and other preventive measures to reduce the risk of sexual transmission of HIV and other sexually transmitted infections
Sexual health services	Providing access to comprehensive sexual health services, including testing, counselling, and treatment for sexually transmitted infections
Access to drug treatment	Ensuring IDUs have access to effective drug treatment programmes, including both pharmacological and psychosocial interventions
Access to HIV treatment	Access to HIV treatment: ensuring timely access to antiretroviral therapy for IDUs living with HIV to suppress viral load and reduce the risk of transmission
Clinical and home-based care	Providing medical care, support services, and adherence support for IDUs living with HIV/AIDS, including both clinical care and community-based support
Outreach and peer education	Mobilising trained outreach workers and peers from affected communities to engage with IDUs directly, providing them with information on harm reduction, HIV prevention, and available services

NEEDLE EXCHANGE SCHEMES

Syringe exchange schemes offer paraphernalia such as syringes, citric and vitamin C sachets, water ampoules, Stericups, and Sterifilts, along with educational resources on safer drug use, safer sexual practices, overdose prevention, and first aid. These interventions aim to empower injecting drug users to protect themselves and their communities by adopting safer injection practices and harm reduction methods. Needle and syringe programmes (NSPs) have been found effective in reducing HIV transmission and injection-related risk behaviours (IRB) among people who inject drugs (PWID) (Fernandes et al., 2017). However, the evidence regarding a reduction in hepatitis C virus (HCV) infection is mixed. Comprehensive harm reduction interventions implemented at the structural level and within multi-component programmes, coupled with high coverage rates, have shown greater effectiveness in achieving positive outcomes for PWID (Fernandes et al., 2017). The WHO (2004) report stresses that providing access to sterile needles and syringes is crucial for effective HIV prevention among people who inject drugs (PWID). It states that needle exchange programmes do not escalate drug use or the frequency of injection. However, it highlights the necessity of customising harm reduction efforts to address the unique requirements of populations with prevalent cocaine injection. Cocaine injectors often inject more frequently than do heroin users, necessitating greater quantities of sterile equipment.

Syringe dispensing machines and mobile vans are innovative components of needle exchange schemes, providing sterile injecting equipment to hard-to-reach and high-risk groups of injecting drug users (Islam & Conigrave, 2007). Dispensing machines, which exchange new for used syringes or provide sterile equipment for a fee or free of cost, offer access to services outside of traditional business hours, addressing the needs of individuals who require equipment in the evening, at night, or on weekends. Mobile vans, while not completely anonymous, offer outreach services to vulnerable groups, such as the homeless, chaotic users, young recreational drug users, and individuals from Black and ethnic minority groups. Both dispensing machines and mobile vans cater to diverse patterns of use, thereby enhancing efforts to reduce the spread of HIV and other blood-borne viruses among injecting drug users (Islam & Conigrave, 2007). Despite their versatility, mobile needle and syringe programmes encounter challenges related to service limitations, confidentiality, and constrained interaction duration due to physical space constraints. Evidence suggests that mobile NSPs contribute to reducing injection-related risks (Strike & Miskovic, 2018). Many needle exchange programmes primarily target self-identified injecting drug users and may overlook occasional or recreational drug users, particularly among young people. Therefore, it is essential to develop strategies specifically tailored to address the needs of young individuals who engage in occasional or recreational drug use. The "Nevershare syringe" represents a new technological innovation in the harm reduction approach for injecting drug users. Key features of the Nevershare syringe include plungers in a range of colours, which serve as visual identifiers for individual users. This color-coded system aims to reduce the likelihood of users mistakenly sharing syringes, as each person can easily distinguish their own syringe based on the colour of the plunger. By introducing such innovative syringe designs, harm reduction efforts aim to enhance safety and reduce the transmission of blood-borne infections, such as HIV and hepatitis C, among injecting drug users.

DRUG CONSUMPTION ROOMS

Drug consumption rooms (DCRs), also known as supervised injection facilities or safe injection sites, are designated spaces where individuals can use drugs under the supervision of trained staff. These facilities are designed to provide a safe and hygienic environment for people who use drugs, reducing the risks associated with drug injection, including overdose, transmission of infectious diseases, and public drug use. The primary goals of drug consumption rooms are to reduce the risk of overdose deaths, prevent the transmission of infectious diseases, improve access to healthcare and social services, and ultimately, promote the health and well-being of individuals who use drugs and the broader community. While DCRs have been implemented in various countries around the world, their establishment and operation often involve legal and political challenges, as well as ongoing evaluation and research to assess their effectiveness and impact. Supervised injection sites (SISs) were not found to lead to increased drug injecting, drug trafficking, or crime in their surrounding areas; instead, SISs were associated with a decrease in public drug injections and discarded syringes (Potier et al., 2014).

KEY POINTS

- *Harm reduction* means trying to reduce the harm that people do to themselves, or other people, from their substance use.
- Harm reduction can work alongside approaches that aim for reductions in drug, alcohol, and tobacco consumption.
- Harm reduction focuses on safer drug use and safer sexual practices.
- It provides better outcomes for substance misusers, as a small reduction in alcohol or drug misuse is better than zero reduction.
- Harm reduction programmes include supervised consumption of methadone or other opiate substitutes and needle exchange schemes (pharmacy-based needle exchange or other forms of needle exchange).
- A comprehensive alcohol policy needs population-level interventions, which focus on the availability and accessibility of alcohol and alcohol harm reduction interventions.
- The harm reduction approach to tobacco smoking has remained controversial despite the universal use of tobacco.
- Currently, the tobacco harm reduction strategy is based on supply-and-demand reduction strategies.
- In the context of HIV and other blood-borne diseases, harm reduction strategies aim to reduce the health and social harms of drug injecting.
- There was no evidence that needle exchange programmes increased either the number of people using drugs or the frequency of injecting drug use.
- Many needle exchanges often target self-identified injecting drug users and miss occasional or recreational drug users, especially among young people.
- A *drug consumption room* is a place where problem drug users are allowed to bring their illegally obtained drugs and take them in a supervised, hygienic environment.

Activity 27.3

Questions

- Discuss the benefits and limitations of the harm reduction approach.
- Identify the hierarchy of goals for drug misusers to reach the abstinence stage.
- Discuss the harm reduction approach to drug, alcohol, tobacco, and blood-borne and HIV infections.
- Explain what is meant by safer drug use and safer sex practice.
- Discuss the advantages and limitations of needle and syringe exchange schemes.
- What are the rationale for dispensing machines and mobile vans in the provision of injecting equipment?
- Examine the benefits and limitations of "drug consumption rooms."

References

Bewick, B. M., Trusler, K., Barkham, M., Hill, A. J., Cahill, J., & Mulhern, B. (2008). The effectiveness of web-based interventions designed to decrease alcohol consumption – a systematic review. *Preventive Medicine, 47*(1), 17–26. https://doi.org/10.1016/j.ypmed.2008.01.005.

CASAA. (2024). *Tobacco Harm Reduction*. Consumer Advocates for Smoke-Free Alternatives Association. https://casaa.org/education/#THR (accessed 9 April 2024).

Coye, A. E., Bornstein, K. J., Bartholomew, T. S., Li, H., Wong, S., Janjua, N. Z., Tookes, H. E., & St Onge, J. E. (2021). Hospital costs of injection drug use in Florida. *Clinical Infectious Diseases: An Official Publication of the Infectious Diseases Society of America, 72*(3), 499–502. https://doi.org/10.1093/cid/ciaa823.

Department of Health. (1999). *Drug Misuse and Dependence-Guidelines on Clinical Management*. London: HMSO.

Erickson, P. G. (1999). Introduction: The three phases of harm reduction. An examination of emerging concepts, methodologies, and critiques. *Substance Use & Misuse, 34*(1), 1–7. https://doi.org/10.3109/10826089909035631.

Fernandes, R. M., Cary, M., Duarte, G., Jesus, G., Alarcão, J., Torre, C., Costa, S., Costa, J., & Carneiro, A. V. (2017). Effectiveness of needle and syringe programmes in people who inject drugs – an overview of systematic reviews.

BMC Public Health, 17(1), 309. https://doi.org/10.1186/s12889-017-4210-2.

Harm Reduction. (2022). *Tobacco Tactics*. https://tobaccotactics.org/article/harm-reduction (accessed 9 April 2024).

Harm Reduction Coalition. *Principles of Harm Reduction*. https://harmreduction.org/about-us/principles-of-harm-reduction/ (accessed 8 March 2024).

Islam, M. M., & Conigrave, K. M. (2007). Assessing the role of syringe dispensing machines and mobile van outlets in reaching hard-to-reach and high-risk groups of injecting drug users (IDUs): A review. *Harm Reduction Journal,* 4, 14. https://doi.org/10.1186/1477-7517-4-14.

Kaner, E. F., Beyer, F. R., Garnett, C., Crane, D., Brown, J., Muirhead, C., Redmore, J., O'Donnell, A., Newham, J. J., de Vocht, F., Hickman, M., Brown, H., Maniatopoulos, G., & Michie, S. (2017). Personalised digital interventions for reducing hazardous and harmful alcohol consumption in community-dwelling populations. *The Cochrane Database of Systematic Reviews,* 9(9), CD011479. https://doi.org/10.1002/14651858.CD011479.pub2.

Kim, S. W., Pulkki-Brannstrom, A. M., & Skordis-Worrall, J. (2014). Comparing the cost effectiveness of harm reduction strategies: A case study of the Ukraine. *Cost Effectiveness and Resource Allocation: C/E,* 12, 25. https://doi.org/10.1186/1478-7547-12-25.

Laugesen, M., Glover, M., Fraser, T., McCormick, R., & Scott, J. (2010). Four policies to end the sale of cigarettes and smoking tobacco in New Zealand by 2020. *The New Zealand Medical Journal,* 123(1314), 55–67.

Marlatt, G. A., & Witkiewitz, K. (2002). Harm reduction approaches to alcohol use: Health promotion, prevention, and treatment. *Addictive Behaviors,* 27(6), 867–886. https://doi.org/10.1016/s0306-4603(02)00294-0.

Nassau, T., Kolla, G., Mason, K., Hopkins, S., Tookey, P., McLean, E., Werb, D., & Scheim, A. (2022). Service utilization patterns and characteristics among clients of integrated supervised consumption sites in Toronto, Canada. *Harm Reduction Journal,* 19(1), 33. https://doi.org/10.1186/s12954-022-00610-y.

Potier, C., Laprévote, V., Dubois-Arber, F., Cottencin, O., & Rolland, B. (2014). Supervised injection services: What has been demonstrated? A systematic literature review. *Drug and Alcohol Dependence,* 145, 48–68. https://doi.org/10.1016/j.drugalcdep.2014.10.012.

Puzhko, S., Eisenberg, M. J., Filion, K. B., Windle, S. B., Hébert-Losier, A., Gore, G., Paraskevopoulos, E., Martel, M. O., & Kudrina, I. (2022). Effectiveness of interventions for prevention of common infections among opioid users: A systematic review of systematic reviews. *Frontiers in Public Health,* 10, 749033. https://doi.org/10.3389/fpubh.2022.749033.

Ruiz, M. S., O'Rourke, A., Allen, S. T., Holtgrave, D. R., Metzger, D., Benitez, J., Brady, K. A., Chaulk, C. P., & Wen, L. S. (2019). Using interrupted time series analysis to measure the impact of legalized syringe exchange on HIV diagnoses in Baltimore and Philadelphia. *Journal of Acquired Immune Deficiency Syndromes (1999),* 82(2), S148–S154. https://doi.org/10.1097/QAI.0000000000002176.

Shults, R. A., Elder, R. W., Sleet, D. A., Nichols, J. L., Alao, M. O., Carande-Kulis, V. G., Zaza, S., Sosin, D. M., Thompson, R. S., & Task Force on Community Preventive Services. (2001). Reviews of evidence regarding interventions to reduce alcohol-impaired driving. *American Journal of Preventive Medicine,* 21(Suppl 4), 66–88. https://doi.org/10.1016/s0749-3797(01)00381-6.

Strike, C., & Miskovic, M. (2018). Scoping out the literature on mobile needle and syringe programs-review of service delivery and client characteristics, operation, utilization, referrals, and impact. *Harm Reduction Journal,* 15(1), 6. https://doi.org/10.1186/s12954-018-0212-3.

Surratt, H. L., Otachi, J. K., Williams, T., Gulley, J., Lockard, A. S., & Rains, R. (2020). Motivation to change and treatment participation among syringe service program utilizers in rural Kentucky. *The Journal of Rural Health: Official Journal of the American Rural Health Association and the National Rural Health Care Association,* 36(2), 224–233. https://doi.org/10.1111/jrh.12388.

Tattan-Birch, H., Hartmann-Boyce, J., Kock, L., Simonavicius, E., Brose, L., Jackson, S., Shahab, L., & Brown, J. (2022). Heated tobacco products for smoking cessation and reducing smoking prevalence. *The Cochrane Database of Systematic Reviews,* 1(1), CD013790. https://doi.org/10.1002/14651858.CD013790.pub2.

van der Deen, F. S., Wilson, N., Cleghorn, C. L., Kvizhinadze, G., Cobiac, L. J., Nghiem, N., & Blakely, T. (2018). Impact of five tobacco endgame strategies on future smoking prevalence, population health and health system costs: Two modelling studies to inform the tobacco endgame. *Tobacco Control,* 27(3), 278–286. https://doi.org/10.1136/tobaccocontrol-2016-053585.

Wagenaar, A. C., Tobler, A. L., & Komro, K. A. (2010). Effects of alcohol tax and price policies on morbidity and mortality: A systematic review. *American Journal of Public Health,* 100(11), 2270–2278. https://doi.org/10.2105/AJPH.2009.186007.

WHO. (2004). *Effectiveness of Sterile Needle and Syringe Programming in Reducing HIV/AIDS Among Injecting Drug Users*. Geneva: World Health Organization.

Williams, E. C., Lapham, G. T., Bobb, J. F., Rubinsky, A. D., Catz, S. L., Shortreed, S. M., Bensley, K. M., & Bradley, K. A. (2017). Documented brief intervention not associated with resolution of unhealthy alcohol use one year later among VA patients living with HIV. *Journal of Substance Abuse Treatment,* 78, 8–14. https://doi.org/10.1016/j.jsat.2017.04.006.

Chapter 28

Intoxication and overdose

Health interventions

Learning outcomes

- Define *intoxication* and *overdose*.
- Identify the reasons for emergency medical attention.
- Discuss the effects of acute intoxication.
- Identify the risks associated with alcohol and drug misuse.
- Describe the interventions in acute intoxication.
- Identify the risk factors associated with an increased likelihood of overdose.
- Describe the interventions in overdose.

Activity 28.1 Intoxication and overdose.

Please state whether the following statements are true or false. Reflect on the statements and give reason(s) for choosing a particular option.

Statements	True	False
Intoxication and overdose are the potential consequences of substance misuse.		
Psychoactive substances taken in combination with alcohol or drugs are considered safe.		
Intoxication is a state when there is an intake of more than the normal amount of a psychoactive substance.		
An *overdose* is the accidental or intentional use of a psychoactive substance which exceeds the individual's tolerance.		
Some medical or psychological conditions may mimic or mask the symptoms of alcohol or drug intoxication.		
The cultural and personal expectations regarding the effects of the drug will also influence the level of intoxication.		
Trauma and head injuries increase the risk of seizures.		
Substance misusers have a lower risk of suicide than the general population.		
Drug overdose is the most common method of suicide amongst substance misusers.		

DOI: 10.4324/9781003456674-33

Statements	True	False
Combining heroin with cocaine as a "speedball" can increase the chances of an overdose.		
The use of antidepressants amongst polysubstance users has been found to heighten the risk of fatality.		
The treatment for overdose from opiates is the antidote naloxone hydrochloride.		
Overdose of GHB can be difficult to treat because of its multiple effects on the body.		

Activity 28.2

There is only one correct answer to the following multiple-choice questions.

1. What is the definition of *intoxication*?
   a. Excessive consumption of alcohol or drugs leading to impaired judgement
   b. The state of being completely sober and lucid
   c. Consuming moderate amounts of alcohol or drugs without impairment
   d. Having a high tolerance to alcohol or drugs
   e. None of the above
2. Which of the following are reasons for seeking emergency medical attention in cases of intoxication?
   a. Severe headache
   b. Loss of consciousness
   c. Slurred speech
   d. Difficulty breathing
   e. All of the above
3. What are the effects of acute intoxication?
   a. Increased coordination and alertness
   b. Enhanced decision-making skills
   c. Impaired judgement and coordination
   d. Improved memory and cognitive function
   e. None of the above
4. Which of the following are risks associated with alcohol and drug misuse?
   a. Increased risk of addiction
   b. Liver damage
   c. Accidental injuries
   d. Impaired driving
   e. All of the above
5. What are the interventions in acute intoxication?
   a. Administering naloxone
   b. Providing emotional support
   c. Encouraging the individual to consume more alcohol or drugs
   d. Calling emergency services
   e. None of the above

6. Which of the following are risk factors associated with an increased likelihood of overdose?
   a. Mixing alcohol with prescription medications
   b. Having a low tolerance to drugs
   c. Using drugs alone
   d. Using drugs in a controlled environment
   e. None of the above
7. What interventions should be implemented in cases of overdose?
   a. Providing supportive care
   b. Administering naloxone for opioid overdoses
   c. Monitoring vital signs
   d. Calling emergency services
   e. All of the above
8. *Intoxication* is defined as:
   a. The presence of alcohol or drugs in the body
   b. The state of being completely free from alcohol or drugs
   c. The consumption of excessive amounts of alcohol or drugs, leading to impaired functioning
   d. The ability to consume large quantities of alcohol or drugs without feeling intoxicated
   e. None of the above
9. Which of the following is NOT a reason for seeking emergency medical attention in cases of intoxication?
   a. Loss of consciousness
   b. Severe headache
   c. Difficulty breathing
   d. Slurred speech
   e. All of the above
10. Acute intoxication can result in:
    a. Improved cognitive function
    b. Enhanced decision-making abilities
    c. Impaired judgement and coordination
    d. Increased alertness
    e. None of the above
11. Risks associated with alcohol and drug misuse include:
    a. Decreased risk of addiction
    b. Improved liver function
    c. Accidental injuries
    d. Enhanced driving skills
    e. None of the above
12. Interventions in cases of acute intoxication may include:
    a. Encouraging the individual to consume more alcohol or drugs
    b. Administering naloxone
    c. Providing emotional support
    d. Avoiding contact with emergency services
    e. None of the above
13. Which of the following is a risk factor associated with an increased likelihood of overdose?
    a. Using drugs in a controlled environment
    b. Having a high tolerance to drugs
    c. Using drugs alone
    d. Avoiding mixing alcohol with prescription medications
    e. None of the above

14. Interventions in cases of overdose typically involve:
    a. Providing supportive care
    b. Monitoring vital signs
    c. Administering naloxone for opioid overdoses
    d. Avoiding contact with emergency services
    e. All of the above
15. Overdose occurs when:
    a. An individual consumes a small amount of alcohol or drugs
    b. An individual consumes a large amount of alcohol or drugs
    c. An individual experiences adverse effects from alcohol or drug use
    d. An individual exhibits enhanced cognitive function after consuming alcohol or drugs
    e. None of the above

INTRODUCTION

Intoxication and overdose are the potential consequences of substance misuse whether the psychoactive substance is illicit, prescribed, or over-the-counter. Emergency medical attention is often required by those misusing psychoactive substances as a result of:

- Toxic or adverse effects of the substance
- The route of administration (injecting may lead to blood poisoning and deep vein thrombosis)
- Lifestyle behaviours (poor nutrition, dehydration)
- Risk-taking whilst under the influence of psychoactive substances (accidents, self-harm)

This chapter addresses the dual aspects of substance misuse: intoxication and overdose, highlighting the heightened risks associated with combining psychoactive substances with alcohol or other drugs. *Intoxication* is defined as the consumption of an excessive amount of a psychoactive substance, resulting in behavioural or physical alterations. On the contrary, an overdose occurs when an individual unintentionally or purposefully consumes a psychoactive substance beyond their tolerance level, posing a risk of death. The chapter emphasises the serious long-term consequences of such actions. Additionally, it outlines relevant health interventions aimed at addressing intoxication and overdose.

ACUTE INTOXICATION

Acute intoxication often manifests in individuals with persistent alcohol- or drug-related issues, characterised by temporary disturbances in consciousness, cognition, perception, affect, behaviour, and physiological functions following the consumption of psychoactive substances. Most psychoactive substances affect the central nervous and cardiopulmonary systems, with the type, dose, and individual tolerance level significantly impacting the degree of intoxication. Recognising the symptoms of alcohol or drug intoxication is crucial not only for confirming their presence and severity but also for distinguishing them from other conditions that may mimic or mask these symptoms. The expected effects of psychoactive substances may not always align with the actual symptoms experienced; for instance, depressant drugs like alcohol or GHB may induce agitation, while stimulants like amphetamine or cocaine may result in withdrawn behaviour. Factors such as body weight, tolerance, volume, and concentration of alcohol consumed, duration of consumption, and personal and cultural expectations influence the level of intoxication. Common features of psychoactive intoxication include disinhibition, euphoria, impaired coordination, and judgement. Importantly, alcohol and drug intoxication can affect mental health and may mimic or obscure symptoms of underlying mental or physical disorders. The resulting lack of inhibition and central nervous system depression may elevate the risk of self-harm, harm to others, and suicide.

RISKS OF ALCOHOL AND DRUG INTOXICATION

Individuals in an acute stage of alcohol intoxication are frequently observed in A&E departments, where treatment is rarely required but may be necessary if seizures are precipitated due to the lowering of seizure threshold levels by alcohol. Paradoxically, alcohol withdrawal symptoms, including seizures, may occur during intoxication due to a relative drop in alcohol levels. Vomiting is common among intoxicated individuals, but persistent vomiting may indicate head injury or other serious illness. Alcohol and drugs impair coordination and reactions, increasing the risk of accidents and trauma. Head injuries caused by poor coordination and judgement while intoxicated are prevalent, with head injury also elevating the risk of seizures. Acute alcohol poisoning can lead to respiratory arrest and choking on vomit, especially while asleep. Homeless problem-drinkers are at high risk of hypothermia, and their behaviour may become belligerent, paranoid, or violent, requiring cautious and sensitive approaches. The use, desired effects, and acute intoxication of psychoactive substances are further discussed in Chapters 7 to 12.

INTERVENTIONS IN ACUTE INTOXICATION

Health interventions are based on the urgency and seriousness of the individual with acute intoxication. When an individual is acutely intoxicated, first aid procedures are implemented in relation to:

- A – airway
- B – breathing
- C – circulation/cardiac

The interventions required for an individual with acute intoxication are presented in Table 28.1.

Additional interventions for individuals with alcohol and drug-related issues include monitoring withdrawal syndrome; screening for substance use problems through assessments and testing; referring individuals to appropriate services; providing contact points for further assistance, such as self-help groups; offering harm reduction advice; distributing informational literature on overdose prevention and viral transmission; and fostering close collaboration with drug treatment providers to improve access to treatment. These interventions aim to address various aspects of substance misuse, enhance awareness, promote harm reduction, and facilitate access to comprehensive care and support services.

OVERDOSE

An overdose occurs when an individual consumes or is exposed to an excessive amount of a substance, such as drugs or alcohol, beyond the body's tolerance level. This excessive intake can lead to harmful effects, including severe toxicity, impairment of bodily functions, and in some cases, death. Overdose can result from intentional or unintentional consumption and may involve a single substance or multiple substances. There has been concern about the high prevalence of mortality amongst substance misusers as a result of overdose. Globally, it is estimated that drug-related deaths with overdose account for up to half of all deaths, with opioids involved in most cases (UNDOC, 2016). Worldwide, opioids accounted for nearly 80% of these deaths, with opioid overdose being responsible for around 25% of opioid-related deaths (WHO,

Table 28.1
Health interventions: intoxication

Medical/physical needs	Psychosocial needs
• Place in recovery position – if appropriate. • Assessment of airway, breathing, and circulation. • Assess level of consciousness (Glasgow coma scale). • Monitor vital signs. • Implement seizure safety precautions. • Monitor fluid intake and output. • Implement interventions to decrease systemic absorption of drugs (use of absorbents [activated charcoal], induced diarrhoea, induced vomiting, gastric lavage) if appropriate. • Administration of antidote, if appropriate.	• Orientation. • "Being there." • Non-judgemental approach in interactions. • Create a supportive environment. • Assess for "risk behaviours" (self-harm, potential for violence). • Contact relatives/friends who are best able to support and reassure the patient.

2023). Opioid overdoses that do not lead to death are several times more common than fatal overdoses. Fentanyl is a highly potent synthetic opioid and chemically similar analogues, such as carfentanil, acetylfentanyl, butyrfentanyl, and furanyl, have been linked to a significant increase in opioid overdose deaths (WHO, 2023). Fentanyl potency can lead to respiratory depression, overdose, and death even in small doses, contributing to the opioid crisis worldwide. Prompt medical intervention is essential to address an overdose and prevent further harm or fatalities.

Drug overdose can result in serious health implications, including respiratory or circulatory failure, as well as damage to major organs, like the kidneys or liver. The pattern of drug overdoses has evolved over recent years, influenced by changes in drug availability and accessibility. Substance misusers, particularly those taking prescribed drugs like antidepressants and methadone, are at higher risk of suicide. Drug overdose is the most common method of suicide among substance misusers, especially when drugs are taken by injection. Fatal overdose, resulting in immediate death, is particularly associated with injecting opioid users (Oyefeso et al., 1999). The misuse of combinations of psychoactive substances, such as benzodiazepines and alcohol with opiates, or the combination of heroin with cocaine as a "speedball," can significantly increase the risk of overdose. In a prospective study by Gossop et al. (2002) on mortality among drug misusers, the majority of deaths (68%) were associated with drug overdoses, with opiates being the most commonly detected substances during post-mortem examinations. Polydrug use, particularly heavy drinking, benzodiazepine use, and amphetamine use, were identified as risk factors for mortality. Additionally, the use of antidepressants among polysubstance users has been found to further heighten the risk of fatality (Oyefeso et al., 2000). Several risk factors are associated with an increased likelihood of overdose, including:

- Administration by injection
- Concomitant use of other depressant drugs
- Loss of tolerance after a period of abstinence
- Injecting in public places or solitary drug use
- Long history of opiate dependence
- Older age
- Unexpected changes in drug purity

There are a number of risk factors for opioid overdose, as depicted in Table 28.2.

These risk factors contribute to the incidence of overdose, particularly when multiple factors are present simultaneously. A summary of the

Table 28.2
Risk factors for opioid overdose

Problem	Descriptions
Having a disorder	Having an opioid use disorder
Injecting	Taking opioids by injection
Abstinence	Resumption of opioid use after an extended period of abstinence (e.g. following detoxification, release from incarceration, cessation of treatment)
Tolerance	High opioid tolerance due to prolonged opioid use
Prescription opioids	Using prescription opioids without medical supervision
High prescribed dosage	High prescribed dosage of opioids (more than 100 mg of morphine or equivalent daily)
Combined psychoactive substances	Using opioids in combination with alcohol and/or other substances or medicines that suppress respiratory function, such as benzodiazepines, barbiturates, anaesthetics, or some pain medications
Concurrent medical conditions	Having concurrent medical conditions, such as HIV, liver or lung diseases, or mental health conditions
Gender, age, and status	Males, people of older age, and people with low socio-economic status at higher risk of opioid overdose than women, people of young age groups, and people with higher socio-economic status
Opioids potency	Using opioids of unknown potency or purity, such as illicitly obtained drugs
Lack of access	Lack of access to overdose reversal medications, like naloxone; lack of access to addiction treatment and harm reduction services

Table 28.3
Predictors of risk associated with overdose

- Injecting drugs (heroin users, high level of dependence)
- Polydrug use (combinations of drugs, such as heroin, methadone, alcohol, and benzodiazepines)
- High tolerance levels (users who have experienced non-fatal overdoses recently)
- Low tolerance levels (using opiates when tolerance is low, particularly after a break in use following imprisonment or detoxification)
- Cocaine and crack (cocaine and crack use among heroin users can play a role in fatal overdoses, as they can temporarily mask the sedative effects of heroin and other depressant-type drugs)
- Poor mental health, depression, hopelessness, and suicidal thoughts
- Not being in treatment (heroin injectors not in methadone treatment are around four times more likely to die in comparison to those in treatment)
- Premature termination of treatment (loss of tolerance, increased polydrug use after detoxification)
- Solitary alcohol or drug use (using drugs alone, especially injecting, places a person at increased risk)

Source: Adapted from Roberts and McVeigh (2004).

predictors of the risk factors associated with incidence of overdose is presented in Table 28.3.

INTERVENTIONS WITH OVERDOSE

Drug overdose among substance misusers is a prevalent and potentially life-threatening emergency, often leading them to seek initial medical care in emergency departments. Immediate intervention is crucial in such cases, with priority given to addressing life-threatening complications, such as respiratory depression, airway obstruction, cardiovascular collapse, and seizures. Treatment should commence promptly upon presentation, focusing on stabilising the individual's vital functions while also addressing the specific drug overdose involved. These interventions aim to mitigate immediate risks and improve outcomes for individuals experiencing drug overdose.

Emergency interventions include:

- Establish a patent airway.
- Provide ventilation support (artificial respiration, respirator).
- Maintain adequate circulatory status (chest compressions, defibrillator, intravenous line).
- Control seizures (safety measures, intravenous diazepam).
- Administer drugs, if appropriate (for example, opiate overdose – naloxone).

After implementing acute interventions to stabilise the individual, a comprehensive assessment is conducted, which includes obtaining a detailed history and performing a physical examination. Information regarding the substance involved in the overdose, including its name, route of administration, amount taken, and timing of ingestion, is gathered. If the individual is unable to provide information, collateral information should be sought from family members, significant others, or past medical records. Routine investigations, such as blood count, chemistry, urinalysis, and toxicological screens of blood and urine, are performed to further evaluate the overdose. Vital signs, including temperature, are monitored regularly, and electrocardiogram (ECG) monitoring is initiated and continued. The level of consciousness is assessed and monitored using the Glasgow coma scale at 15-minute intervals (Teasdale & Jennett, 1974). Continuing interventions for overdose management are outlined in Table 28.4, providing a structured approach to ongoing care and monitoring.

Table 28.4
Continuing interventions in overdose

- Monitor vital signs, including temperature.
- Perform EEG and continue to monitor.
- Check the level of consciousness and continue to monitor at 15-minute intervals using the Glasgow coma scale (Teasdale & Jennett, 1974).
- Maintain hydration and monitor fluid intake and output.
- Safety precautions must be maintained during acute interventions as the individual may show signs of varying levels of consciousness, hallucinations, and seizures.
- Provide reassurance and support.
- Measures to decrease systemic absorption of the substance, such as gastric lavage, induced emesis (vomiting), absorbents (activated charcoal), or induced diarrhoea (magnesium), should be used as appropriate.
- An antidote may be administered depending upon the type of psychoactive substance used.

In cases of loss of consciousness, it is crucial not to assume that alcohol or drugs are the sole cause, as there are various potential underlying factors. Other possible causes include trauma, epilepsy, diabetes, hepatic failure, hypercalcemia, renal failure, cerebral haemorrhage, thrombosis, abscess, tumour, arrhythmias, myocardial infarction, and infections, such as meningitis or encephalitis. After treating the overdose, it is important to assess for depression or self-harm, explore withdrawal management and treatment intervention options, and provide harm reduction interventions and health information, including information about specialist alcohol or drug services.

INTERVENTIONS FOR OPIATE OVERDOSE

Opiate users are prone to accidental overdose because they often overestimate their own tolerance or are unaware of the potency of the drug they use. The presenting features of opiate overdose are:

- Slow respiration (two to seven breaths/minute), usually deep compared with the shallow and more rapid respiration associated with intoxication by barbiturates, etc.
- Pinpoint pupils
- Cyanosis, weak pulse, bradycardia
- Possible pulmonary oedema
- Twitching of muscles
- Subnormal temperature may occur

Naloxone hydrochloride is the antidote for opiate overdose, typically administered intravenously for rapid effect, but also available through intramuscular injection, subcutaneous injection, or nasal spray. A dose of 0.8 to 2 mg intravenously, repeated every 2–3 minutes up to a maximum of 10 mg, is recommended. If intravenous access is unavailable, subcutaneous or intramuscular routes are alternatives. Naloxone is short-acting, necessitating repeated doses or infusion for longer-acting opiates like methadone, which can prolong effects up to 72 hours. Patients should be monitored inpatient for up to 72 hours, especially after high-dose intoxication. Naloxone infusion may be considered for severe cases.

TAKE-HOME NALOXONE

The distribution of naloxone through programmes informally referred to as "take-home naloxone" has emerged as a key intervention to reduce opioid overdose deaths. The World Health Organization (WHO, 2014) recommended that take-home naloxone programmes be expanded to increase accessibility and save the lives of drug users. Many countries have implemented such programmes, allowing naloxone to be supplied to anyone according to Public Health England (2015):

- Currently using illicit opiates, such as heroin
- Receiving opioid substitution therapy
- Leaving prison with a history of drug use
- Those who have previously used opiate drugs (to protect in the event of relapse)

In take-home naloxone programmes, information, advice, and training on naloxone products are provided to people who use drugs, as well as their families, carers, and peers, to equip them to respond effectively to overdose emergencies. Due to the urgency of opiate overdose situations, self-administration of naloxone is unlikely, hence the importance of educating individuals on how to administer it to others. In some countries, naloxone is available only by prescription, necessitating direct prescription to a named patient or special dispensation to an individual or family member.

Research on community-based programmes has consistently shown that drug users, their peers, and other potential first responders are capable of being trained to recognise overdoses and administer naloxone effectively (Clark et al., 2014; Mueller et al., 2015; Williams et al., 2014). A systematic review of take-home naloxone programme's effectiveness revealed that combining naloxone provision with overdose education and first aid training resulted in reduced overdose mortality (EMCDDA, 2016). Take-home naloxone programmes have been shown to effectively decrease overdose mortality both among programme participants and in the broader community, with a minimal incidence of adverse events.

OVERDOSE OF SYNTHETIC OPIOIDS AND CANNABINOIDS

In opioid overdose, the classic symptoms include miosis (pinpoint pupils), respiratory depression, and decreased level of consciousness or coma, known as the "opioid overdose triad" (Schiller et al., 2023). Severe opioid toxicity can lead to respiratory arrest and death, particularly when vomiting occurs, heightening the risk of aspiration. Synthetic opioids may induce further adverse effects, including changes in muscle tone, chest wall rigidity, seizure-like activity, confusion, mood alterations, cough suppression, orthostatic hypotension, urinary issues, folliculitis, dermatitis with hair loss, dry eyes, elevated liver enzymes, and delayed bilateral hearing loss (Helander et al., 2014; Helander et al., 2017; Siddiqi et al., 2015). In opioid overdose, rapid recognition of overdose symptoms and prompt initiation of appropriate medical interventions are crucial to improve outcomes and reduce the risk of mortality. In the initial management of opioid overdose, it is crucial to prioritise protecting the airway and sustaining breathing and circulation, similar to any emergency situation. Naloxone, the antidote for opioid overdose, can be administered via various routes, including intravenous, intramuscular, intranasal, intraosseous, subcutaneous, endotracheal, inhalational, and sublingual routes. However, opioid overdose management requires ongoing monitoring and supportive care to prevent recurrence and address potential complications.

Emergency departments are observing a rising number of overdoses involving synthetic cannabinoids, such as K2 and spice. These overdoses manifest not only with symptoms like agitation, paranoia, anxiety, and confusion but also with medical complications, including palpitations, hypertension, nausea, vomiting, and seizures (Ford et al., 2017). There is also Evidence suggests that cannabis-related emergency department (ED) visits are often due to acute intoxication/overdose, pediatric exposure, cannabinoid hyperemesis syndrome, cannabis withdrawal, e-cigarette or vaping product use-associated lung injury (EVALI), and synthetic cannabinoids (Takakuwa & Schears, 2021). In addition, acute intoxication/overdose of synthetic cannabinoids was related to agitation, central nervous system depression/coma, and delirium/toxic psychosis (Riederer et al., 2016). Management of synthetic cannabinoid overdose involves supportive care to address symptoms such as agitation, anxiety, and cardiovascular effects. Additionally, patients may require sedation, antipsychotic medications, or benzodiazepines to manage severe symptoms. There is an investigation of the use of cannabidiol (CBD) as a potential method to manage overdose and toxicity associated with synthetic cannabinoids (Meredith et al., 2020).

INTERVENTIONS FOR OTHER DRUGS OVERDOSE

In cases of overdose from drugs such as amphetamines, cocaine, cannabis, LSD, ecstasy, barbiturates, and alcohol, no specific antidote exists. Thus, maintaining respiration through artificial means until the drugs are metabolised and removed from the system is crucial. Some drugs may aid in accelerating the excretion of barbiturates. When individuals misuse substances, they may commonly use tricyclic antidepressants. In high doses, these antidepressants can induce coma, cardiac arrhythmias, and anticholinergic effects and pose a high risk of mortality. Treatment interventions for overdose should be directed towards addressing the presenting symptoms and may include:

- Management of the unconscious patient
- Management of hypothermia
- Management of acute psychosis

Overdosing on GHB (gamma-hydroxybutyrate) can be challenging to manage due to its diverse effects on the body. GHB overdose commonly leads to life-threatening respiratory depression, bradycardia, and subsequent heart failure. Additionally, GHB ingestion often induces nausea and vomiting, particularly when combined with alcohol. Consequently, individuals who misuse GHB may experience unconsciousness, vomiting, and convulsions simultaneously (Miotto & Roth, 2001). The most significant risk of death from GHB overdose is aspiration of vomit while unconscious. Individuals are prone to vomiting as they lose consciousness and regain consciousness. This risk can be mitigated by placing them in the recovery position.

KEY POINTS

- Intoxication and overdose are the potential consequences of substance misuse, whether the psychoactive substance is illicit, prescribed, or over-the-counter.
- Psychoactive substances taken in combination with alcohol or drugs increase the risk of death by overdose and can have serious long-term consequences.
- Acute intoxication frequently occurs in persons who have more persistent alcohol- or drug-related problems.

- The type and dose of drug and the individual's level of tolerance have a significant influence on the state of intoxication.
- Alcohol and drug intoxication may influence a person's mental health and may imitate or mask symptoms of an underlying mental or physical disorder.
- Drug-related deaths are deaths where the underlying cause is poisoning, alcohol, or substance use disorder.
- Substance misusers are at higher risk of suicide than the general population, and prescribed drugs, notably antidepressants and methadone, heighten that risk.
- Drug overdose is the most common method of suicide amongst substance misusers, and the likelihood of overdose is increased when drugs are taken by injection.
- Fatal overdose (immediate death) is particularly associated with injecting opioid users.
- Overdose amongst substance misusers is an acute life-threatening emergency.
- The treatment of overdose from opiates is the antidote naloxone hydrochloride (naloxone).
- In take-home naloxone programmes, information of the naloxone products, advice, and training are provided to people who use drugs and to their families, carers, and peers, to enable them to respond in the event of an overdose emergency.
- No antidote exists for the treatment of overdose from other drugs such as amphetamines, cocaine, cannabis, LSD, ecstasy, barbiturates, and alcohol.

References

Clark, A. K., Wilder, C. M., & Winstanley, E. L. (2014). A systematic review of community opioid overdose prevention and naloxone distribution programs. *Journal of Addiction Medicine,* 8(3), 153–163.

EMCDDA. (2016). *Preventing Opioid Overdose Deaths with Take-Home Naloxone.* Luxembourg: The European Monitoring Centre for Drugs and Drug Addiction (EMCDDA), Publications Office of the European Union.

Ford, B. M., Tai, S., Fantegrossi, W. E., & Prather, P. L. (2017). Synthetic pot: Not your grandfather's marijuana. *Trends in Pharmacological Sciences,* 38(3), 257–276. https://doi.org/10.1016/j.tips.2016.12.003.

Gossop, M., Duncan, S., Samantha, T., & Marsden, J. (2002). A prospective study of mortality among drug misusers during a 4-year period after seeking treatment. *Addiction,* 97(1), 39–47.

Helander, A., Bäckberg, M., & Beck, O. (2014). MT-45, a new psychoactive substance associated with hearing loss and unconsciousness. *Clinical Toxicology,* 52(8), 901–904. https://doi.org/10.3109/15563650.2014.943908.

Helander, A., Bradley, M., Hasselblad, A., Norlén, L., Vassilaki, I., Bäckberg, M., & Lapins, J. (2017). Acute skin and hair symptoms followed by severe, delayed eye complications in subjects using the synthetic opioid MT-45. *The British Journal of Dermatology,* 176(4), 1021–1027. https://doi.org/10.1111/bjd.15174.

Meredith, G., DeLollis, M., & Shad, M. U. (2020). Potential treatment for overdose with synthetic cannabinoids. *Medical Cannabis and Cannabinoids,* 3(1), 74–75. https://doi.org/10.1159/000506635.

Miotto, K., & Roth, B. (2001). *Patients with a History of Around-the Clock Use of Gamma Hydroxybutyrate May Present as Disturbing and Difficult to Manage.* UCLA Integrated UTSW Toxicology Substance Abuse Program Training Service.

Mueller, S. R., Walley, A. Y., Calcaterra, S. L., Glanz, J. M., & Binswanger, I. A. (2015). A review of opioid overdose prevention and naloxone prescribing: Implications for translating community programming into clinical practice. *Substance Abuse,* 36(2), 240–253.

Oyefeso, A., Ghodse, H., Clancy, C., & Corkery, J. M. (1999). Suicide among drug addicts in the UK. *The British Journal of Psychiatry: The Journal of Mental Science,* 175, 277–282. https://doi.org/10.1192/bjp.175.3.277.

Oyefeso, A., Valmana, A., Clancy, C., Ghodse, H., & Williams, H. (2000). Fatal antidepressant overdose among drug abusers and non-drug abusers. *Acta Psychiatrica Scandinavica,* 102(4), 295–299. https://doi.org/10.1034/j.1600-0447.2000.102004295.x.

Public Health England. (2015). *Take-Home Naloxone for Opioid Overdose in People Who Use Drugs.* London: Public Health England.

Riederer, A. M., Campleman, S. L., Carlson, R. G., Boyer, E. W., Manini, A. F., Wax, P. M., Brent, J. A., & Toxicology Investigators Consortium (ToxIC). (2016). Acute poisonings from synthetic cannabinoids – 50 U.S. toxicology investigators consortium registry sites, 2010–2015. *MMWR: Morbidity and Mortality Weekly Report,* 65(27), 692–695. https://doi.org/10.15585/mmwr.mm6527a2.

Schiller, E. Y., Goyal, A., & Mechanic, O. J. (2023). *Opioid Overdose.* In StatPearls Treasure Island, FL: StatPearls. Publishing 2024 Jan. https://www.ncbi.nlm.nih.gov/books/NBK470415/

Siddiqi, S., Verney, C., Dargan, P., & Wood, D. M. (2015). Understanding the availability, prevalence of use, desired effects, acute toxicity and dependence potential of the novel opioid MT-45. *Clinical Toxicology,* 53(1), 54–59. https://doi.org/10.3109/15563650.2014.983239.

Takakuwa, K. M., & Schears, R. M. (2021). The emergency department care of the cannabis and synthetic cannabinoid patient: A narrative review. *International Journal of Emergency Medicine,* 14, 10. https://doi.org/10.1186/s12245-021-00330-3.

Teasdale, G., & Jennett, B. (1974). Assessment of coma and impaired consciousness: A practical scale. *The Lancet,* 304(7872), 81–84.

UNODC. (2016). *2016 World Drug Report.* The United Nations Office on Drugs and Crime. www.unodc.org/wdr2016/ (accessed 14 June 2017).

WHO. (2014). *Community Management of Opioid Overdose.* Geneva: WHO.

WHO. (2023). *Opioid Overdose.* https://www.who.int/news-room/fact-sheets/detail/opioid-overdose (accessed 9 April 2024).

Williams, A. V., Marsden, J., & Strang, J. (2014). Training family members to manage heroin overdose and administer naloxone: Randomized trial of effects on knowledge and attitudes. *Addiction,* 109(2), 250–259.

Chapter 29

Drug misuse

Pharmacological and psychosocial interventions

Learning outcomes

- Define the term *detoxification*.
- Describe the management strategies for opioids users.
- Outline the management strategies for polydrug users.
- Describe the management strategies for stimulant users.
- Describe the pharmacological interventions in pregnancy.

Activity 29.1 Pharmacological and psychosocial interventions: drug misuse.

Please state whether the following statements are true or false. Reflect on the statements, and give reason(s) for choosing a particular option.

Statements	True	False
Intervention strategies involve pharmacological and psychosocial interventions and educational and vocational rehabilitation.		
Drug misusers must undergo a detoxification process as part of the initial stage of the treatment plan.		
Detoxification should be a readily available treatment option for people who are opioid-dependent and have expressed an informed choice to become abstinent.		
Heroin, morphine, codeine, and methadone will not produce similar withdrawal signs and symptoms.		
Withdrawal from heroin or morphine begins 8–12 hours after the last dose of the drug.		
Service users with significant comorbid physical or mental health problems are able to undertake community-based detoxification.		
The most rapid methadone regime can be carried out by incremental cuts in dose over 7–21 days.		
Contingency management and behavioural couples therapy are effective in the treatment of drug misuse.		

DOI: 10.4324/9781003456674-34

Statements	True	False
Multiple drug-taking or polydrug use has become a common feature with opiate users.		
The drug naltrexone may not be used to prevent relapse in patients who are opiate-free.		
For clients on therapeutic doses of benzodiazepines, withdrawal is best completed in a community-based service.		
Amphetamine, cocaine, and ecstasy are the most commonly abused stimulants, and they produce a major physiological withdrawal syndrome.		

Activity 29.2

There is only one correct answer to the following multiple-choice questions.

1. Which of the following best defines the term *detoxification*?
   a. A process of removing toxins from the body
   b. A medical intervention to manage withdrawal symptoms
   c. An educational programme for substance users
   d. A psychological therapy for addiction treatment
   e. A method to enhance drug potency
2. What is the primary focus of management strategies for opioid users?
   a. Increasing opioid dosage to achieve desired effects
   b. Providing alternative opioid formulations
   c. Addressing withdrawal symptoms and preventing relapse
   d. Encouraging long-term opioid use for pain management
   e. Ignoring psychological support and counselling
3. Which of the following describes a key aspect of management strategies for polydrug users?
   a. Focusing solely on one drug of choice for treatment
   b. Implementing harm reduction approaches to minimise risks
   c. Isolating users from social support networks
   d. Ignoring the presence of multiple substances in the treatment plan
   e. Administering a single medication to treat all substances
4. What is an essential component of management strategies for stimulant users?
   a. Administering sedatives to counteract stimulant effects
   b. Encouraging increased stimulant consumption for tolerance
   c. Providing behavioural therapies to address craving and relapse
   d. Using stimulants as a substitute for opioids
   e. Avoiding any medication-based interventions
5. What is the recommended approach for pharmacological interventions in pregnancy regarding substance use?
   a. Limiting interventions to psychological counselling only
   b. Avoiding pharmacotherapy due to potential foetal harm
   c. Using a combination of medications to treat addiction
   d. Adjusting medication doses to account for pregnancy-related changes
   e. Administering high doses of medication to counteract maternal drug use

6. Detoxification is primarily aimed at:
   a. Encouraging continued substance use
   b. Removing toxins from the body
   c. Preventing substance withdrawal symptoms
   d. Managing psychological addiction
   e. Enhancing the potency of drugs
7. Which of the following is a recommended management strategy for opioid users?
   a. Prescribing opioids without monitoring
   b. Focusing solely on acute pain management
   c. Addressing withdrawal symptoms and preventing relapse
   d. Disregarding the risk of overdose
   e. Ignoring the potential for dependence
8. What approach is typically employed in managing polydrug users?
   a. Focusing solely on one substance of abuse
   b. Implementing harm reduction strategies
   c. Encouraging increased drug use for tolerance
   d. Avoiding psychological support
   e. Administering a single medication for all substances
9. Which of the following is a crucial aspect of managing stimulant users?
   a. Administering stimulants for pain management
   b. Using sedatives to counteract stimulant effects
   c. Providing behavioural therapies for craving and relapse
   d. Encouraging increased stimulant consumption
   e. Avoiding any form of intervention
10. What is a key consideration in pharmacological interventions for substance use during pregnancy?
    a. Administering high medication doses
    b. Limiting interventions to psychological counselling
    c. Avoiding pharmacotherapy due to foetal harm
    d. Using a single medication to treat addiction
    e. Disregarding pregnancy-related changes in medication doses
11. What is a primary goal in managing opioid users?
    a. Encouraging higher opioid dosages
    b. Providing alternative opioid formulations
    c. Addressing withdrawal symptoms and preventing relapse
    d. Disregarding psychological support
    e. Focusing solely on acute pain management
12. Which approach is commonly used in managing polydrug users?
    a. Isolating users from social networks
    b. Employing harm reduction strategies
    c. Prescribing a single medication for all substances
    d. Ignoring the presence of multiple substances
    e. Focusing solely on one substance
13. What is a crucial aspect of managing stimulant users?
    a. Using sedatives to counteract stimulant effects
    b. Providing behavioural therapies for craving and relapse
    c. Encouraging increased stimulant consumption
    d. Administering stimulants for pain management
    e. Avoiding any form of intervention

14. What is a key consideration in pharmacological interventions for substance use during pregnancy?
    a. Administering high medication doses
    b. Limiting interventions to psychological counselling
    c. Avoiding pharmacotherapy due to foetal harm
    d. Using a single medication to treat addiction
    e. Disregarding pregnancy-related changes in medication doses
15. The ways people can access drug treatment are:
    a. Self-referral
    b. Primary healthcare
    c. Criminal justice system
    d. All of the above
    e. A and C only
16. The time of onset and the duration of the withdrawal syndrome will depend on:
    a. The drug itself
    b. The total intake of the drug
    c. The duration of use
    d. All of the above
    e. None of the above
17. The baseline dose of methadone aims to:
    a. Suppress opioid withdrawal symptoms and cravings
    b. Induce euphoria and sedation
    c. Increase tolerance to opioids
    d. Counteract the effects of other substances
    e. Exacerbate withdrawal symptoms
18. This gradual reduction of methadone can occur at:
    a. 5–10 mg per day
    b. 20–30 mg per week
    c. 2–5 mg per day
    d. 10–20 mg per week
    e. 50–100 mg per week
19. The following substance should be offered as the first-line treatment in opioid detoxification:
    a. Methadone
    b. Naloxone
    c. Buprenorphine
    d. Cocaine
    e. Diazepam
20. The treatment of substance use disorder is focused on:
    a. Addressing underlying psychological issues
    b. Promoting increased substance use
    c. Encouraging social isolation
    d. Ignoring withdrawal symptoms
    e. Implementing comprehensive approaches, including medical, psychological, and social interventions

INTRODUCTION

This chapter aims to outline specific treatment strategies, pharmacological interventions, and detoxification methods for psychoactive substance use disorders. It also includes psychosocial interventions. Various community-based and residential services are available exclusively for individuals struggling with alcohol and drug use, offering structured programmes of care and intervention. These services encompass advice, information, needle exchange facilities, day programmes, community drug and alcohol services, community prescribing services, inpatient services, and residential rehabilitation. Access to drug treatment services can occur through self-referral; referral by general practitioners, social workers, or hospital staff; or involvement in the criminal justice system following a court order. The treatment of drug addiction is focused on three main components:

- Dealing with detoxification and withdrawal effects
- Maintenance (also known as substitution or harm reduction therapies)
- Abstinence

Drug treatment encompasses various interventions, including drug detoxification, methadone maintenance therapy, motivational interviewing, counselling, cognitive behavioural therapies, marital and family therapy, relapse prevention, and 12-step approaches. Additionally, self-help groups like Narcotics Anonymous and Cocaine Anonymous play a role in the treatment journey. Both pharmacological and psychosocial interventions are utilised, often supplemented by educational and vocational rehabilitation efforts.

DETOXIFICATION

Drug misusers typically undergo a detoxification process as the initial stage of their treatment plan. Following detoxification, treatment involves psychosocial approaches and/or substitute medication. Detoxification entails allowing the body to eliminate a psychoactive substance while managing withdrawal symptoms. This process is gradual and may include the use of substitute medication to alleviate physical withdrawal symptoms. Some drug users undergo a stabilisation process, where they are prescribed substitutes for the psychoactive substance, such as methadone for heroin users.

OPIOID DETOXIFICATION AND PSYCHOSOCIAL INTERVENTIONS

Opioid detoxification is the process of safely and effectively eliminating the effects of opioid drugs from dependent opioid users, with the aim of minimising withdrawal symptoms (NICE, 2007a). It should be readily available for individuals who are opioid-dependent and have chosen to become abstinent. Heroin, morphine, codeine, and methadone produce similar withdrawal signs and symptoms, although withdrawal from shorter-acting opiates tends to occur and resolve more quickly. The onset and duration of withdrawal syndrome depend on factors such as the specific drug, total intake, duration of use, and individual health. Withdrawal from heroin or morphine typically begins 8 to 12 hours after the last dose, with symptoms diminishing over 5 to 7 days. Methadone withdrawal symptoms start around 12 hours after the last dose, with peak intensity on the third day of abstinence, and typically subside after 2 to 3 weeks. Common signs and symptoms of opioid withdrawal syndrome are detailed in Chapter 8.

Before the implementation of the detoxification process, there is a need to provide information, advice, and support. Service users should be informed about detoxification and the associated risks (NICE, 2007a), including:

- The physical and psychological aspects of opioid withdrawal, including the duration and intensity of symptoms, and how these may be managed.
- The use of non-pharmacological approaches to manage or cope with opioid withdrawal symptoms.
- The loss of opioid tolerance following detoxification, and the ensuing increased risk of overdose and death from illicit drug use that may be potentiated by the use of alcohol or benzodiazepines.
- The importance of continued support, as well as psychosocial and appropriate pharmacological interventions, to maintain abstinence, treat comorbid mental health problems, and reduce the risk of adverse outcomes (including death).

The detoxification process should be conducted under the supervision of healthcare personnel, as part of either a hospital or community-based programme. However, it is advised that individuals who have not experienced improvement with previous formal community-based detoxification, those requiring medical and/or nursing care due to significant comorbid physical or mental health issues, individuals needing complex polydrug detoxification (e.g. simultaneous detoxification from alcohol or benzodiazepines), and those facing significant social problems should not undergo community-based detoxification (NICE, 2007a).

Once the presence and severity of opioid dependence are established, the detoxification process can commence. Methadone or buprenorphine should be offered as the first-line treatment in opioid detoxification (NICE, 2007a). The baseline dose of methadone aims to minimise withdrawal severity, provide comfort, and reduce the risk of overdose. Dose reduction can be initiated based on assessment results and treatment plans. The speed of methadone dose reduction varies, depending on individual circumstances. Rapid regimes involve incremental dose reductions over 7 to 21 days, while slower regimes may span several months. When complex social or other needs are present, methadone reductions are slower. The general principle is that higher dose levels allow for greater reduction, as they represent a smaller percentage of the total dose.

The pace of methadone dose reduction can vary, occurring daily, every other day, or weekly. Occasionally, holding the reduction steady at a given dose for a few days may alleviate anxiety and increase the individual's sense of control. Delays in reduction rates should be accompanied by psychological support. Progress should be monitored regularly, and the individual's status should be discussed with the multidisciplinary team. All detoxification programmes necessitate relapse prevention strategies and psychological support post-detoxification due to high relapse rates. While some patients may achieve total abstinence from opioids rapidly through detoxification and psychosocial interventions, others may require ongoing support and monitoring. However, others may require a methadone maintenance approach on a medium- to long-term basis, depending on the complex needs of the patient. The aims of the methadone maintenance approach are to:

- Reduce illicit heroin use
- Reduce craving
- Prevent withdrawal
- Eliminate the hazards of injecting
- Reduce criminal behaviour
- Enhance stability to prevent patients returning to previous patterns of drug use

To fully benefit from the overall treatment package, it is essential to provide psychosocial interventions alongside pharmacological interventions for opioid users. Various psychosocial interventions have proven effective in treating drug misuse. These include contingency management and behavioural couples therapy for drug-specific issues, as well as evidence-based psychological interventions, such as cognitive behavioural therapy, for common comorbid mental health problems (NICE, 2007b). Counselling and support are crucial during and after medication withdrawal. Counselling sessions offer an opportunity to explore underlying emotional conflicts and establish mutually agreed-upon goals to help clients remain drug-free and enhance their self-esteem. NICE recommends considering contingency management to reduce illicit drug use during detoxification and for up to three to six months post-detoxification (NICE, 2007b).

Behavioural couples therapy should be considered for individuals who are in close contact with a non-drug-misusing partner and seek treatment for opioid misuse, including those who continue to use illicit drugs while receiving opioid maintenance treatment or after completing opioid detoxification (NICE, 2007b). Psychoeducational interventions, both individual and group-based, should be provided to offer information about lifestyle changes, reducing exposure to blood-borne viruses, and minimising sexual and injection risk behaviours for people who misuse drugs. Relapse prevention programmes should enable patients to identify high-risk situations or "cues" and develop coping skills to prevent relapse. Some patients may require assistance in managing issues like anxiety, sleeplessness, accommodation, homelessness, and unemployment. Support with housing and benefit issues, as well as practical help in finding suitable employment, may be necessary. Facilitating attendance at self-help groups such as Narcotics Anonymous and Cocaine Anonymous is recommended for patients showing interest. For some patients, a period of stay in a residential rehabilitation facility may be necessary to achieve abstinence. For patients with co-existing substance misuse and psychiatric disorders (e.g. depression and anxiety), cognitive behavioural therapy is recommended (NICE, 2007b).

POLYDRUG USERS

Polydrug use, involving the concurrent use of multiple substances, has become common among opiate users. Substances such as benzodiazepines, amphetamines, cocaine, and alcohol are often used either to enhance the effects of opiates or to alleviate withdrawal symptoms. Alcohol detoxification, typically using benzodiazepines like Valium or Librium, can be conducted at community-based services for most cases, except for patients with a history of seizures or serious physical or psychiatric conditions. Benzodiazepine withdrawal usually involves switching to a long-acting drug like Valium and gradually reducing the dose every two to three weeks. It is recommended to withdraw clients from any hypno-sedative drugs before attempting to reduce methadone. Some polydrug users may require hospital admission to stabilise their medication needs or for safer detoxification, particularly if there is a risk of withdrawal seizures.

Healthcare professionals should be mindful that medications used in opioid detoxification are prone to misuse and diversion in all settings, including prisons. Therefore, monitoring medication adherence and implementing methods to limit the risk of diversion, such as supervised consumption, may be necessary (NICE, 2007a). Naltrexone, a drug that blocks the effects of opiates, may be used to prevent relapse in patients who are opiate-free. A small minority of opiate users is prescribed injectable methadone and pharmaceutical injectable heroin (diamorphine) for managing their addiction.

BENZODIAZEPINES

Benzodiazepines carry their own addictive potential and are frequently used in combination with opiates. Abrupt cessation of benzodiazepine use can result in a recognised withdrawal state. Many opiate users engage in polydrug use involving benzodiazepines. Withdrawal symptoms associated with benzodiazepines include anxiety, panic attacks, insomnia, perceptual disturbances, seizures, aches and pains, impaired memory and concentration, difficulty in thinking, and confusion. Discontinuation of benzodiazepine dependence should be conducted under nursing and medical supervision. The two fundamental components of a successful benzodiazepine withdrawal strategy are gradual dosage reduction and anxiety management. While dosage reduction is relatively straightforward, psychological support is equally crucial for achieving a favourable outcome, especially in reducing the incidence and severity of post-withdrawal syndromes (Aston, 1994). Another alternative strategy involves substituting a long-acting benzodiazepine. For patients on therapeutic doses of benzodiazepines, withdrawal is ideally completed in community-based services. However, for individuals who are high-dose and chronic benzodiazepine users, hospital admission may be necessary, allowing for a faster initiation of drug reduction. Withdrawal prescribing should only commence when there is clear evidence of benzodiazepine dependence. The management of benzodiazepine withdrawal involves gradually tapering the dose, which may extend over several weeks, depending on the duration of use and severity of symptoms. The rate of withdrawal should be personalised to the patient's lifestyle, personality, environmental stressors, reasons for benzodiazepine use, and the level of available support (Aston, 1994).

The use of a long-acting benzodiazepine such as diazepam is widely recognised as the most effective method for withdrawing patients because it gradually leaves the system, thereby slowing the onset of withdrawal symptoms. On the contrary, short-acting benzodiazepines may lead to more abrupt and severe withdrawal reactions. A typical withdrawal period lasts six to eight weeks, but it can be extended for several months for patients experiencing severe symptoms. However, excessively prolonged withdrawal programmes may become counterproductive, as some patients may become overly fixated on their symptoms. If the client is also receiving a long-term prescription of methadone for concurrent opiate dependence, the methadone dose should be maintained throughout the benzodiazepine reduction period. Concurrent detoxification of both drugs is not recommended in a community setting.

Many patients undergoing benzodiazepine withdrawal may experience anxiety symptoms and sleep difficulties, regardless of the rate of reduction. These symptoms can be alleviated through counselling, psychological support, and practical advice, such as using relaxation techniques and sleep management strategies. The level of support and intervention required will vary among patients, and additional approaches such as massage, aromatherapy, and physical exercises can also help reduce symptoms (Gafoor, 1998). Patients experiencing more severe withdrawal symptoms, such as panic attacks, agoraphobia, or depression, may require more intensive cognitive behavioural treatment to address their specific needs.

STIMULANTS

Amphetamine, cocaine, and ecstasy are among the most commonly abused stimulants, yet they do not typically produce a significant physiological withdrawal syndrome. There is a lack of consensus regarding the existence of a stimulant withdrawal syndrome, and as such, there is no specific detoxification protocol for stimulant withdrawal (Feigenbaum & Allen, 1996). Regular users of stimulants may experience symptoms such as exhaustion, insomnia, intense dreaming, and depressed mood. These symptoms generally subside over a period of two to four days of abstinence from the drug. However, the nature of withdrawal symptoms may vary between intermittent binge users and chronic users of stimulants. The goal of treatment interventions is to address the complexity of biochemical, psychological, and social factors that perpetuate stimulant use. This may involve a comprehensive approach tailored to the individual's needs.

There is no indication for the prescription of cocaine or methylamphetamine in the treatment of stimulant withdrawal. However, there may be a limited role for the prescription of dexamphetamine sulphate 5 mg in the treatment of amphetamine misuse. After discontinuation of stimulant use, antidepressant drugs are sometimes prescribed. Antidepressants, such as fluoxetine, can be effective in managing major depressive episodes associated with stimulant use, but occasional toxic reactions have been reported when selective serotonin reuptake inhibitors (SSRIs) are prescribed alongside continued stimulant use (Barrett et al., 1996). Ghodes (1995) suggests a treatment plan involving oral or intravenous diazepam to alleviate agitation. In some individuals with a dual diagnosis, abrupt cessation of stimulants may trigger profound transient depression with suicidal thoughts, necessitating hospitalisation or close monitoring (Banerjee et al., 2002).

Studies have found that an abstinence-based psychosocial treatment approach, combining counselling and social support, had the most significant impact on cocaine misuse (Donmall et al., 1995). There is evidence to suggest that contingency management programmes may be beneficial for the treatment of cocaine use disorder among adults who actively use cocaine (Bentzley et al., 2021). Complementary therapies, such as acupuncture, are increasingly used for crack cocaine detoxification (Lipton et al., 1994), although evidence supporting their effectiveness is limited. This alternative treatment may appeal to those with limited contact with drug specialist services. General principles of management, including harm reduction approaches regarding safer injecting practices and safer sex, should be incorporated into the psychosocial and educational programme.

GHB

A GHB withdrawal syndrome, resembling aspects of alcohol and benzodiazepine withdrawal, has been documented. This syndrome typically occurs in individuals who have self-administered GHB every two to three hours and are therefore at increased risk for severe symptoms. GHB withdrawal can manifest after several months of regular use. Management of the withdrawal syndrome often requires the use of high doses of hypno-sedatives and physical restraints to control symptoms such as confusion, delirium, psychosis, and resultant agitation. Due to the potentially severe nature of GHB withdrawal, close monitoring and appropriate medical intervention are essential components of management.

CANNABIS/HALLUCINOGENS/ PHENCYCLIDINE

Recent research has provided evidence indicating that cessation from long-term and regular cannabis use can precipitate a specific withdrawal syndrome, contrary to earlier beliefs. This withdrawal syndrome typically manifests with a range of mood and behavioural symptoms of light to moderate intensity. A systematic review and meta-analysis investigated the prevalence of cannabis withdrawal syndrome (CWS) among regular users of cannabinoids. The findings indicate a significant prevalence of CWS in this population, highlighting the importance for clinicians to be cognisant of this phenomenon (Bahji et al., 2020). There is evidence to suggest that factors such as clinical settings (inpatient and outpatient), concurrent tobacco or other substance use, and daily cannabis use were associated with a higher severity of cannabis withdrawal syndrome (Bahji et al., 2020). There are no acute withdrawal syndromes associated with hallucinogens and phencyclidine (PCP). However, chronic use of PCP may lead to toxic psychosis. Pharmacological treatments for cannabis and stimulant misuse are not well developed. Therefore, psychosocial interventions remain the primary approach for effective treatment in these cases.

PHARMACOLOGICAL TREATMENT FOR DRUG MISUSERS IN PREGNANCY

The use of psychoactive substances such as cocaine and heroin during pregnancy is unfortunately common. The overall aim of antenatal treatment varies depending on the type of drug being misused. Methadone remains the drug of choice for opiate/opioid substitution, offering proven medical and social benefits by stabilising drug use and lifestyle and facilitating contact with services. Compared to illicit heroin use, methadone maintenance is associated with greater access to antenatal care and thus better maternal and infant outcomes. These benefits include a reduced risk of preterm delivery and low birth weight (Jarvis & Schnoll, 1995). However, it is important to note that neonatal abstinence syndrome may be more common in infants whose mothers took methadone rather than heroin (Chasnoff et al., 1990).

Antenatal detoxification should only be undertaken if appropriate and if there is a reasonable prospect of success. Antenatal detoxification from benzodiazepines, aimed at reducing the risk of maternal convulsion, should be conducted under the cover of a short reducing course of diazepam, starting with an initial dose of 10 mg three times daily and reducing by 5 mg each day (with rotation of the dose to be reduced). This approach has been proven safe in practice (Hepburn, 2004). Withdrawal from alcohol during pregnancy can be safely managed with the same regime as used for benzodiazepine withdrawal. However, there is no evidence to support substitution therapy during pregnancy for any other type of drug.

KEY POINTS

- Services for alcohol and drug users include advice and information, needle exchange facilities, day programmes, community drug and alcohol services, community prescribing services, inpatient services, and residential rehabilitation.
- The treatment of drug addiction is focused on three main components: dealing with detoxification and withdrawal effects, maintenance (also known as "substitution" or "harm reduction" therapies), and abstinence.
- Drug misusers must undergo a detoxification process as part of the initial stage of the treatment plan.
- The treatment's journey is followed by treatment with psychosocial approaches and/or substitute medication.
- *Opioid detoxification* refers to the process by which the effects of opioid drugs are eliminated from dependent opioid users in a safe and effective manner, such that withdrawal symptoms are minimised.
- Service users should be informed about detoxification and the associated risks.
- Methadone or buprenorphine should be offered as the first-line treatment in opioid detoxification.
- All detoxification programmes require relapse-prevention strategies and psychological support after detoxification because relapse rates are high.
- The aims of the methadone maintenance approach are to reduce illicit heroin use, reduce craving and prevent withdrawal, eliminate the hazards of injecting, reduce criminal behaviour, and enhance stability to prevent patients from returning to previous patterns of drug use.
- A range of psychosocial interventions is effective in the treatment of drug misuse; these include contingency management and behavioural couples therapy for drug-specific problems.
- Cognitive behavioural therapy is effective for common comorbid mental health problems.
- Many opiate users use benzodiazepines as part of polydrug use.
- Concurrent detoxification of both heroin and benzodiazepines is not recommended in a community setting.
- There is no specific detoxification protocol for stimulant withdrawal.
- After cessation of stimulant use, antidepressant drugs are sometimes prescribed.
- A GHB withdrawal syndrome that has aspects of alcohol and benzodiazepine withdrawal has been reported.
- A valid cannabis withdrawal syndrome has been established.
- The overall aim of antenatal treatment varies according to the type of drug being misused.
- Methadone remains the drug of choice for opiate/opioid substitution with proven medical and social benefits.

References

Aston, H. (1994). The treatment of benzodiazepine dependence. *Addiction,* 89(11), 1535–1541. https://doi.org/10.1111/j.1360-0443.1994.tb03755.x.

Bahji, A., Stephenson, C., Tyo, R., Hawken, E. R., & Seitz, D. P. (2020). Prevalence of cannabis withdrawal symptoms among people with regular or dependent use of cannabinoids: A systematic review and meta-analysis. *JAMA Network Open,* 3(4), e202370. https://doi.org/10.1001/jamanetworkopen.2020.2370.

Banerjee, S., Clancy, C., & Crome, I. (2002). *Co-Existing Problems of Mental Disorder and Substance Misuse (Dual Diagnosis).* London: Royal College of Psychiatrists' Research Unit.

Barrett, J., Meehan, O., & Fahy, T. (1996). SSRI and sympathomimetic interaction. *British Journal of Psychiatry,* 168(2), 253. https://doi.org/10.1192/bjp.168.2.253.

Bentzley, B. S., Han, S. S., Neuner, S., Humphreys, K., Kampman, K. M., & Halpern, C. H. (2021). Comparison of treatments for cocaine use disorder among adults: A systematic review and meta-analysis. *JAMA Network Open,* 4(5), e218049. https://doi.org/10.1001/jamanetworkopen.2021.8049.

Chasnoff, I. J., Landress, H. J., & Barrett, M. E. (1990). The prevalence of illicit-drug use during pregnancy and discrepancies in mandatory reporting in Pinellas County, Florida. *New England Journal of Medicine,* 322(17), 1202–1206. https://doi.org/10.1056/NEJM199004263221706.

Donmall, M., Seivewright, N., Douglas, J., Draycott, T., & Millar, T. (1995). *National Cocaine Treatment Study: The Effectiveness of Treatments Offered to Cocaine/Crack Users.* A Report to the Task Force. London: Department of Health.

Feigenbaum, J. C., & Allen, K. M. (1996). Detoxification. In K. M. Allen (Ed.), *Nursing Care of the Addicted Client.* Philadelphia: Lippincott, pp. 139–175.

Gafoor, M. (1998). Benzodiazepines: Clinical care and nursing interventions. In G. H. Rassool (Ed.), *Substance Use and Misuse: Nature, Context and Clinical Interventions.* Oxford: Blackwell Science.

Ghodes, H. (1995). *Drugs and Addictive Behaviour: A Guide to Treatment* (2nd ed.). Oxford: Blackwell Scientific Publications.

Jarvis, M. A., & Schnoll, S. H. (1995). Methadone use during pregnancy. *NIDA Research Monograph,* 149, 58–77.

Hepburn, M. (2004). Substance abuse in pregnancy. *Current Obstetrics & Gynaecology,* 14(6), 419–425.

Lipton, D. S., Brewington, V., & Smith, M. (1994). Acupuncture for crack-cocaine detoxification: Experimental evaluation of efficacy. *Journal of Substance Abuse Treatment,* 11(3), 205–215. https://doi.org/10.1016/0740-5472(94)90077-9.

NICE. (2007a). *Drug Misuse: Opioid Detoxification* (NICE Clinical Guideline 52). London: National Institute for Clinical Excellence. www.nice.org.uk/CG52.

NICE. (2007b). *Drug Misuse Psychosocial Interventions* (NICE Clinical Guideline 51). London: National Institute for Clinical Excellence. www.nice.org.uk/CG51.

Chapter 30

Alcohol misuse

Pharmacological and psychosocial interventions

Learning outcomes

- List the screening instruments for identifying alcohol problems.
- Describe the management and treatment of harmful and hazardous drinkers.
- Describe the management and treatment of moderate and severe dependent drinkers.
- Discuss the advantages and limitations of community detoxification.
- Discuss the pharmacological management of withdrawal.
- Discuss the psychosocial interventions in management and treatment of alcohol problems.

Activity 30.1

There is only one correct answer to the following multiple-choice questions.

1. Which of the following is a commonly used screening instrument for identifying alcohol problems?
   a. Beck Depression Inventory (BDI)
   b. Alcohol Use Disorders Identification Test (AUDIT)
   c. Hamilton Anxiety Rating Scale (HARS)
   d. Brief Psychiatric Rating Scale (BPRS)
   e. Zung Self-Rating Depression Scale
2. What is the recommended management approach for harmful and hazardous drinkers?
   a. Immediate referral to residential rehabilitation
   b. Prescribing benzodiazepines for withdrawal symptoms
   c. Brief interventions and motivational interviewing
   d. Initiating long-term pharmacotherapy
   e. Providing self-help literature only
3. Which treatment modality is typically recommended for moderate and severe dependent drinkers?
   a. Outpatient detoxification only
   b. Self-help groups only
   c. Residential rehabilitation
   d. Brief interventions
   e. Prescription of benzodiazepines without supervision

DOI: 10.4324/9781003456674-35

4. What are the advantages of community detoxification?
   a. Round-the-clock medical supervision
   b. Access to specialised psychiatric care
   c. Reduced risk of social isolation
   d. Enhanced continuity of care post-detoxification
   e. Limited access to supportive services
5. Which of the following psychosocial interventions is often used in the management and treatment of alcohol problems?
   a. Electroconvulsive therapy (ECT)
   b. Dialectical behaviour therapy (DBT)
   c. Transcranial magnetic stimulation (TMS)
   d. Relaxation techniques
   e. Eye movement desensitisation and reprocessing (EMDR)
6. Which medication is commonly used for the pharmacological management of alcohol withdrawal symptoms?
   a. Opioids
   b. Antidepressants
   c. Antipsychotics
   d. Benzodiazepines
   e. Stimulants
7. What is the primary goal of screening instruments for alcohol problems?
   a. To diagnose alcohol dependence
   b. To assess the severity of withdrawal symptoms
   c. To identify individuals at risk of alcohol-related harm
   d. To measure the effectiveness of treatment interventions
   e. To monitor changes in alcohol tolerance levels
8. What is a commonly used pharmacological agent for managing alcohol withdrawal seizures?
   a. Naloxone
   b. Disulfiram
   c. Acamprosate
   d. Diazepam
   e. Fluoxetine
9. Which of the following is a characteristic feature of moderate alcohol withdrawal syndrome?
   a. Hallucinations and delusions
   b. Seizures
   c. Tremors and agitation
   d. Coma
   e. Bradycardia
10. Which psychosocial intervention focuses on enhancing an individual's motivation to change their alcohol consumption behaviour?
    a. Cognitive behavioural therapy (CBT)
    b. Motivational interviewing (MI)
    c. Family therapy
    d. Group therapy
    e. Psychoeducation
11. What is the primary objective of managing severe alcohol withdrawal syndrome?
    a. Preventing relapse
    b. Alleviating withdrawal symptoms

c. Addressing underlying psychological issues
d. Enhancing social support
e. Encouraging moderate alcohol consumption

12. Which medication is commonly prescribed as a maintenance therapy to prevent relapse in individuals with alcohol dependence?
a. Methadone
b. Buprenorphine
c. Naltrexone
d. Bupropion
e. Modafinil

13. What is the primary focus of community detoxification programmes?
a. Providing long-term residential care
b. Minimising the risk of relapse
c. Promoting social reintegration
d. Reducing the severity of withdrawal symptoms
e. Facilitating access to alcohol supply

14. Which psychosocial intervention emphasises the identification and modification of maladaptive thoughts and behaviours related to alcohol use?
a. Motivational interviewing
b. Rational emotive behaviour therapy (REBT)
c. Solution-focused brief therapy (SFBT)
d. Gestalt therapy
e. Art therapy

15. Which of the following is a limitation of pharmacological management of alcohol withdrawal?
a. High efficacy in preventing relapse
b. Potential for adverse effects and drug interactions
c. Minimal impact on withdrawal symptoms
d. Long-term sustainability of treatment effects
e. Accessibility and affordability issues

INTRODUCTION

The models of care for alcohol misusers (MoCAM) in the UK provides comprehensive guidance for local health organisations in delivering integrated treatment systems for adult alcohol misusers (NTA, 2006). MoCAM categorises alcohol misusers into four main groups: hazardous drinkers, harmful drinkers, moderately dependent drinkers, and severely dependent drinkers. *Hazardous drinkers* consume alcohol above sensible limits but have not yet experienced significant alcohol-related problems. *Harmful drinkers* exhibit clear evidence of alcohol-related harm from drinking above recommended levels. Both groups may benefit from brief interventions and advice. *Moderately* and *severely dependent drinkers* require specialist alcohol treatment, with severe and complex cases needing higher levels of intervention initially. The effectiveness review conducted by Heather et al. (2006) suggests that, for treatment planning purposes, categorising alcohol misusers into "moderate dependence" and "severe dependence" and "dependence with complex needs" is the most useful approach. This is because individuals classified under the latter category, termed as "severe and complex," are likely to require a higher level of intervention at the outset compared to those with moderate dependence. While moderately dependent drinkers may be managed effectively in home or community settings, severely dependent drinkers with complex needs may require inpatient withdrawal support, multiple agency services, and residential rehabilitation.

MoCAM advocates a stepped model of care for alcohol misusers, which includes:

- Provision of brief interventions for those drinking excessively but not requiring treatment for alcohol dependence
- Provision of treatment interventions for those with moderate or severe dependence and related problems

Alcohol misusers typically require specialised treatment from various sources, including community alcohol teams, inpatient detoxification units, and structured day or residential programmes. Additionally, self-help groups like Alcoholics Anonymous (AA) and other voluntary agencies may also contribute significantly to the management of care and treatment interventions. The selection of the appropriate setting for each individual case depends on a variety of factors, such as accompanying physical, psychological, or social issues, as well as the risks posed to the drinker and others from the drinker's behaviour (NTA, 2006). Individuals struggling with alcohol use disorder who engage with healthcare professionals, whether in primary care or specialist units, are often offered a detoxification programme as an initial step before further psychosocial interventions.

SCREENING FOR ALCOHOL PROBLEM

Heather et al. (2006) advocate for the use of several screening tools and methods to effectively identify alcohol problems among individuals. These include:

- *AUDIT (Alcohol Use Disorders Identification Test)*. Recommended for embedding within general health questionnaires, the AUDIT efficiently detects hazardous drinking behaviours.
- *FAST*. A rapid screening tool particularly useful in settings like accident and emergency (A&E) departments for swiftly identifying alcohol misuse.
- *Clinical history and physical examination*. These traditional methods remain valuable for detecting harmful drinking patterns.
- *Laboratory tests*. Tests for liver enzyme gamma-glutamyl transferase (GGT) can reveal underlying alcohol-related issues that may otherwise go unnoticed.
- *Initial or comprehensive assessment*. Essential for determining the nature and severity of drinking problems, which subsequently informs decisions regarding detoxification. This assessment helps in choosing the appropriate setting for detoxification, whether it be at home, in a community facility, or in an inpatient detoxification unit.

WORKING WITH HARMFUL AND HAZARDOUS DRINKER

In both primary healthcare and hospital settings, opportunistic triage screening presents an opportunity to provide health information, advice, and brief interventions to individuals with alcohol-related issues. Standard practice involves offering simple, structured advice to hazardous and harmful drinkers without complex needs, aiming to promote reduced alcohol consumption to safer levels. Brief interventions, effective across various settings, including primary care and A&E departments, are provided to those who do not respond adequately to initial advice and information. Individuals requiring further interventions due to high alcohol consumption levels are referred to specialist alcohol agencies. These interventions, often completed in a single session, may include providing necessary health information, setting sensible drinking limits, offering clear advice on reducing alcohol intake, and encouraging the completion of alcohol diaries. While a follow-up appointment can be beneficial, it is not always necessary. For hazardous and harmful drinkers with complex needs, such as psychiatric issues, learning disabilities, advanced age, or social and housing problems, more intensive or prolonged interventions involving multiple agencies may be required. These interventions address the specific challenges and complexities faced by these individuals, ensuring comprehensive support and care.

WORKING WITH MODERATE TO SEVERE DEPENDENT DRINKERS

For moderately dependent drinkers, community or home detoxification may be considered based on an assessment of associated physical, psychological, and social risks to both the individual and others. However, severely dependent drinkers often present with serious, long-standing issues, including significant alcohol withdrawal symptoms. With thorough risk

Table 30.1
Alcohol: key areas of care plan

Needs or problems	Expected outcome	Interventions
Poor physical health	Improvements in daily intake of nutrition	Assessment of daily intake of nutrients Vitamin supplements
Fear of withdrawal symptoms	Prevention of withdrawal symptoms	Health information and advice
Risk behaviour	Elimination or reduction of risk behaviour	Assessment and monitoring
Low self-esteem	Adoption of more positive attitude	Counselling
Lack of assertive skills	Development of assertive skills	Counselling and cognitive behavioural techniques
Anxiety	Control of anxiety	Anxiety/stress management
Boredom	Reduction of boredom	Encourage participation in alternative leisure activities
Detoxification	Client will not experience any physical distress and discomfort while undergoing detoxification	Explain the role of medication in facilitating detoxification and overcoming withdrawal
Dealing with loss or grief reactions	Facilitating the grieving process Resolution of grieving process	Counselling
Relapse	Prevention of relapse	Relapse prevention

Source: Adapted from Gafoor and Rassool (1998).

assessment and a comprehensive care plan, medically assisted alcohol withdrawal can be safely administered to many severely dependent individuals in community or home settings (NTA, 2006). Yet more severely dependent drinkers may necessitate inpatient assisted detoxification and residential rehabilitation due to the complexity of their needs. These individuals often exhibit multiple substance misuse, complicated alcohol withdrawal symptoms, and co-existing psychiatric disorders or social problems. In such cases, a more structured and intensive treatment approach is required to address their diverse challenges effectively. The comprehensive alcohol assessment encompasses various domains, including patterns of alcohol use, withdrawal symptoms, psychological history, physical health issues, self-harm tendencies, and levels of risk related to both mental health and alcohol consumption. Additionally, it involves evaluating a history of trauma and addressing social factors, such as childcare responsibilities, relationships, domestic violence, housing, employment, financial status, and involvement with legal or forensic services (Royal College of Psychiatrists, 2005).

In terms of mental health needs, targeted questioning focuses on cues such as stress, anxiety, low mood, and psychological distress. For dependent drinkers with psychiatric issues, immediate risk assessment guides the intervention of psychiatric services, determining the timing, manner, and location of intervention. Individualised care plans are developed based on assessment findings, integrating both mental health and alcohol use aspects. These plans include tailored treatments and strategies that address psychosocial functioning, with consideration given to risk factors (Moore, 2006). Key areas of a care plan are presented in Table 30.1.

DETOXIFICATION

Alcohol-induced physical withdrawal syndromes often necessitate detoxification as a treatment intervention, which can be administered in both community and inpatient settings. Community detoxification operates on the principle of allowing individuals to remain in their familiar environments, rooted in social learning theory (Gafoor & Rassool, 1998). This approach recognises that alcohol consumption is often a learned response to environmental and social cues. Detoxification serves as an initial step toward further social and psychological interventions aimed at motivating individuals to alter their behaviours (Gafoor & Rassool, 1998). By undergoing detoxification in their own surroundings, individuals can potentially benefit from the support and resources available in their community. The potential advantages of community detoxification are outlined in Table 30.2.

Table 30.2
Potential benefits and limitations of community detoxification

Benefits	Limitations
• Interventions in a familiar environment. • Support of family network and significant others. • Client able to resist environmental cues to drinking and develop new coping strategies. • Stigma of admission to hospital or specialist unit is disengaged. • A more accessible and flexible service. • Enabling service user to seek help at an early stage of their drinking career. • Client remains at work during treatment interventions. • More dependent drinkers can be recruited for detoxification rather than being on a waiting list for inpatient detoxification. • Cost-effective.	• Clients remain in an environment which might be perpetuating alcohol misuse. • Family or carers do not have any respite. • Some clients may not view their problems as severe. • Not suitable for those with complex needs or history of mental health problems and severe withdrawal.

Source: Adapted from Gafoor and Rassool (1998).

Stockwell et al. (1991) provide evidence supporting the notion that home detoxification can be just as safe and effective as hospital-based care, given adherence to appropriate standards and policies. However, a critical condition for considering home detoxification is the absence of any prior history of alcohol withdrawal seizures or delirium tremens. Clients experiencing moderate or severe withdrawal symptoms may necessitate inpatient detoxification instead. Table 30.3 outlines the indications warranting inpatient detoxification.

Table 30.3
Indications for inpatient detoxification

- Alcohol delirium or seizures present at the time of assessment
- A history of seizures or alcoholic delirium and high alcohol consumption
- A history of high-dose polydrug use
- Pyrexia greater than 38.5°C
- A history of recent head injury with loss of consciousness
- Illnesses requiring medical or surgical treatment
- Wernicke's encephalopathy
- Conditions requiring psychiatric admission (self-harm, severe anxiety or depression, psychotic disorders)

MANAGEMENT OF WITHDRAWAL

The primary goals of pharmacological interventions in alcohol withdrawal include alleviating subjective withdrawal symptoms, preventing and managing more severe complications, and preparing individuals for further psychosocial and educational interventions. Typically, the alcohol withdrawal syndrome persists for approximately five days, with the highest risk of severe withdrawal occurring within the initial 24 to 48 hours. Chlordiazepoxide or diazepam loading regimens are commonly employed to shorten the detoxification period, enhance safety, and mitigate the indiscriminate use of medications (Wasilewski et al., 1996). Diazepam, in particular, possesses anticonvulsant properties, which help mitigate the risk of seizures. A standard prescribing regimen is outlined in Table 30.4.

Table 30.4
Specimen prescribing regime for diazepam

Dosage	Duration
10 mg tds	1 day
5 mg qds	1 day
5 mg tds	1 day
5 mg bd	1 day
5 mg nocte	1 day

Table 30.5
A framework for supportive care for alcohol withdrawal

Needs	Interventions
Environmental stimuli	Nursing in quiet area, with only one staff in contact.
Body temperature	Control body temperature: apply or remove bed clothing when necessary.
Blood pressure	Monitor blood pressure.
Foods and fluids	Offer fluids every 60 minutes and record fluid intake.
Rest and sleep	Allow rest or sleep between monitoring of vital signs.
Elimination	Assist to bathroom and record output.
Epigastric distress	Deep breathing and relaxation.
Physical comfort	Change position if necessary.
Reality orientation	Time, place, and person.
Providing positive reinforcement	Reinforce positive elements of the intervention.
Visitors	No visitors during supportive care.

Source: Adapted from Shaw et al. (1981).

The management of alcohol detoxification involves several key principles, including monitoring for signs of dehydration; blood pressure; dietary intake; orientation to time, place, and person; as well as sleep patterns. A framework outlining the management of alcohol withdrawal, as proposed by Shaw et al. (1981), is presented in Table 30.5.

Preparation plays a crucial role in building the confidence of service users and maximising the benefits of the detoxification process (Heather et al., 2006). It is essential to create a non-stimulating and non-threatening environment with low lighting at night to help reduce perceptual disturbances. Although detoxification primarily involves physical aspects, nurses are adept at recognising and managing various psychological elements, such as hallucinations, delirium, altered mental states, hyper-vigilance, anxiety, paranoia, depression, tactile hallucinations, and levels of risk (Moore, 2006). Evidence suggests that therapeutic interventions, coupled with closely monitored medication, play a significant role in the treatment of alcohol withdrawal syndrome (Bennie, 1998). This integrated approach addresses both the physical and psychological aspects of withdrawal, promoting a comprehensive and effective treatment outcome.

PSYCHOSOCIAL INTERVENTIONS

Psychosocial interventions serve to complement pharmacological approaches, aiding in detoxification or relapse prevention, while facilitating clients in achieving stability and adopting healthier lifestyles. Brief interventions, as outlined in Chapter 26, have proven effective in assisting harmful or hazardous drinkers in reducing or ceasing alcohol consumption and in motivating moderate or severe alcohol-dependent individuals to engage in long-term treatment. Motivational interviewing represents a primary psychological intervention in specialised settings for clients with moderate or severe dependence who may initially be resistant to change. This approach enhances the efficacy of subsequent psychological treatments (Heather et al., 2006). Table 30.6 provides examples of motivational interviewing questions aligned with the stage of change model and interviewing strategies, facilitating discussions tailored to individuals' readiness to change (Burge & Schneider, 1999; Rollnick et al., 1992).

Psychological interventions, particularly cognitive behavioural approaches, have demonstrated effectiveness in reducing or halting alcohol use. For instance, contingency management (CM) has shown significant effectiveness in encouraging behaviour change in individuals grappling with substance use disorder (Proctor, 2022). Studies by Petry et al. (2000) and Silverman et al. (1996) provide strong evidence of CM's efficacy in addressing specific illicit drug use. Social behaviour and network therapy focuses on modifying and maintaining changes in alcohol consumption by helping clients develop positive social networks (Copello et al., 2002). Coping and social skills training are effective for those

Table 30.6
Stage of change model and interviewing strategies

Stage of Change	Strategies	Description
Pre-contemplation	Lifestyle, stresses, and alcohol use	Discuss lifestyle and life stresses. "Where does your use of alcohol fit in?"
Pre-contemplation	Health and alcohol use	Ask about health in general. "What part does your drinking play in your health?"
Pre-contemplation	A typical day	"Describe a typical day, from beginning to end. How does alcohol fit in?"
Contemplation	"Good" things and "less good" things	"What are some good things about your use of alcohol?" "What are some less good things?"
Contemplation	Providing information	Ask permission to provide information. Deliver information in a non-personal manner. "What do you make of all this?"
Contemplation	The future and the present	"How would you like things to be different in the future?"
Preparation or action	Exploring concerns	Elicit the patient's reasons for concern about alcohol use. List concerns about changing behaviour.
Preparation or action	Helping with decision-making	"Given your concerns about drinking, where does this leave you now?"

Source: Adapted from Burge and Schneider (1999); Rollnick et al. (1992).

with moderate alcohol dependence. Marital therapy, grounded in cognitive behavioural principles, has shown efficacy in improving interpersonal relationships and reducing drinking problems (Heather et al., 2006).

Treating individuals with co-existing alcohol and anxiety issues presents challenges, and there is no universally validated treatment package (Oei & Loveday, 1997). However, various psychological therapies, such as relaxation training, stress management, and skills training, can be utilised alongside pharmacological treatments to address both alcohol misuse and anxiety (Oei & Loveday, 1997). Identifying and effectively managing anxiety is crucial, as it can help prevent relapse into alcohol use (Petrakis et al., 2002). Nonetheless, the complexity of treating co-existing anxiety disorders and alcohol misuse underscores the importance of individualised treatment approaches tailored to the unique needs and circumstances of each person.

Relapse prevention, a crucial component of psychosocial interventions, helps individuals identify high-risk situations and develop coping strategies (Gafoor & Rassool, 1998). Medications like disulfiram, naltrexone, and acamprosate can aid in relapse prevention. Vitamin deficiency, common in alcoholism, can lead to conditions like Wernicke's encephalopathy, necessitating thiamine and vitamin B supplementation during detoxification (Royal College of Physicians, 2001). Continued assistance through structured aftercare programmes, including psychological interventions like counselling or marital therapy and participation in self-help groups like AA, enhances long-term outcomes (Ito & Donovan, 1986; Heather et al., 2006). A multidimensional approach involving pharmacological and psychosocial interventions, along with a multi-professional team, is essential for optimal outcomes in individuals with alcohol-related problems.

KEY POINTS

- Four main categories of alcohol misusers who may benefit from some kind of intervention or treatment: hazardous drinkers, harmful drinkers, moderately dependent drinkers, and severely dependent drinkers.
- Both hazardous and harmful drinkers may benefit from advice, health information, and brief interventions.
- The main groups of alcohol users who clearly may benefit from specialist alcohol treatment are those who are moderately and severely dependent.

- Alcohol misusers require specialist treatment from community alcohol teams, inpatient detoxification units, and structured day or residential programmes.
- A number of screening tools are available to identify current or potential alcohol problems among service users.
- Community or home detoxification can be offered to moderately dependent drinkers.
- Severe dependent drinkers have complex needs, including multiple substance misuse, complicated alcohol withdrawal, co-existing psychiatric disorders, or social problems.
- Where alcohol causes physical withdrawal syndromes, detoxification is a treatment intervention.
- There is evidence that therapeutic interventions, combined with carefully monitored medication, are an important factor in the treatment of alcohol withdrawal syndrome.
- Motivational interviewing increases the effectiveness of more extensive psychological treatment.
- Social behaviour and network therapy can also be used with service users in modifying and maintaining changes in alcohol consumption.
- Other interventions, such as coping and social skills training, are effective with service users with moderate dependent alcohol use.
- Psychosocial interventions for service users with alcohol and psychiatric disorders require clear and consistent approaches, across multiple agencies, with realistic time frames for interventions to work.
- Relapse prevention should be incorporated in all specialist treatment for alcohol problems, and there is good evidence of its effectiveness.
- There is evidence that a planned and structured aftercare is effective in improving outcome following the initial treatment of service users with severe alcohol problems.

References

Bennie, C. (1998). A comparison of home detoxification and minimal intervention strategies for problem drinkers. *Alcohol and Alcoholism,* 33(2), 157–163. https://doi.org/10.1093/oxfordjournals.alcalc.a008372.

Burge, S. K., & Schneider, F. D. (1999). Alcohol-related problems: Recognition and intervention. *American Family Physician,* 59(2), 361–372.

Copello, A., Orford, J., Hodgson, R., Tober, G., Barrett, C., & UKATT Research Team. United Kingdom Alcohol Treatment Trial. (2002). Social behaviour and network therapy basic principles and early experiences. *Addictive Behaviors,* 27(3), 345–366. https://doi.org/10.1016/s0306-4603(01)00176-9.

Gafoor, M, & Rassool, G. H. (1998). Alcohol: Community Detoxification and Clinical Care. In G. H. Rassool (Ed.), *Substance Use and Misuse: Nature, Context and Clinical Interventions.* Oxford: Blackwell Science.

Heather, N., Raistrick, D., & Godfrey, C. (2006). *A Review of the Effectiveness of Treatment for Alcohol Problems.* London: National Treatment Agency.

Ito, J. R., & Donovan, D. M. (1986). Aftercare in alcoholism treatment: A review. In W. R. Miller & N. Heather (Eds.), *Treating Addictive Behaviours: Processes of Change.* New York: Plenum Press.

Moore, K. (2006). Alcohol and dual diagnosis. In G. H. Rassool (Ed.), *Dual Diagnosis Nursing.* Oxford: Blackwell Publications.

NTA. (2006). *Models of Care for Alcohol Misusers (MoCAM).* Department of Health and National Treatment Agency for Substance Misuse (Gateway Ref: 5899). London: Department of Health.

Oei, T. P., & Loveday, W. A. (1997). Management of co-morbid anxiety and alcohol disorders: Parallel treatment of disorders. *Drug and Alcohol Review,* 16(3), 261–274. https://doi.org/10.1080/09595239800187441.

Petrakis, I. L., Gonzalez, G., Rosenheck, R., & Krystal, J. H. (2002). Comorbidity of alcoholism and psychiatric disorders: An overview. *Alcohol Research & Health,* 26(2), 81–89.

Petry, N. M., Martin, B., Cooney, J. L., & Kranzler, H. R. (2000). Give them prizes, and they will come contingency management for treatment of alcohol dependence. *Journal of Consulting and Clinical Psychology,* 68(2), 250–257. https://doi.org/10.1037//0022-006x.68.2.250.

Proctor, S. L. (2022). Rewarding recovery: The time is now for contingency management for opioid use disorder. *Annals of Medicine,* 54(1), 1178–1187. https://doi.org/10.1080/07853890.2022.2068805.

Rollnick, S., Heather, N., & Bell, A. (1992). Negotiating behaviour change in medical settings: The development of brief motivational interviewing. *Journal of Mental Health,* 1(1), 25–37. https://doi.org/10.3109/09638239209034509.

Royal College of Physicians. (2001). *Report on Alcohol: Guidelines for Managing Wernicke's Encephalopathy in the Accident and Emergency Department.* London: The Royal College of Physicians.

Royal College of Psychiatrists. (2005). *Alcohol: Our Favourite Drug.* Fact Sheet. London: Royal College of Psychiatrists.

Shaw, J. M., Kolesar, G. S., Sellers, E. M., Kaplan, H. L., & Sandor, P. (1981). Development of optimal treatment tactics for alcohol withdrawal, assessment and effectiveness of supportive care. *Journal of Clinical Psychopharmacology,* 1(6), 382–388.

Silverman, K., Higgins, S. T., Brooner, R. K., Montoya, I. D., Cone, E. J., Schuster, C. R., & Preston, K. L. (1996). Sustained cocaine abstinence in methadone maintenance patients through voucher-based reinforcement therapy. *Archives of General Psychiatry,* 53(5), 409–415. https://doi.org/10.1001/archpsyc.1996.01830050045007.

Stockwell, T., Bolt, L., & Russel, G. (1991). Home detoxifi cation from alcohol: Its safety and efficacy in comparison to inpatient care. *Alcohol and Alcoholism*, 26, 645–650.

Wasilewski, D., Matsumoto, H., Kur, E., Dziklińska, A., Woźny, E., Stencka, K., Skalski, M., Chaba, P., & Szelenberger, W. (1996). Assessment of diazepam loading dose therapy of delirium tremens. *Alcohol and Alcoholism,* 31(3), 273–278. https://doi.org/10.1093/oxfordjournals.alcalc.a008147.

Chapter 31

Smoking cessation

Health interventions

Learning outcomes

- Describe the features of a smoking cessation service.
- Discuss the benefits of smoking cessation.
- Identify the psychological interventions used in smoking cessation.
- Identify the nicotine and non-nicotine replacement therapy used in smoking cessation.
- Discuss the assessment and interventions to enable smokers to quit.

Activity 31.1

Please state whether the following statements are true or false. Reflect on the statements, and give reason(s) for choosing a particular option.

Statements	True	False
The dependence of nicotine is classified as a psychiatric disorder in ICD-10 and *DSM-V*.		
Smokers quit rates are still higher among people in routine and manual groups.		
An evaluation of NHS Stop Smoking Service shows that the majority of those setting a quit date for smoking cessation received both NRT and bupropion.		
There is evidence that NRT doubles the chances of a smoker successfully quitting compared to someone using no therapy.		
Using modern technology, the service can now measure the carbon monoxide levels and the chronological age of the lungs.		
Many smokers will need to make multiple attempts to quit before achieving long-term success.		
The aim of nicotine replacement therapy is to reduce withdrawal symptoms associated with stopping smoking.		
Some smokers may prefer a treatment that is not nicotine-based.		
Bupropion is recommended for smokers under the age of 18 years.		

DOI: 10.4324/9781003456674-36

Statements	True	False
There is current evidence to recommend the use of an NRT and bupropion in combination.		
Varenicline (Champix, Pfizer) has been recommended as an option for smokers.		

Activity 31.2

There is only one correct answer to the following multiple-choice questions.

1. Which of the following best describes the features of a smoking cessation service?
   a. Providing free cigarettes to smokers
   b. Offering counselling and support to help smokers quit
   c. Encouraging smokers to increase their tobacco consumption
   d. Promoting the benefits of smoking to the community
   e. None of the above
2. What are the benefits of smoking cessation?
   a. Increased risk of developing lung cancer
   b. Improved cardiovascular health
   c. Reduced risk of respiratory infections
   d. Increased risk of stroke
   e. None of the above
3. Which psychological interventions are commonly used in smoking cessation?
   a. Relaxation training
   b. Cognitive behavioural therapy
   c. Music therapy
   d. Acupuncture
   e. Aromatherapy
4. Which of the following is a nicotine replacement therapy used in smoking cessation?
   a. Meditation
   b. Nicotine gum
   c. Yoga
   d. Reflexology
   e. Herbal supplements
5. What is an example of a non-nicotine replacement therapy used in smoking cessation?
   a. Nicotine patch
   b. Chewing tobacco
   c. Bupropion (Zyban)
   d. Nicotine lozenge
   e. None of the above
6. Which assessment method is commonly used to evaluate smokers' readiness to quit?
   a. Blood pressure measurement
   b. X-ray imaging
   c. Self-report questionnaire
   d. Electrocardiogram (ECG)
   e. Bone density scan

7. Which intervention is aimed at helping smokers quit by increasing their motivation and confidence?
   a. Providing free cigarettes
   b. Counselling and support
   c. Encouraging increased tobacco consumption
   d. Ignoring the smoker's habits
   e. None of the above
8. How does nicotine replacement therapy (NRT) help smokers quit?
   a. By providing a substitute source of nicotine
   b. By blocking nicotine receptors in the brain
   c. By increasing cravings for cigarettes
   d. By inducing withdrawal symptoms
   e. None of the above
9. What is the primary goal of a smoking cessation service?
   a. To promote smoking among individuals
   b. To discourage smokers from quitting
   c. To provide support and resources to help smokers quit
   d. To encourage non-smokers to start smoking
   e. None of the above
10. Which of the following is NOT a psychological intervention commonly used in smoking cessation?
    a. Cognitive behavioural therapy
    b. Hypnotherapy
    c. Yoga
    d. Relaxation techniques
    e. Mindfulness meditation
11. Which of the following is a nicotine replacement therapy (NRT) used in smoking cessation?
    a. Bupropion (Zyban)
    b. Varenicline (Chantix)
    c. Nicotine gum
    d. Acupuncture
    e. None of the above
12. How do non-nicotine replacement therapies aid in smoking cessation?
    a. By reducing withdrawal symptoms
    b. By blocking nicotine receptors in the brain
    c. By providing a substitute source of nicotine
    d. By increasing cravings for cigarettes
    e. None of the above
13. What role does counselling play in smoking cessation?
    a. It helps individuals increase their tobacco consumption.
    b. It provides support and guidance to help individuals quit smoking.
    c. It promotes the benefits of smoking to the community.
    d. It encourages non-smokers to start smoking.
    e. None of the above is correct.
14. Which assessment tool is commonly used to assess the readiness of smokers to quit?
    a. X-ray imaging
    b. Blood pressure measurement
    c. Carbon monoxide (CO) breath test
    d. Electrocardiogram (ECG)
    e. None of the above

15. What is the primary goal of nicotine replacement therapy (NRT) in smoking cessation?
    a. To increase cravings for cigarettes
    b. To provide a substitute source of nicotine
    c. To discourage smokers from quitting
    d. To promote smoking among individuals
    e. None of the above
16. A variety of methods to assist smokers in quitting include:
    a. Identifying high-risk smoking situations
    b. Developing alternative coping strategies
    c. Managing stress
    d. All of the above
    e. A and C only
17. The assessment of nicotine dependence and motivation to quit is based on the:
    a. Model of change
    b. Fagerstrom test
    c. Assessment interview
    d. Counselling
    e. Self-reports
18. The ECO level is undertaken to measure:
    a. Carbon dioxide levels
    b. Carbon monoxide levels
    c. Smoke inhalation
    d. Inhaled nicotine
    e. Recent exercise
19. ECO levels can also be affected by:
    a. Recent exercise
    b. Depth of inhalation
    c. Frequency of inhalation
    d. All of the above
    e. A and B only
20. The main forms of pharmacological treatment covered:
    a. Nicotine replacement therapy
    b. Antidepressant therapy
    c. Counselling therapy
    d. None of the above
    e. All of the above
21. NRT is available as:
    a. Skin patches
    b. Chewing gum
    c. Nasal spray
    d. All of the above
    e. A and B only

INTRODUCTION

In *DSM-V* (APA, 2013), the primary diagnostic term for problematic tobacco use is *tobacco use disorder*, characterised by a problematic pattern of tobacco use leading to clinically significant impairment or distress, as manifested by at least 2 of the 11 symptoms occurring within a 12-month period. Key features of tobacco use disorder include failed attempts to abstain, powerful urges to use nicotine, and withdrawal symptoms upon cessation. According to the World Health Organization (WHO, 2008) report on the status of global efforts against tobacco, only 5% of the global population is protected by comprehensive national smoke-free legislation. Additionally, 40% of countries still allow smoking in hospitals and schools, and services to treat tobacco dependence are fully available in only nine countries, covering 5% of the world's population.

An important strategy in addressing smoking is the establishment of smoking cessation services, recognising that many smokers desire to quit but find it challenging. In England, the NHS (National Health Service) Stop Smoking Service offers counselling and support to smokers aiming to quit, in conjunction with "stop smoking" aids, such as nicotine replacement therapy (NRT) and bupropion (Zyban). However, despite successful outcomes for many individuals, quit rates remain lower among those in routine and manual groups compared to higher-socio-economic groups (Willis, 2007). Evaluation of the NHS Stop Smoking Services programme (Bauld et al., 2005) indicates that these services contribute to a modest reduction in health inequalities. Long-term quit rates show that approximately 15% of individuals remain smoke-free at 52 weeks, and the services are deemed cost-effective in aiding smoking cessation. Smokers utilising the NHS Stop Smoking Service alongside NRT/Zyban are up to four times more likely to succeed in quitting compared to relying on willpower alone. A Cochrane review (Stead et al., 1996) on NRT suggests that it roughly doubles the chances of successful smoking cessation compared to no therapy. Additionally, a systematic review covering studies from 1990 to 2007 (Bauld et al., 2010) suggests that intensive NHS treatments for smoking cessation are effective. Group treatment may be more effective than one-to-one treatment, and the impact of "buddy support" varies depending on the treatment type.

It is acknowledged that in the future of smoking cessation, innovative technologies are expected to play a crucial role in revolutionising the process. Artificial intelligence (AI)–driven interventions will play a pivotal role in analysing individuals' smoking patterns, triggers, and cravings with meticulous precision. These interventions will offer real-time, adaptive support through chatbots and virtual coaches, providing personalised guidance and motivational messages tailored to each individual's needs to enhance their efforts to quit smoking (Abo-Tabik et al., 2021; Onwuzo et al., 2024).

SMOKING CESSATION SERVICE

A comprehensive smoking cessation service incorporates both psychological (motivational) and pharmacological treatment interventions. The NHS Stop Smoking Service typically integrates behavioural support, offered in group or individual settings, with pharmacotherapy, such as nicotine replacement therapy or bupropion. The primary objectives of the service are to provide accessible and effective smoking cessation counselling to staff, patients, and the local community, as well as to deliver training on smoking cessation to healthcare professionals (Mills, 1998). Referrals to the clinics are commonly made by general practitioners, other healthcare professionals, or smokers who have contacted the service via a free-phone helpline. Upon initial contact with the smoking cessation service, individuals may attend an information session to learn about available services, receive brief intervention advice, and gather information on treatment options for smoking cessation. Service users attending smoking clinics receive assistance and advice in preparation for their quit date, along with ongoing motivational support and encouragement during their first month of quitting.

All service users undergo an assessment interview, followed by either group therapy sessions or individual therapy. The duration of individual therapy sessions may vary based on the patient's needs and progress. Group session durations are flexible and depend on local services and the needs of service users. Some services offer specialised smoking cessation courses tailored for heavily addicted smokers who wish to quit. Drop-in services are available for individuals without the need for an appointment. Partnerships with maternity services have been established in some smoking cessation schemes to encourage pregnant women to access the service. Utilising modern technology, the service can now measure carbon monoxide levels and calculate the chronological age of the lungs. This feedback, along with identified benefits, serves as a motivating factor for pre-contemplators to move towards contemplation or action.

Psychological interventions are important in smoking cessation, whether used alone or alongside medication. They encompass various methods to aid smokers in quitting effectively. Key aspects include coaching individuals to recognise high-risk situations, develop coping strategies, manage stress, and enhance problem-solving skills. Additionally, increasing social support is essential, encouraging

Table 31.1
Benefits of quitting smoking (time lapse)

Time	Changes
20 minutes	Blood pressure drops to normal. Pulse rate drops to normal. Temperature of hands and feet increase to normal.
8 hours	Carbon monoxide level in blood returns to normal. Oxygen level in blood returns to normal.
24 hours	Immediate risk of heart attack starts to fall.
48 hours	Nerve endings start to regrow. Ability to taste and smell enhanced.
14 days	Circulation improves. Walking becomes easier. Lung function increases up to 30%.
1 month	Most nicotine withdrawal symptoms disappear.
3 months	Lung function improves. Nagging cough disappears. Cilia regrow in the lungs, increasing their ability to handle mucus, clean themselves, and reduce infection.
9 months	Risk of pregnancy complications and foetal death reduced to level of non-smoker.
1 year	Excess risk of coronary heart disease half that of a smoker. There is no safe point beyond which relapse will not occur. It continues at a much slower rate beyond one year of abstinence.
5 years	Risk of lung cancer decreases by half. Stroke risk same as non-smoker. Risk of mouth, throat, and oesophageal cancer half that of a smoker.
10 years	Lung cancer death rate same as non-smoker. Pre-cancerous cells replaced.
15 years	Risk of coronary heart disease same as non-smoker.

Source: Adapted from www.quitsmokingsupport.com/benefits.htm.

individuals to seek support from various sources. Self-help materials complement these interventions, offering educational resources and ongoing support. Overall, psychological interventions in smoking cessation treatment encompass a comprehensive approach aimed at empowering individuals with the skills, strategies, and support needed to successfully quit smoking and maintain long-term abstinence.

HEALTH GAINS AND BENEFITS OF SMOKING CESSATION

Quitting smoking is a paramount action for improving health, irrespective of age or duration of smoking. Improvement in overall health and health gains will be gained through smoking cessation (CDC, 2023).

- Enhances health status and quality of life
- Reduces the risk of premature death, potentially adding up to ten years to life expectancy
- Lowers the risk of various adverse health effects, including cardiovascular diseases, chronic obstructive pulmonary disease (COPD), cancer, and poor reproductive health outcomes
- Benefits individuals already diagnosed with coronary heart disease or COPD
- Positively impacts the health of pregnant women, foetuses, and babies
- Alleviates the financial burden on smokers, healthcare systems, and society as a whole

Quitting smoking yields significant health benefits at any age, even for long-term heavy smokers (CDC, 2023). Additionally, it is the most effective way to protect loved ones and others from the health risks associated with second-hand smoke exposure. A summary of the key benefits of quitting smoking is presented in Table 31.1.

ASSESSMENT AND INTERVENTIONS

The assessment of nicotine dependence and motivation to quit is based on the Fagerstrom test for

Table 31.2
Taking a smoking history

- Number of years as a smoker?
- How soon after waking is the first cigarette?
- Does the client crave a cigarette when in a no-smoking area or situation?
- Examine any previous attempts to quit.
- Assess suitability for nicotine replacement therapy (NRT), for example, no contraindications (in certain cases, written permission from the client's GP may need to be obtained).
- Ensure the client has realistic expectations of the efficacy of the treatment.
- Discuss concerns, for example, withdrawal discomfort.
- Measure expired carbon monoxide levels (ECO).

nicotine dependence (Heatherton et al., 1991). The taking of a smoking history is presented in Table 31.2.

The assessment interview, lasting 20 to 30 minutes, is a crucial step for all potential quitters. During this session, individuals may opt for group counselling or one-on-one sessions. A "quit date" is established, and ground rules or contracts are discussed upon admission to the clinic. This allows patients to voice any anxieties about quitting and explore past failed attempts. Determining the type of nicotine replacement therapy (NRT) is essential, whether it is patches or gum, and explaining its use and limitations to the patient. Carbon monoxide levels are measured using the ECO (exhaled carbon monoxide) test, serving as an indicator of smoke inhalation. While ECO measurement is quick and non-invasive, levels can be influenced by factors like time since last cigarette, exercise, and inhalation patterns. Afternoon readings are often more accurate than morning ones. Carbon monoxide levels decrease rapidly after smoking cessation, and displaying this change with an ECO monitor can motivate patients to quit. Follow-up sessions can be scheduled for ongoing support, counselling, and ECO measurements. Telephone support is offered as an alternative for patients unable to attend in-person sessions regularly. ECO levels are typically measured four weeks from the quit date for most quitters. Since many smokers require multiple attempts to quit successfully, it is essential for services to remain committed to providing support for those motivated to make new quit attempts after relapse. Brief interventions for smokers are important components of this support.

When discussing options to help individuals stop smoking, it is essential to consider various factors to tailor the approach to their preferences, health, and social circumstances (NICE, 2023). Some individuals may prefer behavioural interventions like counselling or support groups, while others may lean towards pharmacological aids, such as nicotine replacement therapy (NRT), prescription medications (e.g. bupropion, varenicline), or a combination of both. Considerations such as the individual's daily routine, stress levels, social support network, and financial constraints should also be taken into account. It is important to evaluate if the individual is already taking any medications and assess potential interactions with stop-smoking aids. For example, some medications may interact with NRT or prescription drugs used for smoking cessation. In such cases, alternative options may need to be explored. Before recommending any stop-smoking aids, it is important to assess if there are any contraindications based on the individual's medical history or current health status.

Certain medical conditions or medications may make some stop-smoking aids unsuitable or increase the risk of adverse effects. For instance, individuals with cardiovascular problems may need to avoid nicotine replacement therapy in certain forms. Inquire about the individual's previous attempts to quit smoking and their experiences with different stop-smoking aids. Understanding what has worked or not worked for them in the past can guide the selection of appropriate options. If they have had adverse effects from previous attempts, alternative strategies may be needed. By taking into account these factors and engaging in open communication with individuals seeking to quit smoking, healthcare professionals can develop personalised cessation plans that maximise effectiveness and minimise potential risks or barriers to success.

BRIEF INTERVENTIONS FOR SMOKERS

The psychological technique of brief interventions involves opportunistic advice, discussion, negotiation, or encouragement (see Chapter 26) and is delivered in range of primary and community service provisions. For smoking cessation, brief interventions (NICE, 2006) typically take between 5 and 10 minutes and may include one or more of the following:

- Simple opportunistic advice to stop
- Assessment of the patient's commitment to quit
- Pharmacotherapy and/or behavioural support
- Provision of self-help material and referral to more intensive support, such as the NHS

General practitioners and nurses in primary and community care should advise smoking patients to quit and offer a referral to an NHS Stop Smoking Service. Other healthcare professionals, including hospital clinicians, pharmacists, dentists, and community workers, should refer smokers to intensive support services, such as NHS Stop Smoking Services. Figure 31.1 illustrates brief interventions for smokers.

PHARMACOLOGICAL INTERVENTIONS

The main forms of pharmacological treatment covered are nicotine replacement therapy (NRT) and

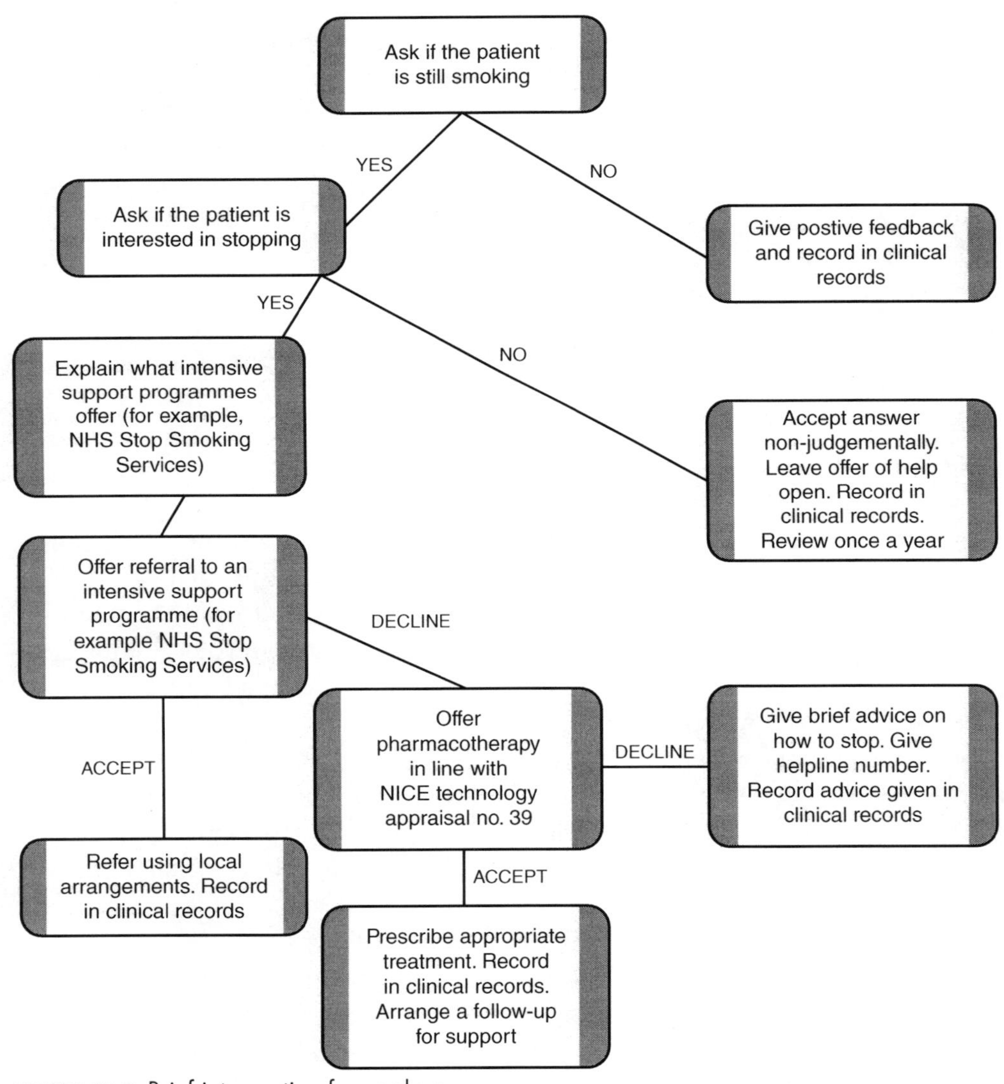

FIGURE 31.1 Brief intervention for smokers.
Source: NICE (2006).

the antidepressant bupropion. NICE (2002) has recommended that in deciding which therapies to use and in which order they should be prescribed, practitioners should take into account:

- Intention and motivation to quit, and likelihood of compliance
- The availability of counselling or support
- Previous usage of smoking cessation aids
- Contraindications and potential for adverse effects
- Personal preferences of the smoker

NICOTINE REPLACEMENT THERAPY

Nicotine replacement therapy (NRT) serves the purpose of alleviating withdrawal symptoms that arise when individuals stop smoking, by providing a controlled dose of nicotine. NRT comes in various forms, including skin patches, chewing gum, nasal spray, inhalers, and lozenges/tablets. Each form delivers nicotine to the body at different rates, offering flexibility in addressing individual preferences and needs. NRT is currently produced as:

- Transdermal patch (varying doses, 16-hour and 24-hour duration)
- Gum (2 mg and 4 mg)
- Sublingual tablet (2 mg)
- Nasal spray (0.5 mg per dose, usually administered two doses at a time)
- Inhalator/inhaler
- Lozenge (1, 2, and 4 mg).

NRT offers a safer alternative to tobacco-based systems, containing nicotine without harmful carcinogens and gases, and posing little abuse potential due to its lack of pleasurable effects. The effectiveness of NRT in aiding smoking cessation is widely recognised and supported by robust evidence. According to a Cochrane review (Stead et al., 1996), all forms of NRT significantly increase the likelihood of successful smoking cessation attempts, boosting the chances of quitting by 50 to 70%. This efficacy holds true regardless of whether additional counselling is utilised, with heavier smokers possibly requiring higher doses for optimal results. Many clinical guidelines now advocate for NRT as a primary treatment option for individuals seeking pharmacological assistance to quit smoking. This acknowledgement underscores the importance of NRT in supporting individuals in their efforts to overcome nicotine dependence and achieve successful cessation (Le Foll et al., 2005). Nicotine preloading, also known as pre-cessation or pre-quitting NRT, involves the use of nicotine replacement therapy for several weeks before the planned quit date. This approach allows individuals to gradually reduce their nicotine dependence and withdrawal symptoms before completely stopping smoking (Wadgave & Nagesh, 2016). By using NRT prior to quitting, individuals can adjust to lower nicotine levels, making the transition to cessation smoother and potentially increasing the likelihood of long-term success in quitting smoking

NON-NICOTINE-BASED PHARMACOLOGICAL MEDICATION

In addition to nicotine replacement therapy (NRT), several non-nicotine-based pharmacological medications have been developed to aid in smoking cessation. These medications target different aspects of nicotine dependence and withdrawal symptoms, offering alternative options for individuals who may not respond well to or prefer not to use nicotine-containing products. Some examples include the following.

Bupropion (Zyban/Wellbutrin). Bupropion is an effective intervention and should be offered as a treatment option for patients requesting help with smoking cessation, unless any of the contraindications apply. Bupropion has been shown to improve quit rates compared to placebo and is often recommended as a first-line treatment option. When used to aid in smoking cessation, bupropion may provide both anti-craving and anti-withdrawal effects by inhibiting the reuptake of dopamine (Hays et al., 2001). Bupropion therapy for smoking cessation typically begins before the patient's planned quit day. A "target quit date" should be set within the first 2 weeks of treatment, and patients can continue smoking during this time as it does not significantly impact the drug's effectiveness. Steady-state blood levels of bupropion are usually reached after 1–2 weeks of treatment. If the patient is unable to quit by the target date, smoking cessation can be delayed until the third or fourth week of treatment or until abstinence is achieved (U.S. Department of Health and Human Services, 2020). However, bupropion is unsuitable for some patient groups (for example, pregnant women and people with a history of seizures or eating disorders), for which nicotine replacement may be considered (Lingford-Hughes et al., 2004). Bupropion is not recommended for smokers under the age of 18 years, as its safety and efficacy have not been evaluated for this group. Bupropion should normally only be prescribed as part of an abstinent-contingent treatment (ACT), in which the smoker makes a commitment to stop smoking on or before a particular date (target stop date) (NICE, 2002). There is currently insufficient evidence to recommend the use of an NRT and bupropion in combination.

Varenicline (brand names Champix or Chantix) is a prescription medication specifically developed to aid in smoking cessation. It works by targeting nicotine receptors in the brain, acting both as a partial agonist and antagonist. This dual action reduces both the pleasurable effects of smoking and withdrawal symptoms, making it easier for individuals to quit smoking. The findings from a meta-analysis from Cahill et al. (2013) showed that varenicline significantly increased the odds of quitting smoking compared to placebo or other pharmacotherapies. The study concluded that varenicline was the most effective pharmacotherapy for smoking cessation. The Evaluating Adverse Events in a Global Smoking Cessation Study (EAGLES) (Anthenelli et al., 2016) was a large, randomised, double-blind trial comparing the safety and efficacy of varenicline, bupropion, nicotine patch, and placebo for smoking cessation. The trial found that varenicline was more effective than bupropion, nicotine patch, or placebo in achieving abstinence from smoking. According to various clinical guidelines and recommendations, including those by the National Institute for Health and Care Excellence (NICE) in the UK and the US Public Health Service, varenicline should not be offered to individuals under the age of 18 due to safety concerns and insufficient evidence of effectiveness in this age group. These medications are typically recommended for use in adults only. Instead, alternative cessation strategies and support should be considered for younger individuals, including behavioural interventions, counselling, and support groups. However, it is important to recognise that like all medications, bupropion and varenicline may have potential side effects and contraindications. Therefore, individuals considering these medications should discuss their options with a healthcare professional to determine the most suitable treatment plan based on their individual needs and medical history. This ensures that they receive appropriate guidance and support throughout their smoking cessation journey.

Researchers are investigating various non-nicotine medications for treating tobacco addiction, including antidepressants, anti-hypertensive drugs, and a nicotine vaccine. These medications aim to reduce cravings and withdrawal symptoms or block nicotine's effects on the brain.

Some antidepressant medications, such as nortriptyline, have shown effectiveness for smoking cessation independent of their antidepressant effects (NIDA, 2021). Nortriptyline has been found to be equally effective as NRT in some small studies, with no reported side effects specifically related to smoking cessation. However, selective serotonin reuptake inhibitors (SSRIs), such as fluoxetine, paroxetine, and sertraline, have not shown any significant impact on smoking cessation when used alone or in combination with NRT (NIDA, 2021).

STOP SMOKING IN PREGNANCY AND FOLLOWING CHILDBIRTH

From a public health perspective, smoking during pregnancy poses a preventable risk for adverse birth and health outcomes. Pregnant women should be informed about the significant perinatal risks associated with tobacco use, including orofacial clefts, foetal growth restriction, placenta-related complications, preterm birth, low birth weight, and increased perinatal mortality (ACOG, 2020). Evidence-based strategies should be integrated into routine pre-natal care for all pregnant women (NICE, 2010). Clinicians should advise cessation of all tobacco products and provide tailored interventions, including counselling, behavioural support, and pharmacotherapy. Regular discussions about available cessation resources, including digital tools, should occur at pre-natal and postpartum visits to support women in quitting smoking.

Quitting smoking, even late in pregnancy, can reduce health risks for the baby and complications during delivery, while also benefiting the woman's long-term health. A five-step intervention programme, known as the "5 As" model, is recommended for assisting pregnant women in quitting smoking (Melvin et al., 2000; ACOG, 2010). The 5 As include: Ask about smoking status. Advise to quit. Assess readiness to quit. Assist with quitting. and Arrange follow-up support. A brief, five-step intervention programme, referred to as the "5 As" model, is recommended in clinical practice to help pregnant women quit smoking. The 5 As include the following:

- Ask about tobacco use.
- Advise to quit.
- Assess willingness to make a quit attempt.
- Assist in quit attempt.
- Arrange follow-up.

NICE (2010) provides recommendations for supporting smoking cessation in pregnant women and following childbirth. Healthcare professionals should:

- Assess the woman's exposure to tobacco smoke through discussion and use of a CO test.
- Provide health information about the risks of smoking during pregnancy for the unborn child and the hazards of second-hand smoke exposure for both mother and baby.
- Explain the health benefits of quitting smoking for the woman and her baby.
- Advise the woman to quit smoking completely, rather than just cutting down.
- Refer all women who smoke, or have stopped smoking within the last weeks, to Stop Smoking Services.
- Encourage the woman's partner or other household members who smoke to contact Stop Smoking Services for support in quitting.

HARM REDUCTION APPROACH

NICE (2013), in relation to the harm reduction approach to smoking, has recommended the following actions:

- Raise public awareness of the harm caused by smoking and second-hand smoke.
- Provide information on how to obtain and use licensed nicotine-containing products.
- Provide self-help materials in a range of formats and languages, tailored to meet the needs of groups where smoking prevalence and tobacco dependency is high.
- Identify people who smoke, and advise them to stop smoking in one step as the best approach.
- Find out about the person's smoking behaviour and level of nicotine dependence by asking how many cigarettes they smoke – and how soon after waking.
- Reassure people who smoke that licensed nicotine-containing products are a safe and effective way of reducing the amount they smoke.
- Offer all types of licensed nicotine-containing products to people who smoke, as part of a harm reduction strategy (either single or in combination). Take into account their preference and level of dependence. As an example, patches could be offered with gum or lozenges.
- Follow up with people to see whether they have achieved their goal(s). If those who set out to reduce the amount they smoke (or to abstain temporarily) have been successful, assess their motivation to maintain that level, to further reduce the amount they smoke or to stop smoking.
- Offer people who want (or need) to abstain temporarily on a short-, medium-, or longer-term basis advice on how to do this (include information about the different types of licensed nicotine-containing products and how to use them). Where possible, prescribe them.
- Incorporate management of smoking in the care plan of people in closed institutions who smoke.

KEY POINTS

- The Stop Smoking Service provides counselling and support to smokers wanting to quit, complementing the use of stop smoking aids nicotine replacement therapy (NRT) and bupropion (Zyban).
- An evaluation of NHS Stop Smoking Service shows that the majority of those setting a quit date for smoking cessation received NRT.
- A smoking cessation service should include both psychological (motivational) and pharmacological treatment interventions.
- Brief intervention advice and information on treatment interventions to aid smoking cessation are provided.
- The assessment of nicotine dependence and motivation to quit is based on the Fagerstrom test for nicotine dependence.
- NICE has provided a care pathway for smokers who wish to quit tobacco smoking.
- NICE has recommended that everyone who smokes should be advised to quit.
- The aims of NRT are to reduce withdrawal symptoms associated with stopping smoking by replacing the nicotine from tobacco smoking.

- Some smokers may prefer a treatment that is not nicotine-based.
- The atypical antidepressant bupropion has been well studied and is the only non-nicotine medication licensed as an aid to smoking cessation.
- Bupropion is unsuitable for some patient groups (e.g. pregnant women, people with a history of seizures or eating disorders), for which nicotine replacement may be considered.
- Varenicline (Champix, Pfizer) has also been recommended as an option for smokers who have expressed a desire to quit smoking.
- Varenicline may be associated with nausea and other gastrointestinal disorders, such as vomiting.
- Several other non-nicotine medications are being investigated for the treatment of tobacco addiction, including other antidepressants and an antihypertensive medication.
- Scientists are also investigating the potential of a vaccine that targets nicotine for use in relapse prevention.
- Evidence-based smoking cessation strategies should be integrated into routine pre-natal care for every pregnant woman.
- The harm reduction approach may cause some smokers to eventually quit smoking. This approach may or may not include temporary or long-term use of nicotine-containing products.

Activity 31.3

Questions

- Describe the features of a smoking cessation service.
- Discuss the benefits of smoking cessation.
- Identify the psychological interventions used in smoking cessation.
- Identify the nicotine and non-nicotine replacement therapy used in smoking cessation.
- Discuss the assessment and interventions to enable smokers to quit.
- Examine the intervention strategies used with pregnant women and following childbirth.
- Discuss the advantages and limitations of the harm reduction approach to tobacco smoking.

References

Abo-Tabik, M., Benn, Y., & Costen, N. (2021). Are machine learning methods the future for smoking cessation apps? *Sensors,* 21(13), 4254. https://doi.org/10.3390/s21134254.

ACOG (American College of Obstetricians and Gynecologists). (2010). Smoking cessation during pregnancy. ACOG Committee Opinion #471. *Obstetrics and Gynecology,* 166, 1241–1244.

ACOG (American College of Obstetricians and Gynecologists). (2020). *Tobacco and Nicotine Cessation During Pregnancy.* https://www.acog.org/clinical/clinical-guidance/committee-opinion/articles/2020/05/tobacco-and-nicotine-cessation-during-pregnancy (accessed 13 April 2024).

American Psychiatric Association. (2013). *Diagnostic and Statistical Manual of Mental Disorders* (5th ed.). Arlington, VA: American Psychiatric Publishing, p. 571.

Anthenelli, R. M., Benowitz, N. L., West, R., St Aubin, L., McRae, T., Lawrence, D., Ascher, J., Russ, C., Krishen, A., & Evins, A. E. (2016). Neuropsychiatric safety and efficacy of varenicline, bupropion, and nicotine patch in smokers with and without psychiatric disorders (EAGLES): A double-blind, randomised, placebo-controlled clinical trial. *Lancet,* 387(10037), 2507–2520. https://doi.org/10.1016/S0140-6736(16)30272-0.

Bauld, L., Bell, K., McCullough, L., Richardson, L., & Greaves, L. (2010). The effectiveness of NHS smoking cessation services: A systematic review. *Journal of Public Health,* 32(1), 71–82. https://doi.org/10.1093/pubmed/fdp074.

Bauld, L., Coleman, T., Adams, C., Pound, E., & Ferguson, J. (2005). Delivering the English smoking treatment services. *Addiction,* 100(Suppl 2), 19–27. https://doi.org/10.1111/j.1360-0443.2005.01024.x.

Cahill, K., Stevens, S., Perera, R., & Lancaster, T. (2013). Pharmacological interventions for smoking cessation: An overview and network meta-analysis. *The Cochrane Database of Systematic Reviews,* 2013(5), CD009329. https://doi.org/10.1002/14651858.CD009329.pub2.

CDC. (2023). *Benefits of Quitting.* Centers for Disease Prevention and Control. https://www.cdc.gov/tobacco/quit_smoking/how_to_quit/benefits/index.htm (accessed 12 April 2024).

Hays, J. T., Hurt, R. D., Rigotti, N. A., Niaura, R., Gonzales, D., Durcan, M. J., Sachs, D. P., Wolter, T. D., Buist, A. S., Johnston, J. A., & White, J. D. (2001). Sustained-release bupropion for pharmacologic relapse prevention after smoking cessation: A randomized, controlled trial. *Annals of Internal Medicine,* 135(6), 423–433. https://doi.org/10.7326/0003-4819-135-6-200109180-00011.

Heatherton, T. F., Kozlowski, L. T., Frecker, R. C., & Fagerström, K. O. (1991). The Fagerström test for nicotine dependence: A revision of the Fagerström tolerance questionnaire. *British Journal of Addiction,* 86(9), 1119–1127. https://doi.org/10.1111/j.1360-0443.1991.tb01879.x.

Le Foll, B., Melihan-Cheinin, P., Rostoker, G., Lagrue, G., & Working Group of AFSSAPS. (2005). Smoking cessation guidelines: Evidence-based recommendations of the French health products safety agency. *European Psychiatry: The Journal of the Association of European Psychiatrists,* 20(5–6), 431–441. https://doi.org/10.1016/j.eurpsy.2004.12.008.

Lingford-Hughes, A. R., Welch, S., Nutt, D. J., & British Association for Psychopharmacology. (2004). Evidence-based guidelines for the pharmacological management of substance misuse, addiction and comorbidity: Recommendations from the British association for psychopharmacology. *Journal of Psychopharmacology,* 18(3), 293–335. https://doi.org/10.1177/0269881104018003211.

Melvin, C. L., Dolan-Mullen, P., Windsor, R. A., Pennington Whiteside, J., Goldenberg, R. L., Whiteside, H. P., & Melvin, D. (2000). Recommended cessation counselling for pregnant women who smoke: A review of the evidence. *Tobacco Control,* 9, iii80–iii84.

Mills, C. (1998). Nicotine addiction: Health care interventions. In G. H. Rassool (Ed.), *Substance Use and Misuse: Nature, Context and Clinical Interventions.* Oxford: Blackwell Publications.

NICE. (2002). *Guidance in the Use of Nicotine Replacement Therapy (NRT) and Bupropion for Smoking Cessation* (Summary, TA39). London: National Institute for Clinical Excellence.

NICE. (2006). *Brief Interventions and Referral for Smoking Cessation in Primary Care and Other Settings* (Public Health Guidance No. 1). London: National Institute for Clinical Excellence. This Guideline Has Been Updated and Replaced by the NICE Guideline on *Tobacco: Preventing Uptake, Promoting Quitting and Treating Dependence* (NG209) (2023).

NICE. (2010). *How to Stop Smoking in Pregnancy and Following Childbirth* (Public Health Guidance 26). London: National Institute for Clinical Excellence.

NICE. (2013). *Smoking: Harm Reduction.* (Public Health Guideline.nice.org.uk/guidance/ph45). London: National Institute for Clinical Excellence.

NICE. (2023). *Tobacco: Preventing Uptake, Promoting Quitting and Treating Dependence* (NICE Guideline NG209). London: National Institute for Clinical Excellence.

NIDA. (2021). *What Are Treatments for Tobacco Dependence?* https://nida.nih.gov/publications/research-reports/tobacco-nicotine-e-cigarettes/what-are-treatments-tobacco-dependence (accessed 13 April 2024).

Onwuzo, C. N., Olukorode, J., Sange, W., Orimoloye, D. A., Udojike, C., Omoragbon, L., Hassan, A. E., Falade, D. M., Omiko, R., Odunaike, O. S., Adams-Momoh, P. A., Addeh, E., Onwuzo, S., & Joseph-Erameh, U. (2024). A review of smoking cessation interventions: Efficacy, strategies for implementation, and future directions. *Cureus,* 16(1), e52102. https://doi.org/10.7759/cureus.52102.

Stead, L. F., Perera, R., Bullen, C., Mant, D., & Lancaster, T. (1996). Nicotine replacement therapy for smoking cessation. *Cochrane Database of Systematic Reviews,* 1996(3), Article ID CD000146. https://doi.org/10.1002/14651858.CD000146.pub3.

U.S. Department of Health and Human Services. (2020). *Smoking Cessation: A Report of the Surgeon General.* Atlanta, GA: U.S. Department of Health and Human Services, Centers for Disease Control and Prevention, National Center for Chronic Disease Prevention and Health Promotion, Office on Smoking and Health. https://www.hhs.gov/sites/default/files/2020-cessation-sgr-full-report.pdf (accessed 13 April 2024).

Wadgave, U., & Nagesh, L. (2016). Nicotine replacement therapy: An overview. *International Journal of Health Sciences,* 10(3), 425–435.

WHO. (2008). *Global Efforts Against Tobacco.* Geneva: World Health Organization.

Willis, N. (2007). *NHS Stop Smoking Services – Service and Monitoring Guidance 2007/08.* London: Crown Copyright.

Chapter 32

Epilogue

Alcohol and drug use is a complex and persistent issue that cannot be fully eradicated overnight. Healthcare professionals must remain committed to the ongoing task of understanding, addressing, and mitigating the impact of substance misuse on individuals and society. This commitment involves staying engaged and proactive in efforts to prevent and treat substance misuse, even in the face of challenges and setbacks. As the field of healthcare evolves and new developments emerge in the understanding and treatment of alcohol and substance use disorders, healthcare professionals must continuously update their knowledge and skills. Ongoing education and training programmes are essential to ensure that healthcare professionals remain equipped to provide effective care and support to individuals affected by substance misuse. The goal of education and training in alcohol and drug use would be to:

- *Increase awareness and understanding*. Educate health and social care professionals about the prevalence, patterns, and consequences of alcohol and drug use and misuse, including the impact on physical health, mental health, and social well-being.
- *Enhance assessment skills*. Provide training on how to effectively screen individuals for alcohol and drug use, identify signs of misuse or dependence, and conduct comprehensive assessments to determine the severity of the problem.
- *Develop intervention strategies*. Equip professionals with the knowledge and skills to deliver brief interventions and motivational interviewing techniques to support individuals in reducing or quitting substance use, as well as providing appropriate harm reduction strategies.
- *Foster collaboration*. Encourage collaboration between health, social care, and criminal justice professionals to ensure a holistic approach to addressing substance misuse, including effective referral pathways and coordination of care.
- *Promote cultural competence*. Recognise and address the cultural and contextual factors that influence alcohol and drug use, ensuring that interventions are tailored to the needs and preferences of diverse populations.
- *Support self-care and resilience*. Provide education on self-care strategies for professionals working with individuals with substance misuse issues, including strategies for managing stress, compassion fatigue, and burnout.

Overall, the goal is to empower health and social care professionals with the knowledge, skills, and confidence to effectively respond to alcohol and drug use, promote health and well-being, and support individuals in accessing appropriate treatment and services.

Addressing substance misuse requires collaboration among various stakeholders, including healthcare professionals, policymakers, educators, and community organisations. By working together, these stakeholders can leverage their respective expertise and resources to develop comprehensive strategies for prevention, intervention, and treatment. Collaboration fosters a more holistic and coordinated approach to addressing substance misuse and maximises the impact of interventions. Recognising addiction as an ongoing challenge underlines the

DOI: 10.4324/9781003456674-37

need for a long-term perspective in addressing this issue. While immediate interventions are crucial for individuals in need of assistance, long-term strategies are necessary to address the root causes of substance misuse and promote sustainable change. This long-term perspective encourages healthcare professionals to remain vigilant and committed to their efforts, even when progress may seem slow or incremental.

The book highlights alcohol and drug misuse as one of today's most critical public health challenges, emphasising the need for urgent action. It stresses the importance of nurturing compassion, integrity, and equity as guiding principles in addressing substance misuse with empathy, honesty, and fairness. Essentially, the book serves as a call to action for healthcare and social professionals to uphold these core values in their efforts to combat alcohol and drug misuse. It underlines the collaborative nature of this undertaking and the pressing need for decisive action, while also offering a framework for informed decision-making aimed at achieving positive outcomes.

Index

Printed in the United States
by Baker & Taylor Publisher Services